NUFD 499

Medical Nutrition Applications

Professor Lauren Dinour

Montclair State University

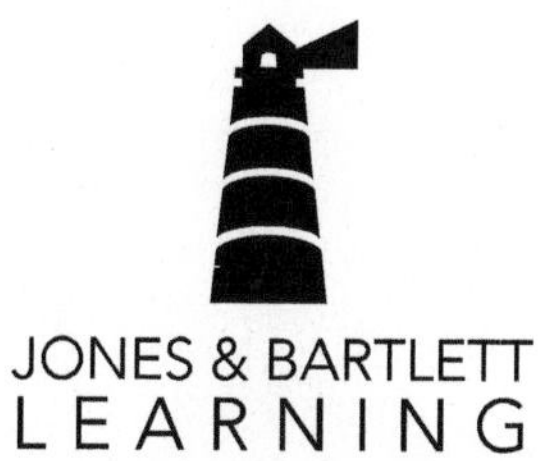

World Headquarters
Jones & Bartlett Learning
5 Wall Street
Burlington, MA 01803
978-443-5000
info@jblearning.com
www.jblearning.com

Jones & Bartlett Learning books and products are available through most bookstores and online booksellers. To contact Jones & Bartlett Learning directly, call 800-832-0034, fax 978-443-8000, or visit our website, www.jblearning.com.

This book is produced through PUBLISH – a custom publishing service offered by Jones & Bartlett Learning. For more information on PUBLISH, contact us at 800-832-0034 or visit our website at www.jblearning.com.

Disclaimer

This publication is sold with the understanding that the publisher is not engaged in rendering medical, legal, accounting, or other professional services. If medical, legal, accounting, or other professional service advice is required, the service of a competent professional should be sought. The authors, editor, and publisher have designed this publication to provide accurate information with regard to the subject matter covered. However, they are not responsible for errors, omissions, or for any outcomes related to the use of the contents of this publication and make no guarantee and assume no responsibility or liability for the use of the products and procedures described, or the correctness, sufficiency, or completeness of stated information, opinions, or recommendations. Treatments and side effects described in this publication are not applicable to all people; required dosages and experienced side effects will vary among individuals. Drugs and medical devices discussed herein are controlled by the Food and Drug Administration (FDA) and may have limited availability for use only in research studies or clinical trials. Research, clinical practice, and government regulations often change accepted standards. When consideration is being given to the use of any drug in the clinical setting, the health care provider or reader is responsible for determining FDA status of the drug, reading the package insert, and reviewing prescribing information for the most current recommendations on dose, precautions, and contraindications and for determining the appropriate usage for the product. This is especially important in the case of drugs that are new or seldom used. Any references in this publication to procedures to be employed when rendering emergency care to the sick and injured are provided solely as a general guide; other or additional safety measures might be required under particular circumstances. This publication is not intended as a statement of the standards of care required in any particular situation; circumstances and the physical conditions of patients can vary widely from one emergency to another. This publication is not intended in any way to advise emergency personnel concerning their legal authority to perform the activities or procedures discussed. Such local determination should be made only with the aid of legal counsel. Some images in this publication feature models; these models do not necessarily endorse, represent, or participate in the activities represented in the images.

Cover Image: © Ivan Mikhaylov/Dreamstime.com

6048
Printed in the United States of America
24 23 22 21 20 10 9 8 7 6 5 4 3

Contents

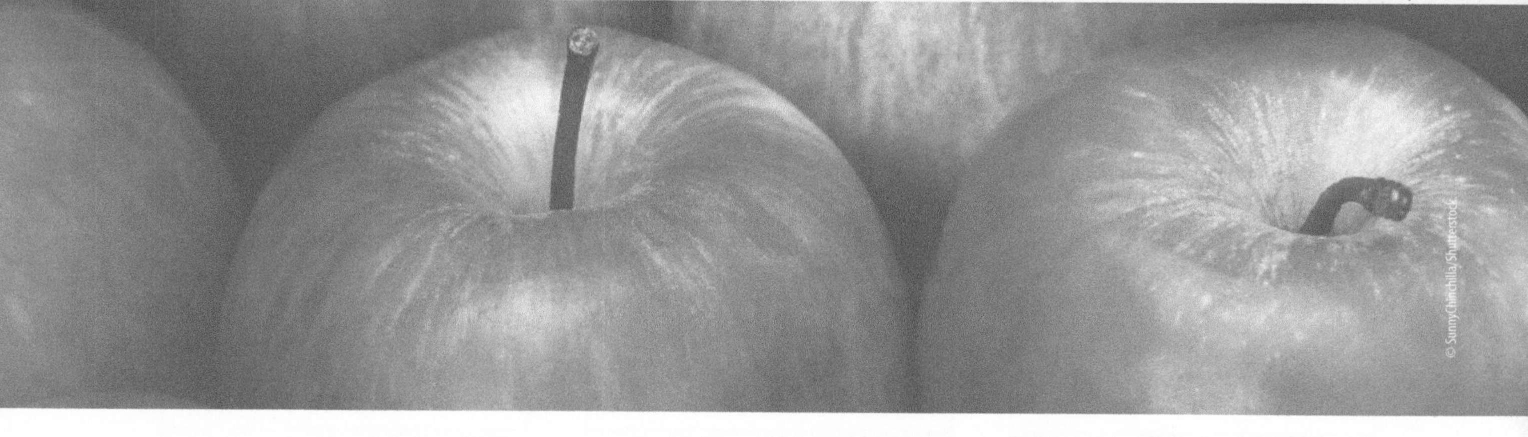

Nutritional Assessment

Nancy Munoz, DCN, MHA, RDN, FAND
Mary Dean Coleman-Kelly, PhD, MS, RDN

CHAPTER OUTLINE

LEARNING OBJECTIVES

After completing this chapter, the reader should be able to:

1. Describe the historic evolution of nutrient deficiency diseases, the role of nutrition with chronic disease, and the screening and diagnosis of malnutrition in the clinical setting.
2. Differentiate between screening and assessment for nutritional risk.
3. Understand the different methods of collecting nutrition assessment data.
4. Recognize the different components of the nutrition care process.
5. Examine the role of nutrition assessment in the prevention and treatment of chronic disease.

▸ Introduction

Nutritional imbalances are a severe public-health problem that has been associated with a significant increase in the risk of mortality and morbidity. An individual's nutritional status is influenced by factors such as consuming food in sufficient amounts, selecting the right foods to promote adequate nutrient intake, and the individual's eating pattern. A sedentary lifestyle and a poor-quality eating pattern have been identified as risk factors for the development of chronic diseases such as hypertension, cardiovascular disease, diabetes mellitus (DM), stroke, and cancer. Adverse outcomes such as disability, poor quality of life, and high rates of low-birthweight babies occur as a result of poor eating patterns and malnutrition in both developed and underdeveloped countries. Identifying the impact of poor eating patterns on chronic diseases and assessing the nutritional status of individuals, families, and communities are important tasks in promoting population health.[1,2]

In the United States, approximately 50% of the adult population suffers from one or more avoidable

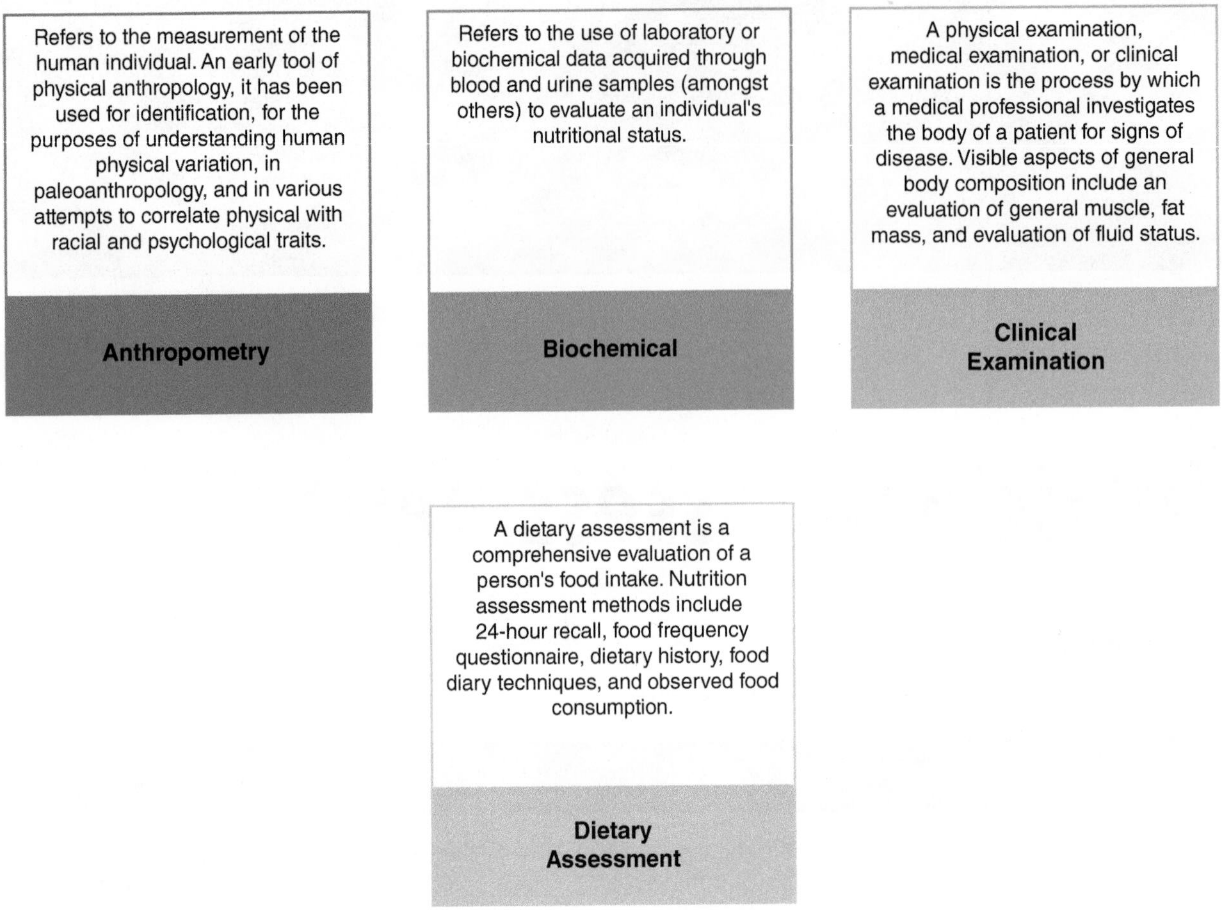

Refers to the measurement of the human individual. An early tool of physical anthropology, it has been used for identification, for the purposes of understanding human physical variation, in paleoanthropology, and in various attempts to correlate physical with racial and psychological traits.

Anthropometry

Refers to the use of laboratory or biochemical data acquired through blood and urine samples (amongst others) to evaluate an individual's nutritional status.

Biochemical

A physical examination, medical examination, or clinical examination is the process by which a medical professional investigates the body of a patient for signs of disease. Visible aspects of general body composition include an evaluation of general muscle, fat mass, and evaluation of fluid status.

Clinical Examination

A dietary assessment is a comprehensive evaluation of a person's food intake. Nutrition assessment methods include 24-hour recall, food frequency questionnaire, dietary history, food diary techniques, and observed food consumption.

Dietary Assessment

FIGURE 1 ABCDs of nutritional assessment

chronic disease. More than two-thirds of adults and approximately one-thirds of children and youth are overweight or obese. These extreme rates of overweight, obesity, and chronic disease have been a public-health concern for more than two decades and contribute not only to increased health risks but also to associated high medical costs.[3] In 2008, the medical costs connected with obesity were assessed at $147 billion. In 2012, the total estimated cost of diagnosed diabetes was $245 billion, including $176 billion in direct medical costs and $69 billion in decreased productivity.[4]

The evaluation of the nutrition status of different segments of the population helps in measuring the prevalence of nutritional disorders, and also to plan counteractive strategies (see **FIGURE 1**).

Nutrition and Health

Preview Nutritional assessment is the first step to identify nutrition-related problems that arise from nutrient deficiency and lead to chronic disease or result in malnutrition.

Nutrient Deficiency Diseases: A Historical Perspective

Good health and quality of life are desired by all individuals living in a society. Access to safe drinking water, nutritious food, and quality medical care are essential to the well-being of any person. Undernutrition and hunger are prevalent in underdeveloped as well as developed countries. An estimated 870 million adults and children worldwide have inadequate food intakes.[5] Chronic undernutrition leads to the onset of deficiency diseases, and physical signs of such diseases emerge when the intake of essential nutrients is inadequate and prolonged.

Keen observations by physicians in the early 1700s identified that in some instances the cause of human illness was related to the absence of certain foods; they proposed that those foods contained specific compounds whose absence led to the signs and symptoms of disease. One of the earliest known discoveries of the curative effects of foods with deficiency diseases was by Scottish physician James Lind in the mid-1700s. British sailors taking long voyages were developing **scurvy** and becoming severely ill or dying on the voyage. Observational research has progressed over time to the current

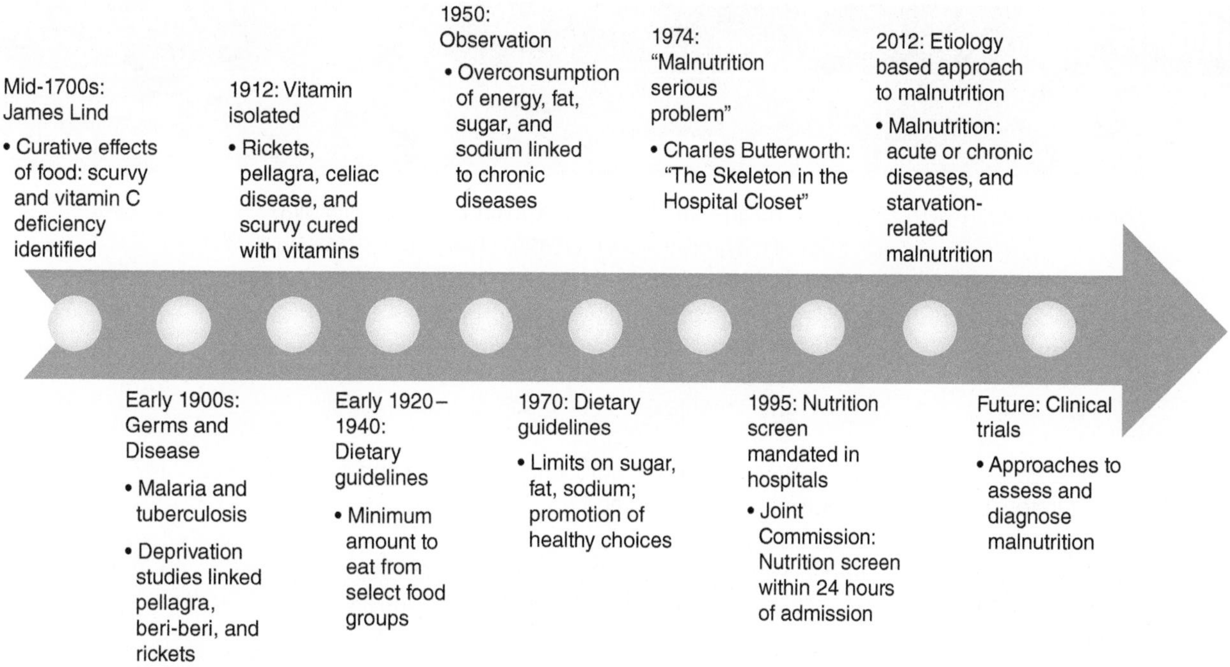

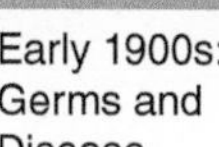
Mid-1700s: James Lind
• Curative effects of food: scurvy and vitamin C deficiency identified
Early 1900s: Germs and Disease
• Malaria and tuberculosis
• Deprivation studies linked pellagra, beri-beri, and rickets
1912: Vitamin isolated
• Rickets, pellagra, celiac disease, and scurvy cured with vitamins
Early 1920–1940: Dietary guidelines
• Minimum amount to eat from select food groups
1950: Observation
• Overconsumption of energy, fat, sugar, and sodium linked to chronic diseases
1970: Dietary guidelines
• Limits on sugar, fat, sodium; promotion of healthy choices
1974: "Malnutrition serious problem"
• Charles Butterworth: "The Skeleton in the Hospital Closet"
1995: Nutrition screen mandated in hospitals
• Joint Commission: Nutrition screen within 24 hours of admission
2012: Etiology based approach to malnutrition
• Malnutrition: acute or chronic diseases, and starvation-related malnutrition
Future: Clinical trials
• Approaches to assess and diagnose malnutrition

FIGURE 2 Nutrition and health: A historical perspective

Data from Rosenfeld, L. (1997). "Vitamine—vitamin. The early years of discovery". *Clin Chem.* 43 (4): 680–5. Semba R. The Discovery of Vitamins. *Int J Vitamin Nutrition Research*. 2012;5:310-315. Funk C. The etiology of the deficiency diseases. Beri-beri, polynueritis in birds, epidemic dropsy, scurvy, experience scurvy in animals, infantile scurvy, ship beri-beri, pellagra. *J State Med*. 1912;20:341. Davis C, Saltos E. *Dietary Recommendations and How They Have Changed Over Time*. Ch. 2. America's Eating Habits: Changes and Consequences. http://purl.umn.edu/33604. Accessed January 24, 2017. Butterworth C. The Skeleton in the Hospital Closet. *Nutrition Today* 1974;March/ April:436. Dougherty D, et al. Nutrition care given new importance in JCAHO standards. *Nutr Clin Pract*. 1995;10(1):26-31. White JV, Guenter P, Jensen G, et al. Consensus Statement: Academy of Nutrition and Dietetics and American Society for Parenteral and Enteral Nutrition: Characteristics Recommended for the Identification and Documentation of Adult Malnutrition (Undernutrition). *Journal of Parenteral and Enteral Nutrition*. 2012;36(3):275-283.

dietary guidelines. **FIGURE 2** shows a short historic timeline of nutrition and health.[6,7]

Leading Causes of Death and Chronic Diseases

The interest in modifying diet to prevent chronic disease in Americans began when deficiency diseases and infectious diseases were eradicated. In addition, the implementation of government-mandated enrichment and fortification of food staples and the use of vaccinations to reduce deaths from infectious diseases also contributed to increased awareness of the American diet.[8]

TABLE 1 ranks the 10 leading causes of death in the United States today. Four of the ten—heart disease, cancer, stroke, and diabetes mellitus[9]—are linked to diet and either can be prevented or have their onsets delayed by implementing healthy eating practices and making positive lifestyle choices.

Nutritionists today are challenged to find the optimal food pattern and nutrient profile that will optimize the quality of life and prevent chronic disease for their clients. Conducting nutritional assessment in the community setting is important when identifying early risks for chronic disease. Novel approaches such as evaluating the genetic profile of individuals to identify genetic determinates that lead to chronic disease are being researched as a potential added "tool" that registered dietitian nutritionists (RDNs) can use along with traditional assessment measures. Understanding genomics in relationship to nutritional management of complex diseases is in its infancy, so routine genetic testing to provide dietary advice is not ready for practical application. The prospect for using nutritional genomics in the future, however, is exciting. It has the potential to offer RDNs and healthcare professionals the tools to create "genetically" personalized diet plans that are specific to any individual's genetic makeup.

History of Diagnosing Malnutrition in the Clinical Setting

Identifying malnutrition and offering nutrition support to malnourished patients is relatively new in the clinical setting. In 1974, Dr. Charles Butterworth wrote a landmark paper, "The Skeleton in the Hospital Closet," in which he exposed malnutrition in the hospital as a serious problem.[10] In 1995, the Joint Commission (a US nonprofit healthcare accrediting organization), working with input from the American Society of Clinical Nutrition and the American Dietetic Association (now the Academy of Nutrition and Dietetics), created the standard requirement that hospitals provide a nutrition screening of each patient within 24 hours of admission.[11] Although this requirement offered a

TABLE 1 Leading causes of death in the United States

Rank	Disease	Contributing Risk Factors	Number of Deaths Annually
1	Heart disease	Increasing age, family history, smoking, poor-quality diet, obesity, hypertension, increased cholesterol, stress, physical inactivity	614,348
2	Cancer	Increased age, smoking, excessive consumption of alcohol, excessive exposure to sun, obesity, family history, presence of some chronic conditions such as ulcerative colitis	591,699
3	Chronic lower-respiratory diseases	Exposure to tobacco smoke, chemicals, dust and burning fuel; advanced age and genetics	147,101
4	Accidents (unintentional injuries)	Motor-vehicle accidents most common; contributing factors include inexperience, teenage drivers, distractions	136,053
5	Stroke (cerebrovascular diseases)	Hypertension, tobacco use, diabetes, increased cholesterol, obesity, inactivity, coronary disease, excessive alcohol intake	133,103
6	Alzheimer's disease	Conditions that damage the heart and blood vessels such as diabetes, high cholesterol, and hypertension	93,541
7	Diabetes	Family history, dietary factors such as low vitamin D consumption, increased weight, obesity, inactivity, race, hypertension, increased cholesterol, polycystic ovarian syndrome, gestational diabetes, increased age	76,488
8	Influenza and pneumonia	Chronic disease, smoking, being immunocompromised	55,227
9	Nephritis, nephrotic syndrome, and nephrosis	Medical conditions that cause kidney injury such as diabetes, side effects of certain medications such as nonsteroidal anti-inflammatory drugs, infections such as HIV and malaria	48,146
10	Intentional self-harm (suicide)	Depression, previous self-harm	42,773

Modified from Health United States. Table 19 (data are for 2014). 2015. www.cdc.gov. Accessed January 24, 2017.

framework for early identification of malnutrition, there has been considerable variance in the nutrition screening tools used and the procedures needed to follow and implement the rest of the nutrition care plan.[12] Many screening tools have used albumin as the primary indicator to identify malnutrition in patients. It is well documented, however, that albumin is a poor diagnostic indicator for malnutrition given the fact that it fluctuates in the presence of inflammation that could be induced by external factors such as trauma, surgery, or inflammatory diseases. The American Society for Parenteral and Enteral Nutrition (ASPEN) and the European Society for Clinical Nutrition and Metabolism has created an etiology-based approach to diagnose adult malnutrition in the clinical setting. This approach identifies malnutrition in the context of acute illness, chronic diseases, and starvation-related malnutrition.[13] This approach has been widely adopted by clinical dietitians across the United States. Clinical trials are currently underway to validate this approach to assessing and diagnosing malnutrition in the hospital setting.

Recap Nutrition has played an integral role in maintaining optimal health and quality of life for individuals in the United States and elsewhere in the world. A paradox exists in the United States where healthcare professionals need to have the knowledge and skills to address the health-related problems associated with over nutrition (obesity and chronic diseases) and undernutrition (frailty and wasting diseases). Nutritional assessment is the first step to implementing a nutrition care plan that assists individuals in successfully implementing dietary and lifestyle changes to improve their quality of life, lower their risks for disease, and help prevent or overcome malnutrition.

▸ Nutritional Screening and Nutritional Assessment Tools

Preview Nutritional screening tools are designed to quickly evaluate nutritional risk in individuals. Nutritional assessment tools identify malnutrition in individuals.

Nutritional Screening Tools

The Academy of Nutrition and Dietetics (the Academy) recommends the use of nutrition screening to identify individuals who are at nutritional risk. This ensures that those patients who are at risk, are given high priority for a thorough nutritional evaluation by an RDN. **Nutrition screening** is defined as "the process of identifying patients, clients, or groups who may have a nutrition diagnosis and benefit from nutritional assessment and intervention by a registered dietitian."[14] Nutritional screening tools should be quick, easy-to-use tools that can be completed by any member of a healthcare team with minimal nutrition expertise (e.g., diet technicians, nurses, and physician assistants). Furthermore, screening tools should be validated to ensure that they accurately identify nutritional risks for the population and setting for which they are intended. Screening forms have use in both community and clinical settings. In community settings, for example, forms can be used to identify risk for chronic diseases such as diabetes, heart disease, and high blood pressure in adults. These are typically used at community events such as health fairs and workplace wellness fairs. When the results identify individuals at risk for a chronic disease, they are often referred to their primary care physicians for extensive evaluation to determine whether a chronic disease is present. They may also be referred to an RDN who will offer recommendations for making dietary and lifestyle changes to the individual that, depending on the diagnosis, will either ward off the onset of the disease or will help the individual manage the newly diagnosed disease. Screening forms are also offered to the elderly living in the community setting or assisted living to identify risks for malnutrition, osteoporosis, and other chronic diseases. The criteria on the screening form varies by facility; key criteria that are commonly included are shown in **TABLE 2**.

TABLE 2 Nutrition screening key criteria
Height and weight
History of weight gain or loss (intentional or unintentional)
Changes in appetite
Lifestyle habits (tobacco use, physical activity, alcohol consumption)
Digestive disorders (constipation, diarrhea, nausea, vomiting)
Laboratory measures (blood, urine, or both)
Family history, previous medical history, or both

Modified from Field LB, Hand RK. Differentiating malnutrition screening and assessment: a nutrition care process perspective. *J Acad Nutr Diet.* 2015;15:824-828.

In the clinical and long-term care setting, screening forms are designed to identify risks of malnutrition (undernutrition), determine the need for more-in-depth nutritional assessment, and ultimately offer an early detection of malnutrition so that nutrition support is provided in a timely manner. In the United States, an estimated 30% to 50% of adult hospital patients are malnourished. Few patients, however receive the formal diagnosis of malnutrition at discharge, and only an estimated 3.2% of discharged patients are diagnosed with malnutrition.[15] It has been well documented that patients who enter the hospital malnourished and are not given nutrition support have increased morbidity and mortality, decreased function and quality of life, and increased length of hospital stays.[16,17] This leads to increased healthcare costs expenses that can cost hospitals millions of dollars.[18]

It is critical for clinical, long-term care, and community facilities to use validated screening tools to identify patients for malnutrition risk or use validated screening tools to diagnose patients with malnutrition—and sometimes both. Using a validated screening tool ensures that (1) the individual who is identified at risk for malnutrition is indeed malnourished (high sensitivity), and (2) the individual who is not identified at risk for malnutrition is likely to be well nourished (high specificity).[14]

The Academy has identified several validated nutritional screening tools that have been researched for their ability to help identify malnutrition risk in individuals in community and clinical settings.[19] These tools largely use the same screening parameters to determine scores and risk levels. Commonly used risk-assessment parameters include recent weight loss, recent poor intake or appetite, and body mass index (BMI).[20] **TABLE 3** summarizes the most commonly used validated screening tools available and a description of their target populations when screening for malnutrition risk.

Nutrition Assessment Tools

Nutritional assessment is defined by the Academy as "identifying and evaluating data needed to make decisions about a nutrition-related problem/diagnosis."[21] In essence, the difference between nutritional screening and nutritional assessment is that a screen identifies the "risk" for a nutrition problem or malnutrition, while the assessment "identifies the presence of or diagnosis" of a nutrition problem or malnutrition. Once identified, the practitioner creates an intervention to resolve the nutrition problem.[14] Validated nutritional assessment tools have been designed to allow RDNs and other healthcare professionals who are trained to use the tool to quickly and cost-effectively diagnose malnutrition in the acute care setting. The **subjective global assessment (SGA)** form initially started as a screening tool that has evolved as a validated diagnostic tool for malnutrition. When administrated

TABLE 3 Commonly used nutrition screening tools

Nutrition Screening Tool	Patient Population	Risk-Screening Parameters	Measures for Malnutrition Risk
Malnutrition screening tool	Acute-care hospitalized adults, oncology patients	▪ Recent weight loss ▪ Recent poor intake	▪ Score 0–1 for recent intake ▪ Score 0–4 for recent weight loss ▪ Total score: ≥2 = at risk for malnutrition
Mini Nutritional Assessment (MNA): Short Form	Subacute and ambulatory elderly patients	▪ Recent intake ▪ Recent weight loss ▪ Mobility ▪ Recent acute disease or psychological stress ▪ Neuropsychological problems ▪ BMI	▪ Score 0–3 for each parameter ▪ Total score: <11 = at risk for malnutrition
Malnutrition Universal Screening Tool (MUST)	Acute-care medical adults, medical surgical hospitalized adult patients	▪ BMI ▪ Weight loss (%) ▪ Acute disease	▪ Score 0–3 for each parameter ▪ Total score: >2 = high risk 1 = medium risk
Nutrition Risk Screening (NRS 2002)	Medical-surgical hospitalized, acute-care hospitalized patients	▪ Recent weight loss (%) ▪ BMI ▪ Severity of disease ▪ Elderly (>70 years of age) ▪ Food intake or eating problems, skipping meals	▪ Score 0–3 for each parameter ▪ Total score: >3 = start nutrition support

Data from The Academy of Nutrition and Dietetics. *The Nutrition Care Manual*. https://www.nutritioncaremanual.org/. Accessed January 15, 2017.

by a trained professional, it is recognized as a validated method to diagnose malnutrition and predict postoperative complications, longer length of stay in postoperative patients and patients in the intensive care unit, readmission to the intensive care unit, and mortality.[22,23]

Recap Nutritional screening tools are designed to quickly evaluate nutritional risk in individuals. Nutritional assessment tools are used to identify the presence of malnutrition in individuals. It is important that the RDN use validated screening and assessment tools to ensure that the results are correct for the population being evaluated.

TABLE 4 Calculating body mass index

BMI Formula	Weight (kilograms) ÷ height (meters^2)
Interpretation	BMI values <18.5 = Underweight BMI values 18.5–24.9 = Normal or desirable BMI values 25.0–29.9 = Overweight BMI values 30.0–34.9 = Obese (class I) BMI values 35.0–39 = Obese (class II) BMI values > 40.0 = Extreme obesity

Data from National Institutes of Health. Clinical guidelines on the identification, evaluation, and treatment of overweight and obesity adults. 1988. Report no. 98-4083. https://www.ncbi.nlm.nih.gov/books/NBK2003/. Accessed December 3, 2016.

Standard Methods of Evaluating Nutritional Status

Preview The use of nutrition assessment methods such as anthropometry, biochemical, and clinical dietary methods are essential tools to determine the health of individuals and groups.

Although the type of data collected to conduct nutritional assessments varies by clinical setting, the process and goal are the same. The evaluation of an individual or population nutritional status involves the interpretation of anthropometric, biochemical, clinical, and dietary data to define whether an individual or a group of individuals are well nourished or suffer from malnutrition. Malnutrition includes both overnutrition and undernutrition.

Anthropometric Measures Method

Anthropometry is defined as the study of the measurement of the human body. It includes dimensions of bone, muscle, and adipose tissue. The area of anthropometry is a noninvasive process for determining body fat mass that incorporates several human body dimensions. Weight, standing height, horizontal length, skinfold thicknesses, limb lengths, wrist breadths, and head, chest, and waist circumferences are just a few examples of the different human body measurements that fall under anthropometric measures.[24]

Many indexes and ratios can be calculated from anthropometric measurements. One common indicator calculated from anthropometric measurements is the **body mass index (BMI)**. BMI is a measure of body fat utilizing height and weight for adult men and women. The National Academies of Science Engineering and Medicine (NASEM)—Health and Medicine Division, the Centers for Disease Control and Prevention (CDC), and many other organizations that conduct research on the health risks associated with excess weight and obesity use BMI as a measure.[25] **TABLE 4** shows the formula used to calculate BMI as well as the parameters used to interpret measures.

Anthropometry is a significant element in the nutrition assessment of individual children and adults, as well as segments of the population. Through the use of the National Health and Nutrition Examination Survey (NHANES), data collected through anthropometric measurements have been used to monitor growth and weight trends in the American population for more than 50 years.[26]

The anthropometric data for infants and children reveal general health status and dietary adequacy and are used to track trends in growth and development over time. The data collected have been used to produce national reference standards or growth charts.[27] Researchers from different health disciplines, for example, cardiovascular health, gerontology, nutrition, and occupational health, use anthropometric data to examine health status and healthcare utilization trends in U.S. adults.[24]

Biochemical Measures Method

Variations in the quantity and composition of a person's diet are reflected in the concentration of chemical substances in tissue and body fluids and the appearance of different metabolites. The nutrition gamut ranges from an extreme of malnutrition because of deficiency, to optimal nutrition, to malnutrition because of overnutrition at the other end. Biochemical measures serve to identify nutritional status at any stage along the nutrition spectrum.

Although used commonly for identifying malnutrition, current literature is inconsistent for showing the validity of biochemical markers as determinants of individuals' nutritional status. The main consensus in the literature is that laboratory markers are not reliable as a stand-alone assessment.[28] The analysis of laboratory data can be difficult, and results are not always connected to clinical or nutrition findings. Biochemical results can be influenced by nonnutritional factors such as medications, hydration status, disease state, and stress.[28]

Not all content of body nutrients can be assessed by biochemical methods. Common deficiencies identified via biochemical or laboratory methods include[9]:

- Blood-forming nutrients such as iron, folacin, and vitamins B_6 and B_{12}
- Water-soluble vitamins such as thiamine, riboflavin, niacin, and vitamin C
- All of the fat-soluble vitamins (A, D, E, and K)
- Minerals such as iron, iodine, and trace elements; and
- Levels of blood lipids, including cholesterol, triglycerides, glucose, and enzymes linked to heart disease

The results of anthropometric, clinical, and dietary assessment methods can guide decisions concerning the need for biochemical or laboratory data.

Clinical Method: History and Physical

A comprehensive look at an individual's or a group's nutrition assessment takes into account their history. A clinical history coupled with a physical examination is essential to identify signs and symptoms of malnutrition. A clinical history usually includes information such as medical diagnosis, recent hospital admissions, medications, changes in intake of food and fluids, food supply and preparation ability, and weight changes.

Once a history is obtained, a **nutrition-focused physical exam (NFPE)** should be conducted. An NFPE is a systematic way of evaluating an individual from head to toe, paying attention to his or her physical appearance and function to discover signs and symptoms related to malnutrition, nutrient deficiency, and toxicity.[29]

The presence of weight loss is an indicator of an individual's nutritional status.[30] In 2012, the Academy and the American Society for Parenteral and Enteral Nutrition put out a consensus statement defining malnutrition as the presence of two of the following symptoms: inadequate energy intake, weight loss, loss of muscle mass, loss of subcutaneous fat, localized or generalized accumulation of fluid, or decreased functional status as measured by handgrip strength.[12] Many of these characteristics are easily evaluated via an NFPE. See **TABLE 5** to review some of the signs and symptoms that can be identified as a result of conducting a systems-focused assessment.

Dietary Methods

Dietary assessment methods are used to collect an individual's and group information on food supply and nutrients consumed. For groups of individuals (population groups), statistical databases such as the **Food and Agriculture Organization of the United Nations (FAO)** and the **Bureau of Labor Statistics Consumer expenditure survey data** provide information on food supply and purchasing habits. Actual food-intake data are obtained through the use of dietary surveys, food diaries, 24-hour recall, food-frequency questionnaires, food-habit questionnaires, or a combination of any of these methods. The NHANES is an example of a national survey program in the United States that has been designed to assess the health and nutritional status of adults and children.[26] This survey is unique in combining interviews and physical examinations.

A food diary requires that a participant report all food and fluids consumed for a specified period of time. A 24-hour recall involves listing all food and fluids consumed in the previous 24 hours. Foods and quantity consumed are recalled from memory with the assistance of a trained interviewer to facilitate the process. A food-frequency questionnaire is a structured listing of individual foods or groups of foods. For each food item or group, the participant must define the frequency in which the food is consumed in a specified time frame. This can be the number of times the food or group is consumed in a day, a week, or even a month. Diet histories are used to determine the usual intake of a specific individual. Food-habit questionnaires are used to collect either general information or specific details such as food perceptions and beliefs. Food likes and dislikes, food-preparation methods, and social surroundings related to meals are collected using this method. Combined dietary assessment methods can be pooled to improve accuracy and enable interpretation of the dietary data.[31]

Like all self-reported data, the complete accuracy of information obtained from dietary assessment methods such as surveys can be questioned. A study designed to evaluate the validity of the data reported by NHANES on caloric intake reported that in the 39 years of the history of the survey, data reported by the majority of participants were not physiologically reasonable.[32] These findings suggest that the ability to estimate population trends in caloric intake

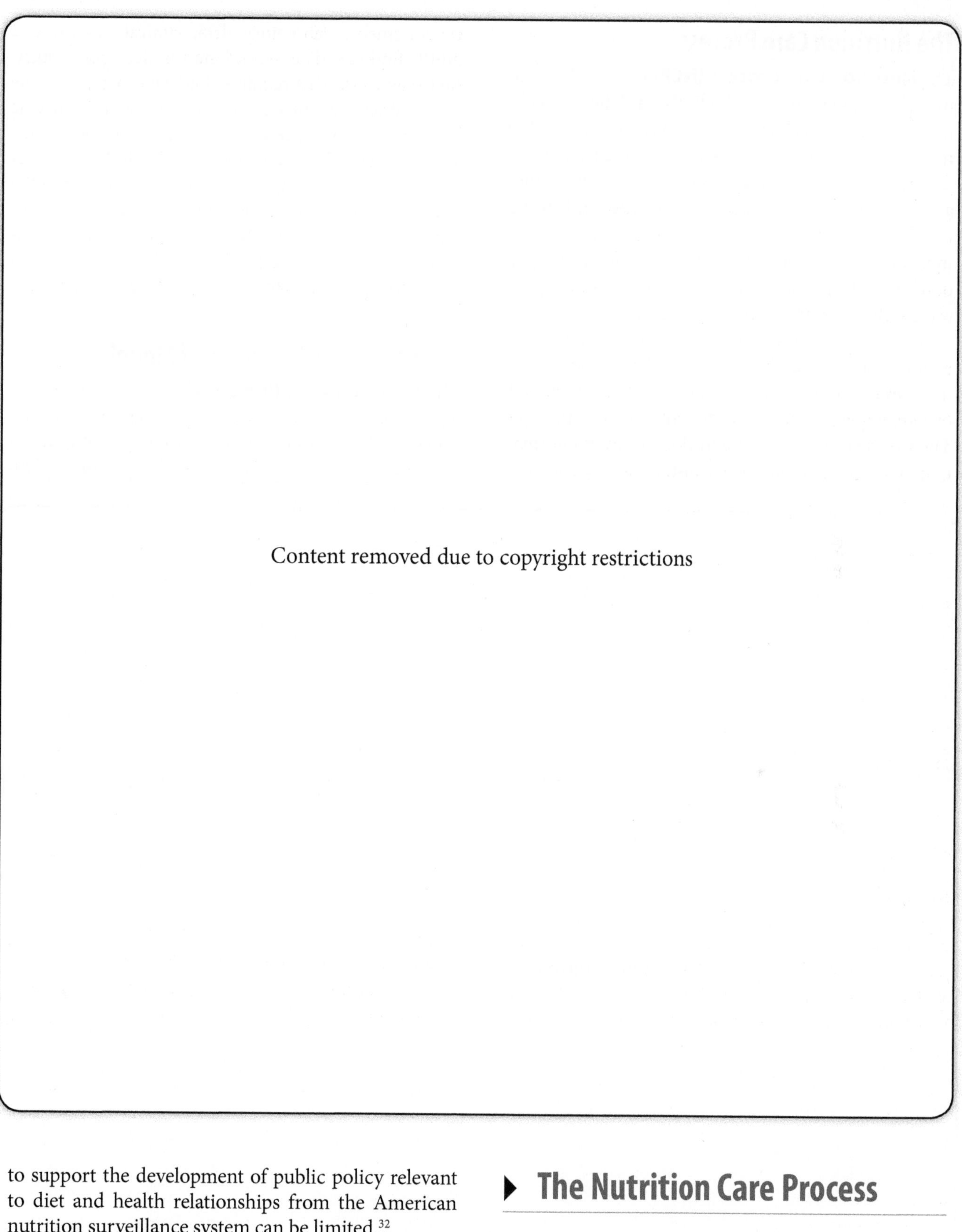

Content removed due to copyright restrictions

to support the development of public policy relevant to diet and health relationships from the American nutrition surveillance system can be limited.[32]

Recap The use of the different nutrition assessment methods are valuable, simple, and practical tools used to describe nutrition problems in individuals as well as groups within the community.

The Nutrition Care Process

Preview The Nutrition Care Process is a tool used by nutrition and dietetics professionals to improve the consistency and quality of individualized care for patients, clients, or groups.

The Nutrition Care Process

The **Nutrition Care Process (NCP)** is a standardized model developed to assist the RDNs and dietetic technicians, registered (NDTR), in delivering high-quality nutrition care.[33] This process provides the framework for the RDN and NDTR to customize care, taking into account the individual's needs and values, while using the best scientific evidence at the time care decisions must be made. In 2003, the Academy endorsed the use of the NCP to afford nutrition specialists a strategy for critical thinking and decision making.

The NCP involves the use of unique yet interdependent—that is, distinct but interrelated—steps. This includes the completion of a nutrition assessment. Part of completing a nutrition assessment involves four steps. The first step is collecting and documenting information such as nutrition-related history, anthropometric measurements, laboratory data, clinical history, and NFPE findings. The second step is defining a nutrition diagnosis. This requires the RDN to evaluate the collected assessment information and name a specific problem that can be resolved through nutritional interventions. The third step requires the RDN to select nutrition interventions that will address the root of the nutrition diagnosis to resolve or control signs and symptoms. The last step of the NCP is monitoring and evaluation to determine whether the individual has achieved or is making progress toward the predetermined goal.[33]

Nutrition Care Process and Model

The **Nutrition Care Process and Model (NCPM)** is a pictorial conception that shows the steps of the Nutrition Care Process as well as internal and external factors that influence application of the NCP (**FIGURE 3**).

Content removed due to copyright restrictions

The relationship between the RDN and the individual or groups of individuals is at the center of the model, which defines the four steps of the NCP—nutrition assessment, diagnosis, intervention, and monitoring and evaluation. The NCP helps to identify external factors such as skill and ability of the RDN, application of evidence-based practice, application of the code of ethics, and knowledge of the RDN as some of the external factors influencing the process. This set of factors defines how individuals and groups of individuals receive nutrition information.

Other factors that impact the ability of individuals and groups to take advantage of the RDN services includes the healthcare system, socioeconomics, and the practice setting. The practice setting reveals rules and regulations that guide a practice and include the age and conditions qualifying for services and how the nutrition and dietetics professional apportions his or her time. The healthcare system defines the amount of time available for the nutrition and dietetics professional–patient interaction, the kind of services offered, and who provides the services. Social components reflect the health-related knowledge, values, and the time devoted to improving nutritional health of both individuals and groups. The economic aspect integrates resources assigned to nutrition care, including the value of a food and the nutrition professional's time expressed in the form of salary and reimbursement.[34]

The screening and referral process as well as outcomes management complete the components of the NCP. The NCPM offers a consistent structure and framework for nutrition and food professionals to use when providing nutrition care. The model is intended for use with individuals and groups of individuals of all ages with any healthcare condition and in all care settings.[13]

Nutrition Care Process: Standardized Language

RDNs utilize **Nutrition Care Process Terminology (NCPT)** to describe all activities performed in the four steps of the NCP.[21] The NCPT is a controlled vocabulary used to depict the distinctive activities of nutrition and dietetics in completing the nutrition assessment, nutrition diagnosis, nutrition intervention, and nutrition monitoring and evaluation. It is intended to enable clear and reliable narratives of the services provided by RDNs.[35] Aside from facilitating communication, the NCPT enables researchers to define the types of nutrition problems observed in patient populations (nutrition diagnoses), the interventions to put in place, and the outcomes obtained.

The NCPT contains more than 1,000 terms and was developed with contributions from practitioners and researchers. Many of the terms have been matched for incorporation into the Systematized Nomenclature of Medicine—Clinical Terms and Logical Observation Identifiers Names and Codes. These are clinical terms in use worldwide for electronic health records. The NCPT's specific vocabulary allows for data gathering for nutrition research and documentation of quality measures.

The NCPT includes specific language for nutrition diagnosis. These statements help describe nutrition problems that the RDN can treat. The unique language developed to identify nutrition interventions helps outline actions intended to change a nutrition-related behavior, environmental condition, or aspect of health status for an individual or a group.[35] The NCPT also includes nomenclature to identify nutrition monitoring and evaluation parameters that can be used to determine changes in outcomes as they relate to nutrition diagnosis and intervention.

Nutrition Care Process: Assessment

Nutrition assessment is a systematic method for obtaining, verifying, and interpreting data needed to identify nutrition-related problems, their causes, and their significances.[36] It is a continuous, nonlinear, and dynamic procedure that includes initial data gathering as well as recurrent reassessment and analysis of the individual's status compared to identified standards. Through the evaluation of the data collected for the nutrition assessment, the RDNs is able to determine whether a nutritionally diagnosable problem exists.[36]

The nutrition assessment terms are identified and grouped into five domains: food/nutrition-related history, anthropometric measurements, biochemical data, medical tests, and procedures.

A nutrition assessment commences after an individual is referred, as a consequence of an at-risk nutrition screen, or when an individual can benefit from nutrition care. Nutrition assessment allows the nutrition practitioner to determine if a nutrition diagnosis or problem exists. When that is the case, the RDN properly diagnoses the problem and generates a *problem, etiology, signs* or *symptoms* (PES) statement. This is step two of the NCP. In addition, RDNs create a plan to put in place interventions to resolve the nutrition diagnoses. In some instances, a plan of care identifies the need for further information or testing. If the initial completed assessment or reassessment shows that a nutrition problem is not present or that current problems cannot be improved by supplementary nutrition care, discharge from nutrition care services is appropriate.[21]

Data to complete a nutrition assessment of individuals is obtained from the person through interviews, observation, measurements, medical records, and information provided by the referring healthcare provider. For population groups, data from surveys, administrative data sets, and epidemiological or research studies are used to collect assessment information. The use of standardized language enables effective comparison of nutrition-assessment findings. When conducting the assessment, the RDN must determine which are the most appropriate data to collect, assess the need for additional data, select assessment tools and procedures that match the situation, and apply assessment tools in a reliable manner. The assessor must determine which data are relevant, important, and valid for inclusion in the nutrition assessment.[21]

NCP: Nutrition Diagnosis

Defining a nutrition diagnosis is an important step between nutrition assessment and defining nutrition interventions. The purpose of a standardized nutrition diagnosis language is to designate nutrition problems reliably so that they are clear for all professionals. A **nutrition diagnosis** is used to identify and define a particular nutrition problem that can be solved or whose symptoms can be managed through nutrition interventions by a nutrition and food professional. A nutrition diagnosis (such as inadequate sodium intake) is different from a medical diagnosis (such as congestive heart failure). Unlike a nutrition diagnosis, a medical diagnosis defines a disease process or pathology such as congestive heart failure. It is not within the scope of nutrition and dietetics professionals to determine or assign medical diagnoses. The standardized language improves communication and documentation of nutrition care, and it offers a minimum data set and consistent data foundations for future research. The nutrition diagnosis falls into three domains: intake, clinical, and behavioral or environment. **TABLE 6** shows examples of nutrition diagnostic terminology that fall under each domain. A designation of "no nutrition diagnoses" can be used for individuals whose documented nutrition assessment indicate no nutritional problem requiring nutrition intervention and treatment.[21]

The outcome of the nutrition-diagnosis step of the NCP is the creation of a diagnosis statement, or **PES statement**, which has three elements: the problem (P), its etiology (E), and its signs and symptoms (S). The elements of the PES statement are joined by the phrases "related to" and "as evidenced by." The data collected and analyzed during the nutrition assessment are used to generate the PES statement.[21] **FIGURE 4** shows how the standardized language is used to create a nutrition diagnosis and PES statement.

TABLE 6 Nutrition diagnostic terminology

Domain	Problem
Intake	Inadequate energy intake Malnutrition
Clinical	Impaired nutrient utilization Unintended weight loss
Behavioral/ Environmental	Not ready for diet or lifestyle change Limited access to food or water

Data from Academy of Nutrition and Dietetics. *Nutrition Terminology Reference Manual (eNCPT): Dietetics Language for Nutrition Care.* 2016. http://ncpt.webauthor.com/. Accessed December 8, 2016.

NCP: Intervention

The third step of the NCP is determining the most appropriate intervention to resolve the nutrition problem. A **nutrition intervention** is the action taken by the nutrition and dietetics professional to correct or manage a nutrition problem. Its purpose is to target and resolve the diagnosis by eliminating signs and symptoms related to nutrition-related behaviors, environmental conditions, or conditions that affect nutrition and health. Nutrition interventions need to be individualized to meet the specific needs of each person.[21,36]

The NCP nutrition intervention has two distinct steps: planning and implementation. Planning involves selecting and prioritizing the nutrition diagnosis, collaborating with other caregivers, involving the patient and his or her representative, and reviewing evidence-based practice guidelines. With the patient at the center of the care, the FDN should work toward the expected outcome for the nutrition diagnosis, outline nutrition interventions, identify the frequency of the treatment, and identify the resources needed. The implementation step involves communicating and carrying out the care plan developed for the individual. Plan implementation involves monitoring the plan for acceptance (by the individual) and effectiveness. If the expected outcome for the individual is not being obtained, the interventions must be changed.[21,36]

Most often the nutrition intervention is designed to correct the etiology component of the PES statement.

Patient Information

Mrs. Smith is a 66-year-old female who was referred to your office by her primary care provider. The reason for the referral is outlined weight loss in the past 3 months.

Mrs. Smith's diagnosis includes diabetes, hypertension, and arthritis. Her height is 5'4". Her weight in the past three months: month 1 = 135 lbs, month 2= 127 lbs, month 3 = 122 lbs. Her usual body weight fluctuates between 137 and 134 lbs. Her current BMI = 20.9. This value is within the range for normal BMI.

Mrs. Smith's medical history is significant for diabetes and arthritis. During your interaction with the Mrs. Smith, you determine that overall her blood sugars are well controlled. She understands her medication regime and the importance of following her medication schedule. She reports that she has been "a bit out of sorts" since her husband died four months ago. Mr. Smith had been a world-renowned chef who had retired and turned his energy to shopping for and preparing every meal at home. Since his death, Mrs. Smith has not had the desire to shop for food or cook meals. This just does not seem important to her.

As the nutrition assessment is completed, you conclude that Mrs. Smith has poor intakes of calories and protein. Her intake is related to changes in her living situation following the death of her husband, who had supported her by preparing all meals. The poor intake has resulted in a 13-lb weight loss in three months.

Focusing on the poor intake as the key problem, the PES statement can be written as:

> Inadequate protein-energy intake (NI-5.3) related to poor meal intake and loss of support for preparing meals as evidenced by a 13-lb weight loss in three months.

To address the weight loss, the PES statement can be written as:

> Unintended weight loss (NC-3.2) related to poor meal intake and loss of support for preparing meals as evidenced by a 13-lb weight loss in 3 months.

FIGURE 4 Using standardized language to create a PES statement

Data from Academy of Nutrition and Dietetics. *Nutrition Terminology Reference Manual (eNCPT): Dietetics Language for Nutrition Care.* 2016.http://ncpt.webauthor.com/. Accessed December 8, 2016.

Four domains are used when creating nutrition interventions: (1) food or nutrient delivery, (2) nutrition education, (3) nutrition counseling, and (4) coordination of care. The food or nutrient delivery domain encompasses provision of meals, snacks, and enteral and parenteral nutrition. Education and counseling tactics can help operationalize food and nutrient delivery efforts and guide individuals to make food choices that promote healthy eating patterns and optimize health. Nutrition education varies by care setting, desired outcome, and whether the person has a chronic or acute disease process. For instance, for home-dwelling individuals, food safety might be the focus of their nutrition education; therefore, counseling goes beyond understanding healthy eating patterns. It requires influencing and coaching individuals to foster lifestyle changes. Coordination of care is an **interprofessional** collaboration to identify the individual's needs and identify resources.[21,36]

NCP: Monitoring and Evaluation

Nutrition monitoring and evacuation is the fourth step of the NCP. The purpose of this step is to measure the progress made by the individual in achieving the predetermined outcome. The individual's outcomes that are relevant to the nutrition diagnosis and interventions are monitored and measured. Data sources to aid in this step include self-monitoring information and material collected through records such as forms, spreadsheets, and computer programs. Information from anthropometric measurements, biochemical data, tests, and procedures also help to evaluate progress from current status to desired state. Data from pretests, questionnaires, surveys, and mail or telephone follow-up can also be used to measure the level of success of the plan of care.[21,36]

Outcomes associated with food and nutrient intake, nutrition-related physical signs and symptoms, and nutrition-related patient- and individual-centered outcomes are usually monitored by the nutrition and dietetics professional.[21,36]

The NCP's nutrition monitoring and evaluation step incorporates three unique and interconnected processes: monitoring process, measuring outcomes, and evaluating outcomes. Monitoring process involves ensuring that the client, patient, or individual understands and complies with the plan. This includes determining if the interventions were implemented as prescribed, providing evidence of how the plan is helping the patient to meet (or not meet) their goals, detecting other positive or negative outcomes, collecting information, identifying causes for absence of progress, and aggregating data that support the lack of progress as well as support conclusions with evidence. Measuring outcomes involves identifying markers that are relevant to the nutrition diagnosis or signs and symptoms, nutrition goals, medical diagnosis and outcomes, and quality-management goals. Evaluating outcomes requires that the nutrition care provider evaluate the change between the outcomes obtained to the individual's status at the beginning of the care process.[21,36]

Recap The use of standardized indicators and criteria helps nutrition and dietetics professionals communicate using a common language understood inside and outside the profession. Data collected are used to promote continued development of the outcome data's validity and reliability.

Emerging Opportunities for Nutritional Assessment and Evaluation

Preview Micronutrient deficiencies are no longer the leading public-health priority in the United States. It is important to monitor individual and groups of individuals' diet and body weight as part of health-promotion and disease-prevention programs.

For more than a century, the role of nutrition in promoting health and preventing disease was overshadowed by great achievements in medicine. In the same time frame, science and research increased our knowledge and understanding of micronutrient requirements and their role in supporting health. Changes in the food industry supporting the enrichment and fortification of food products have contributed to eradicating micronutrient deficiencies in some segments of the population. As a result, micronutrient deficiencies are no longer the highest public-health priority. Currently, a better understanding of the complex relationship between nutrition and health has placed the conduct of nutrition assessments as a key indicator in the surveillance of population health. Conducting population nutrition assessments provides data that help to continue advance healthcare practices.

Healthy People 2020 Nutrition Objectives

One of the goals of the Healthy People 2020 initiative is to reduce the proportion of adults who are obese. The goal is to decrease this rate from a 2020 baseline of 33.9% to 30.5% by 2020. The 2011–2014 data reflecting rate of obesity per race are shown in Figure 4. These data show that the obesity rate for the white non-Hispanic or Latino rate is 34.4%. The obesity rate for African Americans is 47.9%. There is a 13.5 percentage-point difference between the groups with the best and worst obesity rates. This type of information is important for healthcare providers regardless of the practice setting. For the researcher interested in public health, this type of information is essential to demonstrate the need for additional research involving this segment of the population. **FIGURE 5** shows obesity disparities by race and ethnicity.

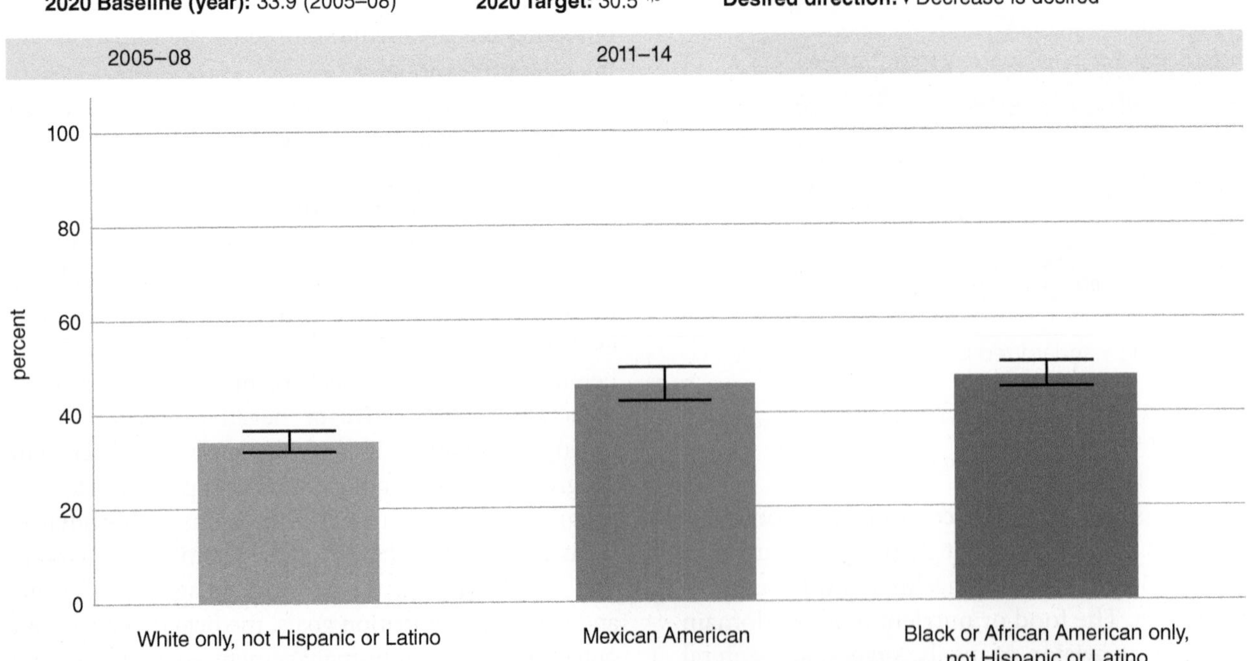

FIGURE 5 Disparities details by race and ethnicity for 2011–2014: Obesity among adults (age adjusted, percent, 20+ years)

Reproduced from Healthy People 2020. Disparities Details by Race and Ethnicity for 2011-14: Obesity among adults (age adjusted, percent, 20+ years) https://www.healthypeople.gov/2020/data/disparities/detail/Chart/4968/3/2014 Accessed 7/1/2017.

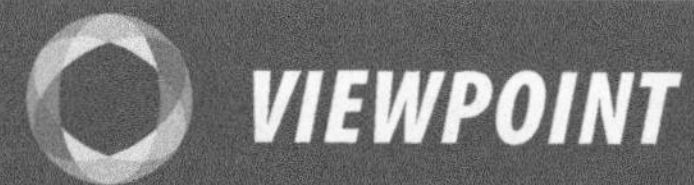

Health Initiatives

Robin S. Rood, MA, MEd, RD, LD

A health initiative is a strategy, action plan, or approach offered by an agency of the federal government, private business, or nonprofit organization to inform and direct people toward better health. In March 2010, the Affordable Care Act (ACA) was enacted into law, expanding access to health care to millions of people who had previously been unable to get health care because of preexisting conditions or simply because they could not afford it (**FIGURE A**).[1] One of the ACA's most popular features is that it allows children to remain on their parents' insurance until age 26 years.[2] In addition, preventive care services such as free flu shots, birth control, and annual physicals are more easily accessed.

In September 2010, First Lady Michelle Obama and National Football League (NFL) Commissioner Roger Goodell launched the "Let's Move" Campaign. Although the website is still available for public viewing, it is no longer being updated.[3] The "Play 60" campaign is now called the "Fuel Up to Play 60" and is an in-school nutrition and physical-activity program sponsored by the National Dairy Council, the NFL, and partners with the U.S. Department of Agriculture.[4] These programs encourage children, teens, and adults to engage in physical activity every day. The goal is to create a public and private partnership to combat childhood obesity.

The Presidential Active Lifestyle Award (PALA+) was created by the National Foundation on Fitness, Sports, and Nutrition to promote physical activity and good nutrition, and encourage Americans to meet the Physical Activity Guidelines and Dietary Guidelines for Americans. To win this award you can register at www.supertracker .usda.gov/PALAplus.aspx and log in to track foods and exercise for five weeks to earn a PALA+, or sign up at the

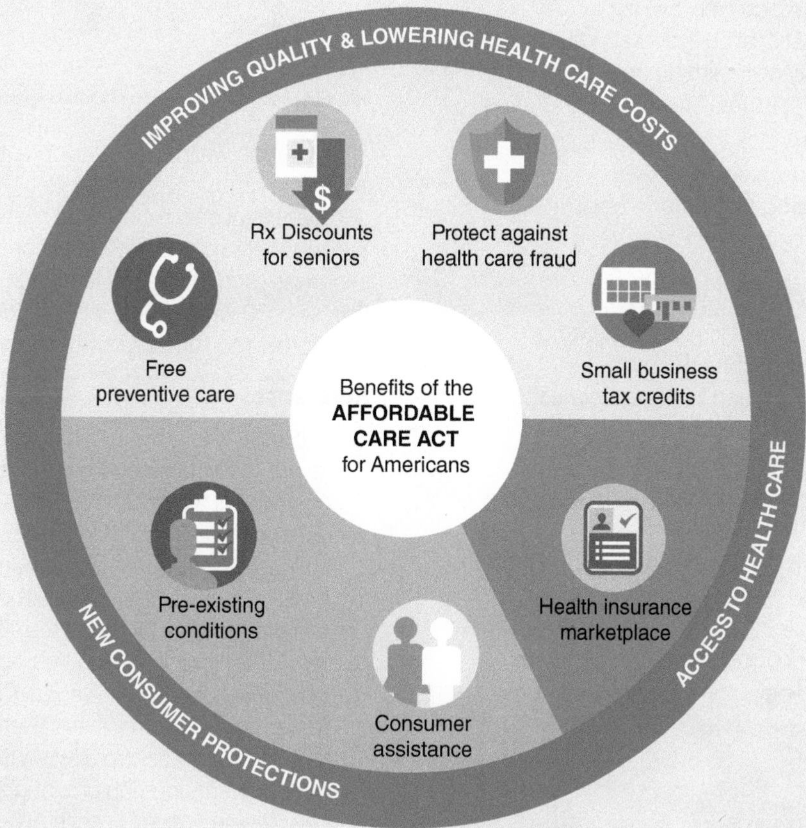

Benefits for women	**Your adult coverage**	**Strengthening Medicare**	**Holding insurance companies accountable**
Providing insurance options, covering preventing service, and lowering costs.	Coverage available to children up to age 26 years.	Yearly wellness visit and many free preventing services for some seniors with Medicare.	Insures must justify any premium increase of 10% or more before the rate takes effect.

FIGURE A Benefits of the Affordable Care Act

Reproduced from Issues: Affordable Care Act. United States Congressman Gene Green. https://green.house.gov/issues/affordable-care-act.

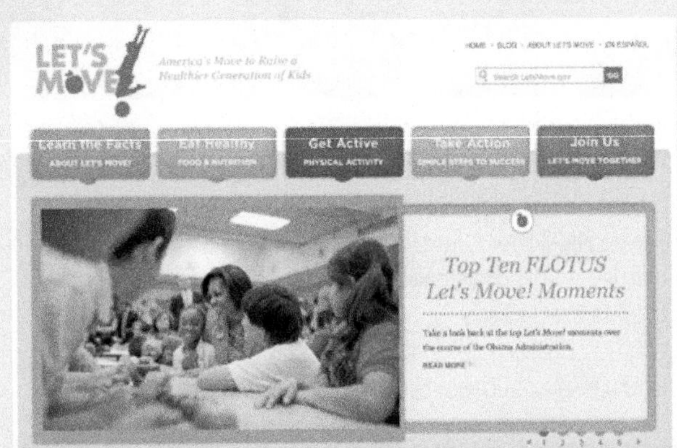

Reproduced from Let's Move! https://letsmove.obamawhitehouse.archives.gov.

National Fitness Foundation (www.fitness.foundation/pala), the only nonprofit officially chartered by Congress. Anyone who extends the challenge to weeks 6–8 will achieve a Presidential Active Lifestyle Premium Award.[5,6]

In December 2010, a health initiative called Healthy People 2020 was launched to assess the current health of Americans and offer health education programs targeted to their needs so that every population can live healthy lives.[7]

Now in its third decade, Healthy People 2020 is a science-based set of national objectives aimed at improving the health of all Americans. Healthy People 2020 reflects the need to address current issues in health care, including:

- Adolescent health
- Blood disorders and blood safety
- Dementias, including Alzheimer's disease
- Early and middle childhood
- Genomics
- Global health
- Health-related quality of life and well-being
- Healthcare-associated infections
- Lesbian, gay, bisexual, and transgender health
- Older adults
- Preparedness
- Sleep health
- Social determinants of health

The results of this ongoing collection of information can be found at www.healthypeople.gov. At this time, Healthy People 2030 is in development to project what areas of health are of concern to future generations.

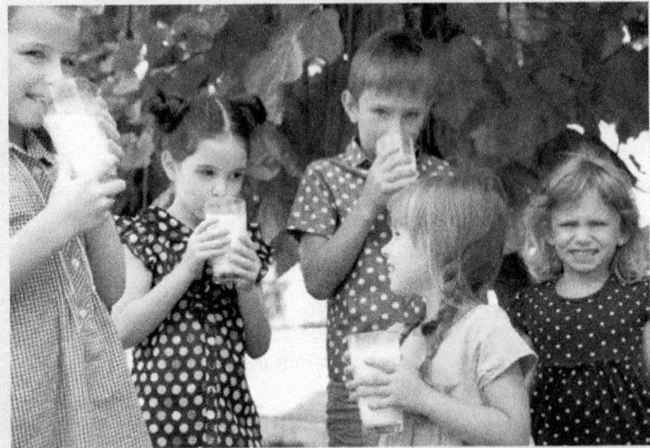
© Africa Studio/Shutterstock.

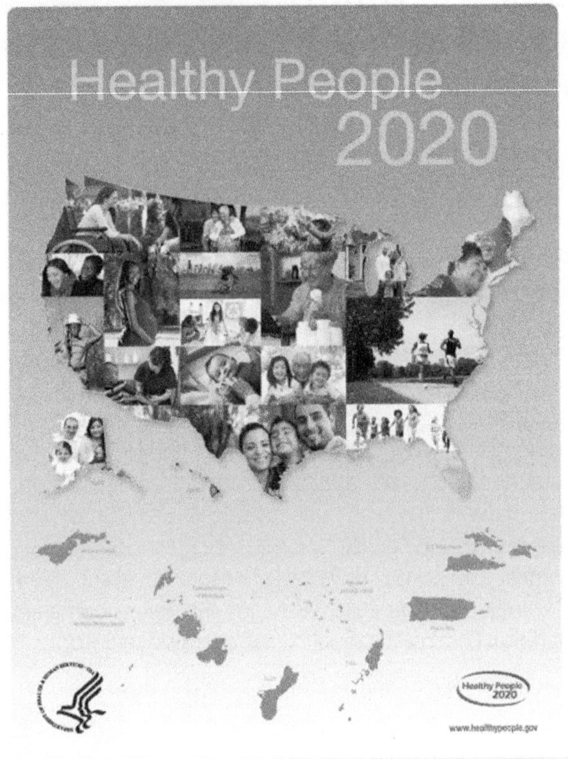

Reproduced from Healthy People 2020. U.S. Department of Health and Human Services. https://www.healthypeople.gov/.

A nation with a healthy population means a stronger and more productive society. Healthy minds and bodies also benefit economically from diet and physical exercise. Because health care costs have continued to increase, initiatives such as Healthy People 2020 and Healthy People 2030 will help keep costs down, create a healthier workforce, and stimulate the economy.

References

1. HHS.gov. About the ACA [online]. (2017). Available at https://www.hhs.gov/healthcare/about-the-aca/index.html. Accessed July 10, 2017.
2. Healthcare.gov. Health Insurance Coverage for Children and Young Adults Under 26 [online]. (2017). Available at https://www.healthcare.gov/young-adults/children-under-26/. Accessed July 10, 2017.
3. Let's Move! [online]. (2017). Available at https://letsmove.obamawhitehouse.archives.gov/. Accessed July 10, 2017.
4. Fueluptoplay60.com. What Is Fuel Up to Play 60? [online]. (2017). Available at https://www.fueluptoplay60.com/funding/nutrition-equipment-grant.
5. Presidential Active Lifestyle Award (PALA+). [online]. (2017). Available at https://www.supertracker.usda.gov/PALAPlus.aspx. Accessed July 10, 2017.
6. President's Council on Fitness, Sports, and Nutrition. PALA+. [online]. (2017). Available at: https://www.hhs.gov/fitness/programs-and-awards/pala/. Accessed July 10, 2017.
7. Office of Disease Prevention and Health Promotion. Healthy People 2020. [online]. (2017). Available at: https://www.healthypeople.gov/. Accessed July 10, 2017.

Healthy People 2020 (HP 2020) is a set of goals and objectives with 10-year targets that are designed to guide national health-promotion and disease-prevention efforts to improve the health of all people in the United States. Released by the U.S. Department of Health and Human Services each decade, the Healthy People initiatives reflect the idea that setting objectives and providing science-based benchmarks to track and monitor progress can motivate and focus action. HP 2020 represents the fourth generation of this initiative, building on three decades of previous work.[38]

HP 2020 is a tool used for strategic management by the federal government, states, communities, and many other public- and private-sector partners. Its comprehensive set of objectives and targets is used to measure progress for health issues in specific populations as well as serve as a foundation for prevention and wellness activities across various sectors and within the federal government. It also serves as a model for measurement at the state and local levels. HP 2020 is committed to the vision of "a society in which all people live long, healthy lives." The initiative has four predominant goals:[38]

1. Help Americans have higher-quality and longer lives that are free of preventable diseases, disabilities, injuries, and premature death.
2. Help Americans achieve health equity, eliminate disparities, and improve the health of all groups.
3. Create social and physical environments that promote good health for all.
4. Promote quality of life, healthy development, and healthy behaviors across all life stages.

HP 2020 monitors approximately 1,200 objectives organized into 42 topic areas, each of which represents an important public-health area.[38] See **TABLE 7**.

The goal of the nutrition and health-status objective is to promote health and reduce chronic-disease risk through the consumption of healthful diets and achievement and maintenance of healthy body weights.[39]

The nutrition and weight status objectives for HP 2020 reflect strong science supporting the health benefits of eating a healthful diet and maintaining a healthy body weight. The objectives also emphasize that efforts to change diet and weight should address individual behaviors as well as the policies and environments that support these behaviors in settings such as schools, work sites, healthcare organizations, and communities.[39]

The goal of promoting healthy diets and healthy weight includes increasing household food security and eliminating hunger. A healthy diet includes a variety of nutrient-dense foods within and across the food groups, especially whole grains, fruits, vegetables, low-fat or fat-free milk or milk products, and lean meats and other protein sources. Individuals are also encouraged to limit the intake of saturated and *trans* fats, cholesterol, added sugars, sodium, and alcohol, as well as limit overall intake to meet caloric needs.[40]

Monitoring population diet and body weight is an important part of any health-promotion and disease-prevention program. Good nutrition is especially important to the growth and development of children. A healthy diet also helps Americans reduce their risks for many health conditions, including overweight and obesity, malnutrition, iron-deficiency anemia, heart disease, hypertension, dyslipidemia, type 2 diabetes, osteoporosis, oral disease, constipation, diverticular disease, and some forms of cancer.[22,39]

Diet reflects the variety of foods and beverages consumed over time in the home and in settings such as work sites, schools, and restaurants. Interventions that support the consumption of a healthier diet help ensure that individuals will have the knowledge and skills to make healthier choices.

Because weight is influenced by the balance between number of calories consumed versus calories expended, interventions put in place to improve weight should support changes in diet as well as physical activity. As new and innovative policies and environmental interventions to support diet and physical activity are implemented, it will be important to identify which are most effective. A better understanding of how to prevent unhealthy weight gain is also needed.[39] HP 2020 includes 22 objectives[21] as shown in **TABLE 8**.

Diabetes Mellitus

Diabetes mellitus is perhaps one of the oldest disorders known to medicine. Clinical descriptions describing what we now call DM were portrayed 3,000 years ago by the ancient Egyptians.[41] See **FIGURE 6** for a quick history of DM.

Because DM is so widespread, it is now considered a 21st-century global emergency. An estimated 415 million adults worldwide live with DM. In addition, 318 million adults suffer from impaired glucose tolerance, thus increasing their risk for developing DM.[24] In the United States, 29.1 million people—9.3% of the American population—have diabetes, out of which only 21 million individuals have been diagnosed. During 2008–2009, an estimated 18,436 people younger than 20 years in the United States were newly diagnosed with type 1 diabetes annually, and 5,089

TABLE 7 Healthy People 2020 topic areas

	Public-Health Area		
	Access to Health Services	**Genomics***	**Nutrition and Weight Status**
Topic Areas	Adolescent health*	Global health*	Occupational safety and health
	Arthritis, osteoporosis, and chronic back conditions Blood disorders and blood safety*	Healthcare-associated infections* Health communication and health information technology	Older adults* Oral health
	Cancer	Health-related quality of life and well-being*	Physical activity
	Chronic kidney disease	Hearing and other sensory or communication disorders	Preparedness*
	Dementias, including Alzheimer's disease*	Heart disease and stroke	Public-health infrastructure
	Diabetes	HIV	Respiratory diseases
	Disability and health	Immunization and infectious diseases	Sexually transmitted diseases
	Early and middle childhood*	Injury and violence prevention	Sleep health*
	Educational and community-based programs	Lesbian, gay, bisexual, and transgender health*	Social determinants of health*
	Environmental health	Maternal, infant, and child health	Substance abuse
	Family planning	Medical product safety	Tobacco use
	Food safety	Mental health and mental disorders	Vision

*These topics were not included in HP2010 and are new to HP2020.

Data from Centers for Disease Control and Prevention. *HP 2020.* https://www.cdc.gov/nchs/healthy_people/hp2020.htm. 2015. Accessed December 17, 2016.

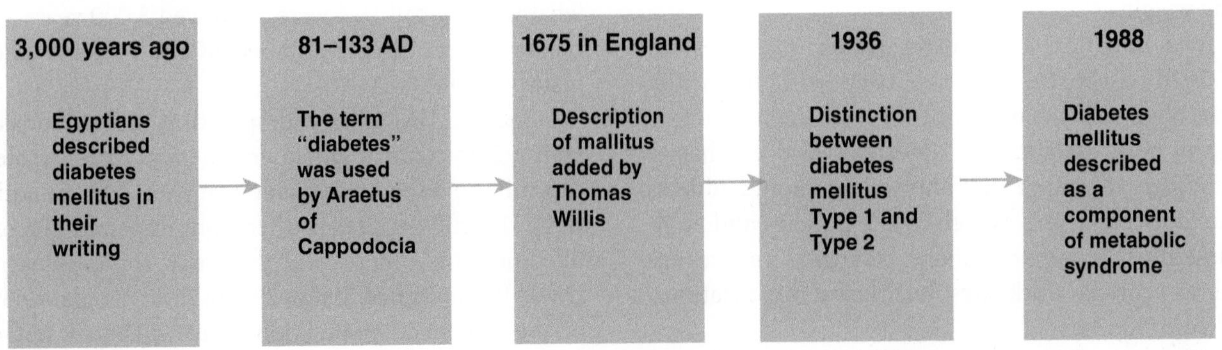

FIGURE 6 History of diabetes mellitus

Data from Ahmed AM. History of diabetes mellitus. *Saudi Med J.* 2002. Apr;23(4):373-378.

TABLE 8 HP 2020 nutrition and weight status objectives	
Area	**Objectives**
Healthier Food Access	Increase the number of states with nutrition standards for foods and beverages provided to preschool-aged children in childcare
	Increase the proportion of schools that offer nutritious foods and beverages outside of school meals ■ Increase the proportion of schools that do not sell or offer calorically sweetened beverages to students ■ Increase the proportion of school districts that require schools to make fruits or vegetables available whenever other food is offered or sold
	Increase the number of states that have state-level policies that incentivize food retail outlets to provide foods that are encouraged by the *Dietary Guidelines for Americans*
	Increase the proportion of Americans who have access to a food retail outlet that sells a variety of foods that are encouraged by the *Dietary Guidelines for Americans*
Health Care and Work-Site Settings	Increase the proportion of primary care physicians who regularly measure their patients' body mass index (BMI) ■ Increase the proportion of primary care physicians who regularly assess BMI in their adult patients ■ Increase the proportion of primary care physicians who regularly assess BMI for age and gender in their child or adolescent patients
	Increase the proportion of physician office visits that include counseling or education related to nutrition or weight ■ Increase the proportion of physician office visits made by patients with a diagnosis of cardiovascular disease, diabetes, or hyperlipidemia that include counseling or education related to diet or nutrition ■ Increase the proportion of physician office visits made by adult patients who are obese that include counseling or education related to weight reduction, nutrition, or physical activity ■ Increase the proportion of physician visits made by all child or adult patients that include counseling about nutrition or diet
	Increase the proportion of work sites that offer nutrition or weight-management classes or counseling
Weight Status	Increase the proportion of adults who are at a healthy weight
	Reduce the proportion of adults who are obese
	Reduce the proportion of children and adolescents who are considered obese ■ Reduce the proportion of children ages 2 to 5 years who are considered obese ■ Reduce the proportion of children ages 6 to 11 years who are considered obese ■ Reduce the proportion of adolescents ages 12 to 19 years who are considered obese ■ Reduce the proportion of children and adolescents ages 2 to 19 years who are considered obese
	Prevent inappropriate weight gain in youth and adults ■ Prevent inappropriate weight gain in children ages 2 to 5 years ■ Prevent inappropriate weight gain in children ages 6 to 11 years ■ Prevent inappropriate weight gain in adolescents ages 12 to 19 years ■ Prevent inappropriate weight gain in children and adolescents ages 2 to 19 years ■ Prevent inappropriate weight gain in adults ages 20 years and older
Food Insecurity	Eliminate the worst food insecurity among children
	Reduce household food insecurity and thus reduce hunger

(*continues*)

TABLE 8 (continued)	
Area	**Objectives**
Food and Nutrient Consumption	Increase the contribution of fruits to the diets of the population age 2 years and older ▪ Increase the variety and contribution of vegetables to the diets of the population age 2 years and older ▪ Increase the contribution of total vegetables to the diets of the population age 2 years and older
	Increase the contribution of dark green vegetables, red and orange vegetables, and beans and peas to the diets of the population age 2 years and older
	Increase the contribution of whole grains to the diets of the population age 2 years and older
	Reduce consumption of calories from solid fats and added sugars in the population age 2 years and older ▪ Reduce consumption of calories from solid fats ▪ Reduce consumption of calories from added sugars ▪ Reduce consumption of calories from solid fats and added sugars
	Reduce consumption of saturated fat in the population age 2 years and older
	Reduce consumption of sodium in the population age 2 years and older
	Increase consumption of calcium in the population age 2 years and older
Iron Deficiency	Reduce iron deficiency among young children and females of childbearing age ▪ Reduce iron deficiency among children ages 1 to 2 years ▪ Reduce iron deficiency among children ages 3 to 4 years ▪ Reduce iron deficiency among females ages 12 to 49 years
	Reduce iron deficiency among pregnant females

Data from US Department of Health and Human Services. (2015), *Heathy People 2020*. https://www.healthypeople.gov/. Accessed December 17, 2016.

people younger than 20 years were newly diagnosed with type 2 diabetes annually (see **FIGURE 7**).[42]

Diabetes was the seventh-leading cause of death in the United States in 2010 based on the 69,071 death certificates that listed diabetes as the underlying cause of death. Studies have found that only 35% to 40% of deceased people with diabetes had death certificates that listed diabetes; 10% to 15% had diabetes listed as the underlying cause of death. From 2003–2006, after adjusting for population age differences, death rates from all causes were 1.5 times higher among adults 18 years of age and older with diagnosed diabetes than among adults without diagnosed diabetes.[42]

Managing DM

Diabetes can be treated and managed when someone adopts a healthy eating pattern, engages in regular physical activity, and takes prescribed medications to lower blood glucose levels. Another critical part of diabetes management is reducing cardiovascular disease risk factors such as high blood pressure, high lipid levels, and the use of tobacco. Patient education and self-care practices also are important aspects of

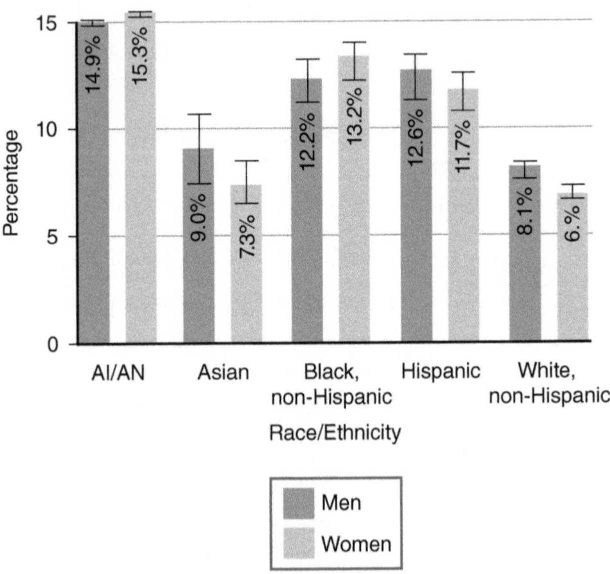

FIGURE 7 New cases of DM in individuals younger than 20 years of age-2013–2015

Reproduced from Center for Disease Control and Prevention, *National Diabetes Statistics Report, 2014*. http://www.thefdha.org/pdf/diabetes.pdf.

disease management that help people with diabetes stay healthy. Nutritional assessment has been vital in identifying risks and diagnosing symptoms and comorbidities associated with DM.[42] Medical nutrition therapy is key to preventing DM, managing individuals who have been diagnosed with DM, and preventing—or at least reducing—the development of DM comorbidities.[43]

Weight Management

From 2011–2014, 36.5% of adult Americans were considered obese. Overall, the prevalence of obesity among middle-aged adults ages 40 to 59 years (40.2%) and older adults ages 60 years and older (37.0%) was higher than among younger adults ages 20 to 39 years (32.3%). The prevalence of obesity among women (38.3%) was higher than among men (34.3%).[44] In 2015, the rate of obesity by state was higher in states such as Texas, Oklahoma, Missouri, and South Carolina. Obesity increases the risk for morbidity because of higher risks for; or the presence of hypertension, dyslipidemia, diabetes, coronary heart disease, stroke, gallbladder disease, osteoarthritis, sleep apnea and respiratory problems, and some cancers. Obesity is also related to increased risks of mortality. The biomedical, psychosocial, and economic effects of obesity have significant repercussions for the health and well-being of the US population.[45] **FIGURE 8** shows the rate of obesity and the rate of coronary heart disease by state for 2015.

The worldwide rate of obesity has more than doubled since 1980. In 2014, more than 1.9 billion adults ages 18 and older (39% of the world's population) were classified as overweight. Of these, more 600 million (13%) were deemed obese. Sadly, most of the world's population lives in countries where being overweight or obese kills more people than being underweight. In 2014, 41 million children over the age of five years fell into the category of overweight or obese. The silver lining in this epidemic is that obesity is preventable.[46]

The World Health Organization (WHO) defines overweight and obesity as "abnormal or excessive fat accumulation that presents a risk to health."[47] Different measuring indexes are used to capture weight measurements, depending on the age group. For children up to 5 years of age, the WHO's child growth standards introduced in April 2006 are recommended. For individuals 5 to 19 years of age, the WHO has developed growth reference data. The data are a reconstruction of the 1977 National Center for Health Statistics (NCHS) and WHO reference and uses the original NCHS data set supplemented with data from the WHO child growth standards sample for young children up to age 5 years. Body mass index is the most frequently used measure of overweight and obesity in adults. BMI is calculated by dividing an individual's weight in kilograms by the square of his or her height in meters ($kg \div m^2$).[47] See **TABLE 9** for a list of BMI ranges and corresponding weight classifications.

The BMI provides the most useful population-level measure of overweight and obesity, as it is the same for both genders and for all ages of adults. It is important to note that one of the limitations of BMI measurement is that it may not correspond to the same body-fat percentage in different individuals.[47]

Globally, increased BMI is a risk factor for noncommunicable diseases such as cardiovascular disease, DM, musculoskeletal disorders (such as osteoarthritis), and cancer (particularly endometrial, breast, ovarian, prostate, liver, kidney, and colon). The risk for these noncommunicable illnesses rises for individuals with higher BMIs. Childhood obesity is linked with a higher chance of adult obesity, premature death, and adult disability. Aside from health risks in their future, obese children suffer from breathing problems and have higher risks for fractures, hypertension, cardiovascular disease, insulin resistance, and attendant psychological consequences.[46]

What Is Being Done About the Obesity Epidemic?

In 2004, the World Health Organization implemented the "WHO Global Strategy on Diet, Physical Activity and Health" program, which outlines the steps needed to promote healthy diets and active lifestyles. This initiative challenges all stakeholders to get involved at global, regional, national, and local levels to improve diet and physical-activity patterns for all members of the population. The WHO has also put in place its "Global Action Plan for the Prevention and Control of Non-Communicable Diseases 2013–2020." Endorsed by heads of state and government in September 2011, this program seeks a 25% reduction in premature mortality from noncommunicable diseases by 2025. In 2016, the World Health Assembly requested a plan from the director general of the WHO's Commission on Ending Childhood Obesity to address the obesogenic environment and critical periods in the life course to tackle childhood obesity.[46] In the United States, HP 2020 addresses nutrition and weight status as one of its topic areas.

Heart Disease

Every 42 seconds, someone somewhere in the United States has a heart attack. Every minute, an American

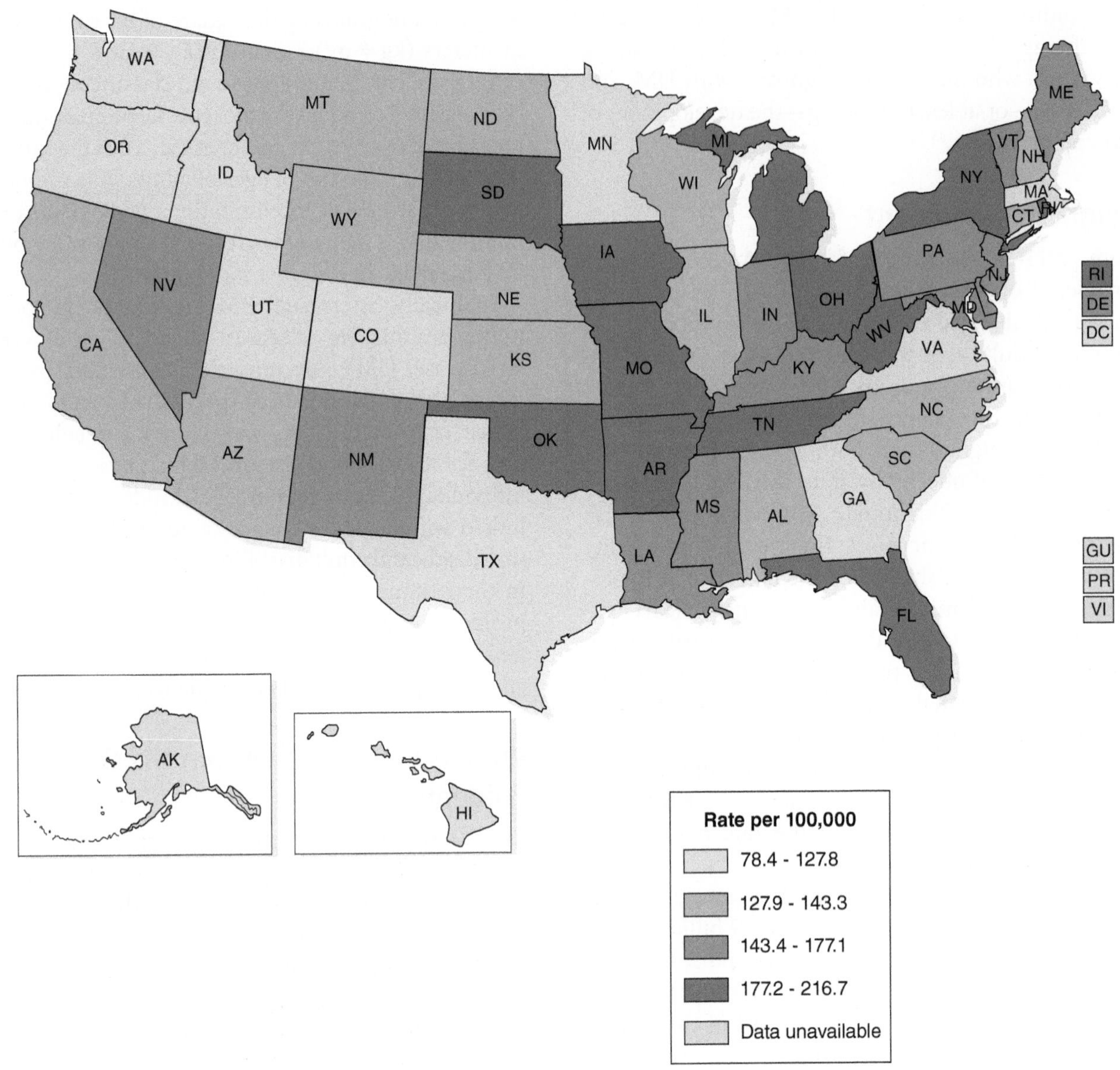

FIGURE 8 Coronary heart disease and obesity rate, 2015 (a) Rate of coronary heart disease (b) Prevalence of obesity

Data from CDC Data Trend Interactive Maps. https://www.cdc.gov/dhdsp/maps/dtm/index.html Accessed July 3, 2017. Map developed by Nancy Munoz using CDC interactive data tools

dies from a condition related to heart disease.[48] In fact, heart disease is the leading cause of death for both men and women. More than half of those who died from heart disease in 2009 were men. In the United States, one out of every four deaths results from heart disease, and approximately 610,000 Americans die from heart disease every year.[49] Heart disease includes several types of heart conditions such as coronary artery disease, heart attacks, and related conditions such as angina. The most common type of heart disease in the United States is coronary artery disease, which affects the blood flow to the heart. In 2014, approximately 356,000 people died from coronary artery disease.[49]

Heart disease is the leading cause of death for people of most racial and ethnic groups in the United States, including African Americans, Hispanics, and whites. For Asian Americans or Pacific Islanders and American Indians or Alaska Natives, heart disease is second only to cancer.[50] The United States spends some $207 billion per year in caring for individuals with heart disease when healthcare services,

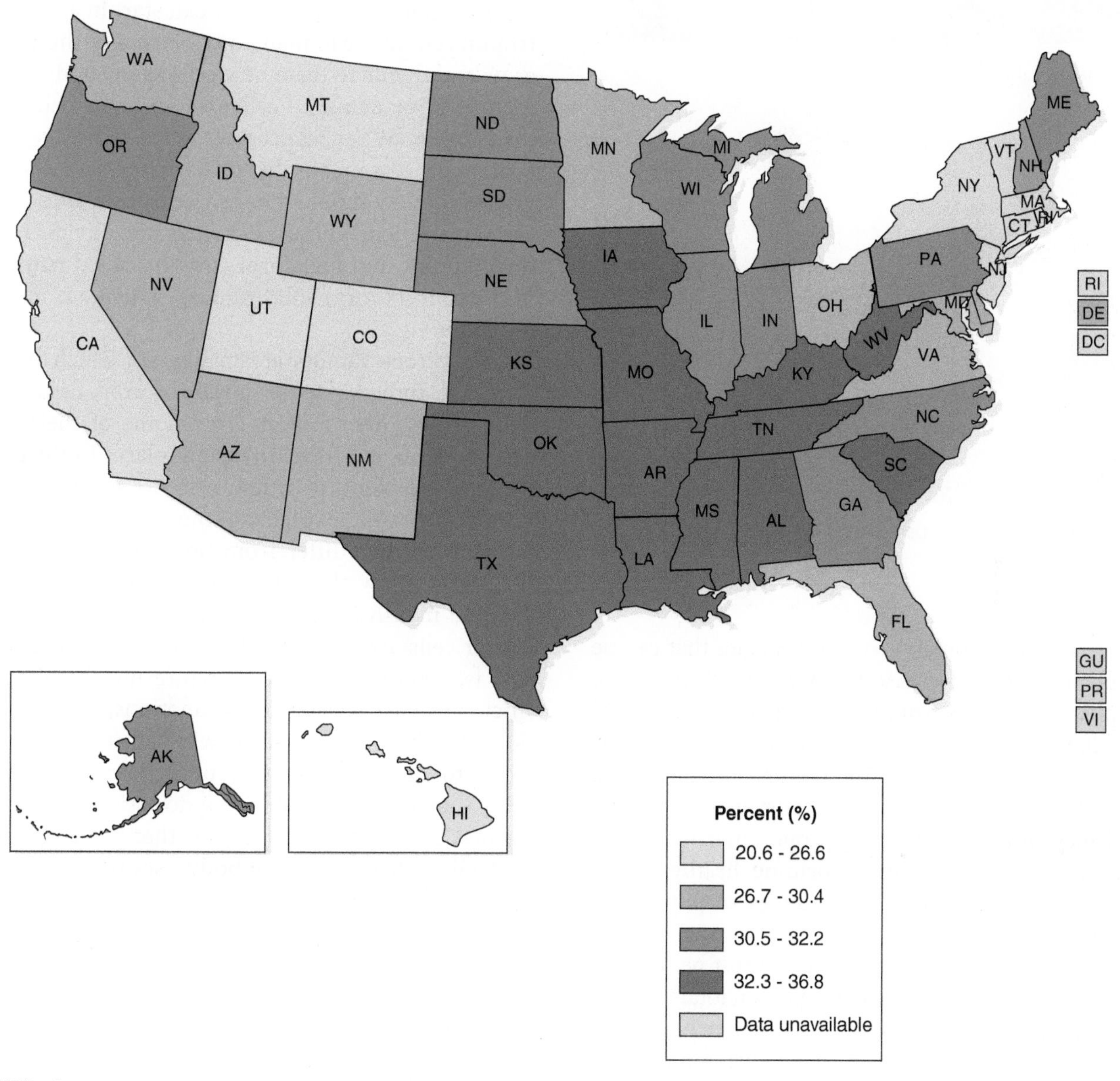

FIGURE 8 *(continued)*

Data from CDC Data Trend Interactive Maps. https://www.cdc.gov/dhdsp/maps/dtm/index.html Accessed July 3, 2017. Map developed by Nancy Munoz using CDC interactive data tools.

medications, and loss of productive time are included in this amount.[49]

Additionally, heart disease is also the leading cause of death around the world. In 2012, 15.5 million people reportedly died from heart disease, accounting for 31% of all worldwide deaths. Of these deaths, 7.4 million died from coronary heart disease and 6.7 million died from strokes. More than three-quarters of the deaths related to heart disease occur in countries with low to middle incomes.[49]

Most cardiovascular diseases can be prevented when an individual focuses on behavioral factors such as the use of tobacco, being obese and overweight, engaging in unhealthy eating patterns, having a physically inactive lifestyle, and consuming alcohol in higher-than-recommended amounts. Individuals with heart disease or who have a high risk for developing heart disease (by having one or more risk factors such as hypertension, diabetes, hyperlipidemia, or a preexisting diagnosis of the disease) need early detection and intervention as appropriate.[51] The WHO has identified both population-wide and individual low-resource interventions that, when used jointly, can help decrease the burden associated with

Classification	BMI Range
Underweight	< 18.5
Normal	18.5–24.9
Overweight	> 25.0
Pre-obese	25–29.9
Obese	> 30.0
Obese I	30–34.9
Obese II	35–39.0
Obese III	> 40

TABLE 9 BMI classification

Data from World Health Organization. (2016). *Global Strategy on Diet, Physical Activity, and Health*. http://www.who.int/dietphysicalactivity/childhood_what/en/. Accessed August 18, 2017.

heart disease. Population-wide strategies that can be implemented to decrease heart disease include the implementation of comprehensive tobacco policies and the use of taxation to decrease the intake of foods that are considered high in sodium, fat, and sugar. Adjusting the environment by constructing walking and bicycling paths, helping people limit their consumption of alcohol, and providing heathy school meals to children are also examples of population strategies.[51]

At the individual level, systems must be in place to identify individuals with overall high total risk factors or single risk factors such as hypertension and hypercholesterolemia. Secondary prevention of heart disease in individuals with a diagnosis of the disease includes the use of medications such as aspirin, beta blockers, angiotensin-converting-enzyme inhibitors, and statins.[51]

Health benefits achieved by implementing these interventions are mostly independent. When smoking cessation is added to these strategies, 75% of recurrent vascular events are preventable.[51]

In 2013, WHO members agreed on global strategies to decrease the avoidable noncommunicable-disease burden. This includes reducing the global prevalence of hypertension by 25% and ensuring that at least 50% of eligible individuals would receive drug therapy and counseling to prevent heart attacks and strokes.[51]

In the United States, one HP 2020 goal is focused on improving the cardiovascular health of all Americans by 20% and reducing deaths from cardiovascular diseases and stroke by 20% by the year 2020.[52]

Cancer

Cancer is the name given to a collection of related diseases. Some types of cancer can start in any of the trillion cells in the human body. Normally, these cells grow and divide to form new cells as the body needs them. Old or damaged cells die, and new cells take their place. When cancer develops, however, this orderly process breaks down. As abnormal cells survive when they should die, new cells form when they are not needed. These extra cells can divide without stopping and may form growths called **tumors**. Many cancers form solid tumors, which are masses of tissue.[53]

Cancerous tumors are malignant, which means they can spread into or invade nearby tissues. In addition, as these tumors grow, some of their cells can break off and travel to distant places in the body through the blood or lymph systems and form new tumors far from the original tumor.[53]

Cancer cells differ from normal cells in many ways that allow them to grow out of control and become invasive. One important difference is that cancer cells are less specialized than normal cells—that is, where normal cells mature into highly distinct cell types with specific functions, cancer cells do not. This is one reason why cancer cells continue to divide without stopping, unlike normal cells. Cancer cells are able to ignore signals that tell normal cells to stop dividing or that begin apoptosis (cell death), which the body uses to rid itself of unneeded cells.[36]

Each year in the United States, more than 1.5 million people are diagnosed with cancer—and more than 500,000 Americans die of cancer. By 2020, the number of new cancer cases is expected to increase to nearly 2 million a year.[54]

More than half of all cancer deaths could be prevented by healthy choices, screening, and vaccinations. Not smoking, drinking alcohol in moderation or not at all, getting enough sleep, eating a diet rich in fruits and vegetables and low in red meat, and getting enough physical activity have been shown to improve overall health and lower the risk of developing some cancers.[54]

Smoking causes approximately 90% of lung cancer deaths in men and almost 80% in women. Smoking also causes cancers of the larynx, mouth, throat, esophagus, bladder, kidney, pancreas, cervix, colon, and stomach, as well as a type of blood cancer called acute myeloid leukemia.[54]

The CDC supports comprehensive efforts at local, state, and national levels to prevent and control cancer for all Americans. To optimize public-health efficiency and effectiveness, the CDC recommends coordinating chronic-disease prevention efforts in four key domains:[54]

1. Epidemiology and surveillance to monitor trends and track progress
2. Environmental approaches to promote health and support healthy behaviors
3. Healthcare system interventions to improve the effective delivery and use of clinical and other high-value preventive services
4. Community programs linked to clinical services to improve and sustain the management of chronic conditions

These four domains help organize and focus the effective work done by the public-health community for many years. At the same time, they help concentrate efforts to strengthen programs and build expertise to address gaps in services. Finally, they help government agencies, state and local grantees, and diverse public and private partners find new ways to work together and support each other's efforts.[54]

Worldwide, cancer is among the leading cause of morbidity and mortality. In 2012, 14 million new cases and 8.2 million cancer-related deaths were reported. New cases of cancer are expected to grow by 70% over the next 20 years. The most-common cancer sites in men were lung, prostate, colon and rectum, stomach, and liver. In women, cancer is most commonly diagnosed in the breast, colon and rectum, lungs, cervix, and stomach. Approximately one-third of cancer-related deaths are associated with lifestyle behaviors such as increased BMI, minimal intake of fruit and vegetables, sedentary lifestyles, and habitual use of tobacco and alcohol.[55]

In excess of 60% of all new annual cases of cancer arise in Africa, Asia, and Central and South America. These regions account for 70% of the world's cancer deaths.[56]

In 2013, the WHO rolled out its Global Action Plan for the Prevention and Control of Non-Communicable Diseases 2013–2020. One aim of the plan includes reducing premature mortality from cancer by 25%.[55]

Nutritional Epidemiology

Epidemiology concerns itself with the causes of diseases in populations and how diseases they develop and spread. The patient is the community, and individuals are viewed collectively. By definition, epidemiology is the scientific, systematic, and data-driven study of the distribution (frequency, pattern) and determinants (causes, risk factors) of health-related states and events (not just diseases) in specified populations (neighborhood, school, city, state, country, global). It is also the application of such study to controlling health problems.[57] Epidemiology is an essential element of public health, offering the basis for guiding practical and appropriate public-health interventions grounded in this science and in causal reasoning.[58]

Results obtained from epidemiologic studies are used to assess a community's health, make individual decisions, complete a clinical picture, and look for causes.[57] Public-health officials accountable for policy development, implementation, and evaluation use epidemiologic data as a factual framework for decision making. Many individuals may not recognize that they use epidemiologic evidence to make daily decisions affecting their health. When someone decides to quit smoking for example, or climbs the stairs rather than wait for an elevator, or eats a salad rather than a cheeseburger with fries for lunch, he or she may be influenced, consciously or unconsciously, by epidemiologists' assessment of risk.[57]

As epidemiologists research illness occurrence, they depend on healthcare providers to determine the correct diagnosis of each individual. On the other hand, epidemiologists offer providers an increased understanding of the clinical presentation and history of the condition being evaluated. A considerable number of epidemiologic studies are focused on finding causal elements that affect any individual's possibility of developing disease.[57]

Nutritional epidemiology is a moderately new field of medical research that looks at the association between nutrition and health. Diet and physical activity are difficult to measure accurately, which may partly explain why nutrition has received less attention than other risk factors for disease in epidemiology.[42]

The rigor of the research associated with nutritional epidemiology varies. Meta-analyses with questionable design and execution have helped to disperse contradictory messages about nutrition and health. One example of this is Flegal et al.,[59] who concluded that being overweight lessens the risk of all-cause mortality. Similarly, a contradicting meta-analysis reported that substituting saturated fat with polyunsaturated fats has no significant effect on cardiovascular risk.[59] These types of conclusion can be dangerous. Misleading or contradicting messages can prevent the public from adopting healthy lifestyles.[60]

Nutritional epidemiology requires design and analysis strategies that are unique to the field of food and nutrition. Appreciating the particulars of nutritional epidemiologic research demands a thorough understanding of nutritional science and its methodological background.[60]

Measuring Nutrition Intake

Although the methods to collect information on nutrient intake have many limitations, numerous procedures have been created to determine nutrient intake from individuals and populations at large. Tools such as food-composition tables, food-frequency questionnaires, and

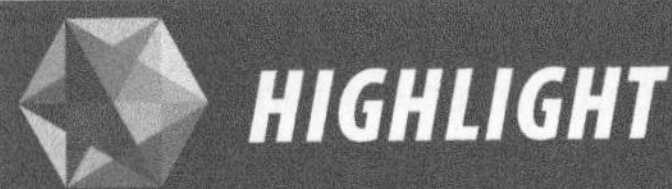

HIGHLIGHT

Understanding Types of Research

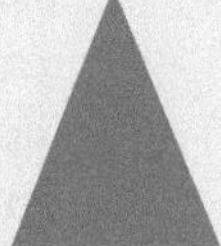

Meta-analysis and systematic review

Summarizes the clinical research that has been performed by independent investigators and researchers. This is critical assessment of all the research that looks at a specific topic.

Randomized controlled trials

Subjects that have a specific condition are randomly (by chance) assigned to one of two groups, eighter a treatment or a control group. While at baseline both groups one similar, the control group receives the standard treatment/intervention and the treatment group receives the treatment/intervention that is newly created.

Cohort study

Groups of people that have a certain condition or receive a specific treatment are followed over time. This group is compared to a similar group of people that do not have the condition or receive the treatment of interest.

Case-control studies

Compares two groups, one with a condition of interest to a similar group that is free from the condition of interest.

Cross-sectional studies

This type of study looks at specific populations at a given point in time to measure the occurrence of a clinical risk factor, outcome, or unique result.

Case reports / Case series

Case reports are published of clinical obsevation. This is a retrospective description of a distinct case that presents differently than projected. A case series is a retrospective report of the outcomes of a group of petients with the condition of intrest that are treated in a similar fashion.

References

1. Aslam S, Georgiev H, Mehta K, Kumar A. Matching research design to clinical research questions. *Indian J Sex Transm Dis.* 2012;33:49–53.
2. Kumar R. *Research Methodology*. 2008. New Delhi, India: APH Publishing.
3. Titler MG. The evidence for evidence-based practice implementation. Chapter 7 in: Hughes RG, editor. *Patient Safety and Quality: An Evidence-Based Handbook for Nurses*. (2008). Rockville, MD: Agency for Healthcare Research and Quality. Available from: http://www.ncbi.nlm.nih.gov/books/NBK2659/.

biomarkers have shown good validity with the use of several criteria. The strengths unique to each method make it appropriate for use in particular applications.

The gold standard for determining nutrient information is the multiple-week diet record. With this tool, individuals document all items they consume over a period of several weeks. The method is different from other data-collection processes because an individual does not have to depend on his or her memory. The high contributor burden as well as the cost of maintaining diet records has reduced their use in large-scale epidemiologic studies. The capacity of these records to convey thorough diet data makes them valuable in validation studies for other dietary assessment techniques. Another drawback of diet records is that the procedure of logging data can alter an individual's diet, thus rendering the data nonrepresentative of actual and usual intake. On the other hand, projected intakes from diet records have shown high correlation with results from multiple 24-hour recalls.[61] In recurrent 24-hour recalls, a participant details all foods eaten in the preceding 24 hours or calendar day to a skilled interviewer in person or over the phone. This technique has been commonly used in dietary-intervention trials. It is also used in national surveys to discover trends in nutritional intake.[60]

Nutritional Epidemiology in Illness Cause and Effect

One of the main reproaches stacked against nutritional epidemiology is that it depends heavily on observational data. This research method is believed to be secondary to experimental data in defining causation. When evidence from randomized controlled trials is not available, nutritional epidemiologists characteristically rely on prospective cohort studies, the strongest observational study design in terms of diminishing bias and deducing causality.[60]

Recap The incidence of obesity is associated with increased risks for morbidity associated with the presence of hypertension, dyslipidemia, diabetes, coronary heart disease, stroke, gallbladder disease, osteoarthritis, sleep apnea, respiratory problems, and some cancers. Obesity has also been linked to increased risk of mortality. Nutritional epidemiology is a moderately new field of medical research that looks at the association between nutrition and health.

Chapter Summary

Consuming healthy foods and living an active lifestyle are basic ways to promote health and well-being. Getting adequate nutrition is particularly important during periods of rapid growth and development. Following an unhealthy eating pattern during pregnancy, infancy, childhood, and adolescence can contribute to underdeveloped physical and mental abilities that have lifelong consequences. Prolonged nutrition deficiency, whether from excessive or inadequate intake, will promote or exacerbate a range of ailments and affect an individual's quality and length of life.

The use of nutrition screening allows for the identification of individuals who are at nutritional risk so that a full nutrition assessment can be completed. The Academy defines a nutrition assessment as "identifying and evaluating data needed to make decisions about a nutrition-related problem/diagnosis."[21] Nutrition-assessment techniques can be classified as one of four types: anthropometric, biochemical, clinical, or dietary.

The increased understanding of the role of nutrition in promoting health and well-being has made the evaluation of individuals, families, and communities key to monitoring public health.

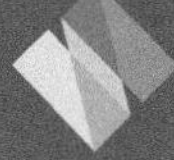

CASE STUDY

In the 21st century, the incidence of chronic disease has displaced the previous prevalence of nutrient deficiency as the primary area of public-health concern as population conditions. Leading causes of death have shifted from infectious diseases to chronic conditions. Approximately one-half of all American adults—117 million individuals—have one or more preventable chronic diseases, many of which are related to poor-quality eating patterns and physical inactivity.

Dr. Jones is a researcher who was just awarded a grant by the National Institute of Health (NIH) to measure the prevalence of diabetes in a selected sector of Camden, New Jersey.

Questions:

1. As you go through the information in this chapter, determine which nutrition assessment methods you would incorporate in your procedure.
2. What drives your assessment-method selection?

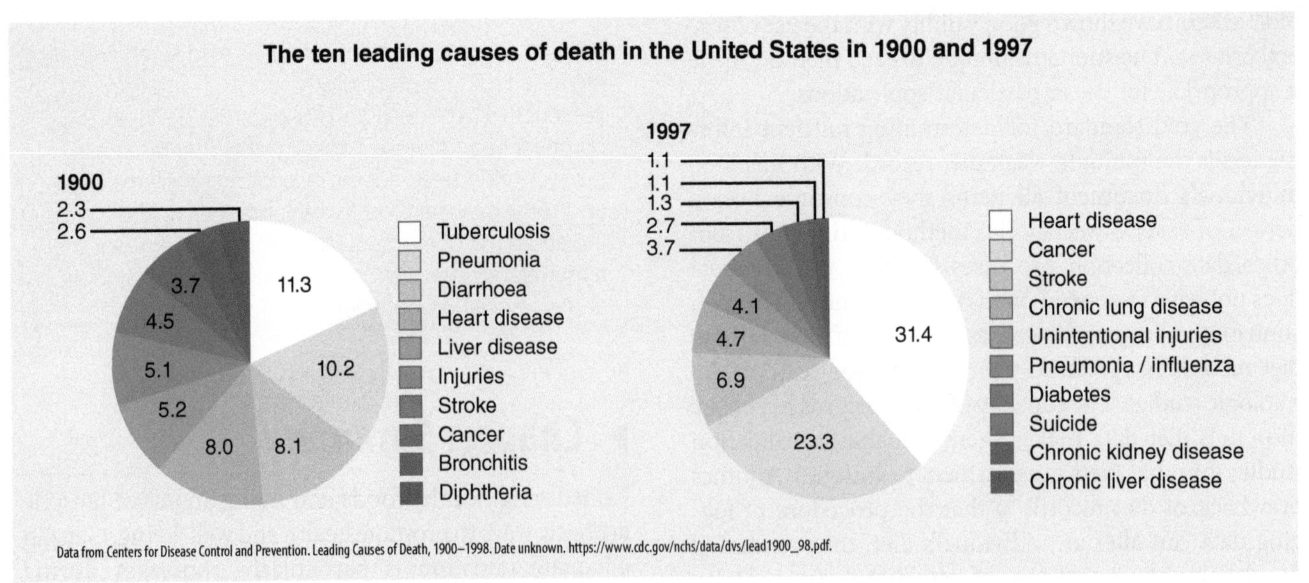

Data from Centers for Disease Control and Prevention. Leading Causes of Death, 1900–1998. Date unknown. https://www.cdc.gov/nchs/data/dvs/lead1900_98.pdf.

Learning Portfolio

Key Terms

Anthropometry
Body mass index (BMI)
Bureau of Labor Statistics Consumer expenditure survey data
Epidemiology
Food and Agriculture Organization of the United Nations (FAO)
Healthy People 2020 (HP 2020)
Interprofessional
Nutrition assessment
Nutrition Care Process (NCP)
Nutrition Care Process Terminology (NCPT)
Nutrition Care Process and Model (NCPM)
Nutrition diagnosis
Nutrition-focused physical exam (NFPE)
Nutrition intervention
Nutrition screening
PES statement
Scurvy
Subjective global assessment (SGA)
Tumors

Study Questions

1. The key difference between a nutrition-screening form and a nutrition-assessment form is:
   a. Screening forms provide a diagnosis for malnutrition
   b. Screening forms determine risk for malnutrition
   c. Screening forms diagnose chronic disease
   d. Screening forms determine risk for weight gain
2. The Academy of Nutrition and Dietetics recommends using the ____________ screening form to assess risk for malnutrition in the adults in the clinical setting.
   a. MUST
   b. SNAQ
   c. Mini SNAQ
   d. Mini MUST

3. When writing PES statements, the section that includes the cause of the nutrition problem is the ________________.
   a. Problem
   b. Etiology
   c. Signs and symptoms
   d. Intervention

4. Which of the following is *not* one of the four steps of the Nutrition Care Process?
   a. Screening and referral
   b. Nutrition assessment
   c. Nutrition intervention
   d. Nutrition diagnosis

5. The part of the Nutrition Care Process that involves data collection, reviewing the data for key factors, and comparing that data against nutrition care criteria is:
   a. Nutrition diagnosis
   b. Nutritional assessment
   c. Nutrition intervention
   d. Nutrition monitoring and evaluation

6. The HP 2020 Nutrition objectives:
   a. Are released by the Food and Drug Administration
   b. Are objectives to measure progress for health concerns in specific populations
   c. Has 10 prominent goals
   d. Provides strategic management for use only at the national level

7. Which of the following is *not* one of the four prominent nutrition goals for HP 2020?
   a. Eliminate all tobacco use by adults, teenagers, and children
   b. Attain high-quality longer lives free of preventable disease, disability, injury, and premature death
   c. Create social and physical environments that promote good health for all
   d. Achieve health equity, eliminate disparities, and improve the health of all groups

8. Which of the following is an objective that falls in the "weight status" category of the HP 2020 objectives?
   a. Reduce the proportion of adults who are at a healthy weight
   b. Reduce the number of women who are morbidly obese
   c. Increase the proportion of adults who are at a healthy weight
   d. Reduce the proportion of men who are underweight

9. Which of the following is *not* one of the objectives for the area of food and nutrient consumption for individuals age 2 years and older?
   a. Increase the consumption of fruits
   b. Increase the consumption of dairy
   c. Reduce the consumption of calories from solid fats
   d. Reduce the consumption of sodium

10. Diabetes is the __________ leading cause of death in the United States.
    a. First
    b. Second
    c. Seventh
    d. 10th

11. The most useful population-level measure of overweight and obesity in adults is:
    a. Ideal body weight
    b. Body mass index
    c. Body fat and lean mass percentages
    d. Growth charts

12. Which of the following is the leading cause of death for Americans?
    a. Diabetes mellitus
    b. Heart disease
    c. Stroke
    d. Osteoporosis

13. Half of all cancer deaths could be prevented by:
    a. Frequent primary care provider visits
    b. Sedentary lifestyle
    c. Polypharmacy
    d. Healthy eating practices and lifestyle choices

14. The strongest observational study design used in nutritional epidemiology is the:
    a. Meta-analysis
    b. Randomized placebo-controlled trial
    c. Prospective cohort
    d. Case control

15. Information included in the clinical history includes all of the following *except*:
    a. Medication
    b. Changes in food intake
    c. Medical diagnosis
    d. Laboratory tests

16. When should the nutrition-focused physical exam be conducted?
    a. After the lab values are in the medical record
    b. At the time of admission
    c. After the history is obtained
    d. Before any procedure is performed

17. According to the consensus statement by the Academy of Nutrition and Dietetics and ASPEN, malnutrition is diagnosed when the following two symptoms are present:
   a. Loss of muscle mass and loss of fluid
   b. Excessive energy intake and excessive subcutaneous fat
   c. Inadequate energy intake and weight loss
   d. Improved handgrip strength and fluid loss

18. Which of the following are two distinct steps in the intervention part of the Nutrition Care Process?
   a. Planning and implementation
   b. Communication and nutrient delivery
   c. Coordinating care and education
   d. Collecting and assessing data

19. Which of the following is a reason why micronutrient deficiency is not as prevalent in the United States today?
   a. Food staples were required by law to be enriched or fortified with important nutrients
   b. More people have access to antibiotics
   c. It is a farm-to-table philosophy
   d. Megadoses of nutrients are frequently used

20. The phrase "inadequate intake" is found in the ______________ part of the nutrition diagnostic statement:
   a. Problem
   b. Signs and symptoms
   c. Etiology
   d. Assessment

21. Measuring weight, height, and body composition are examples of the data collection for the ______________ method.
   a. Biochemical
   b. Anthropometric
   c. Clinical
   d. Dietary

22. Measuring blood nutrient concentrations, urinary metabolites, and blood lipid concentrations are examples of data collected in the ______________ assessment method.
   a. Clinical
   b. Anthropometric
   c. Biochemical
   d. Dietary

23. The dietary data-collection method that uses a structured listing of individual foods or groups of foods that an individual consumes over a period of time is called a ______________.
   a. 24-hour recall
   b. Food-frequency questionnaire
   c. Diet history
   d. Three-day food record

24. In the early 1700s, Dr. James Lind discovered an association between the consumption of citrus fruits and the prevention of which deficiency disease?
   a. Osteoporosis
   b. Rickets
   c. Pellegra
   d. Scurvy

25. During the so-called germ theory era, physicians believed that the cause of frequent illnesses in the general population were from ______________.
   a. Infectious organisms
   b. Nutrient deficiencies
   c. Nutrient toxicity
   d. Nutrient excesses

26. ____________ is the method used to find the causes of health outcomes and diseases in populations.
   a. Assessment
   b. Nutrition-focused physical exam
   c. Epidemiology
   d. Nutrition care process

27. Once micronutrient deficiency diseases were eradicated in the United States, health officials focused their attention on the dietary practices associated with chronic disease. These dietary practices include all of the following *except*:
   a. Excessive sugar intake
   b. Excessive fruit and vegetable intake
   c. Excessive saturated fat intake
   d. Excessive sodium intake

28. The part of the Nutrition Care Process that determines the extent to which intervention goals are met is:
   a. Assessment
   b. Intervention
   c. Diagnosis
   d. Monitoring and evaluation

29. The assessment tool that has been validated to accurately predict poor outcomes and longer length of hospital stay after surgery is the:
   a. Mininutritional assessment form
   b. Mini SNAQ
   c. Malnutrition Universal Screening Tool (MUST)
   d. Subjective global assessment

30. The most reliable indicator of poor nutritional status is:
    a. Weight loss
    b. Low albumin concentrations
    c. Low dietary intake of nutrients
    d. Poor handgrip strength

Discussion Questions

1. How does the obesity rate affect the incidence of chronic disease in the United States?
2. Describe the shift from infectious disease to chronic disease that affects public health.
3. Nutrition screens allow individuals who are at risk of suboptimal nutritional status to be identified. List and describe the most commonly used screening tools. What are the benefits and drawbacks of each screening tool?

Activities

1. Develop a marketing campaign targeting a specific segment of the community you live or study in that introduces population-based intervention strategies to reduce obesity and impact overall health.
2. Type 2 diabetes is widespread in all obese groups and now even in preteen children. Develop an education tool to teach young children the health risks associated with diabetes.
3. Select a chronic condition that is prevalent in the American population. Work with three to four classmates to develop "the top 10 must know topics" by the average person in efforts to prevent or manage the disease. Develop a wiki page to communicate the information. Use videos and graphics on the page to deliver the message.

Online Resources

Food and Agriculture Organization (FAO) of the United Nations

The FAO develops methods and standards for food and agriculture statistics, provides technical assistance services, and disseminates data for global monitoring. It is the world's largest database of food and agriculture statistics:
http://www.fao.org/statistics/en/.

Bureau of Labor Statistics Consumer Expenditure Survey Data

This database provides information on the buying habits of American consumers, including data on their expenditures, income, and consumer unit (families and single consumers) characteristics:
http://www.bls.gov/cex/.

Anthropometric Measurement Videos

This website provides technical videos on how to conduct anthropometric measures:
https://wwwn.cdc.gov/nchs/nhanes/nhanes3/anthropometricvideos.aspx.

The State of Obesity: Adults in the United States

This website provides interactive maps on adult obesity in the United States:
http://stateofobesity.org/adult-obesity/.

Malnutrition Universal Screening Tool (MUST)

This website provides the background for the MUST tool, online calculator, and videos.
http://www.bapen.org.uk/screening-and-must/must.

Mini Nutritional Assessment Tool (MNA)

This website provides an overview of the MNA tool and videos and provides access to the required forms:
http://www.mna-elderly.com/.

References

1. Herder R, Demmig-Adams B. The power of a balanced diet and lifestyle in preventing cardiovascular disease. *Nutr Clin Care.* 2004;7:46-55.
2. Price S. Understanding the importance to health of a balanced diet. *Nurs Times.* 2005;2005;101:30.

3. Centers for Disease Control and Prevention. What we eat in America. DHHS-USDA Dietary Survey Integration. 2015.https://www.cdc.gov/nchs/nhanes/wweia.htm. Accessed February 3, 2017.
4. Centers for Disease Control and Prevention. Adult obesity causes and consequences. 2016. https://www.cdc.gov/obesity/adult/causes.html. Accessed February 3, 2017.
5. Academy of Nutrition and Dietetics. Nutrition security in developing nations: sustainable food, water, and health. *J Acad Nutr Diet*. 2013;113:581-595.
6. Funk C. The etiology of the deficiency diseases. Beri-beri, polyneuritis in birds, epidemic dropsy, scurvy, experience scurvy in animals, infantile scurvy, ship beri-beri, pellagra. *J State Med*. 1912;20:341.
7. Semba R. The discovery of vitamins. *Int J Vit Nutr Res*. 2012;5:310-315.
8. Davis C, Saltos E. Dietary recommendations and how they have changed over time. Ch. 2 in *America's Eating Habits: Changes and Consequences*. 1999. http://purl.umn.edu/33604. Accessed January 24, 2017.
9. Centers for Disease Control and Prevention. Leading causes of death. 2016. https://www.cdc.gov/nchs/fastats/leading-causes-of-death.htm. Accessed January 22, 2017.
10. Butterworth C. The skeleton in the hospital closet. *Nutrition Today*. 1974 (March–April):436.
11. Dougherty D, Bankhead R, Kushner R, Mirtallo J, Winkler M. Nutrition care given new importance in JCAHO standards. *Nutr Clin Pract*. 1995;10(1):26-31.
12. White JV, Guenter P, Jensen G, et al. Consensus statement: Academy of Nutrition and Dietetics and American Society for Parenteral and Enteral Nutrition: characteristics recommended for the identification and documentation of adult malnutrition (undernutrition). *J Parenter Enteral Nutr*. 2012;36(3):275-283.
13. Lacey K, Pritchett E. Nutrition care process and model: ADA adopts road map to quality care and outcomes management. *J Am Diet Assoc*. 2003;103:1061-1071.
14. Field LB, Hand RK. Differentiating malnutrition screening and assessment: A nutrition care process perspective. *J Acad Nutr Diet*. 2015;15:824-828.
15. Donini LM, De Felice MR, Savina C, et al. Predicting the outcome of long-term care by clinical and functional indices: the role of nutritional status. *J Nutr Health Aging*. 2011;15:586-592.
16. Donini LM, Bernardini LD, De Felice MR, et al. Effect of nutritional status on clinical outcome in a population of geriatric rehabilitation patients. *Aging Clin Exp Res*. 2004;16:132-138.
17. National Alliance for Infusion Therapy, American Society for Parenteral and Enteral Nutrition Public Policy Committee and Board of Directors. Disease-related malnutrition and enteral nutrition therapy: a significant problem with a cost-effective solution. *Nutr Clin Pract*. 2010;25:548–554.
18. Jensen GL, Bistrian B, Roubenoff R, Heimburger DC. Malnutrition syndromes: a conundrum vs continuum. *J Parenter Enteral Nutr*. 2009;33:710-716.
19. Academy of Nutrition and Dietetics Evidence Analysis Library. Nutrition screening (NSCR) (2009–2010). 2010. http://www.andeal.org/topic.cfm?menu=3584. Accessed November 16, 2016.
20. Watterson C, Fraser A, Banks MI, et al. Evidence based practice guidelines for the nutritional management of malnutrition in adult patients across the continuum of care. *Nutr Diet*. 2009;66 (suppl):S1-S34.
21. Academy of Nutrition and Dietetics. International Dietetics and Nutrition Terminology (IDNT) 2008; Reference Manual. ISBN-13: 978-0880914451.
22. Detsky A, Smalley P, Change J. Is this patient malnourished? *JAMA*. 1994;271:54-58.
23. Lew C, Yandell R, Fraser RJ, Chua AP, Chong MF, Miller M. Association between malnutrition and clinical outcomes in the intensive care unit: a systematic review. *J Parenter Enteral Nutr*. 2016;41(5):744-758.
24. Centers for Disease Control and Prevention. *National Health Nutrition Examination Surveys (NHANES)*. 2013. http://www.cdc.gov/nchs/data/nhanes/nhanes_13_14/2013_Anthropometry.pdf. Accessed December 3, 2016.
25. National Institutes of Health. *Clinical Guidelines on the Identification, Evaluation, and Treatment of Overweight and Obesity Adults*. 1998; Report no. 98-4083. https://www.ncbi.nlm.nih.gov/books/NBK2003/. Accessed December 3, 2016.
26. National Center for Health Statistics. *National Health and Nutrition Examination Survey*. 2016; https://www.cdc.gov/nchs/nhanes/. Accessed December 16, 2016.
27. National Center for Health Statistics. *Growth Charts*. 2010. https://www.cdc.gov/growthcharts/. Accessed December 3, 2016.
28. Bharadwaj S, Ginoya S, Tandon P, et al. Malnutrition: laboratory markers vs nutritional assessment. *Gastroenterol Rep*. 2016; 4(4):272-280.
29. Lichford M. Putting the nutrition-focused physical assessment into practice in long-term care. *Ann Longterm Care*. 2013;21(11):38-41.
30. Jensen GL Hsiao PY, Wheeler D. Adult nutrition assessment tutorial. *J Parenter Enteral Nutr*. 2012;36:267-274.
31. Frank-Stromborg M, Olsen SJ. *Instruments for Clinical Health-care Research*. 3rd ed. 2004. Sudbury, MA: Jones and Bartlett.
32. Archer E, Hand GA, Blair SN. *Validity of U.S. Nutritional Surveillance: National Health and Nutrition Examination Survey Caloric Energy Intake Data, 1971–2010*. Johannsen D, ed. PLoS ONE. 2013. 8(10):e76632.
33. Academy of Nutrition and Dietetics. NCP 101. 2016. http://www.eatrightpro.org/resources/practice/nutrition-care-process/ncp-101. Accessed December 4, 2016.
34. Bueche J, Charney P, Pavlinac J, Annalynn S, Thompson E, Meyers E. Nutrition care process and model part I: The 2008 update. *J Am Diet Assoc*. 2008; 108(7):1113-1117. https://www.ncbi.nlm.nih.gov/pubmed/18589014.
35. Bueche J, Charney P, Pavlinac J, Annalynn S, Thompson E, Meyers E. Nutrition care process and model part II: the 2008 update. *J Am Diet Assoc*. 2008;108(8):1113-1117. http://jandonline.org/article/S0002-8223(08)01203-0/references.
36. Academy of Nutrition and Dietetics. *Nutrition Terminology Reference Manual (eNCPT): Dietetics Language for Nutrition Care*. 2016. http://ncpt.webauthor.com/. Accessed December 8, 2016.
37. Healthy People 2020. Disparities details by race and ethnicity for 2011–14. 2017. https://www.healthypeople.gov/2020/data/disparities/detail/Chart/4968/3/2014. Accessed July 1, 2017.
38. Centers for Disease Control and Prevention. Healthy People 2020.2015.https://www.cdc.gov/nchs/healthy_people/HP2020.htm. Accessed December 17, 2016.
39. US Department of Health and Human Services. Heathy People 2020. 2016. https://www.healthypeople.gov/. Accessed December 17, 2016.
40. US Department of Health and Human Services. *Dietary Guidelines for Americans*. 2005. Washington, DC: US Government Printing Office.
41. Ahmed AM. History of diabetes mellitus. *Saudi Med J*. 2002;23(4):373-379.
42. Centers for Disease Control and Prevention. *National Diabetes Statistics Report, 2014*. 2015. http://choosehealth.utah.gov

/documents/pdfs/factsheets/national-diabetes-report-web.pdf. Accessed December 17, 2016.

43. American Diabetes Association. Nutrition recommendations and interventions for diabetes: a position statement of the American Diabetes Association. *Diabetes Care.* 2008;31(suppl 1):S61-S78.
44. Ogden CL, Carroll MD, Fryar CD, Flegal KM. Prevalence of obesity among adults and youth: United States, 2011–2014. NCHS Data brief, No. 219. 2015. https://www.cdc.gov/nchs/data/databriefs/db219.pdf. Accessed December 17, 2016.
45. US Department of Health and Human Services. *Managing Overweight and Obesity in Adults: Systematic Review from the Obesity Expert Panel—2013.* 2014. Washington, DC: National Heart, Lung, and Blood Institute. https://www.nhlbi.nih.gov/sites/www.nhlbi.nih.gov/files/obesity-evidence-review.pdf. Accessed December 17, 2016.
46. World Health Organization. Obesity and overweight. 2016. http://www.who.int/mediacentre/factsheets/fs311/en/. Accessed December 18, 2016.
47. World Health Organization. *Global Strategy on Diet.* 2016. http://www.who.int/dietphysicalactivity/childhood_what/en/. Accessed August 18, 2017.
48. Mozzafarian D, Benjamin EJ, Go AS, et al. Heart disease and stroke statistics—2015 update: a report from the American Heart Association. *Circulation.* 2015;131:e29–e322.
49. Mozzafarian D, Benjamin EJ, Go AS, et al. Heart disease and stroke statistics—2016 update: a report from the American Heart Association. *Circulation.* 2016; 133(4):e38-e360.
50. Heron M. Deaths: leading causes for 2008. *Natl Vital Stat Rep.* 2012; 60. https://www.cdc.gov/nchs/data/nvsr/nvsr60/nvsr60_06.pdf. Accessed December 18, 2016.
51. World Health Organization. Cardiovascular diseases (CVDs). 2016. http://www.who.int/mediacentre/factsheets/fs317/en/. Accessed December 18, 2016.
52. American Heart Association and American Stroke Association. Heart disease and stroke statistics—at-a-glance. 2015. http://www.onebraveidea.com/submissions/ucm_470704.pdf. Accessed December 18, 2016.
53. National Cancer Institute. What is cancer? 2015. https://www.cancer.gov/about-cancer/understanding/what-is-cancer. Accessed December 19, 2016.
54. Centers for Disease Control and Prevention. Preventing one of the nation's leading causes of death at a glance 2016. 2016. https://www.cdc.gov/chronicdisease/resources/publications/aag/dcpc.htm. Accessed December 19, 2016.
55. World Health Organization. Cancer. 2015. http://www.who.int/mediacentre/factsheets/fs297/en/. Accessed December 19, 2016.
56. International Agency for Research in Cancer. *World Cancer Report 2014.* 2015. http://publications.iarc.fr/Non-Series-Publications/World-Cancer-Reports/World-Cancer-Report-2014. Accessed December 19, 2016.
57. Centers for Disease Control and Prevention. What is epidemiology? 2016. https://www.cdc.gov/careerpaths/k12teacherroadmap/epidemiology.html. Accessed December 21, 2016.
58. Cates W. Epidemiology: applying principles to clinical practice. *Contemp Ob/Gyn.* 1982;20:147–161.
59. Chowdhury R, Warnakula S, Kunutsor S, et al. Association of dietary, circulating, and supplement fatty acids with coronary risk: a systematic review and meta-analysis. *Ann Intern Med.* 2014;160:398-406.
60. Satija A, Yu E, Willett WC, Hu FB. Understanding nutritional epidemiology and its role in policy. *Adv Nutr.* 2015;1(5):5-18.
61. Hebert JR, Hurley TG, Chiriboga DE, Barone J. A comparison of selected nutrient intakes derived from three diet assessment methods used in a low-fat maintenance trial. *Public Health Nutr.* 1998;1:207-214.

Nutrition Assessment

V. Paige Murphy
Kelly Kane

Chapter Outline

CORE CONCEPTS

1. The purpose of nutrition assessment is to identify malnutrition via assessment of various domains—anthropometrics, biochemical, clinical, dietary, energy expenditure, and functional.
2. The registered dietitian is the most competent professional to assist in selecting or developing the screening method used in acute care, particularly when the screening is to be completed by a nondietetics clinician.
3. A wide variety of nutrition screening questions or tools are employed in clinical settings across the United States. Several well-validated screening tools exist with the goal of identifying nutritional status or predicting poor clinical outcomes related to malnutrition.
4. Different screening tools may be better or worse predictors in specific patient populations.
5. Nutrition screening tools should have acceptable validity, be simple to administer, have wide applicability across the various populations, and use commonly available information.

Learning Objectives

1. Describe the purpose of nutrition assessment as part of the Nutrition Care Process and Model.
2. Define and differentiate between nutrition screening and nutrition assessment.
3. Identify the screening tools applicable to clinical practice.
4. Explain the components of anthropometric assessment and their purposes, and recognize which have greater relevance to clinical practice and which should be used with caution.
5. Describe appropriate components of a clinical assessment and why that information may be pertinent to the overall nutrition assessment.
6. State the benefits and limitations of dietary assessment and the dietary recall methods.
7. Identify the purpose and relevant components of a functional assessment of muscle strength.

Nutritional status affects virtually every individual's response to illness.[1] Those in a malnourished state benefit most if malnutrition is quickly identified. The importance of thorough and appropriate nutrition assessment is critical in both the prevention and treatment of illness. The process of assessment will provide the foundation from which any necessary nutrition-related intervention is built. The purpose of this chapter is to identify the specific components of recognizing and evaluating at-risk adult patients as the integral backbone of dietetics practice.

Overview of the Nutrition Care Process

In order to facilitate the provision of the highest quality of care, the Academy of Nutrition and Dietetics (AND; formerly known as the American Dietetic Association, or

CASE STUDY INTRODUCTION

Mary is a 73-year-old female who presents to her primary care physician with weakness and reduced oral intake for the past 3 months. Mary is admitted to the medical inpatient unit. Due to her recent admission, there is limited information in the medical record.

Anthropometric Data:

Height: 160 cm (63")
Weight: 65 kg (143 lbs)
BMI: 25.4 kg/m^2
Weight history
66.5 kg (145 lbs) 1 month ago
70 kg (154 lbs) 3 months ago
77 kg (169 lbs) 6 months ago (usual body weight)

Biochemical Data:

Sodium 149 (135-145 mEq/L)
Potassium 3.4 (3.6-5.0 mEq/L)
Blood urea nitrogen 28 (6-24 mg/dL)
Creatinine 0.5 (0.4-1.3 mg/dL)
Glucose 105 (70-99 mg/dL)
Albumin 2.9 (3.5-5.0 g/dL)
Total cholesterol 150 mg/dL (Desirable<200 mg/dL)

Clinical Data:

Past Medical History: Hypertension, osteoporosis
Medications: Lisinopril, alendronate
Vital Signs: Blood pressure 100/70 mm Hg, Temperature 99°F, Heart rate 85 beats/min

Questions

1. To determine whether Mary warrants immediate nutrition assessment, what additional information from the patient or the medical record would you like to consider?
2. What validated screening tool(s) would be appropriate to use to determine Mary's nutrition risk?
3. What specific information do you need to determine whether Mary has malnutrition?

ADA) adopted the **Nutrition Care Process and Model (NCPM)** as a systematic framework to recognize, diagnose, and intervene upon nutrition-related problems for which a nutrition intervention is the primary treatment. The NCPM (**Figure 1**) was designed to provide a methodical structure for critically assessing patients across the wide spectrum of health and disease. The process consists of four steps to be completed in sequence—assessment, diagnosis, intervention, and monitoring and evaluation—each of which is linked to corresponding standardized terminology, called the **Nutrition Care Process Terminology (NCPT)**, for consistent documentation. In all cases, assessment is preceded by screening, a separate but supportive task that triggers the entry of a patient into the NCPM.[2-6]

Nutrition assessment serves as the essential first step that provides a comprehensive evaluation of an individual's nutrition-related history. It is a systematic approach to collecting, recording, and interpreting all relevant data for the purpose of accurately diagnosing a nutrition-related problem. As part of the NCPM, nutrition assessment is organized into five domains: anthropometric measurements; biochemical data, medical tests, and procedures; client history; nutrition-focused physical exam; and food/nutrition-related history. This information may be obtained from a number of sources, including, but not limited to, the patient, family members, caregivers, medical care team, or medical record, depending upon the specific situation. The process of assessment is not stagnant; instead, it should be viewed as an ongoing and continual analysis of an individual's nutritional status.[2,4,6]

The Purpose of Nutrition Assessment

The purpose of nutrition assessment is straightforward: to identify the presence of any nutrition-related problems, particularly malnutrition. However, over the past several decades, the topic of assessment has been surrounded by ongoing discussion, research, reworking, and redefining. Although researchers, clinicians, and public policy makers have invested significant energy into a unified approach for the identification and evaluation of malnutrition, no universally accepted approach has been determined. This may be attributed to the wide variation in existing definitions of the malnourished state.[8-10]

Defining Malnutrition

A clear definition of the components of clinical malnutrition is imperative to the assessment process. It would be difficult to identify the malnourished state without a

Content removed due to copyright restrictions

known set of risk factors and/or manifestations for which to probe. One may assume that defining such a common and well-researched phenomenon would be relatively simple. Unfortunately, the nutrition community lacks a universal agreement; every organization, every publication, and every practitioner claims its own (slightly different) definition of the state.[11-13]

The relationship between malnutrition and nutrition assessment is critical. Any elements that influence the development of malnutrition and the manifestations that result should both comprise the steps of assessment and provide reliable identifiers for nutrition screening. Solidifying a transparent definition of the malnourished state is vital to understanding what and why specific signs and symptoms are assessed.

Consider the general concept of nutritional adequacy—the state of equilibrium in which an individual's dietary intake matches his or her requirements. In theory, malnutrition will occur when intake falls below (or exceeds) what is required. In practice, this process is significantly more complex. It is marked by a resulting succession of metabolic abnormalities, physiologic changes, reduced organ and tissue function, and loss of critical body mass. For these reasons, malnutrition can be identified as any alteration in physiology, composition, or function attributable to a diet or to a disease that affects nutritional outcomes. Malnutrition for the purposes of nutrition assessment in the clinical setting refers to a disease-related malnutrition that differs dramatically from that associated with natural disaster, conflict, or deprivation in the public health arena.[8,9,11,14]

Box 1

Nutrition Screening versus Nutrition Assessment

Although not a direct component of the NCPM, nutrition screening is the critical antecedent step to identify patients who require additional assessment. This distinction is best illustrated using the definitions provided by the American Society for Parenteral and Enteral Nutrition (A.S.P.E.N.). This interprofessional organization defines nutrition screening as "a process to identify an individual who is malnourished or who is at risk for malnutrition to determine if detailed nutrition assessment is indicated." In contrast, the longer, more detailed nutrition assessment process evaluates the patient in detail to identify a nutrition-related problem. In other words, screening determines the *risk* of a problem and assessment determines the *presence* of a problem.[5,7]

Current research indicates that varying degrees of acute or chronic inflammation as part of the disease state are key factors in the pathogenesis of malnutrition. In clinical practice, malnutrition should be considered within one of three subcategories as defined by a joint International Guidelines Committee of A.S.P.E.N. and the European Society for Clinical Nutrition and Metabolism (ESPEN):

1. Chronic starvation without inflammation (e.g., anorexia nervosa)
2. Chronic disease–associated malnutrition, when inflammation is chronic and of mild-to-moderate degree (e.g., organ failure, pancreatic cancer)
3. Acute disease- or injury-associated malnutrition, when inflammation is acute and of severe degree (e.g., sepsis, burns, trauma, or closed head injury)[11-13,15,16]

With these considerations in mind, one definition serves as a solid framework for the purposes of identifying and assessing clinical malnutrition: "**Malnutrition** is a subacute or chronic state of nutrition, in which a combination of varying degrees of overnutrition or undernutrition and inflammatory activity has led to a change in body composition and diminished function."[17]

Identifying Malnutrition

Identification of malnutrition and the entire purpose of the nutrition assessment process require a general understanding of its risk factors and manifestations.[16,18] Because it is estimated that malnutrition affects between 30% and 55% of hospitalized patients, many of whom are malnourished at baseline, nutrition assessment is fundamental to the evaluation of the acutely ill adult.[5,19-21]

Parameters used for the identification of malnutrition within the screening and assessment processes should encompass both nutrition intake and severity of disease. Since no single clinical parameter is indicative of the malnourished state, data must be collected from a variety of domains.[7,16] Per consensus recommendations published by AND and A.S.P.E.N.,[10] certain data are useful in the identification of malnutrition (Table 1).

This consensus statement provides further guidance for the identification and documentation of malnutrition in adults. AND and A.S.P.E.N. propose specific diagnostic criteria that can be identified within the aforementioned domains:

- Insufficient energy intake, established by determining the percentage of needs consumed
- Unintended weight loss over a specific period of time
- Indications of muscle mass and/or subcutaneous fat loss identified upon physical exam or fluid accumulation (generalized or localized) that may mask any recent weight loss
- Diminished functional status as measured by handgrip strength

TABLE 1 DATA USEFUL IN THE IDENTIFICATION OF MALNUTRITION	
Domain	**Specific Data**
Anthropometric	Standard measures of height, weight, and body composition, with particular focus on unintended weight loss
Biochemical	Biochemical assessment involves use of laboratory tests of patients' blood, urine, feces, and tissue samples to help determine nutritional status and organ function
Clinical	Nutrition-focused past medical history and clinical diagnosis, as well as a nutrition-focused physical exam that may reveal the presence of several diagnostic characteristics of malnutrition
Dietary	Information regarding food and nutrient intake will indicate the presence of any inadequacies or imbalances
Energy	Estimation of energy requirements and comparison to current intake; determining ability to meet needs, particularly when increased by disease state
Functional	Declines in function measured via muscle strength and/or physical performance

A positive finding of any two characteristics indicates malnutrition. Purposeful examination for these features should be present in every nutrition assessment.[10,12]

Consequences of Malnutrition

The importance of an appropriate assessment for the identification of malnutrition can be attributed to prevention of its far-reaching and damaging clinical impacts. It has long been understood that patients with poor nutritional status have inferior outcomes compared to their well-nourished counterparts. In the acute care setting, malnutrition is a major contributor to increased morbidity and mortality, increased lengths of stay and rates of readmission, decreased function and quality of life, and higher healthcare costs. The presence of malnutrition alters the function and recovery of virtually every organ system, which can manifest as the development of pressure injuries, increased rates of infection, impaired wound healing, surgical complications, and increased ventilatory requirements, among others. Assessment of nutritional status in critically ill patients should evaluate for the presence of malnutrition in its many domains to prevent clinical deterioration.[5,9,10,18,22-25]

CORE CONCEPT 1

The purpose of nutrition assessment is to identify malnutrition via assessment of various domains—anthropometrics, biochemical, clinical, dietary, energy expenditure, and functional.

Nutrition Screening

The Role of Nutrition Screening in NCPM

Prior to the introduction of the NCPM, nutrition screening was recommended by AND as an integral component of care.[26] The process to identify those individuals at nutritional risk who would benefit from further assessment and intervention has evolved into a critical antecedent step of the NCPM. AND currently defines **nutrition screening** as "the process of identifying patients, clients, or groups who may have a nutrition diagnosis and benefit from nutrition assessment intervention by a registered dietitian (RD)."[5] The initial screen may not always be completed by a dietetics practitioner and is not actually considered to be part of the NCPM.[4,12]

AND supports nutrition screening as the preliminary step that triggers entrance into the NCPM. Given the impracticality of conducting a full assessment of all patients, practitioners rely upon an appropriate screen to identify individuals who are either already malnourished or at risk of becoming malnourished. The goal in this case is not necessarily to *diagnose* malnutrition, but instead to identify the known characteristics associated with the malnourished state or other nutritional issues that would warrant a more thorough evaluation and potential intervention.[5,12,27]

Screening in Acute Care

The Joint Commission (JC) is the independent entity responsible for the accreditation and certification of healthcare organizations in the United States. In 1995, the JC mandated that the nutrition screen be performed when warranted by the patient's needs and conditions based upon organizational criteria. When applicable to a patient's condition, the screen must be completed within 24 hours of an inpatient admission.[7,28] The JC does not require that a specific tool or criteria be used; the guidelines instead specify that each organization must have "defined criteria that identify when nutritional plans are developed."[28] In other words, there are no clear standards that dictate the screening tool itself, only that each organization screens within the designated time frame. As such, the methods used between sites vary considerably.[5,28,29]

The vast majority of acute care centers have incorporated screening into the admission process in order to help prioritize hospital resources, although the screening methods used to meet JC's mandate will vary from center to center. Several common denominators prevail among the multitude of tools utilized: validity and reliability, ease of use and convenience, speed (typically requiring less than 5 minutes), avoidance of complicated calculations or laboratory data, minimal expense, and noninvasiveness. In order to meet each of these characteristics, initial screening in most hospitals is based, at least in part, on height and weight collected upon admission.[5,12,26,28,30]

Any screening tool a hospital employs will be unable to account for the extreme variability seen in patients within an acute care setting. Other aspects of the disease state must be considered, in addition to nutritional measurements, to determine if and when intervention is warranted or is likely to be beneficial. Screening is not meant to replace the training and clinical judgment of the RD, but instead to assist in initiating the NCPM.[7,20]

Selecting a Screening Method

A number of existing screening tools are available for use as is or with slight modification in the clinical setting. These tools, which will be described in detail in the following sections, serve as exceptional resources for implementing a new, or revamping an existing, screening method. When selecting the tool or criteria to be used in acute care, there are two important considerations:

1. The screening of patients in the clinical setting differs greatly from that of the community setting. The primary purpose in this context is to identify those patients who will require further assessment of need for nutrition support. Given that many of the developed tools were intended for use in the community setting, it is important to ensure that the tool selected has been validated within the specific inpatient population in which it will be used.[5]
2. Given the complexity of the malnourished state, there is no single parameter that is both sensitive and specific for malnutrition. Screening patients in acute care must be ongoing and should consider the routes for development of malnutrition (deficient intake, excessive losses, increased metabolic demand, etc.) in order to identify those who increase in risk over time.[5,19,30]

Overall, the screening tool selected should identify all individuals at risk. In order to ensure this validity, a screening tool will have a high sensitivity (meaning that patients identified as at risk of malnutrition are actually generally malnourished) *and* a high specificity (patients not identified as at risk are, in fact, not malnourished). Furthermore, a screening tool should be reliable in that it consistently reproduces the same or similar results. The use of an inappropriate tool—or one that has not been validated or has been validated in a different population than the one for which it is currently being used—will negatively influence patient care and risk misdiagnosis of malnutrition.[5,30]

CORE CONCEPT 2

The registered dietitian is the most competent professional to assist in selecting or developing the screening method used in acute care, particularly when the screening is to be completed by a nondietetics clinician.[12]

Nutrition Screening Tools

Nutrition screening allows all patients at risk to receive the appropriate individualized nutrition care they require. The consensus of literature and clinical practice demonstrates that when appropriate screening leads to appropriate intervention, outcomes are dramatically improved including reduced readmissions, shorter lengths of hospital stays, and lower mortality rates.[12] Given this insight, a number of screening tools have been developed and validated for use in the acute care setting. Most validated tools will address four basic areas of nutrition risk: recent weight loss, recent dietary intake, current body mass index (BMI), and current disease state. Depending on the tool, various other measurements of nutritional status may be included to further assist in the prediction of malnutrition risk.[20,31,32]

Although some screening tools have been endorsed by international nutrition societies, there is no universal or empirical agreement on a single best tool. The four most well-known and widely used examples include Nutritional Risk Screening (NRS-2002), Malnutrition Universal Screening Tool (MUST), Short Nutritional Assessment Questionnaire (SNAQ), and Malnutrition Screening Tool (MST). Please note that while some of these tools were developed by professional groups outside of the United States, they are used widely across clinical practice.[20,28]

Nutritional Risk Screening (NRS-2002)

When the **Nutritional Risk Screening (NRS-2002)** tool was developed by a working group of ESPEN, the goal was to establish a screening system based on the nutrition criteria or characteristics used in the current clinical trials. The developers relied on the assumption that nutritional status and indication for nutrition support (based on undernutrition and/or increased nutritional requirements) relate directly to severity of disease. The tool measures disease impact in addition to the markers of current or potential malnutrition. It has been validated to identify not only patients who are malnourished at the time of screening, but also those at risk for malnutrition secondary to the disease state or associated treatment, thus emphasizing the need for preventing further deterioration of nutritional status as the clinical course progresses.[21,30-32]

The purpose of the NRS-2002 system is to detect either existing or anticipated malnutrition in the hospital setting. The initial screening tool consists of four simple, but strategic, questions (Figure 2) that consider weight loss, BMI, and dietary intake history in the setting of illness. If there is a positive response to any of the questions in the initial screen, a second, more detailed screen is conducted. This final screen calculates two scores: one for current nutritional status and another for severity of disease as a reflection of the increase in metabolic demand it may cause. These scores are then combined and adjusted for age (with age older than 70 years as a risk factor) to result in a final evaluation of nutrition risk. Ultimately, this score is linked to an example intervention, although the content of the nutrition care plan is determined by the clinician.[9,12,18,20,28,30]

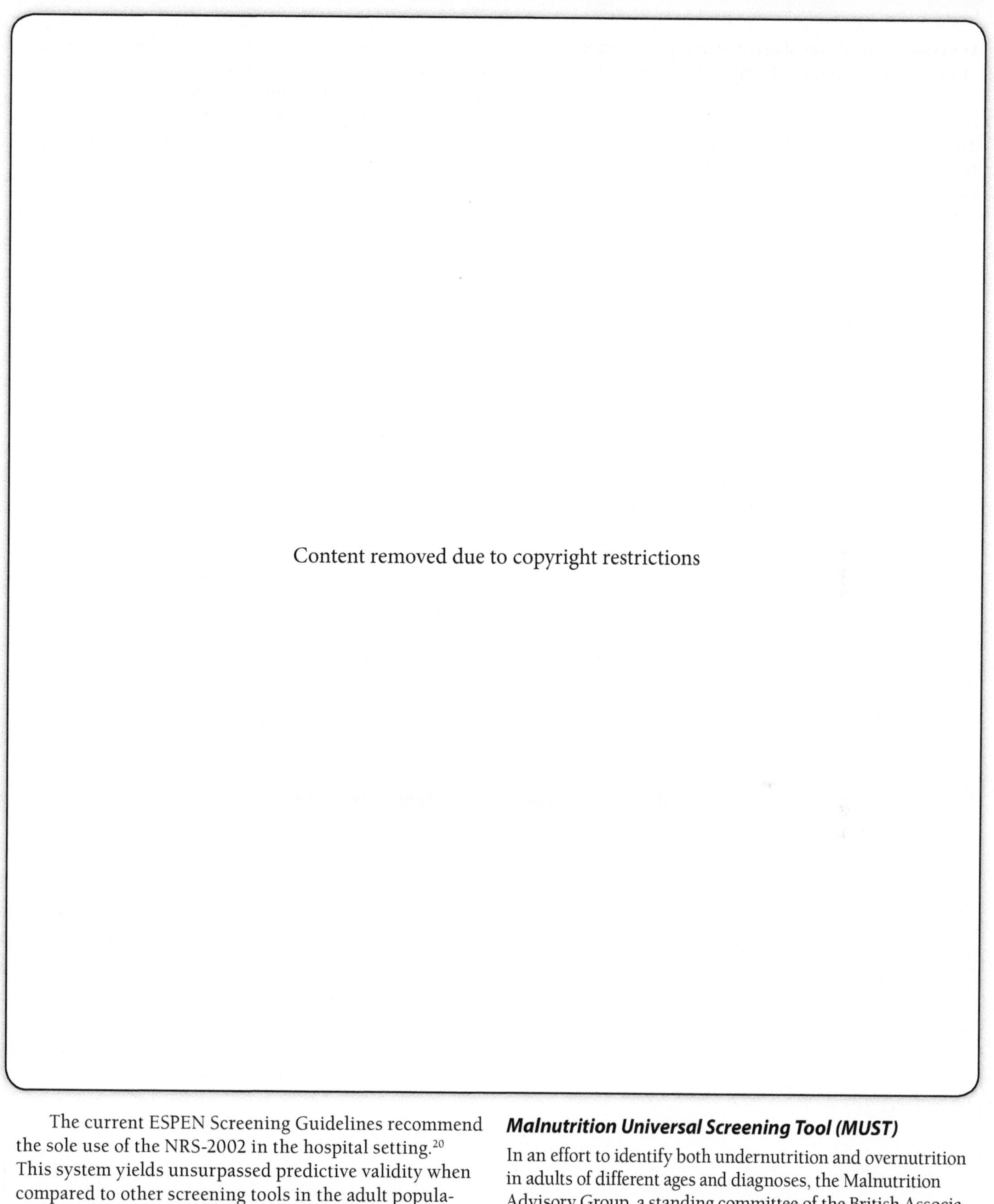

The current ESPEN Screening Guidelines recommend the sole use of the NRS-2002 in the hospital setting.[20] This system yields unsurpassed predictive validity when compared to other screening tools in the adult population. A number of studies have validated the NRS-2002 across a range of hospitalized patients—from surgical to cardiovascular to gastrointestinal—with strong inter-rater reliability (i.e., can be used by various professionals with similar results). This system can be applied in the acute care setting without concern for impracticality or inaccuracy.[9,20,30,32-37]

Malnutrition Universal Screening Tool (MUST)

In an effort to identify both undernutrition and overnutrition in adults of different ages and diagnoses, the Malnutrition Advisory Group, a standing committee of the British Association for Parenteral and Enteral Nutrition (BAPEN), convened to develop the **Malnutrition Universal Screening Tool (MUST)**. Similar to the NRS-2002, the MUST tool considers current weight status as BMI, unintentional changes in weight, and the presence of an acute disease that influences, or is likely to influence, dietary intake. Each of these three components can individually influence clinical outcome, serving as a powerful predictor of nutrition risk when combined. To assess these variables, the MUST framework utilizes a simple five-step process to arrive at an overall score for risk of malnutrition—either low, medium, or high risk (**Figure 3**). The tool then refers clinicians to management, which can be modified according to the specific healthcare setting and patient population.[12,24,27,28,30,31,38]

MUST has been deemed valid and reliable across a wide spectrum of adult patients, even among those requiring special interpretation for fluid disturbances, amputations, or inability to be measured for height and weight. In these situations, the MUST framework supplies instructions for alternative measurements that ensure reliability nearly identical to that of the original tool. Although originally developed

Content removed due to copyright restrictions

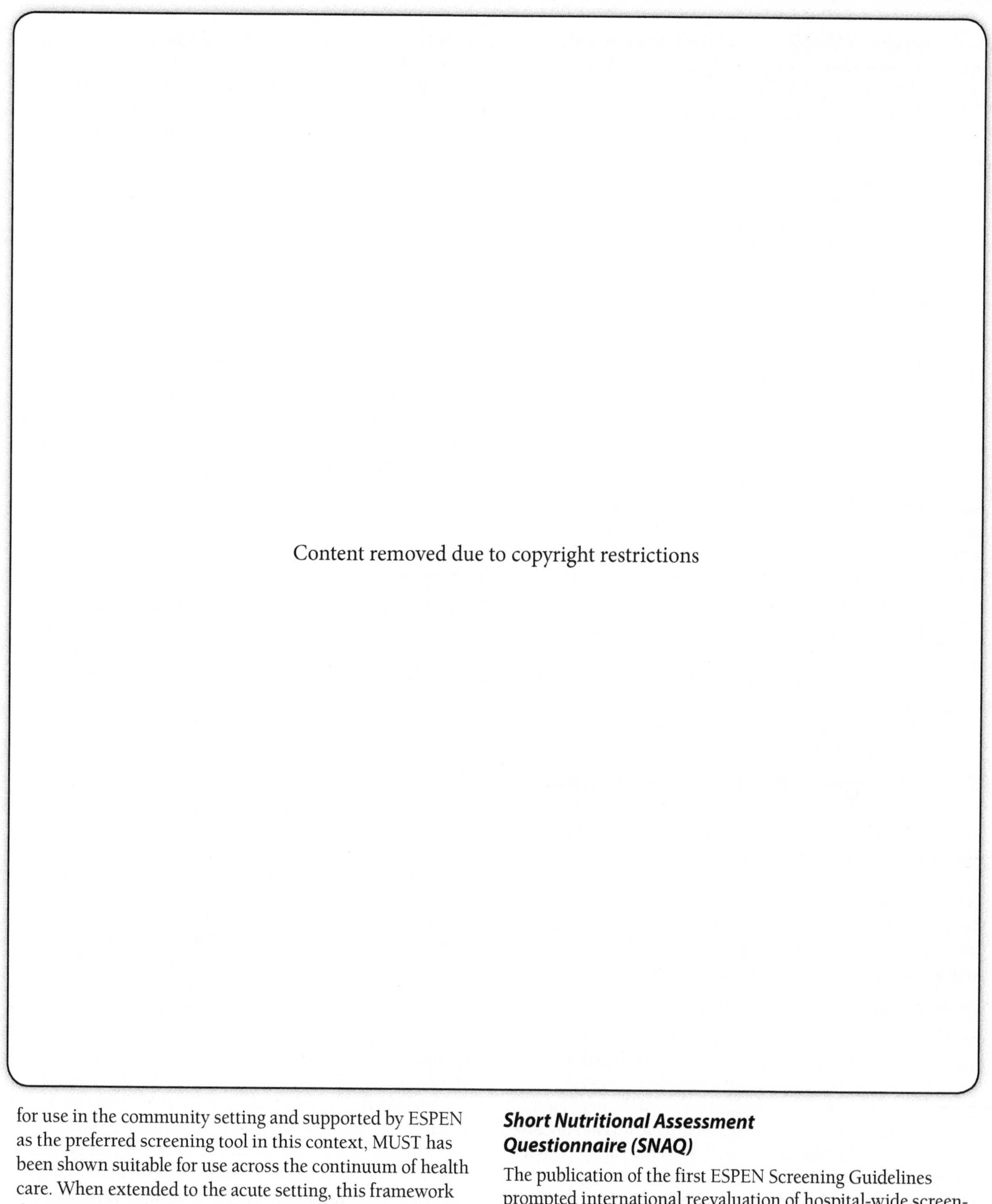

for use in the community setting and supported by ESPEN as the preferred screening tool in this context, MUST has been shown suitable for use across the continuum of health care. When extended to the acute setting, this framework demonstrates concurrent validity with other tools and strong predictive validity in terms of lengths of hospital stay, discharge destination, and mortality. MUST can be utilized by all members of the interdisciplinary team without concern for inter-rater variation. Overall, this tool is simple, evidence-based, valid, and reliable, with a practicability supported by literature and clinical practice.[12,20,30,38-43]

Short Nutritional Assessment Questionnaire (SNAQ)

The publication of the first ESPEN Screening Guidelines prompted international reevaluation of hospital-wide screening processes. Upon assessment of the tools available for use, many nations found that their current frameworks failed to meet the criteria recommended by the guidelines. In response, a committee of dietitians in the Netherlands developed the **Short Nutritional Assessment Questionnaire (SNAQ)**, a "quick and easy" screening tool intended for use during admission to an acute care facility. The development of

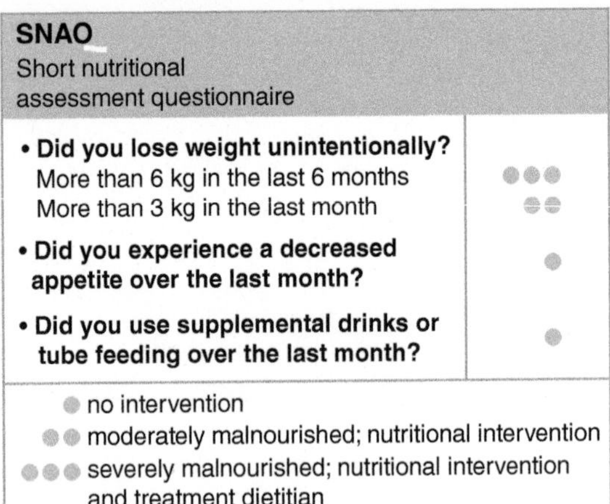

SNAQ
Short nutritional assessment questionnaire
• Did you lose weight unintentionally?
More than 6 kg in the last 6 months
More than 3 kg in the last month
• Did you experience a decreased appetite over the last month?
• Did you use supplemental drinks or tube feeding over the last month?
no intervention
moderately malnourished; nutritional intervention
severely malnourished; nutritional intervention and treatment dietitian

FIGURE 4 The Short Nutritional Assessment Questionnaire

Reproduced from Dutch Malnutrition Steering Group. SNAQ tools in english. Fight Malnutrition Web site. www.fightmalnutrition.eu. Updated 2017. Accessed February 10, 2017.

SNAQ was based on an evaluation of mixed hospitalized medical and surgical adult patients. Following a statistical analysis of 26 questions related to nutritional status and disease state, the 3 questions identified with the highest predictive validity were included in the tool (see Figure 4 for the complete tool):[30,31]

1. Did you lose weight unintentionally? (scored according to the amount of weight loss)
2. Did you experience a decreased appetite over the last month?
3. Did you use supplemental drinks or tube feeding over the last month?

Based on response, the tool then classifies patients as well nourished, moderately malnourished, or severely malnourished. Using the validated tool, malnourished patients are recognized on admission and receive necessary intervention at an early stage. This early identification and intervention has been associated with reduced length of hospital stay. The SNAQ screening tool has been validated in both outpatient and inpatient populations, with a simplicity that allows easy inclusion into the admission process.[12,30,44-48]

Malnutrition Screening Tool (MST)

Similar in concept to the SNAQ, the **Malnutrition Screening Tool (MST)** is a three-question tool that was developed and validated for use based on general medical and surgical hospitalized patients. It was created based on the need for a framework that used routinely available data, was noninvasive and convenient for nondietetics staff, and could be employed across a heterogeneous adult population. In a process similar to that used for the development of SNAQ, 21 screening questions were selected based on the literature and clinical experience. Those with the highest sensitivity and specificity in predicting nutrition status were included in the final tool.[30]

Two questions—"Have you lost weight recently without trying?" and "Have you been eating poorly because of a decreased appetite?"—were deemed the best predictors of nutrition risk. In addition, a third question was incorporated to assess the degree of weight loss, if present. A score is allocated based on patient or caregiver response, which will categorize the patient as "not at risk" or "at risk" (Figure 5). The scoring system can then be used to prioritize patient care, with those receiving the highest scores requiring the earliest intervention.[28,49,50]

The MST is an attractive choice when selecting a screening tool due to its simplicity and ability to be completed without additional calculations. Despite its minimal nature, the MST is an acceptable screening tool secondary to its relative validity, inter-rater reliability, sensitivity, and specificity. In the literature and in practice, the tool is lauded as a strong predictor of nutritional status.[12,28,30,31,49,51,52]

CORE CONCEPT 3

A wide variety of nutrition screening questions or tools are employed in clinical settings across the United States. Several well-validated screening tools exist with the goal of identifying nutritional status or predicting poor clinical outcomes related to malnutrition.[28]

Assessment Tools Confused For Screening Tools

Two additional tools—the Subjective Global Assessment (SGA) and the Mini-Nutritional Assessment (MNA)—are often grouped with the list of screening tools previously discussed. These tools, however, function as a means of nutrition assessment. In other words, the SGA and MNA should most readily be used as to assess, not to screen, because they combine data on nutritional status with clinical observations, disease status, and/or biochemical values.[5,31]

Final Comparison of Screening Tools for Acute Care

As previously mentioned, there is no universal agreement on a "gold standard" in terms of nutrition screening tools. Comprehensive tools, like NRS-2002 and MUST, will require slightly more time and skill from the screening clinician because of the need for measurements, calculations, and evaluation of disease severity. In many studies, these tools (particularly the NRS-2002) outperform all others in the clinical population.[53,54] Conversely, the "quick and easy" tools, such as SNAQ and MUST, are often supported in the literature due to the adequate availability of screening components. The questions used in these tools are not only simple to complete, but have been shown to identify malnutrition risk with similar accuracy as the comprehensive tools without the need for additional calculations.[48,55] Yet another study found each of the four tools to be adequate for screening malnutrition at a nearly identical level. The bottom line is that each of the four screening tools may be employed based on individual hospital or clinical preferences (Table 2). Because each is well validated and considered reliable, the RD must be careful to recommend the most appropriate tool for the specific setting, patient population, and/or screening goals.[11,18,30,55]

Content removed due to copyright restrictions

TABLE 2 COMPARISON OF MALNUTRITION RISK SCREENING TOOLS*

Screening Tool	NRS-2002	MUST	SNAQ©	MST
Complexity	Comprehensive	Comprehensive	Abbreviated	Abbreviated
Intent	Developed for use in acute care settings.	Developed for use in the community setting.	Developed for use during admission to acute care facility.	Developed based on general medical and surgical inpatients.
Brief Description	Two-part tool that relates nutritional status to existing disease state.	Five-step framework that scores nutritional status in the setting of acute illness.	Three question tool that assesses simple and common indicators of malnutrition.	Two question tool that requires no measurements or additional calculations.
Parameters	• Unintentional weight loss • BMI • History of dietary intake • Disease acuity • Age	• Unintentional weight loss • BMI • Presence of an acute illness that may affect dietary intake	• Unintentional weight loss • Decreases in appetite • Need for supplemental or enteral nutrition	• Unintentional weight loss • Decreases in appetite

Modified from Jensen GL, Compher C, Sullivan DH, Mullin GE. Recognizing malnutrition in adults: Definitions, characteristics, screening, assessment, and team approach. *JPEN J Parenter Enteral Nutr*. 2013;37(6):802-807.

CASE STUDY REVISITED

After completing a nutrition screen, Mary is identified as being at high nutrition risk. You initiate a nutrition assessment for Mary, who is now on bedrest. When you seek to confirm Mary's height, she states that she used to be 5'3" tall, but she is now shorter than that and is uncertain of her actual height.

Questions

1. **Given the discrepancy in Mary's reported height, how do you proceed with your anthropometric evaluation?**
2. **Calculate Mary's percent usual body weight and percent weight loss.**
3. **What are Mary's nutritional risk factors?**
4. **Based on the information you have gathered so far, how would you describe Mary's nutritional status?**

CORE CONCEPT 4

Different screening tools may be better or worse predictors in specific patient populations.

CORE CONCEPT 5

Nutrition screening tools should have acceptable validity, be simple to administer, have wide applicability across the inpatient population, and use commonly available information.

Nutrition Assessment

Following the identification of nutrition risk via screening, a thorough assessment of a patient's nutrition status is the critical next step in identifying malnutrition. As there is neither a single parameter nor gold standard that can determine nutritional status or the degree of malnutrition in an individual, a comprehensive nutrition assessment includes a review of the nutrition "ABCDEFs"—anthropometrics, biochemical, clinical, dietary, energy, and functional assessment. The remainder of this chapter will discuss the components of nutrition assessment as they are subdivided by the NCPM terminology. AND defines nutritional assessment as the process "to obtain, verify, and interpret data needed to identify nutrition-related problems, their causes, and significance."[5] It establishes the foundation for all other steps of the NCPM by providing the information necessary for determining a nutrition diagnosis and its etiology. The true purpose of the nutrition assessment is to collect all relevant information to identify nutrition-related problems and their causes[5,8,12,16,56]

Anthropometric Measurements

One of the most obvious and indispensible components of nutrition assessment is the use of **anthropometry**, the assessment of measures and proportions of the human body.[57] Regardless of the setting, anthropometric assessment will involve obtaining and interpreting physical measurements as part of a comprehensive evaluation of nutritional status. These measures are essential to either determining the need for or monitoring the progress of an intervention. In this context, all anthropometric measures obtained should be compared to both of the following:

1. Population-specific standards that help reflect the current condition of the patient
2. The patient's previous measures to identify the loss or gain of body components

PRACTICE POINT

Trending anthropometric data points provide the most useful information. A patient whose measurements begin above or at the upper end of the normal range may still be considered "normal" by comparative standards despite significant individual change.

Height, weight, skinfold measures, and circumferences provide the most readily used data points, although there are a number of additional assessment methods available for use. It is up to the clinician to determine which measures are most appropriate to the individual circumstance.[13,14,58,59]

PRACTICE POINT

Anthropometric measurements are only one piece of the nutrition assessment puzzle. Although changes in these measures are reliable predictors of nutritional outcome,[22] they should always be considered in the context of the overall status of the patient.

Assessing Height

Measures of **height** (stature) are not particularly useful for assessing nutritional status without context. Body height remains an essential measure because it provides a necessary variable for calculating other useful parameters (including ideal body weight and BMI). Several important decisions, both nutrition related (i.e., the estimation of energy needs) and not nutrition related (i.e., medication dosing), depend on the collection of an accurate measure of height.[19,59-62]

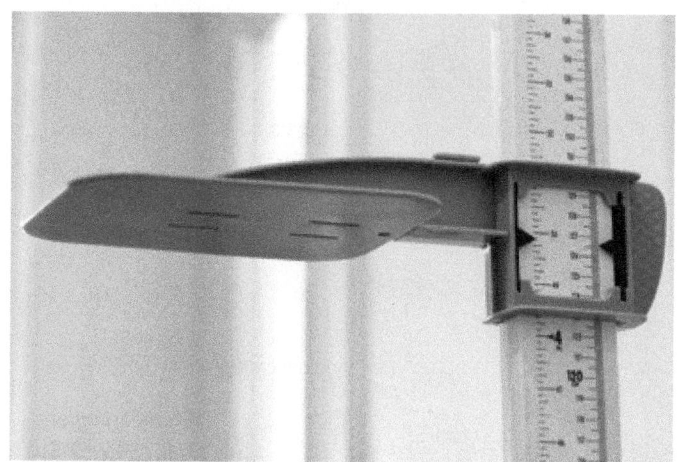

FIGURE 6 **Stadiometer**

Ideally, height is measured with the patient in the standing position using either a wall-mounted or freestanding calibrated **stadiometer**, a piece of equipment designed to measure height constructed of a ruler and sliding horizontal headpiece adjusted to rest on the top of the head (Figure 6). Upright measures are not always feasible in the critical care setting due to the limitations of bed confinement or difficulties in maintaining the erect position. Obtaining an accurate measurement of the hospitalized patient who remains in the supine position attached to several intravenous lines, for example, must instead rely upon an alternate technique.[13,59-62]

PRACTICE POINT

For those able, height is measured in the upright position. To be most accurate, the individual should stand with bare feet flat on the floor and heels together; arms should hang loosely to the side with legs and back straight. The head should be in the Frankfort plane (i.e., outer corners of the eyes and tops of the ears parallel to the floor); height is measured after a deep in-breath, ensuring that the head remains in the correct position. Three points of contact—heels, scapula, and buttocks—should be touching the wall.[13,59] (Figure 7)

Alternate Measures to Assess Height For all patients, an accurate measure of height must be obtained. Given the impracticability of the upright measure because of a number of conditions, such as immobility due to contractures, kyphosis, amputations, or quadriplegia, alternatives for estimating this value are often employed in the clinical setting. These surrogate measures use the length of other body segments in order to predict or estimate standing height.[60,61,63-65]

A large percentage of adult height records in the acute setting are based on verbal information provided by the patient instead of an actual measurement. Although this

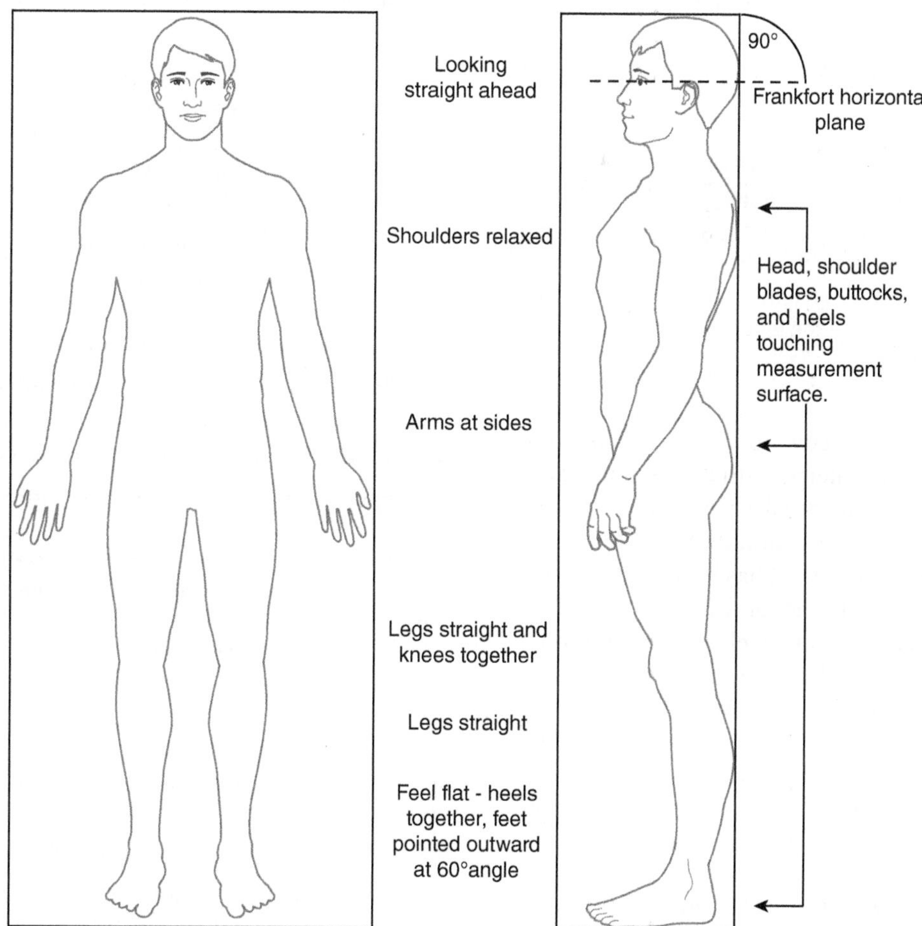

FIGURE 7 **Upright Position for Accurate Measure of Adult Body Height**

Reproduced from Center for Disease Control and Prevention (CDC). National health and nutrition examination survey (NHANES): Anthropometry procedures manual. 2007.

may appear to be an inaccurate substitute for assessing height, several studies have illustrated that the reliability of **self-reported height** (SRH) is comparable to, or often surpasses, other alternative measures. Given the ease and practicably of obtaining a SRH, it is much more likely to see this surrogate measure than any other in the clinical setting. Despite the significant room for error, clinicians can feel comfortable using SRH as long as it is taken with the caveat that most individuals tend to overestimate height.[59,60,66,67]

When neither standing height nor SRH is available (or in an effort to confirm an unlikely SRH), height can be estimated using one of the three most common surrogate measures—knee height, arm span, or arm length. These methods rely on the measurement of one or more long bones that do not lose length with aging in the same manner as the spine. Thereafter, a predictive equation specific to the body segment measured can be used to arrive at an estimate of stature. The available literature is in strong support of the use of any of these three measures; each has been shown to have a reproducible and reliable correlation to standing height.[64,68]

Knee-Height Measurement Of the many available alternate measures of stature, measurement of **knee-height** using a caliper device is perhaps the most acceptable and widely used in the clinical setting.[13,61] Due to its high correlation with upright height, this technique is often selected to assess the critically ill patient given the ability to complete the measure while the patient is recumbent. The measurement itself is easily taken from the sole of the foot to the anterior surface of the thigh while the lower limb is flexed (Figure 8).[19,60]

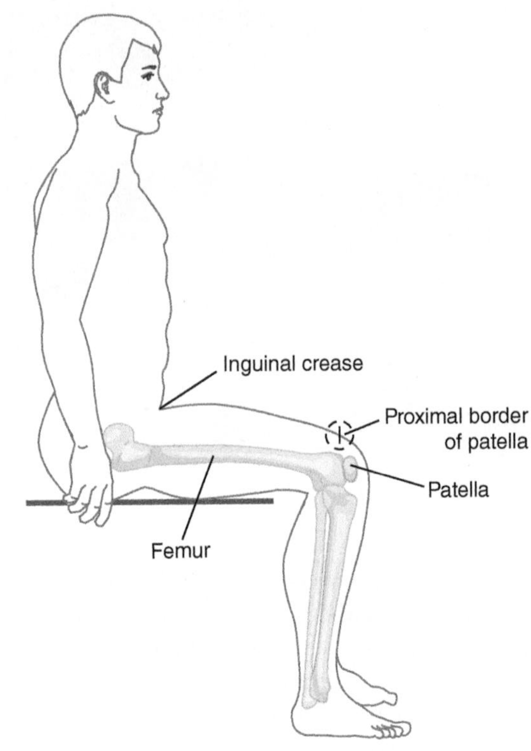

FIGURE 8 **Positioning for the Measurement of Knee-Height**

Reproduced from Center for Disease Control and Prevention (CDC). National health and nutrition examination survey (NHANES): Anthropometry procedures manual. 2007.

PRACTICE POINT

Measurement of knee-height requires positioning of the patient's lower limb at a 90° angle (i.e., the ankle and thigh must be flexed to this degree). Using the caliper device, measure the distance from the sole of the foot (under the heel) to the anterior surface of the thigh—above the level of the condyles of the femur and proximal to the patella.[19,68]

The most accurate predictive equation for estimating standing height from knee-height is that originally developed for use in nonambulatory elderly patients by Chumlea et al., otherwise known as the Chumlea method.[69] Despite its original intention, this method has been cross-validated for use in acute care patients and for those of other ethnic and age groups (such as the Korean elderly and/or immobile patient populations).[61,62,68,70] The original predictive equations are outlined in Table 3. Since its development, variations of the Chumlea equation(s) have been published that allow for its use in a number of populations. Before applying this method, consult current literature for the most appropriate equation specific to the individual patient.[69,71]

Total and Half Arm Span Measurements For those adults who cannot safely stand and are unable to position the lower limb in the angle necessary for measurement of knee-height, measurement of arm span can be used as a surrogate marker of standing height at maturity. Depending on the capacity of the patient, one of two measures can be taken:

1. With the patient's arm horizontal and in line with the shoulders, the length between the middle of the sternal notch and tip of the middle finger for each side is measured and then combined; this is called the **total arm span** (TAS).
2. With one of the patient's arms extended horizontally, measure the extension from the tip of the middle finger to the sternal notch, maintaining the superior limb at a 90° angle to the body; this is called the **half arm span** (HAS; or arm length).

These measures, which are appropriate for use in adolescents, adults, and the elderly, can be accurately obtained whether the patient is standing, sitting, or recumbent.[13,62,65]

PRACTICE POINT

To achieve the most accurate TAS measurement, both of the patient's arms must be spread in a straight line; the fingertips of each hand must be equidistant from and parallel to the floor. For measuring HAS, only one arm must remain extended horizontally in a 90° angle.[65]

Similar to the knee-height estimate, the accuracy of an arm length or span measurement is dependent on the use of a predictive equation.[65,66] When TAS is measured, the following predictive equation can be used to estimate standing height[62]:

Females: Standing height (cm) = [1.35 × total arm span (cm)] + 60.1*

Males: Standing height (cm) = [1.40 × total arm span (cm)] + 57.8*

TABLE 3 EQUATIONS FOR PREDICTING STATURE FROM KNEE-HEIGHT*

White Men	Predicted height (cm) = [knee height (cm) × 1.88] + 71.85
Black Men	Predicted height (cm) = [knee height (cm) × 1.79] + 73.42
White Women	Predicted height (cm) = [knee height (cm) × 1.87] − [0.06 × age (y)] + 70.25
Black Women	Predicted height (cm) = [knee height (cm) × 1.86] − [0.06 × age (y)] + 68.10

*For use in those aged 18 to 60 years

Data from Chumlea WC, Guo SS, Steinbaugh ML. Prediction of stature from knee height for black and white adults and children with application to mobility-impaired or handicapped persons. *J Am Diet Assoc.* 1994;94(12):1385-1388.

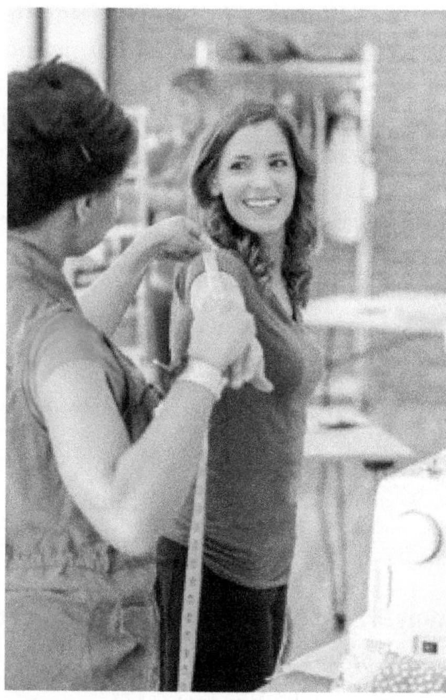

FIGURE 9 **Measurement of Armspan**

HAS (arm length) is recommended by the World Health Organization (WHO) for estimating the height of non-ambulatory patients (Figure 9). The value obtained from this measure can either be multiplied by two to provide an estimate of TAS (and then plugged into the TAS predictive equation mentioned above) *or* can be used to estimate stature using the WHO equation[60]:

WHO Equation: Standing height (cm) = 0.43 + [0.73 × (2 × HAS (cm))]*

Overall, practicality is a critical factor in determining the alternate measure of standing height to be used: While some patients may have difficulty raising one or both arms, which would suggest knee-height as the most appropriate method, others may be unable to bend the lower limb in the necessary angle and would be better assessed using an arm measurement. Given that the literature does not support one surrogate measure over the other, clinicians are advised to consider all estimates of height and select the most appropriate for the individual circumstance.[59]

PRACTICE POINT

In all cases, when standing height cannot be obtained, the clinician must use the SRH, a surrogate measure, or both. Supine length measurement, which uses a flexible measuring tape to determine the length between the vertex of the head and the heel, has been proven inaccurate and unreliable (and as such should be used as a last resort).[61,62] Instead, utilize TAS, HAS, or knee-height, depending on the individual circumstance.

Assessing Weight

The assessment of **actual body weight (ABW)** or body cell mass measurement, which represents the unadjusted sum of all body compartments without distinction between fat and fat-free mass, is fundamental to determining nutritional status. From a nutritional standpoint, an individual weight value provides limited information. Ideally, the value will be contextualized using an additional parameter. This may include the identification of individual trends, as in percent changes from a usual body weight, or relation to appropriate standards, like ideal body weight. Given that ABW is representative of muscle, fat, and fluid combined, the true value of the measure is found in its comparison to other criteria in the setting of the whole medical picture. A number of conditions, such as those that induce fluid retention, will complicate the assessment of an ABW.[58,59] The various adjustments to or calculations that involve ABW measures will be discussed throughout this section.

Weight should be measured upon admission to any acute and chronic care facility and monitored throughout the length of stay. Serial measures are necessary for tracking trends in weight that may relate to nutritional and/or overall clinical status. The most accurate measure of current ABW is that obtained from actually weighing the patient (Figure 10) instead of relying upon self-reported values, which tend to be underestimated. For those in the inpatient setting, this often requires the use of bed scales for those unable to transfer to the standing scale.[10,13,16,67]

*Of note, both the TAS and HAS equations may overestimate height when used in the elderly population. This occurs because arm measurements tend to give an estimate of maximal height rather than current height, which may change as in the aging process progresses.[60,64]

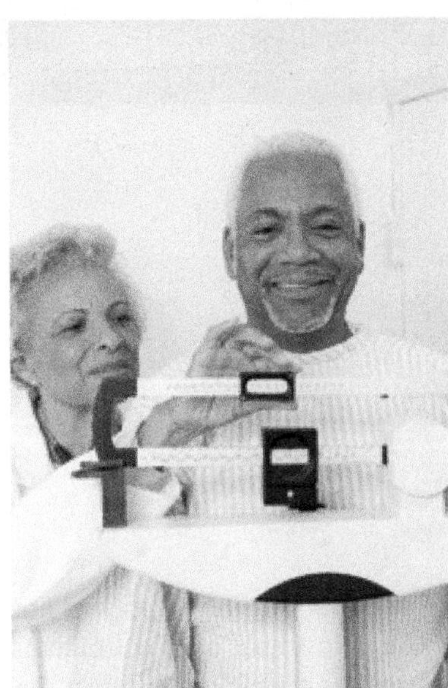

FIGURE 10 **Measurement of Weight**

PRACTICE POINT

Height and weight should never be visually estimated; an inaccurate weight may compromise application of effective medical nutrition therapy when used to assess energy and protein needs. Instead, employment of one of the surrogate measures to provide the best approximation is recommended.

PRACTICE POINT

Patients who can stand should be weighed on a standing digital or balanced-mechanism scale without overgarments or shoes. To obtain an accurate ABW measure, the patient should first remove all outer garments and empty pockets of loose change and/or keys. The patient will then step onto the digital or balanced mechanism scale with feet together in the center and arms hanging loosely at each side.[16,59]

PRACTICE POINT

For hospitalized patients, an appropriately calibrated bed scale may be utilized instead of a standing scale. Standardized procedures (i.e., all of the bedding be removed except for the bottom sheet and one pillow, along with any catheter bags, etc.) are often difficult to maintain for patients in acute care.[16,59]

Usual Body Weight (UBW) In order to identify weight trends, it is necessary to have an understanding of a patient's normal weight range to compare to the current ABW. This value, which can be obtained during the patient interview or estimated using serial measures documented in the medical record, is referred to as **usual body weight (UBW)**. In most cases, the UBW value is a self-reported measure of what the individual has weighed for the majority of his or her adult life. This is a critical comparison used to determine whether any change in weight has occurred. The deviation is quantified as percent UBW and/or percent weight change.

PRACTICE POINT

The majority of patients can respond appropriately to the question, "What have you weighed for most of your adult life?" It may also be helpful to speak with family members or refer to documentation from primary care or past hospital admissions. If weight change is evident, always note the time frame in which the deviation from UBW occurred and if the change was intentional versus unintentional.

Percent Usual Body Weight (%UBW) and Percent Weight Change (%Weight Change) Obtaining repeated body weight measurements over time and/or comparing an ABW measure to UBW are recommended for the identification of weight changes. In the clinical setting, these comparisons are made with specific attention to any losses that occurred unintentionally. Although any unintentional weight loss is concerning, it must be quantified as either **percent usual body weight (%UBW)** or **percent weight change (%weight change)** in order to be used as a nutrition assessment parameter; %UBW and %weight change can be calculated using the following equations[10,16]:

%UBW = (actual body weight/usual body weight) × 100%

For example, a male with a UBW of 91 kg is weighed as 85 kg upon admission to the hospital:

%UBW = (85 kg/91 kg) × 100% = 93.4% UBW

%weight change = (amount of weight lost or gained/usual body weight) × 100%

For this same patient, who has lost 6 kg:

% weight change = (6 kg/91 kg) × 100% = 6.6% weight loss

These values as measures of unintentional weight loss are the best-validated indicators for both the recognition of weight changes and malnutrition. Clinical significance of these values can be determined by the degree and duration of weight loss. The time frame in which the loss occurred is necessary for interpretation of the data. For example, a 5% unintentional weight loss over 1 year may not be considered significant, but a 5% weight loss over the course of 1 month certainly would be. One of the six key indicators of the AND/A.S.P.E.N. consensus statement for malnutrition identification is interpretation of %weight loss in the context of the patient's clinical status and a specified length of time (Table 4).[10,13,18]

Additional parameters exist for the interpretation of %UBW alone:

- 85% to 90% UBW: mild malnutrition
- 75% to 84% UBW: moderate malnutrition
- <74% UBW: severe malnutrition[72]

As with any nutrition-related parameter, the interpretation of weight loss must also be considered in the context

TABLE 4 INTERPRETATION OF %WEIGHT LOSS AS KEY INDICATOR OF MALNUTRITION

	Malnutrition in the Context of							
	Acute Illness or Injury				Chronic Illness			
	Nonsevere (Moderate) Malnutrition		Severe Malnutrition		Nonsevere (Moderate) Malnutrition		Severe Malnutrition	
Interpretation of Weight Loss	%	Time	%	Time	%	Time	%	Time
	1–2	1 week	>2	1 week	5	1 month	>5	1 month
	5	1 month	>5	1 month	7.5	3 months	>7.5	3 months
	7.5	3 months	>7.5	3 months	10	6 months	>10	6 months
	–		–		20	1 year	>20	1 year

Data from White JV, Guenter P, Jensen G, et al. Consensus state of the Academy of Nutrition and Dietetics/American Society of Parenteral and Enteral Nutrition: Characteristics recommended for the identification and documentation of adult malnutrition (undernutrition). *JPEN J Parenter Enteral Nutr*. 2012;36(3):275–283.

of the overall clinical picture. Weight changes often reflect more than just nutritional status. Loss may be an indication of the severity of underlying disease or inflammatory condition, while gains often represent a positive fluid status. This will be important beyond the assessment period when later determining the appropriate intervention.[16]

Ideal Body Weight (IBW) In the clinical setting and beyond, comparisons of weight-to-height measures are the most commonly used anthropometric parameters. **Ideal body weight (IBW)**, a metric that adjusts weight-for-height for comparison of weight status and/or weight-associated health risks, was originally defined according to the weights associated with lowest mortality for the respective heights. Ideal body weight was first based on historical data that compared the relative disease risk and life expectancy of individuals of different height-weight combinations. IBW has historically been the weight-for-height that correlated with the lowest mortality. Today, there are numerous formulas and published height-weight tables available for the determination of IBW. These algorithms are based on the notion that height defines weight as a linear function.[58,73,74]

Ideal body weight is determined using either a predictive equation (most often the Hamwi method) or via a height-weight table (as in the Metropolitan Life Ideal Weight Tables). There is controversy as to which provides the most appropriate or accurate calculation, although an equation is often selected for ease of use.[14,58]

Height-Weight Tables Although a number of height–weight tables exist for the estimation of IBW, the most recognized and widely used are the Metropolitan Life Ideal Weights Tables, which were initially developed by the Metropolitan Life Insurance Company in 1943 based on data obtained from policy holders between the ages of 25 and 59 years. The most recent update of the table, published in 1983, reports IBW as a range for respective height and frame size. The frame size must first be deemed small, medium, or large based on elbow breadth measurements taken from National Health and Nutrition Examination Survey (NHANES) data. Note that this method of assessment is largely outdated and is not routinely used in clinical practice.[58,73]

PRACTICE POINT

The use of height-weight tables (like those developed by Metropolitan Life Insurance Company) is not recommended due to their limited sample size, lack of applicability to a number of age and/or ethnic groups, and inconvenience. These data should not be considered representative of the entire population.[19]

Predictive Equations Given the impracticality of calculating IBW using height–weight tables, equations for predicting weight as a linear function of height have been developed (Table 5). The most frequently used is the Hamwi method; this equation is generally thought to be the "rule of thumb" in calculating IBW. The Hamwi method is often described as the most appropriate measure for use in the clinical setting.[19,58,75,76]

The Hamwi Method:

Females: IBW = 100 lbs for a height of 5 feet plus 5 lbs for each additional inch

Male: IBW = 106 lbs for a height of 5 feet plus 6 lbs for each additional inch

Adjust for large (+10%) and small (–10%) frames to derive the final IBW calculation

TABLE 5 SUMMATION OF IDEAL BODY WEIGHT EQUATIONS FOR MEN AND WOMEN[58,75]

Source	Equation
Broca (1871)	IBW (kg) = height (cm) – 100
Hamwi (1964)*	IBW (females) = 100 lbs+ 5 lbs/inch over 5 feet IBW (males) = 106 lbs + 6 lbs/inch over 5 feet
Devine (1974)	IBW (females) = 45.5 kg + 2.3 kg/inch over 5 feet IBW (males) = 50 kg + 2.3 kg/inch over 5 feet
Robinson et al. (1983)	IBW (females) = 49 kg + 1.7 kg/inch over 5 feet IBW (males) = 52 kg + 1.9 kg/inch over 5 feet
Miller et al. (1983)[†]	IBW (females) = 53 kg + 1.33 kg/inch over 5 feet IBW (males) = 55.7 kg + 1.39 kg/inch over 5 feet
Hammond (2000)*	IBW (females) = 45 kg for 150 cm + 0.9 kg/cm IBW (males) = 48 kg for 150 cm + 1.1 kg/cm
Peterson et al. (2016)	IBW (kg) = 2.2 × BMI + 3.5 × BMI (Height (m) – 1.5 m)

*For Hamwi and Hammond methods, the calculated weight may be subtracted by 10% to account for a small frame or increased by 10% for a large frame.

[†]The Miller et al. formula is calculated for a medium frame.

Data from Shah B, Sucher K, Hollenbeck CB. Comparison of ideal body weight equations and published height-weight tables with body mass index tables for healthy adults in the United States. *Nutr Clin Pract.* 2006;21(3):312–319; Peterson CM, Thomas DM, Blackburn GL, Heymsfield SB. Universal equation for estimating ideal body weight and body weight at any BMI. *Am J Clin Nutr.* 2016;103(5):1197–1203.

TABLE 6 IDEAL BODY WEIGHT DETERMINED FROM BMI OF 22 KG/M²

Height	IBW
58 in/147 cm	105 lbs/47.7 kg
59 in/150 cm	109 lbs/49.5 kg
60 in/152 cm	112 lbs/50.9 kg
61 in/155 cm	116 lbs/52.7 kg
62 in/158 cm	120 lbs/54.5 kg
63 in/160 cm	124 lbs/56.4 kg
64 in/163 cm	128 lbs/58.2 kg
65 in/165 cm	132 lbs/60 kg
66 in/168 cm	136 lbs/61.8 kg
67 in/170 cm	140 lbs/63.6 kg
68 in/173 cm	144 lbs/65.5 kg
69 in/175 cm	149 lbs/67.7 kg
70 in/178 cm	153 lbs/69.5 kg
71 in/180 cm	157 lbs/71.4 kg
72 in/183 cm	162 lbs/73.6 kg
73 in/185 cm	166 lbs/75.5 kg
74 in/188 cm	171 lbs/77.7 kg
75 in/191 cm	176 lbs/80 kg
76 in/193 cm	180 lbs/81.8 kg
IBW = BMI 22 kg/m² × [height in m]²	

Data from Shah B, Sucher K, Hollenbeck CB. Comparison of ideal body weight equations and published height-weight tables with body mass index tables for healthy adults in the united states. *Nutr Clin Pract.* 2006;21(3):312-319.

IBW can be determined using an equation based on the BMI that is associated with the lowest morbidity (22 kg/m^2, the middle value within the normal range). Current literature suggests that estimates made using BMI [i.e., 22 kg/m^2 × height in meters^2] are comparable to what is determined from other predictive equations and is desirable in the clinical setting due to the simplicity of the calculation.[58] Refer to **Table 6** for a reference table generated using this calculation.

Applications of Ideal Body Weight Similar to the use of %UBW as an indicator of weight status, **percent ideal body weight (%IBW)** can be used to compare current ABW to the IBW value specific to the patient's height.

$$\%IBW = (\text{actual body weight}/\text{ideal body weight}) \times 100\%$$

For example, a male who measures as 183 cm (72 in) tall would have an IBW of 81 kg (178 lbs) based on the Hamwi method. If this patient actually weighs 97 kg (213 lbs), %IBW is calculated as:

$$\%IBW = (97\ \text{kg}/81\ \text{kg}) \times 100\% = 120\%\ IBW$$

Because IBW was standardized using healthy adult populations, %IBW should never be used as the sole basis for determination of nutritional status. Percent IBW is used much more infrequently in the clinical setting when compared to the use of %UBW. Instead, IBW can be useful when assessing the energy needs of an obese patient requiring nutrition support. It is important to recognize how the different anthropometric parameters can be applied within the nutrition care process.[74]

Adjusted Body Weight (Adjusted BW) In addition to assessment of body weight as a measure of nutritional status, weight is an important component in the determination of energy expenditure. A body weight at the extremes (i.e., obese) complicates this calculation by resulting in a possible underestimation or overestimation of needs. Although this practice is significantly less common now, utilizing **adjusted body weight** (adjusted BW) was a common method of preventing under- or overfeeding in the past. Adjusted BW can be calculated for those with an ABW greater than 115% of the calculated IBW.[77-79]

Adjusted BW = [(actual body weight – ideal body weight) × 0.25] + IBW[79]

For example, consider a 170 cm (67 in) female with an IBW of 61 kg (135 lbs; per Hamwi method) and an ABW of 95.5 kg (210 lbs):

Adjusted BW = [(95.5 kg – 61 kg) × 0.25] + 61 kg = 70 kg

Use of adjusted BW was first recommended in order to account for the percentage of obese weight that is most metabolically active (i.e., lean mass) instead of feeding based on ABW. The underlying rationale is that subcutaneous fat is significantly less metabolically active than lean tissue and thus using ABW to calculate needs will result in overprediction. It is important to note that adjusted BW, although sometimes used in practice, is *not* an evidence-based assessment. Recent studies have illustrated that utilizing adjusted BW actually results in a vast underestimation of energy needs. A.S.P.E.N. and AND both urge against the use of adjusted BW despite its previous longstanding use in the clinical setting, recommending instead the use of ABW and IBW based on the severity of obesity.[78,80,81]

Body Weight Modifications for Special Circumstance As previously mentioned, body weight must always be considered in the setting of the overall clinical picture. There are two notable (and common) conditions that require special assessment of body weight measures: amputations and chronic fluid retention.

Adjusting Body Weight for Amputations For those with extremity amputation(s), special weight adjustments are necessary in order to account for the body compartment that has been lost. An adjusted BW is calculated based on an estimate of the proportion of total body weight that the lost body segment represents (Figure 11). Using this technique, known as the Osterkamp method, the proportion that represents the missing limb is added back to the individual's current ABW. This new adjusted BW can be used in other calculations or for comparison to population targets, such as body mass index (BMI).[19,82,83]

Adjusted BW (Osterkamp) = actual body weight/(100 – %amputation) × 100

Content removed due to copyright restrictions

For example, consider a male who weighs 91 kg (200 lbs) with a total leg amputation:

Adjusted BW (Osterkamp) = 91 kg/(100 – 16) × 100 = 108 kg

The Osterkamp method, when completed correctly, will yield an adjusted BW that provides a better basis for most nutritional assessments when compared to the use of post-amputation ABW. Some measures (most notably the calculation of energy requirements) will be best completed using the new ABW and not the adjusted BW.[82,84]

Calculating Dry Weight for Chronic Fluid Overload For many hospitalized patients, including those with liver disease, renal failure, or malignancy, fluid overload precludes the use of ABW. Increases in weight will often reflect overhydration, edema, ascites, or dialysate in the abdomen, instead of providing an accurate picture of actual body compartments. An estimate of **dry weight** is used to represent an individual's ABW without the excess fluid. For those with chronic and fluctuating retention, dry weight may be estimated based on the UBW of the patient prior to onset of fluid retention *or* based on other clinical parameters, like the achievement of a normotensive blood pressure.[14,85]

Calculating Body Mass Index (BMI)

The Quetelet's Index, better known as **body mass index (BMI)**, is the most common anthropometric comparison of body weight to body height independent of frame size. Defined by the equation weight (kg)/(height [m])^2, BMI offers a simple measure of body composition that can be read (with caution) as an indirect measure of fat mass. The BMI classifications for interpretation of the adult patient population are outlined in Table 7, although all clinicians should be aware of the many caveats associated with this measure. Although sex, body type, and ethnicity influence

TABLE 7 BODY MASS INDEX (BMI) CATEGORIES	
BMI (kg/m²)	Classification
<18.5	Underweight
18.5–24.9	Normal
25.0–29.9	Overweight
30.0–34.9	Obese Class I
35.0–39.9	Obese Class II
>40.0	Obese Class III

Data from National Heart, Lung, and Blood Institute. Classification of Overweight and Obesity by BMI, Waist Circumference, and Associated Disease Risks. https://www.nhlbi.nih.gov/health/educational/lose_wt/BMI/bmi_dis.htm.

BMI results, these factors are neither taken into account nor reflected in the measure. For example, BMI will often overestimate body fat for the muscular athlete and underestimate fat stores in the elderly. As with any method of nutrition assessment, interpretation of the measure should be made in the context of the individual situation.[16,18,19]

Despite the known limitations of BMI, it remains widely used due to both its efficiency and its relatively high correlation with estimates of body fatness.[59] Although malnutrition can occur in individuals of any BMI, measures at either extreme represent an increased likelihood of poor nutritional status and are associated with increased risk of mortality. This phenomenon is represented by a J-shaped relationship between mortality and BMI. Relative to normal weight, BMI values categorized as overweight or obese are associated with increased risk of cardiovascular disease and some cancers, while measures representing the underweight classification are associated with increased postsurgical complications, infection rates, and length of hospital stay.[10,59,86,87]

PRACTICE POINT

Interpretation of BMI should involve consideration of age, sex, body type, and common confounders of body weight in the clinical setting, such as edema or ascites.

PRACTICE POINT

Use caution when applying BMI to patients with amputations. Refer to the Osterkamp method (as previously mentioned) for a more appropriate weight assessment.

Body Composition Measures

Classic anthropometric measurements, such as height, weight, and BMI, are extremely useful in the clinical setting but are unable to accurately represent body composition. As understanding of body composition and its impact on health risk and clinical outcome increases, so does the importance of obtaining its accurate measure. Clinicians turn to skinfold anthropometry and circumference measures for the most feasible representation of an individual's fat and muscle stores.[13,16,59]

Skinfold Anthropometry Skinfold anthropometry, often referred to as skinfold thickness, involves the measure of one or more anatomical sites using a skinfold caliper device to estimate body fat stores. The measures of skinfold thickness are representative of subcutaneous fat stores in the triceps, biceps, subscapular, and suprailiac regions (Figure 12). This measure is the most widely used method of indirectly estimating body fat percentage and, when used in an additional calculation, can provide an approximation of muscle stores.[59,88]

PRACTICE POINT

A "skinfold" measure represents the subcutaneous fat layer. Clinicians should take caution to avoid including the underlying muscle in this measure. Anatomic sites often used in this context are the biceps, triceps, subscapular, and suprailiac regions.

The procedure itself requires noncomplex portable equipment and can be applied to most clinical and public health settings. A variety of calipers—ranging from precision-engineered to plastic and disposable—are available for use. Validity of skinfold thickness depends less on the caliper used and more on the measurement technique

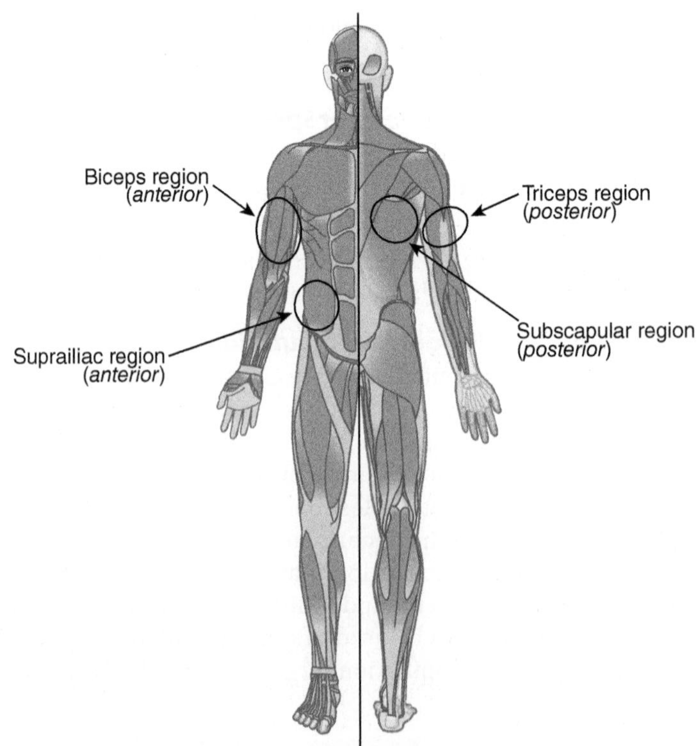

FIGURE 12 **Common Body Sites for Skinfold Anthropometry**

and repetition over time. As with any anthropometric measure, differences in equipment can account for differences in measures. When used for serial measurements of the same individual, the same caliper tool should be used for each measure to best represent any changes (or lack thereof) in body composition.[59,89]

PRACTICE POINT

Follow the procedures that accompany the skinfold caliper for the most accurate instructions on use. In general, at the given site, a lengthwise skinfold should be grasped and slightly lifted between the index and thumb of the hand (without including underlying muscle). The caliper is applied approximately 1 cm below the finger grasping the skinfold. All measurements should be repeated three times and averaged for the final value.

PRACTICE POINT

Accuracy of the skinfold measure decreases with increasing obesity. This technique is more useful in lean individuals (i.e., those with smaller fat stores) because skinfold caliper devices are unable to assess intra-abdominal adipose tissue.[59]

Triceps Skinfold For clinicians in the inpatient and outpatient settings, triceps skinfold (TSF) is the most common skinfold measure used for nutritional assessment. As with any other anatomic location mentioned above, TSF measures the amount of subcutaneous body fat, which represents ~50% of total body fat stores. TSF is the site found to be most reflective of actual body fatness when performed with strict adherence to measurement protocols by a trained professional. This site is not only the most convenient and accessible, but can be accurately measured in the supine position for patients unable to sit or stand (Figure 13).[19,59,89-91]

PRACTICE POINT

Triceps skin fold measurements are taken using skinfold calipers on the nondominant arm of the individual, midway between the olecranon process and the acromion process (i.e., midway between the shoulder and the elbow). This measure may be difficult to implement in the critically ill if, for example, impeded by wound dressings or edema.[19,91]

TSF measurements are interpreted in one of two ways: the measure can be compared against population standards due to abundant reference table availability or (preferably) by using serial measurements to assess change in the individual. Serial measures allow for estimates in body fat store changes and are more useful for assessment purposes than population comparisons. Depletion of this compartment can reflect chronic inadequate intake or nutrient depletion, which would be a critical consideration in determining future interventions. As with any other measure of assessment, TSF will be impacted by fluid retention; if edema is present, TSF measures cannot be considered reliable.[59,89]

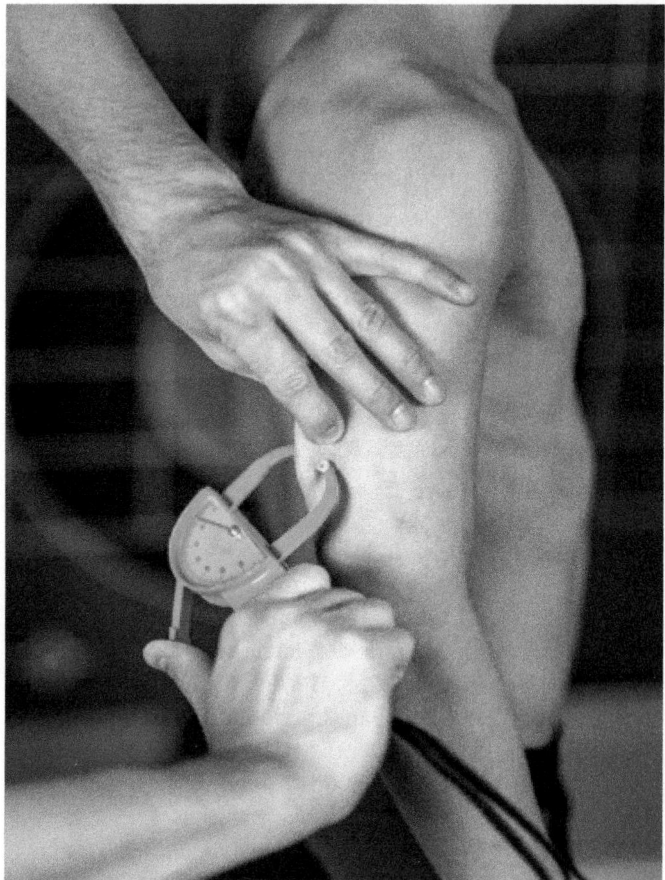

FIGURE 13 **Measurement of Triceps Skinfold**

Circumference Measurements Depending on the anatomic location where the value is obtained, circumference measurements are used to measure skeletal muscle and/or fat mass. For example, mid-upper arm circumference can be used as an index of somatic protein stores (particularly when compared to other measures, like the TSF), whereas waist circumference provides a measure of central adiposity that is considered to be a significant marker of metabolic and cardiovascular risk.[89,92]

Mid-Upper Arm Circumference (MUAC) Mid-upper arm circumference (MUAC) is a measure of total arm circumference and provides a measure of both muscle and fat area (Figure 14). Measures of limb circumference, such as the MUAC, are used as indicators of nutrition status; in other words, MUAC is most often used to estimate malnutrition risk rather than as a marker of obesity. The measure is simple, noninvasive, and feasible (even in the acutely ill patient population) because it can be completed in the supine position (if necessary) using only a tape measure. MUAC becomes particularly useful when height and weight measurements are inappropriate or impossible to obtain on a consistent basis.[1,19,93-95]

PRACTICE POINT

To measure MUAC, a nonstretch tape measure is used at the midpoint between the acromion and olecranon processes.[96]

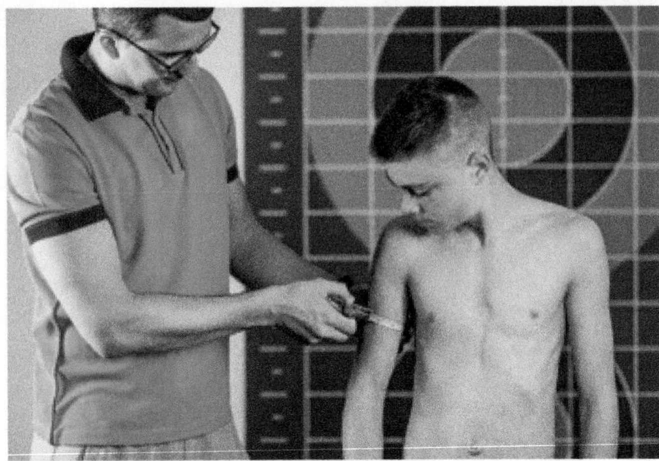

FIGURE 14 **Measurement of Mid-Upper Arm Circumference**

For the critically ill patient unable to assume the supine position for other anthropometric measures, MUAC provides an alternative index of nutritional status that is accurate and comparable to BMI.[89,96-98] MUAC can be used to calculate an estimate of an individual's BMI through a predictive equation; in general, MUAC measures of <25 cm for males and <24 cm for females will correlate with a BMI <20 kg/m^2, providing a substitute measure of potential adult undernutrition. Similarly, if a serial measure of MUAC changes by >10%, it can be assumed that the BMI has also changed by >10%. This solidifies the applicability of MUAC in identifying chronic energy deficiency and as a predictor of mortality in the acutely ill.[95,99,100]

Predicting BMI with MUAC:

Males: BMI (kg/m^2) = 1.01 × MUAC (cm) – 4.7

Females: BMI (kg/m^2) = 1.10 × MUAC (cm) – 6.7

MUAC can be used in combination with a TSF measure to calculate **mid-arm muscle circumference (MAMC)**, a surrogate measure of lean body mass. MAMC cannot be measured directly by anthropometry but is instead obtained from the predictive equation: MAMC (cm) = MUAC (cm) – [TSF (mm) × 0.3142]. The value obtained provides an indication of muscle mass. Note that the equation provided will include the bone as well as the muscle; this should be considered in your assessment. MAMC equations that do correct for bone are available, although these are not routinely used due to inherent issues with adjusting for bone size. Similar to other measures of body composition, interpretation of MAMC requires either comparison to reference standards specific to age, sex, and ethnicity or in the context of changes in serial measures. In general, lower MAMC values (MAMC <90% the reference value for the specific individual)[101] are associated with adverse outcomes including increased risk of mortality.[14,59,89]

Waist Circumference In contrast to limb circumference measures like the MUAC, **waist circumference** is utilized as an assessment of excess abdominal fat. This measure provides an indication of central adiposity, which can be interpreted in terms of obesity-related health risk, that is easily obtainable in the general population.[19,59,92] Waist circumference is more strongly associated with visceral adipose tissue and thus cardiometabolic risk than any other anthropometric measure.[102-105]

The literature describes several different anatomical sites for measuring waist circumference. Four measurement sites are common, including the WHO's recommendation for measuring the midpoint between the iliac crest and costal margin of the lowest rib (WC-mid) and the National Institutes of Health's (NIH) recommendation for measuring in the horizontal plane of the superior border of the iliac crest (WC-IC). Other cited locations include the level of the umbilicus and the minimal waist, regardless of where on the abdomen it occurs. Studies indicate that a waist circumference measured mid-abdominally (WC-mid) is the most accurate measure available for defining central obesity (Figure 15).[106] Because the various sites will yield drastic differences in interpretation of the measure, the clinician must be sure to document the location utilized in order to obtain accurate serial changes in the long term.[59,92,102,106,107]

PRACTICE POINT

Waist circumference is measured using nonstretch tape placed directly on the skin, midway between the iliac crest and costal margin of the lowest rib at end expiration.[19,59,92]

Abdominal obesity is associated with significantly greater health risks than fat deposited below the abdomen. For those with an android ("apple") body shape, a waist measurement >40 inches (102 cm) for males and >34 inches (88 cm) for females has been illustrated to be an independent risk factor for type 2 diabetes mellitus, hypertension, and cardiovascular disease—even for individuals who are of normal weight by BMI standards. This risk has not been demonstrated for those with a gynoid ("pear") shape, indicating fat deposits below the

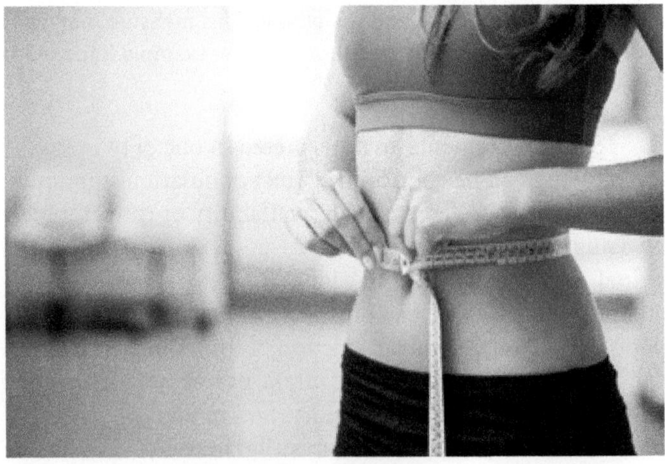

FIGURE 15 **Measurement of Waist Circumference**

Clinical Controversy

Is BMI a reliable indicator of cardiometabolic risk across various racial and ethnic groups?

Obesity as measured by BMI is associated with increased cardiometabolic risk, such as increased risk of cardiovascular disease and type 2 diabetes mellitus. BMI is an imperfect tool; it is limited in its ability to differentiate body composition or body fat distribution. The applicability of BMI as a disease risk indicator across different racial and ethnic groups has been more closely examined. In a study of a cardiometabolic risk phenotype described as "metabolic abnormality but normal weight" (MAN), Gujral et al. conducted a cross-sectional analysis of two community-based normal-weight cohorts to evaluate the prevalence of MAN in five racial/ethnic groups. BMI classification cut-offs can be noted in Table 7. BMI for South Asian and Chinese American participants was classified according to WHO Asian cut-off points: normal weight BMI 18.5 to 22.9 kg/m^2; overweight BMI 23.0 to 24.7 kg/m^2; obese BMI ≥27.5 kg/m^2. The authors found that Indians and other South Asians had more than double the prevalence of MAN, followed by Hispanics, Chinese Americans, and African Americans, who had greater prevalence of MAN compared to whites. It was estimated that the BMI values at which the expected equivalent numbers of metabolic abnormalities would equal those among whites at an overweight BMI of 25 kg/m^2, after adjusting for age, sex, and race-BMI interactions, were as follows:

1. >22.9 kg/m^2 for African Americans
2. 21.5 kg/m^2 for Hispanics
3. 20.9 kg/m^2 for Chinese Americans
4. 19.6 kg/m^2 for South Asians

These findings suggest that standard BMI categories may not be a useful screen for cardiometabolic risk in the non-white population.

Questions

1. How might BMI confound cardiometabolic screening in racial/ethnic minority groups?
2. What metabolic differences could be hypothesized to account for some of these risk variations?
3. How might these findings influence a clinician's ability to utilize BMI classification of overweight and obesity to identify cardiometabolic risk in a racially and ethnically diverse population?

References

1. Gujral UP, Vittinghoff E, Mongraw-Chafflin M, et al. Cardiometabolic abnormalities among normal-weight persons from five racial/ethnic groups in the United States: a cross-sectional analysis of two cohort studies. *Ann Intern Med.* 2017;166:628–636.
2. WHO Expert Consultation. Appropriate body-mass index for Asian populations and its implications for policy and intervention strategies. *Lancet.* 2004;363:157–163.

waist (Figure 16).[19,59,108–111] The measurement of waist circumference has evolved into a key diagnostic criterion for metabolic syndrome; according to the U.S. National Cholesterol Education Program and the International Diabetes Federation, the aforementioned sex-specific thresholds (>102 cm for males and >88 cm for females) are practical indicators of elevated risk.[107,109]

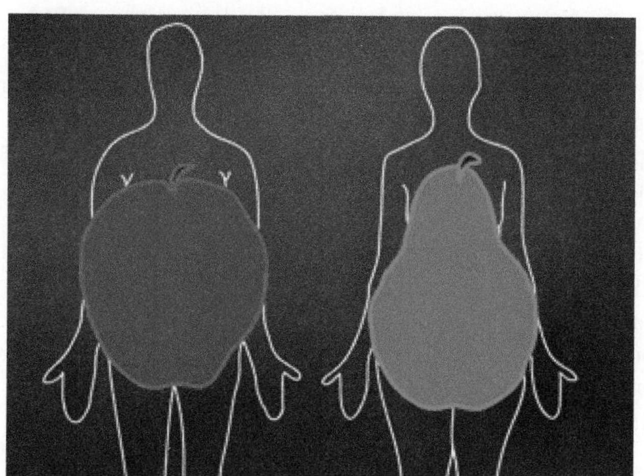

FIGURE 16 **Android ("apple") versus Gynoid ("pear") Body Shapes**

Hip Circumference Similar to waist circumference, hip circumference will also provide an indication of adiposity, although its value in predicting disease risk and/or mortality is of significantly less importance. Although some studies do indicate a significant and inverse relationship between hip circumference and cardiometabolic disease risk, this protective effect is not present in all ethnicities. Instead of using a direct measure of hip circumference as a marker of nutritional status, this value is typically interpreted as part of a **waist–hip ratio (WHR)**. WHR, the waist circumference value divided by the hip circumference value, provides an additional measure of body fat distribution as an index of both subcutaneous and intra-abdominal adipose tissue. In general, a WHR value ≥0.90 in men and ≥0.85 in women is associated with increased risk of cardiometabolic complications, although ethnic-specific cutoffs do exist. While these cutoffs are not well researched, they may provide a general guideline for assessing different patient populations (examples of those acceptable for use are outlined in Table 8).[59,103,108,112,113]

TABLE 8 SUGGESTED WAIST-TO-HIP RATIO ETHNIC CUTOFFS FOR CENTRAL OBESITY[113]

Ethnicity	Male	Female
Asian	≥0.90	≥0.80
African American	≥0.90	≥0.85
European	≥0.90	≥0.85
Hispanic	≥0.90	≥0.85
Middle Eastern	≥0.90	≥0.85

Data from Lear SA, James PT, Ko GT, Kumanyika S. Appropriateness of waist circumference and waist-to-hip ratio cutoffs for different ethnic groups. *Eur J Clin Nutr*. 2010;64:42-61

PRACTICE POINT

When measuring hip circumference, the measuring tape should be positioned at the widest part over the buttocks and below the iliac crest. The subject should be asked not to contract his or her gluteal muscles before the measurement is taken.[59,108]

Imaging Technologies Imaging techniques represent the most precise and reliable assessments of muscle mass when determining body composition; however, these methods are rarely applicable in the clinical setting.[16] The most common methodologies—bioelectrical impedance analysis, dual-energy x-ray absorptiometry, computerized tomography, and magnetic resonance imaging—will be discussed briefly in this section.

Computed Tomography (CT) A **computed tomography (CT)** scan utilizes x-ray technology to provide quantitative data on muscle composition and distribution (Figure 17). CT scans are valuable due to the ability to measure fat and muscle content within a single abdominal cross-sectional slice; thereafter, the images obtained can be used to distinguish between fat mass, fat-free mass, and skeletal muscle, and even further between visceral and subcutaneous fat. The CT scan will provide an accurate quantification of whole body composition. Although this technique may be routinely used for diagnosis and evaluation of a number of medical conditions, its application for nutrition assessment in the clinical setting is limited. CT scans are *not* recommended for the sole purpose of determining body composition due to expense and radiation exposure.[114,115]

Magnetic Resonance Imaging (MRI) Body composition analysis can also be accomplished using **magnetic resonance imaging (MRI)**, utilizing what is referred to as a free-ionizing radiation technique. Following either a whole-body or regional scan, an MRI will illustrate

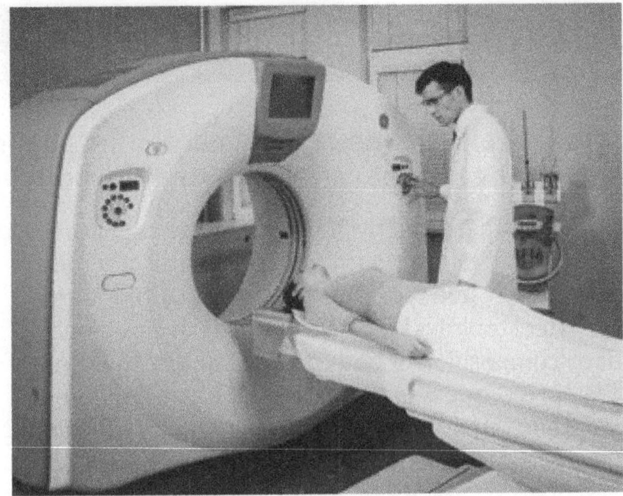

FIGURE 17 **Computed Tomography Machine**

adipose tissue and lean mass (including skeletal muscle) distribution. Although widely used in research, the utility of MRI for assessing body composition in the clinical setting is limited due to long scan duration and extreme expense.[115,116]

Bioelectrical Impedance Analysis (BIA) Of the available technologies, **bioelectrical impedance analysis (BIA)** is perhaps the most widely used for body composition estimation. By measuring the resistance of a high-frequency, low-amplitude electrical current passed through the body, BIA allows for the distinction between fat-free mass (through determination of total body water) and fat mass. The scientific basis for this two-compartment model is based on conductivity of an electrical current, which is greater in compartments rich in fluid and electrolytes such as the fat free mass. Conversely, bone and fat have poor conductivity and greater resistance to the electrical signal. Through conductivity and resistance, fat and fat-free mass can be differentiated. These values can be converted into body fat percentages using a variety of available regression equations. Within the realm of body composition analysis, this method can also be used to assess hydration status. BIA can only be applied to those without significant fluid or electrolyte abnormalities; in addition, a valid BIA equation appropriate to age, sex, and race must be available for the specific patient. When compared to other methods, BIA is attractive due to its relative simplicity, low cost, and portability (Figure 18). Previous research also suggests that changes in body composition as measured by BIA correlate directly with levels of energy and protein intake.[117] BIA cannot be recommended for use in the acutely ill patient population, for subjects at either BMI extreme, or for those with an abnormal hydration status (including renal disturbances).[14,18,117-123]

Dual Energy X-ray Absorptiometry (DXA) Developed originally for the measurement of bone density and bone mass, **dual energy x-ray absorptiometry (DXA)** has quickly

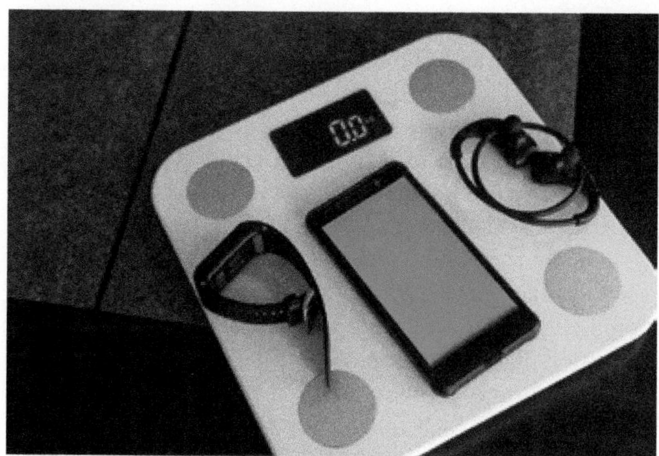

FIGURE 18 **Bioelectrical Impedance Machine**

become a reference method for body composition assessment. Due to technological advancements, DXA can now be used to quantify soft-tissue composition, thus introducing the possibility for measuring total and regional body composition. In sum, the DXA scan divides the body into three compartments: bone, lean body mass, and fat mass. This method relies on the attenuation characteristics of tissues exposed to radiation at two peak energies, which are then converted into body assessment percentages using a number of available equations. Although DXA is not widely used in clinical practice for the assessment of body composition, DXA remains the method of choice for measuring bone mineral density, which, if available, may be an important consideration in a complete nutrition assessment.[14,18,114,115,121,123]

PRACTICE POINT

Although often cited in current literature and research papers, imaging techniques are generally not applicable to the clinical setting for nutrition assessment.

Biochemical Data, Medical Tests, and Procedures

A number of critical biochemical values are important to consider as part of a complete nutrition assessment. Note that a variety of other tests and procedures, including gastric emptying time and resting metabolic rate, may also fall into this category of assessment.

Client History

A patient's nutritional status must be considered in the context of the overall clinical status. For that reason, a thorough nutrition assessment should always include an evaluation of client history, which includes personal as well as familial past medical history.

Nutrition-Focused Past Medical History

The relevance of the clinical picture to nutrition assessment cannot be overstated. Knowledge of an individual's medical and/or surgical history and current disease state(s) are particularly helpful in identifying a nutritional concern. Begin with an overview of the clinical diagnosis and its accompanying symptoms, particularly those that may affect intake. Note that any ongoing complaints or relevant past medical history (PMH) may represent a significant metabolic stressor or provide etiology behind poor appetite, decreased oral intake, or weight loss, all of which can indicate risk of malnutrition.[10,16,18] As a general guideline, a nutrition-focused PMH may include the following factors:

1. Demographic data: age, sex, occupation, family history, education level, any other personal history the clinician deems relevant
2. Chief complaint: a subjective statement of the problem, including onset and duration
3. History of present illness: note all nutritionally relevant data, including recent diet and/or weight changes, UBW, appetite changes, gastrointestinal symptoms (nausea, vomiting, diarrhea, and/or constipation), abdominal pain, etc.
4. PMH: surgical history, previous acute or chronic illnesses, allergies, eating disorders, disease or complication risk, psychosocial health, and/or cognitive disabilities
5. Medication history: evaluate for medications with strong nutrition interactions (such as drugs that may promote anorexia or interfere with the absorption, metabolism, or excretion of nutrients), including steroids, immunosuppressants, chemotherapy

CASE STUDY REVISITED

As you continue your interview, you learn that Mary is a retired school teacher who lives alone in her single-family home since her husband died 6 months ago.

Questions

1. **How might Mary's social history impact her nutritional status?**
2. **What further information might you seek to obtain from Mary?**

agents, antibiotics, diuretics, etc.; this section should also include any herbal or dietary supplement use
6. Family medical history: note the presence of any familial or genetic disorder that may impact nutritional status (cardiovascular disease, diabetes mellitus, cancer, etc.)
7. Social history: socioeconomic status, social and medical support, relevant cultural and religious beliefs, and/or living situation

In general, note any chronic disease state, episode of acute critical illness, and/or surgical procedure that may affect the nutritional status of the patient. Any number of conditions may increase the likelihood that the individual is malnourished. This may take the form of significantly increased metabolic demand, decreased appetite, comprised ability to ingest food by mouth (PO), and/or impaired nutrient absorption.[10,13,16,18,19]

PRACTICE POINT

A number of conditions, injuries, and/or complications cause significant metabolic demands.

Nutrition-Focused Physical Findings

Although often underused in clinical practice, a **nutrition-focused physical exam (NFPE)** is an instrumental and informative component of nutrition assessment. The NFPE is a system-based examination of each region of the body that aids in the evaluation of nutrition status by identifying markers of malnutrition and/or nutrient deficiencies. The goal is to identify whether the fat, muscle, fluid, and/or micronutrient status of a patient has diminished due to inflammation, chronic disease, and/or poor nutrient intake. Because physical signs tend to be nonspecific, any findings should be considered in the context of other clinical parameters (including biomarkers) and the patient interview. Although the NFPE is only one component of a comprehensive nutrition assessment, it can provide the necessary supportive data to identify and/or diagnose malnutrition.[56,124-127]

To assist the clinician in clinical practice, AND/A.S.P.E.N. have published a joint consensus statement with recommended characteristics for the identification and documentation of malnutrition. When diagnosing adult malnutrition, four out of the six necessary components include an evaluation of muscle and fat stores as part of the NFPE. In addition, the NFPE is included as part of the Standards of Practice for dietitians working in both adult and pediatric populations. If the NFPE is not performed, the nutrition assessment is incomplete.[126,127]

Techniques of the NFPE

The NFPE is performed following the review of the PMH and any pertinent laboratory data using four techniques: inspection, palpation, percussion, and auscultation. The bulk of the examination employs the technique of **inspection**, which involves the visual observation of color, shape, texture, and size. **Palpation** is used to evaluate and assess texture, size, temperature, tenderness, and mobility; here, the tips and pads of the fingers should be used to assess pulsations and areas of sensitivity, whereas the back of the hand is used to assess temperature. **Percussion** describes the tapping of fingers against body surfaces for sounds that reflect solids, fluids, or gas. This technique provides minimal nutrition information but is important for abdominal assessment and/or feeding tube placement for advanced practice dietetics. **Auscultation** involves the assessment of sounds that reflect

CASE STUDY REVISITED

As you continue your interview, you complete a nutrition-focused physical examination on Mary. Your findings are as follows:

Mary is alert but appears pale and tired. Her hair is thin, dry, and easily plucked. Her face is notable for dark circles under both eyes, narrow facial appearance, and temporal muscle depression. Her eyes appear normal. Mary's oral exam is notable for dry oral mucosa and angular stomatitis. She has good dentition with no missing teeth and normal tongue. She has evident clavicular muscle wasting. Her biceps reveal muscle wasting and triceps demonstrate subcutaneous fat loss with loose and slightly hanging arm skin. Rib fat loss is evident. Mary's skin is dry with poor skin turgor. No wounds are evident. Abdominal exam is unremarkable. No lower extremity or pedal edema is evident. Nails are thin with slow capillary refill. Interosseous muscle is mildly wasted.

Questions

1. **How would you assess Mary's nutrition-focused physical exam findings?**
2. **Can you corroborate your findings with Mary's anthropometric data and diet history?**
3. **Based on the nutrition-focused physical exam findings, what specific nutrients are of concern for Mary?**
4. **Based on these findings, how would you describe Mary's nutritional status?**

movement of fluid or air through organs and viscera using a stethoscope. Auscultation may provide useful information about the dietary status of the patient (for example, bowel sounds in the intestines as an indication of return of function following a postoperative ileus).[56,128]

PRACTICE POINT

The examination techniques most commonly used for identifying malnutrition as part of the NFPE include observation and palpation.[56]

Using these techniques, the physical examination should begin with observation (i.e., inspection) of the general appearance of the patient, including body type, mobility, skin color, and hair condition. Before initiating any hands-on assessment, the clinician should explain what the assessment will entail and request permission from the patient or healthcare proxy (if applicable) before proceeding. As previously mentioned, the clinician will look to identify any signs of poor nutritional status, including any physical manifestation of deficiency or malnutrition. Any notable observations are then compared to the nutrition-related concerns that were identified when reviewing the patient's PMH.[124,125]

PRACTICE POINT

In order to complete a thorough NFPE, it is recommended that the clinician follow a systematic approach. For example, the cephalocaudal order of examination is a guide to head-to-toe physical examination and includes these nutritionally relevant areas:

- **Head, eyes, ears, nose, throat (HEENT)**
- **Neck**
- **Upper extremities**
- **Chest and back**
- **Breast and axillae**
- **Abdomen**
- **Lower extremities**

Note: Skin is checked throughout the assessment.

Components of the NFPE

A system-based evaluation of body should include the following regions: general inspection, skin, hand and nails, head and hair, eyes and nose, oral cavity, neck and upper body, and musculoskeletal and lower extremities. Although the sections to follow will offer helpful hints on inspecting each region, refer to Table 9 for general guidelines on the NFPE components and to Table 10 for the specific deficiency that can be associated with physical findings.[128]

TABLE 9 COMPONENTS OF THE NUTRITION-FOCUSED PHYSICAL EXAM[56,128]

General Inspection	Observe overall appearance. Evaluate level of consciousness, demeanor, facial expression, body positioning, alterations in motor skills, body habitus, contractures, and/or amputations. Observe for wasting, cachexia, or obesity.
Skin	Observe for redness, pallor, cyanosis, jaundice or yellowing, bruising, and/or dark areas. Monitor for dry/moist skin, sweating, and temperature. Assess texture, thickness or hyperkeritosis, wounds or lesions, and turgor.
Hand and Nails	Inspect the hand and nails for color, texture, shape, and/or presence of lesions. Assess for transverse ridge, koilonychia. Observe and palpate the interosseous muscle for fullness and distribution.
Head and Hair	Inspect the scalp and hair for quantity, distribution, texture, and color. Evaluate for thinning, dryness, depigmentation, and corkscrew appearance. Assess temporalis muscle.
Eyes and Nose/Face	Interview to assess for changes in dryness of eyes or night vision. Observe the color of the sclera and conjunctiva. Evaluate corners of eyes for fissures or redness. Assess fullness and color around the orbital region.
Oral Cavity	Evaluate lips for pallor, dryness, or redness. Inspect corners of the mouth for dryness or redness. Observe tongue for inflammation and atrophic lingual papilla. Assess mucous membranes for moisture or dryness. Observe gums for swelling or bleeding. Evaluate teeth for caries, loose/missing teeth, discoloration, or eroded dentition.
Neck and Upper Body	Inspect the neck for distention or masses. Assess for muscle and subcutaneous fat loss in these regions: clavicles, shoulders, scapula, fat overlying the ribs, and triceps. Note sagging skin. Evaluate for edema.
Musculoskeletal and Lower Extremity	Observe overall muscle appearance. Note size and shape of quadriceps and calf muscles. Rate fluid accumulation around ankles. Assess for atrophy.

Data from Pogatshnik C, Hamilton C. Nutrition-focused physical examination: Skin, nails, hair, eyes, and oral cavity. *Support Line*. 2011;33(2):7-13; and Esper DH. Utilization of nutrition-focused physical assessment in identifying micronutrient deficiencies. *Nutr Clin Pract*. 2015;30(2):194-202.

TABLE 10 PHYSICAL ASSESSMENT NUTRIENT CHART

Region	Abnormal Findings	Possible Deficiency or *Excess* (*in italics*)
Skin	Pallor: paleness Cyanosis: bluish discoloration	Iron Folate or vitamin B_{12} Biotin Copper
	Yellowing of skin	*Carotone or bilirubin (excess related)*
	Dermatitis Follicular hyperkeratosis: rough, cone-shaped, elevated papules around hair follicles	B-complex vitamins Vitamin A Vitamin C Zinc
	Poor wound healing	Vitamin A Vitamin C Zinc
	Xerosis: abnormal dryness	Vitamin A Essential fatty acid
	Perifolliculosis: pigmented plaques (thorax, abdomen, thighs, legs)	Vitamin C
	Pellagrous dermatitis: dermatitis with hyperpigmentation of areas exposed to sunlight	Niacin Tryptophan
	Flaky paint dermatitis: hyperpigmented patches, usually on backs of thighs/buttocks, that peel to reveal hypopigmented skin	Protein
	Edema (Figure 19) Poor turgor or tenting (Figure 20)	*Fluid (hydration) in excess* Fluid (hydration)
	Acanthosis nigricans: dark patches of skin	*Insulin excess due to insulin resistance*
Hand and Nails	Clubbing (Figure 21) Raised edges (spoon-shape) Koilonychia: thin, concave nails	Iron
	Excessive dryness Dark color of nails Curved nail ends	Vitamin B_{12}
	Lackluster or dull nails Pallor or white coloring Ridging, transverse on 2+ extremities	Protein
	Mottled, pale, poor blanching	Vitamin A Vitamin C
	Splinter hemorrhages on distal ends of nails	Vitamin C

(continues)

TABLE 10 PHYSICAL ASSESSMENT NUTRIENT CHART (*continued*)		
Region	**Abnormal Findings**	**Possible Deficiency or *Excess* (in italics)**
Head and Hair	Dull, lackluster color or depigmentation	Protein Copper
	Easily plucked Thinness Sparseness Alopecia	Protein Biotin Copper Essential fatty acids
	Scaly and/or flaky scalp	Essential fatty acids
	Corkscrew, coiled hairs	Vitamin C Copper
Eyes and Nose/Face	Vision changes, particularly at night Excessive dryness Bitot spots: shiny gray spots on conjunctiva Keratomalacia: hazy, dry, softened cornea	Vitamin A
	Itching Burning Corneal inflammation	Riboflavin Niacin
	Pallor conjunctiva	Iron Folate Vitamin B_{12}
	Yellowish icterus (Figure 22)	*Bilirubin in excess*
	Diffuse pigmentation	Protein Energy
	Nasolabial seborrhea: scaling around nostrils	Riboflavin Niacin Vitamin B_6
	Temporal wasting (bilateral)	Protein Energy
Oral Cavity	Angular stomatitis (swollen corners of the mouth)	Riboflavin Niacin Vitamin B_6 Iron
	Glossitis (beefy red tongue, magenta color) (Figure 24) Atrophied papillae	Riboflavin Niacin Folate Vitamin B_{12} Iron (severe)

(continues)

TABLE 10 PHYSICAL ASSESSMENT NUTRIENT CHART (*continued*)

Region	Abnormal Findings	Possible Deficiency or *Excess* (in italics)
Oral Cavity	Pallor and generalized inflamed mucosa	Iron Vitamin B_{12} Folate B-complex
	Bleeding gums and poor dentition	Vitamin C
	Dysgeusia: distorted taste Hypogeusia: diminished taste	Zinc
	Cheilosis: dry, swollen, or ulcerated lips	Riboflavin Vitamin B_6 Niacin Iron (severe)
	Stomatitis: general inflammation of oral mucosa	B-complex Iron Vitamin C
	Edematous tongue	Niacin
	Atrophic filiform papillae: tongue is smooth or slick	Niacin Folate Riboflavin Iron Vitamin B_{12}
	Mottled teeth: whitish opaque-to-severe brown discoloration	*Fluoride excess*
	Caries: tooth decay	Fluoride Vitamin C
Neck and Upper Body	Enlarged thyroid	Iodine
	Enlarged parotid	Protein Bulimia
	Muscle and fat wasting with prominent bony chest region	Calorie and protein depletion
Musculoskeletal and Lower Extremity	Poor muscle control (ataxia) Numbness or tingling	Thiamin Vitamin B_{12} Copper
	Rickets, bowed legs	Vitamin D Calcium Phosphate
	Pitting edema	Protein Thiamin Vitamin C *Fluid excess*
	Swollen, painful joints	Vitamin C

Data from Pogatshnik C, Hamilton C. Nutrition-focused physical examination: Skin, nails, hair, eyes, and oral cavity. *Support Line*. 2011;33(2):7-13;

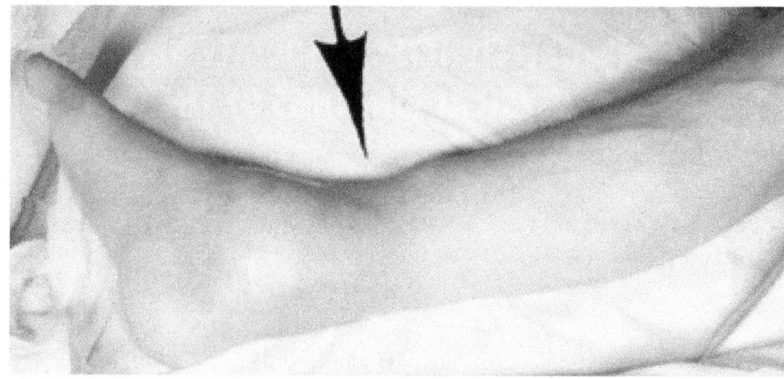

FIGURE 19 **Lower Extremity Edema**

Skin

Findings of the skin examination are considered to be accurate reflections of nutrient deficiencies because rapidly proliferating tissues, such as the skin, are thought to change simultaneously with developing nutritional abnormalities. Although a number of factors may affect the appearance of the skin, alterations in nutrition are often the culprit behind changes in fluid distribution (Figure 19), pigmentation, poor wound healing, development of dermatitis, and changes in turgor (Figure 20). These manifestations may be noted on the trunk or extremities, or on less obvious locations (as in the lips, mucous membranes, fingernails, and/or palms of hands and feet).[56,128]

PRACTICE POINT

When observing the skin, inspect the entire skin surface for changes in color, texture, temperature, moisture, lesions, mobility, and turgor.[128]

Hands and Nails A healthy nail plate should be firmly adhered to the nail bed, feel smooth to the touch, and appear uniformly thick and symmetric. The nail itself should be flat or slightly convex with translucent with a pink hue that is derived from the capillary system located underneath the nail plate. When palpating the nail by gently squeezing between the thumb and forefinger, the nail should blanch white and return to its pink color almost immediately (indicating normal capillary refill time indicating adequate hydration and blood flow to tissue). Any abnormalities in color or structure may represent nutritional deficiency and/or dehydration and should be considered in the context of the overall clinical picture.[56]

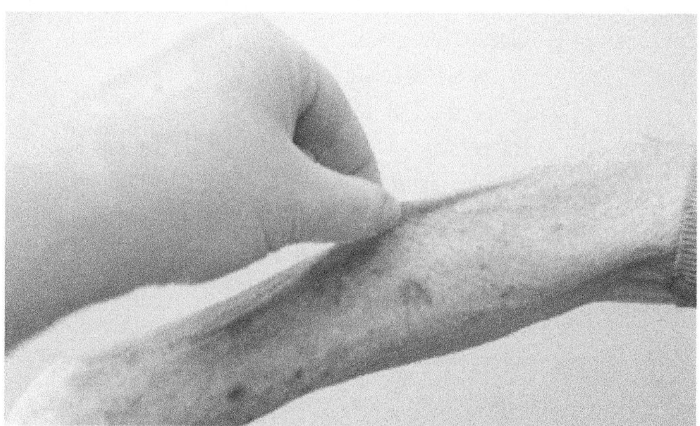

FIGURE 20 **Poor Skin Turgor (Tenting)**

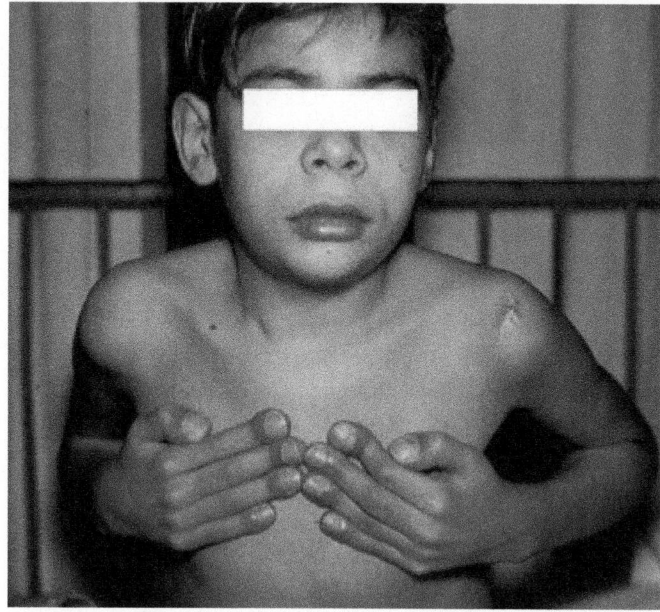

FIGURE 21 **Child with Cyanosis and Clubbing of Fingernails**

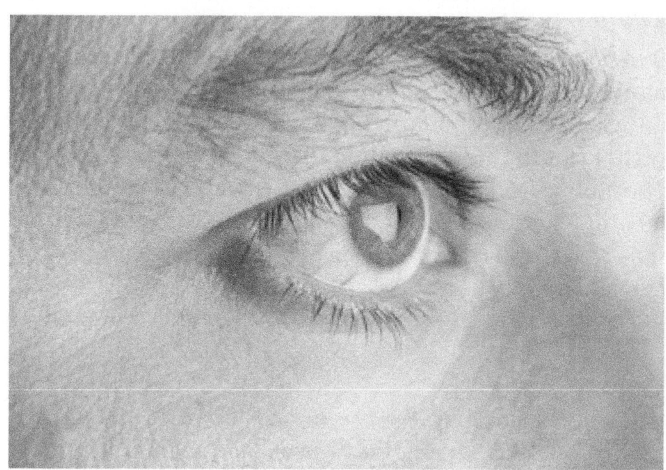

FIGURE 22 **Scleral Icterus**

PRACTICE POINT

Inspect the nails for color, length, configuration, symmetry, and cleanliness; nail hygiene often reflects a patient's self-care and emotional order.[56]

Head and Hair Inspection and palpation of the head, scalp, and hair should be performed to assess for shape, quantity, distribution, and texture. Healthy scalp hair is shiny, smooth, resilient, and not easily plucked. Any abnormalities may indicate nutrient deficiency.[56]

PRACTICE POINT

Inspect the hair for color, pigmentation, distribution pattern, shine, texture, and quantity.[56]

Eyes and Nose/Face In general, the structure of the face should appear symmetric. Facial shape, particularly in regard to the temporal region, can also indicate deficiency in the form of protein-energy malnutrition. Be sure to note any temporal wasting upon inspection.[56]

The most common variations in eye health secondary to nutritional etiology include vitamin A deficiency, which manifests as night blindness or may be observed as Bitot spots in the eye conjunctiva (shiny gray spots). During the patient interview, note changes in night vision, dryness, and/or inability to produce tears.[56]

Oral Cavity The oral cavity is a critical region for identifying malnutrition. Due to the rapid turnover (3 to 5 days) of cells in the oral mucosa, deficiencies often manifest in the lips, tongue, gingiva, or mucosa. NFPE of the oral cavity should also include assessment of the teeth. Prior to the oral examination, note any patient report of taste changes, pain or bleeding gums, and/or burning sensations. Refer to Table 11 for specific locations of the oral cavity to inspect and the associated deficiencies.[56,125]

PRACTICE POINT

A small penlight, tongue depressor, and disposable gloves are recommended for the oral examination. Start by examining the lips, then assess the inside of the mouth, including the tongue, gums, and teeth.[56,125]

Neck and Upper Body, Musculoskeletal and Lower Extremities The most important physical finding to identify on the trunk and extremities is that of muscle and/or fat wasting as an indicator of malnutrition. Incorporating the characteristics of malnutrition into the NFPE requires the evaluation of physical changes, including overt weight loss, shifts in body composition, loss of subcutaneous fat, and muscle wasting. Note that fluid retention in the form of edema or ascites may mask weight loss for many acutely ill patients. In addition, note that the AND/A.S.P.E.N. Consensus Statement on Identifying Adult Malnutrition[10] refers to several specific body areas that require assessment of fat, muscle, and/or fluid status. Per these guidelines, loss of subcutaneous fat is best identified in the orbital region, triceps, and/or overlying the ribs; muscle mass depletion manifests as wasting of the temples (temporalis muscle, clavicles

TABLE 11 DEFICIENCIES ASSOCIATED WITH PHYSICAL FINDINGS OF THE ORAL CAVITY[125]

Location	Signs/Symptoms	Possible Deficiency
Lips	Cheilosis (dry, swollen, ulcerated)	Vitamin B_6
	Angular cheilosis (fissures in the corners of the mouth)	Folate Riboflavin Niacin Vitamin B_{12} Iron
Mouth	Xerostomia (dry mouth)	Zinc
	Aphthous stomatitis (canker sores) (Figure 23)	Vitamin B_{12} Folate
	Candidiasis (thrush)	Vitamin C Iron
	Pale tissues	Iron
	Stomatopyrosis (painful, inflamed mouth)	Iron
	Dysesthesia (burning mouth syndrome)	Vitamin B_{12} Folate Magnesium
Teeth & Gums	Bleeding Gums	Vitamin C
	Tooth Loss	Vitamin C
	Dental Carries	Fluoride Vitamin C Vitamin B_{12}
Tongue	Glossitis (inflamed) Magenta (red colored) (Figure 24) Edematous Atrophic filiform Papillae (flattened protrusions on tongue, giving it a smooth, slick appearance)	Riboflavin Niacin Folate Vitamin B_6 Vitamin B_{12} Iron

Data from Radler DR, Lister T. Nutrient deficiencies associated with nutrition-focused physical findings of the oral cavity. *Nutr Clin Pract.* 2013;28(6):710-721.

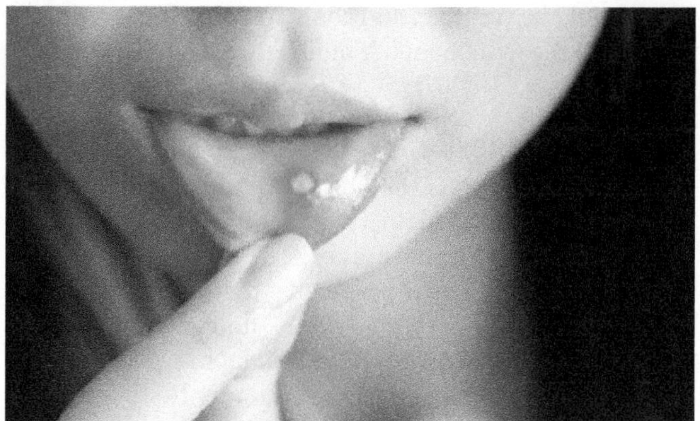

FIGURE 23 **Aphthae on Lip**
© C.PIPAT/Shutterstock.

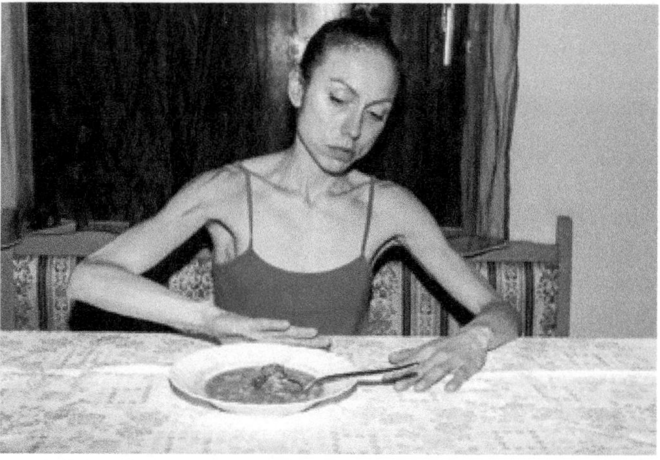

FIGURE 25 **Clavicular Muscle Wasting**
© Bony shoulders/Shutterstock.

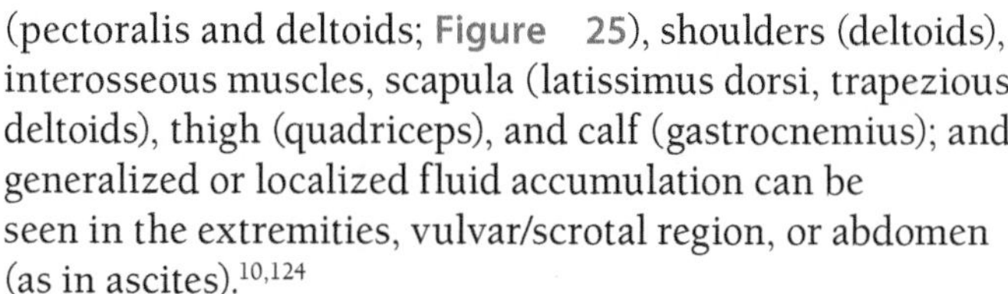

(pectoralis and deltoids; Figure 25), shoulders (deltoids), interosseous muscles, scapula (latissimus dorsi, trapezious, deltoids), thigh (quadriceps), and calf (gastrocnemius); and generalized or localized fluid accumulation can be seen in the extremities, vulvar/scrotal region, or abdomen (as in ascites).[10,124]

Functional Assessment

Advanced malnutrition, often related to a decline in clinical status, is associated with loss of muscle mass and function that leads to measurable declines in strength and/or physical performance. The relationship is reciprocal: malnutrition can impair functioning and impaired functioning can lead to poor nutritional status through a number of avenues (e.g., inability to prepare meals, etc.). A functional assessment can be used to evaluate the degree of baseline impairment and should be repeated regularly thereafter for comparison of improvements with intervention or later declines in status. This assessment may include any abnormalities in body composition that interfere with normal function—including muscle strength and function. The functional assessment becomes particularly important when assessing the geriatric patient population. Both physical performance and the ability to perform **activities of daily living** (ADLs; routine activities that most individuals complete on a daily basis including eating, bathing, dressing, toileting, and walking) have important nutritional implications for older adults.[8,16,17,129]

Muscle Function and Strength: Handgrip Strength Declines in muscle strength will accompany loss of muscle mass—the body's largest protein reserve—that results from advanced malnutrition. The most practical measure for the clinical assessment of muscle strength is that of **handgrip strength** using a simple **handgrip dynamometer** (Figure 26). Other physical performance batteries include measures such as a timed gait, chair stands, and stair steps, although these measures are generally outside the dietetics scope of practice.[16,17,129,130]

Muscle function reacts quickly to nutritional deprivation; changes in muscle function may manifest prior to visual depletions. Because the function most easily measured is muscle force, handgrip strength, which is the simplest to measure and has been correlated with overall muscle strength,[131,132] can be used as a surrogate for voluntary muscle strength. A decline in handgrip strength

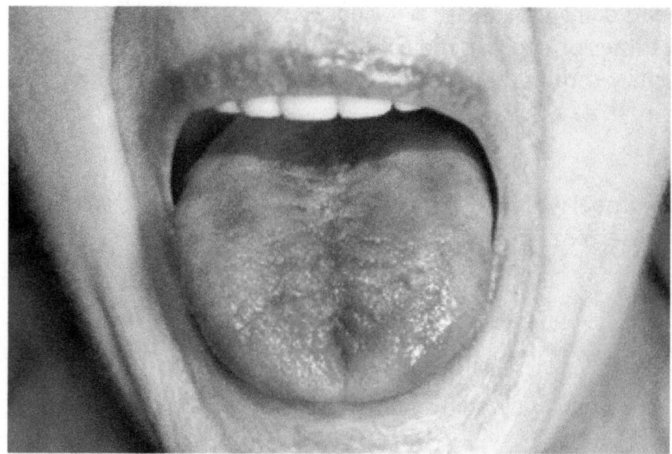

FIGURE 24 **Inflamed, Magenta Tongue**
© Timonina/Shutterstock.

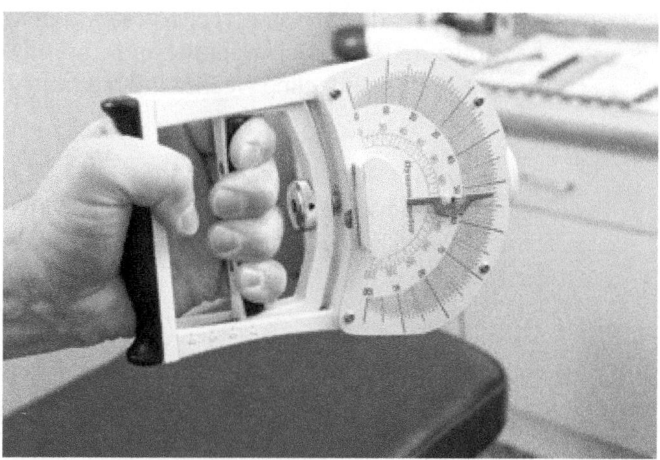

FIGURE 26 **Handgrip Dynamometer**
© BanksPhotos/Getty Images.

has been directly related to declines in nutrition status, especially in the elderly,[30,133] and can be relied upon as a sensitive measurement of short-term response to nutritional therapy.[134] It has also been deemed a relevant predictor of prognosis, hospital length of stay, and re-admission rates. In general, handgrip strength provides information on nutritional status, muscle mass, physical function, and overall health status. Moreover, handgrip dynamometry is rapid, cost-effective, and user-friendly with high test, re-test, and inter-rater reliability.[8,17,129-131,135-140]

PRACTICE POINT

Although handgrip strength has been shown to be a reliable marker of declining nutrition status, for some patients, declines in handgrip strength may be attributable to frailty with old age instead of overt malnutrition.

Procedure In regard to technique, there is some evidence that posture, choice between dominant/nondominant hand, and different dynamometer models produce varying results. These factors can be avoided by following standardized procedures. The patient should perform the test while sitting comfortably with shoulder adducted and forearm neutrally rotated, elbow flexed to 90°, and wrist in a neutral position. Ideally, the patient will be seated on a chair or at the side of the bed with feet on the floor. The grip on the dynamometer should be adjusted for hand size so that the dynamometer rests on the middle of four fingers. The grip should be held for about 3 to 5 seconds with the patient being instructed to perform a maximal isometric contraction and exhaling during grip exertion. The test should be repeated, alternating hands (for example, left hand then right hand then left hand, etc.) with about 15 seconds between each hand with a total of three tests per hand. An average value of the three tests should be recorded and compared to reference ranges specific to the dynamometer model that have been stratified by age and sex.[133,137,140,141]

Food/Nutrition-Related History

Dietary assessment is the portion of nutrition assessment that is used to identify inadequate, excessive, or imbalanced nutrient intakes. The most frequently used method for obtaining dietary history in both acute and outpatient care is the 24-hour dietary recall, although each of the most common techniques will be discussed later in this section. If dietary history cannot be obtained from direct patient interview, then medical records, family members, or caregivers can provide insight. It is not unusual for patients in the clinical setting to have compromised dietary intake for extended periods of time prior to assessment (particularly for those with acute medical events superimposed on chronic health conditions). The diet history can help to identify reasons behind changes in dietary intake, including disease-related symptoms.[13,16]

The diet history is also useful for providing average macronutrient and micronutrient intakes, as well as a depiction of general diet variety and eating patterns. When malnutrition is of concern, the current dietary recall should be compared to a normal dietary recall to provide the current percentage of normal intake. The dietary history will objectivize the contribution of poor dietary intake to the malnourished state.[8,16]

In general, a thorough food and nutrition history should address a number of areas.

Food Intake

Assess for diet composition, adequacy of food and nutrient intake, meal and snack patterns, as well as any allergies or intolerances, food preferences, environmental cues to

CASE STUDY REVISITED

As you continue to interview Mary, you ask about her dietary history. Mary states that she follows a low-sodium diet at home, typically eating three meals daily with one to two snacks, but recently has noticed a decrease in appetite and currently consumes one to two meals and no snacks. She reports that she is feeling weaker and has more difficulty completing her grocery shopping and meal preparation.

24-hour Diet Recall:
Breakfast 8 am: 8 oz coffee black with ½ cup instant oatmeal with 2 oz added skim milk
Lunch 12 pm: ½ low-salt tuna sandwich with mayonnaise, 6 oz water
No dinner

Questions

1. **How is Mary's intake influencing her nutritional status?**
2. **What other assessments can be conducted to assess Mary's functional status?**
3. **Does Mary classify as malnourished?**

eating, and current diets and/or food modifications; note that underreporting or overreporting are both common occurrences. Also note any influences on appetite, which should be assessed as within normal limits or for any relevant changes. Consider the current disease state or medication use as sources for symptoms that affect intake (e.g., taste changes, gastrointestinal symptoms, swallowing ability, requirements for assistance or feeding, etc.). This assessment should also address the use of dietary supplements.[16,18]

Nutrition Support

Assess whether a patient requires nutrition support in the form of oral nutrition supplements, tube feeding, or parenteral support. If so, note the home regimen. In the acute care setting, dietary assessment must continue when nutrition support is initiated in order to monitor adequacy of nutrient provision. If a patient is receiving nutrition support in addition to oral feeding, it is important to track the adequacy of oral feeds in order to adjust the nutrition support provided.[13,16]

Cultural Background

In all settings, assess and consider any cultural or religious influence on eating habits and perception of healthy weight status.

Nutrition and Health Awareness

Assess knowledge and beliefs about nutrition recommendations, including self-monitoring principles and past nutrition experience, particularly in the outpatient setting. Look to identify attitudes toward food or eating patterns.

Food Availability, Economics, Home Life

Food availability and economics will have a significant impact on dietary habits for many patients. Attempt to assess food planning, purchasing, and preparation abilities; limitations; nutrition program utilization; and/or food insecurity. Tailor counseling to income and availability, but always be sensitive to the individual situation.

Within this arena, consider the number of people in the household, the individual who does the shopping and/or cooking, food storage and cooking facilities, and type of housing—each of these factors will certainly impact dietary habits.

Physical Activity and Exercise

Physical activity and exercise habits should be assessed as part of the dietary history. Other pertinent information includes functional status, activity patterns, amount of sedentary time, sleep habits, and occupation. If applicable, also note any handicaps that would impact physical activity and decrease energy need.

Allergies, Intolerances, Food Avoidances

As part of the dietary history, note foods that are avoided and the reason for the avoidance (including allergies and intolerances), description of associated symptoms, length of time of avoidance, and foods used to replace the avoided item.

PRACTICE POINT

When considering the acutely ill inpatient population, assessing dietary intake prior to hospital admission and duration of poor oral intake will be particularly pertinent to the assessment. It is not unusual for patients in acute care to have had compromised dietary intakes for extended periods prior to admission.[13]

Dietary Recall Methods/Methods of Obtaining Intake Data

The accurate assessment of dietary intake is an integral component of nutrition assessment. Self-reporting of intake via 24-hour dietary recalls, food records diary, and/or food frequency questionnaires are the most common methods for assessment. Because diet is inherently complicated to measure, any self-reported data are prone to errors attributed to memory, estimation of portion size, underreporting or overreporting, and distortion to socially desirable responses. These methods may be limited for use in the acutely ill or elderly patients who may be unable to self-report dietary intake. An additional observational method, the calorie count, is useful in the clinical setting but is often cumbersome, reliant on an accurate record, and cannot be applied to the outpatient setting. Despite these difficulties, assessment of nutrient intake is crucial to identifying individuals at risk for malnutrition and to estimating the contribution on decreased oral intake to the malnourished state.[8,17,142-146]

24-Hour Dietary Recall The **24-hour dietary recall** is a retrospective tool that requires the client to recite all food intake during the previous 24 hours. To improve patient recall, a multiple-pass method is often employed; this involves multiple passes through the day ([1] collecting a quick list of foods; [2] assessing time, meal, and place; [3] reviewing a foods forgotten list; [4] revising food details; [5] final review) to provide additional memory cues. This method was developed to minimize underreporting of data by providing respondents with numerous opportunities to recall dietary intake. Visual aids may be used to assist subjects in estimating more accurate portion sizes.[142,144,147-149]

The 24-hour dietary recall is practical, quick, inexpensive, is independent of literacy ability, and has a low respondent burden. With this type of recall, the patient or client is more likely to be honest about their dietary behavior. The known limitations include reliance on respondent memory, tendency to underestimate portion sizes, and high inter-rater variability. The 24-hour recall has several

Clinical Roundtable

Topic: Nutrition Assessment in the Intensive Care Unit (ICU)[13,68,127,154-158]

Background: Patients treated in the intensive care units are some of the highest acuity patients in the hospital. Many of the typical assessment criteria (weight status, dietary intake, biochemical markers, etc.) are difficult to reliably obtain or are confounded by factors like metabolic stress. Anthropometric measurements, which are fundamental to any nutrition assessment, may not be easily acquired from the intubated and sedated critically ill patient who may be both unable to be moved for measurement and unable to provide self-reported data. Other factors related to clinical status, like fluid shifts or edema, will further confound this assessment.

To help clinicians better assess those who are critically ill, Heyland et al.[155] developed and validated a novel risk assessment tool based directly on the ICU patient population. This tool, the NUTrition Risk in the Critically ill (NUTRIC score), is based on variables that are easy to obtain in the critical care setting. Patients receive a score of 1 to 10 based on an algorithm that considers six variables: age; Acute Physiology and Chronic Health Evaluation scores (APACHE II); Sequential Organ Failure Assessment scores (SOFA); number of comorbidities; days from hospital to ICU admission; and serum interleukin-6 (IL-6). The following table outlines the NUTRIC score variables as they apply to the final evaluation:

Variable	Range	Points
Age (years)	<50	0
	50-74	1
	≥75	2
APACHE II	<15	0
	15-19	1
	20-28	2
	≥28	3
SOFA	<6	0
	6-9	1
	≥10	2
Number of Comorbidities	0-1	0
	≥2	1
Days from Hospital to ICU Admission	<1	0
	≥1	1
IL-6	0-399	0
	≥400	1

(continues)

Modified from Heyland DK, Dhaliwal R, Jiang X, Day AG. Identifying critically ill patients who benefit the most from nutrition therapy: the development and initial validation of a novel risk assessment tool. *Crit Care.* 2011;15(6):R268.

To be most clinically applicable, the NUTRIC score provides interpretation guidelines based on whether or not the IL-6 marker is available (the other markers are routinely obtainable from the medical record of an ICU patient):

If IL-6 is available:

- High score (6-10 points): associated with worse clinical outcomes (i.e., mortality); these patients are most likely to benefit from aggressive medical nutrition therapy
- Low score (0-5 points): low malnutrition risk

If IL-6 is *not* available:

- High score (5-9 points): associated with worse clinical outcomes (i.e., mortality); these patients are most likely to benefit from aggressive medical nutrition therapy
- Low score (0-4 points): low malnutrition risk

In general, the higher the sum of the scores from each component, the greater the likelihood of nutritional risk and anticipated benefit of nutrition intervention.

Roundtable Discussion

1. Given the difficulties with nutritional assessment in the critical care setting, how might the NUTRIC score be a valuable tool for clinicians in this setting?
2. Due to its validation, should the NUTRIC score supersede standard nutrition assessment in this setting? Why or why not?
3. What are the advantages and disadvantages of using a nutrition assessment tool, such as the NUTRIC score, in the critical care setting?

limitations to its use in the inpatient clinical setting; be sure to clarify whether the recall depicts a typical day and, if not, determine what makes it atypical. As with any 24-hour recall, engage in a discussion on how that intake compares to usual intake. Bear in mind that this method of recall portrays a snapshot in time; it will be beneficial to combine the information obtained from the recall with information on typical intake to better understand eating habits and any changes in usual patterns. The reliability of dietary assessment increases when 24-hour dietary recalls are repeated on several occasions.[8,17,142,143,150]

Food Records Diary The **food records diary** is applicable only to the outpatient setting. As a prospective tool, this method requires the client to record food intake for a specific time period (usually several days to 1 week). The diary provides greater precision than the 24-hour dietary recall and is not reliant on client memory. It can be considered more reflective of an "actual intake" because it will typically encompass several days, including weekdays and weekend days. The most notable limitation is that participants tend to modify eating behavior based on what they feel is an "acceptable" dietary intake for the duration of the food record. This method has a much higher client burden when compared to the 24-hour dietary recall and is dependent on literacy and numeracy with knowledge of portion sizes.[143]

Food Frequency Questionnaire (FFQ) The **food frequency questionnaire (FFQ)** is utilized most often in the outpatient setting or for national survey data collection, although modified versions may be useful for assessing intake patterns of the hospitalized patient. The FFQ is a retrospective tool that requires the client to complete a survey about food intake over a specific period of time in an attempt to depict "usual" intake. This method has several benefits, including low client burden, ease of administration, low cost, ease of standardization, and ability to examine specific nutrients. The data provided are qualitative. The tool also requires that the client be literate and numerate, and is significantly memory-dependent. The tool may be cognitively difficult because it relies on a foods list and is not meal-based.[143,151,152]

Observation of Food Intake: "Calorie Counts" Observation of food intake in the form of "calorie counts" can only be employed in controlled settings (like an inpatient hospital unit). This method will not represent usual intake, but instead a picture of current intake that is often useful when diagnosing malnutrition or assessing need for nutrition support in the clinical setting. Observation methods have a low client burden (i.e., the client is generally unaware of the dietary assessment) and is not memory or literacy dependent. In addition to increasing staff burden, this tool is intrusive and may be difficult to implement and interpret. This tool should not serve as the first choice for dietary assessment method and should be saved for instances when other dietary recall methods are not feasible.[143,146]

Technological Advancements for Tracking Dietary Intake

Technological advancements have begun to change the way dietary assessment is implemented in the outpatient setting. Innovative dietary assessment technologies using smartphones and web-based platforms have grown in popularity and now tend to replace traditional pen-and-paper versions of dietary assessment. The application of technology in this setting has recently been shown to reduce issues associated with accuracy, client burden, and time of data collection. Being aware of the current technologies and their function may help facilitate better data collection when compared to the traditional methods.[144,145,148,153]

Energy Balance

Assessment of current dietary intake and the influencing factors should be made in the context of energy needs. These needs will vary greatly depending on disease state (among many other factors).

Chapter Summary

Nutrition assessment is an integral part of patient care because it involves obtaining and interpreting information needed to identify and then treat nutrition-related issues, such as malnutrition. It is a multifactorial process that utilizes various data sources including anthropometric, biochemical, clinical, dietary, energy balance, and functional information in order to compare to specific criteria. Although there is a broad range of evaluation parameters, assessment of nutritional status requires interpretation of data compared to standards made within the context, interpreted, and adjusted for the individual clinical situation. Nutrition assessment is supported by, but does not include, nutrition screening, which seeks to identify individuals who would benefit most from a complete assessment.

Key Terms

nutrition care process and model (NCPM), nutrition care process terminology (NCPT), malnutrition, nutrition screening, nutritional risk screening (NRS-2002), malnutrition universal screening tool (MUST), short nutritional assessment questionnaire (SNAQ), malnutrition screening tool (MST), anthropometry, height, stadiometer, self-reported height (SRH), knee-height, total arm span (TAS), half arm span (HAS), actual body weight, usual body weight (UBW), percent usual body weight (%UBW), percent weight change (%weight change), ideal body weight (IBW), percent ideal body weight (%IBW), adjusted body weight, dry weight, body mass index (BMI), skinfold anthropometry, triceps skinfold (TSF), mid-upper arm circumference (MUAC), mid-arm muscle circumference

(MAMC), waist circumference, waist-hip ratio (WHR), computed tomography (CT), magnetic resonance imaging (MRI), bioelectrical impedance analysis (BIA), dual energy x-ray absorptiometry (DXA), nutrition-focused physical exam (NFPE), inspection, palpation, percussion, auscultation, activities of daily living handgrip strength, handgrip dynamometer, 24-hour dietary recall, food records diary, food frequency questionnaire

References

1. Ravasco P, Camilo ME, Gouveia-Oliveira A, Adam S, Brum G. A critical approach to nutritional assessment in critically ill patients. *Clin Nutr.* 2002;21(1):73-77.
2. Charney P, Peterson SJ. Practice papers of the Academy of Nutrition and Dietetics: critical thinking skills in nutrition assessment and diagnosis. *J Acad Nutr Diet.* 2013;115(11):1545-1558.
3. Hammond MI, Myers EF, Trostler N. Nutrition care process and model: an academic and practice odyssey. *J Acad Nutr Diet.* 2014;114(12): 1879-1894.
4. Writing Group of the Nutrition Care Process/Standardized Language Committee. Nutrition care process and model part I: the 2008 update. *J Am Diet Assoc.* 2008;108(7):1113-1117.
5. Field LB, Hand RK. Differentiating malnutrition screening and assessment: a nutrition care process perspective. *J Acad Nutr Diet.* 2015;115(5):824-828.
6. Lacey K, Pritchett E. Nutrition care process and model: ADA adopts road map to quality care and outcomes management. *J Am Diet Assoc.* 2003;103(8):1061-1072.
7. Mueller C, Compher C, Ellen DM. American Society for Parenteral and Enteral Nutrition (A.S.P.E.N.) Board of Directors. A.S.P.E.N. clinical guidelines: nutrition screening, assessment, and intervention in adults. *JPEN J Parenter Enteral Nutr.* 2011;35(1):16-24.
8. Soeters PB, Reijven PLM, van Bokhorst-de van der Schueren MA, et al. A rational approach to nutrition assessment. *Clin Nutr.* 2008;27(5):706-716.
9. Lawson CM, Daley BJ, Sams VG, Martindale R, Kudsk KA, Miller KR. Factors that impact patient outcome: nutrition assessment. *JPEN J Parenter Enteral Nutr.* 2013;37(Suppl 1):30S-38S.
10. White JV, Guenter P, Jensen G, et al. Consensus state of the academy of nutrition and dietetics/american society for parenteral and enteral nutrition: characteristics recommended for the identification and documentation of adult malnutrition (undernutrition). *JPEN J Parenter Enteral Nutr.* 2012;36(3):275-283.
11. Jensen GL, Mirtallo J, Compher C, et al. Adult starvation and disease-related malnutrition: a proposal for etiology-based diagnosis in the clinical practice setting from the international consensus guideline committee. *JPEN J Parenter Enteral Nutr.* 2010;34(2):156-159.
12. Jensen GL, Compher C, Sullivan DH, Mullin GE. Recognizing malnutrition in adults: definitions, characteristics, screening, assessment, and team approach. *JPEN J Parenter Enteral Nutr.* 2013;37(6):802-807.
13. Jensen GL, Wheeler D. A new approach to defining and diagnosing malnutrition in adult critical illness. *Curr Opin Crit Care.* 2012;18(2): 206-211.
14. Jeejeebhoy KN. Nutrition assessment. *J Nutr.* 2000;16(7/8):585-590.
15. Cederholm T, Bosaeus I, Barazzoni R, et al. Diagnostic criteria for malnutrition—an ESPEN consensus statement. *Clin Nutr.* 2015;34(3): 335-340.
16. Jensen GL, Hsiao PY, Wheeler D. Adult nutrition assessment tutorial. *JPEN J Parenter Enteral Nutr.* 2012;36(3):267-274.
17. Soeters PB, Schols AMWJ. Advances in understanding and assessing malnutrition. *Curr Opin Clin Nutr Metab Care.* 2009;12(5):487-494.
18. Alberda C, Graf A, McCargar L. Malnutrition: etiology, consequences, and assessment of a patient at risk. *Best Pract Res Clin Gastroenterol.* 2006;20(3):419-439.
19. Sabol VK. Nutrition assessment of the critically ill adult. *AACN Clin Issues.* 2004;15(4):595-606.
20. Kondrup J, Allison SP, Elia M, Vellas B, Plauth M. ESPEN guidelines for nutrition screening 2002. *Clin Nutr.* 2003;22(4):415-421.
21. Kondrup J, Rasmussen HH, Hamberg O, Stanga Z, an ad hoc ESPEN Working Group. Nutritional risk screening (NRS 2002): a new method based on an analysis of controlled clinical trials. *Clin Nutr.* 2003;22(3):321-336.
22. Hejazi N, Mazloom Z, Zand F, Rezaiazadeh A, Amini A. Nutrition assessment in critically ill patients. *Iran J Med Sci.* 2016;41(3):171-179.
23. Isabel M, Correia TD, Waitzberg DL. The impact of malnutrition on morbidity, mortality, length of hospital stay and costs evaluated through a multivariate model analysis. *Clin Nutr.* 2003;22(3):235-239.
24. Saunders J, Smith T, Stroud M. Malnutrition and undernutrition. *Medicine.* 2011;39(1):45-50.
25. Lim SL, Ong KCB, Chan YH, Loke WC, Ferguson M, Daniels L. Malnutrition and its impact on cost of hospitalization, length of stay, readmission and 3-year mortality. *Clin Nutr.* 2012;31(3):345-350.
26. Skipper A, Ferguson M, Thompson K, Castellanos VH, Porcari J. Nutrition screening tools: an analysis of the evidence. *JPEN J Parenter Enteral Nutr.* 2012;36(3):292-298.
27. Poulia KA, Klek S, Doundoulakis I, et al. The two most popular malnutrition screening tools in light of the new ESPEN consensus definition of the diagnostic criteria for malnutrition. *Clin Nutr.* 2017;36(4): 1130-1135.
28. Phillips W, Zechariah S. Minimizing false-positive nutrition referrals generated from the malnutrition screening tool. *J Acad Nutr Diet.* 2017;117(5):665-669.
29. Patel V, Romano M, Corkins MR, et al. Nutrition screening and assessment in hospitalized patients: a survey of current practice in the united states. *Nutr Clin Pract.* 2014;29(4):483-490.
30. Anthony PS. Nutrition screening tools for hospitalized patients. *Nutr Clin Pract.* 2008;23(4):373-382.
31. van Bokhorst-de van der Schueren MA, Guaitoli PR, Iansma EP, de Vet HCW. Nutrition screening tools: Does one size fit all? A systematic review of screening tools for the hospital setting. *Clin Nutr.* 2014;33(1):39-58.
32. Rasmussen HH, Holst M, Kondrup J. Measuring nutritional risk in hospitals. *Clin Epidemiol.* 2010;21(2):209-216.
33. Gur AS, Atahan K, Aladag I, et al. The efficacy of nutrition risk screening-2002 (NRS-2002) to decide on the nutritional support in general surgery patients. *Bratisl Lek Listy.* 2009;110(5):290-292.
34. Mercadal-Orfila G, Lluch-Taltavull J, Campillo-Artero C, Torrent-Quetglas M. Association between nutritional risk based on the NRS-2002 test and hospital morbidity and mortality. *Nutr Hosp.* 2012;27(4): 1248-1254.
35. Boban M, Laviano A, Persic V, Rotim A, Jovanovic Z, Vcev A. Characteristics of NRS-2002 nutritional risk screening in patients hospitalized for secondary cardiovascular prevention and rehabilitation. *J Am Coll Nutr.* 2014;33(6):466-473.
36. Orell-Kotikangas H, Österlund P, Saarilahti K, Ravasco P, Schwab U, Mäkitie AA. NRS-2002 for pre-treatment nutritional risk screening and

nutritional status assessment in head and neck cancer patients. *Support Care Cancer*. 2015;23(6):1496-1502.

37. Guo W, Ou G, Li X, Huang J, Liu J, Wei H. Screening of the nutritional risk of patients with gastric carcinoma before operation by NRS 2002 and its relationship with postoperative results. *J Gastroenterol Hepatol*. 2010;25(4):800-803.
38. Malnutrition Advisory Group. The 'MUST' report. Nutritional screening of adults: a multidisciplinary responsibility. Development and use of the malnutrition universal screening tool (MUST) for adults. *BAPEN*; 2003. https://www.health.gov.il/download/ng/N500-19.pdf
39. Stratton RJ, Hackston A, Longmore D, et al. Malnutriton in hospital outpatients and inpatients: Prevalence, concurrent validity, and ease of use of the 'malnutrition universal screening tool' ('MUST') for adults. *Br J Nutr*. 2004;92:799-808.
40. Stratton RJ, King CL, Stroud MA, Jackson AA, Elia M. 'Malnutrition universal screening tool' predicts mortality and length of hospital stay in acutely ill elderly. *Br J Nutr*. 2006;95:325-330.
41. Cooper PL, Raja R, Golder J, et al. Implementation of nutrition risk screening using the malnutrition universal screning tool across a large metropolitan health service. *J Hum Nutr Diet*. 2016;29(6):697-703.
42. Rahman A, Wu T, Bricknell R, Muqtadir Z, Armstrong D. Malnutrition matters in Canadian hospitalized patients: malnutrition risk in hospitalized patients in a tertiary care center using the malnutrition universal screening tool. *Nutr Clin Pract*. 2015;30(5):709-713.
43. Boléo-Tomé C, Monteiro-Grillo I, Camilo M, Ravasco P. Validation of the malnutrition universal screening tool (MUST) in cancer. *Br J Nutr*. 2012;108(2):343-348.
44. Dutch Malnutrition Steering Group. SNAQ tools in English. Fight Malnutrition Web site. www.fightmalnutrition.eu. Updated 2017. Accessed February 10, 2017.
45. Kruizenga HM, Seidell JC, de Vet H.C., Wierdsma NJ, van Bokhorst-de van der Schueren, M.A. Development and validation of a hospital screening tool for malnutrition: the short nutritional screening questionnaire (SNAQ©). *Clin Nutr*. 2005;24(1):75-82.
46. Kruizenga HM, de Jonge P, Seidell JC, et al. Are malnourished patients complex patients? Health status and care complexity of malnourished patients detected by the short nutritional assessment questionnaire (SNAQ). *Eur J Intern Med*. 2006;17(3):189-194.
47. Neelemaat F, Kruizenga HM, de Vet HC, Seidell JC, Butterman M, van Bokhorst-de van der Schueren, MA. Screening malnutrtion in hospital outpatients. Can the SNAQ malnutrition screening tool also be applied to this population? *Clin Nutr*. 2008;27(3):439-446.
48. van Venrooij LM, de Vos R, Borgmeijer-Hoelen AM, Kruizenga HM, Jonkers-Schuitema CF, de Mol BA. Quick-and-easy nutritional screening tools to detect disease-related undernutrition in hospital in- and outpatient settings: a systematic review of sensitivity and specificity. *e-SPEN Eur E J Clin Nutr Metab*. 2007;2:21-37.
49. Ferguson M, Capra S, Bauer J, Banks M. Development of a valid and reliable malnutrition screening tool for adult acute hospital patients. *Nutrition*. 1999;15(6):458-464.
50. Abbott Nutrition. Malnutrition screening tool (MST). Abbott Nutrition Web site. https://abbottnutrition.com/tools-for-patient-care/rd-toolkit. Updated 2017. Accessed October 29, 2017.
51. Isenring E, Cross G, Daniels L, Kellett E, Koczwara B. Validity of the malnutrition screening tool as an effective predictor of nutritonal risk in oncology outpatients receiving chemotherapy. *Support Care Cancer*. 2006;14(11):1152-1156.
52. Ferguson ML, Bauer J, Gallagher B, Capra S, Christie DR, Mason BR. Validation of a malnutrition screening tool for patients receiving radiotherapy. *Australas Radiol*. 1999;43(3):325-327.
53. Raslan M, Gonzalez MC, Dias MC, et al. Comparison of nutritinal risk screening tools for predicting clinical outcomes in hospitalized patients. *Nutrition*. 2010;26(7-8):721-726.
54. Kyle UG, Kossovsky MP, Karsegard VL, Richard C. Comparison of tools for nutritional assessment and screening at hospital admission: a population study. *Clin Nutr*. 2006;25(3):409-417.
55. Neelemaat F, Meijers J, Kruizenga H, van Ballegooijen H, van Bokhorst-de van der Schueren, M. Comparison of five malnutrition screening tools in one hospital inpatient sample. *J Clin Nurs*. 2011;20(15-16): 2144-2152.
56. Pogatshnik C, Hamilton C. Nutrition-focused physical examination: skin, nails, hair, eyes, and oral cavity. *Support Line*. 2011;33(2):7-13.
57. Gorstein J, Akré J. The use of anthropometry to assess nutritional status. *World Health Stat Q*. 1988;41(2):48-58.
58. Shah B, Sucher K, Hollenbeck CB. Comparison of ideal body weight equations and published height-weight tables with body mass index tables for healthy adults in the United States. *Nutr Clin Pract*. 2006;21(3):312-319.
59. Madden AM, Smith S. Body composition and morphological assessment of nutritional status in adults: a review of anthropometric variables. *J Hum Nutr Diet*. 2016;29(1):7-25.
60. Beghetto MG, Fink J, Luft VC, de Mello ED. Estimates of body height in adult inpatients. *Clin Nutr*. 2006;25(3):438-443.
61. Cereda E, Bertoli S, Battezzati A. Height prediction formula for middle-aged (30-55 y) Caucasians. *Nutrition*. 2010;26(11-12):1075-1081.
62. Venkataraman R, Ranganathan L, Nirmal V, et al. Height measurement in the critically ill patient: a tall order in the critical care unit. *Indian J Crit Care Med*. 2015;19(11):665-668.
63. Centers for Disease Control and Prevention (CDC). National Health and Nutrition Examination survey (NHANES): Anthropometry procedures manual. https://www.cdc.gov/nchs/data/nhanes/nhanes_07_08/manual_an.pdf Updated January, 2007. Accessed October 29, 2017.
64. Hickson M, Frost G. A comparison of three methods for estimating height in the acutely ill ederly population. *J Hum Nutr Diet*. 2003;16(1):13-20.
65. Brown JK, Whittemore KT, Knapp TR. Is arm span an accurate measure of height in young and middle-age adults? *Clin Nurs Res*. 2000;9(1):84-94.
66. Brown JK, Feng J, Knapp TR. Is self-reported height or arm span a more accurate alternative measure of height? *Clin Nurs Res*. 2002;11(4):417-432.
67. Gorber SC, Tremblay M, Moher D, Gorber B. A comparison of direct vs. self-report measures for assessing height, weight, and body mass index: a systematic review. *Obes Rev*. 2007;8(4):307-326.
68. Berger MM, Cayeux M, Schaller M, Soguel L, Piazza G, Chioléro RL. Stature estimation using the knee height determination in critically ill patients. *e-SPEN Eur E J Clin Nutr Metab*. 2008;3(2):e84-e88.
69. Chumlea WC, Guo SS, Steinbaugh ML. Prediction of stature from knee height for black and white adults and children with application to mobility-impaired or handicapped persons. *J Am Diet Assoc*. 1994;94(12):1385-1388.
70. Hwang IC, Kim KK, Kang HC, Kang DR. Validity of stature-predicted equations using knee height for elderly and mobility impaired persons in koreans. *Epidemiol Health*. 2009;31:e20009004.
71. Chumlea WC, Guo SS, Wholihan K, Cockram D, Kuczmarski RJ, Johnson CL. Stature prediction equations for elderly non-hispanic white, non-hispanic black, and Mexican-American persons developed from NHANES III. *J Am Diet Assoc*. 1998;98(2):137-142.
72. Buchman AL. *Handbook of Nutritional Support*. Baltimore: Williams & Wilkins; 1997.
73. Pai MP, Paloucek FP. The origin of the "ideal" body weight equations. *Ann Pharmacother*. 2000;34(9):1066-1069.

74. Müller MJ. Ideal body weight or BMI: so, what's it to be? *Am J Clin Nutr.* 2016;103(5):1193-1194.
75. Peterson CM, Thomas DM, Blackburn GL, Heymsfield SB. Universal equation for estimating ideal body weight and body weight at any BMI. *Am J Clin Nutr.* 2016;103(5):1197-1203.
76. Hamwi GJ. Changing dietary concepts. In: Donowski TS, ed. *Diabetes mellitus: Diagnosis and treatment.* New York, NY: American Diabetes Association;1964:73-78.
77. Ireton-Jones C. Adjusted body weight, con: Why adjust body weight in energy-expenditure calculations? *Nutr Clin Pract.* 2005;20(4):474-479.
78. Kohn JB. Adjusted or ideal body weight for nutrition assessment? *J Acad Nutr Diet.* 2015;115(4):680.
79. Barak N, Wall-Alonso E, Sitrin MD. Evaluation of stress factors and body weight adjustments currently used to estimate energy expenditure in hospitalized patients. *JPEN J Parenter Enteral Nutr.* 2002;26(4):231-238.
80. Krenitsky J. Adjusted body weight, pro: Evidence to support the use of adjusted body weight in calculating calorie requirements. *Nutr Clin Pract.* 2005;20(4):468-473.
81. McClave SA, Taylor BE, Martindale RG, et al. Guidelines for the provision and assessment of nutrition support therapy in the adult critically ill patient: Society of Critical Care Medicine (SCCM) and American Society for Parenteral and Enteral Nutrition (A.S.P.E.N.). *JPEN J Parenter Enteral Nutr.* 2016;40(2):159-211.
82. Andrews AM, Pruziner AL. Guidelines for using adjusted versus unadjusted body weights when conducting clinical evaluations and making clinical recommendations. *J Acad Nutr Diet.* 2017;117(7):1011-1015.
83. Osterkamp LK. Perspective on assessment of human body proportions of relevance to amputees. *J Am Diet Assoc.* 1995;95(2):215-218.
84. Mozumdar A, Roy SK. Method for estimating body weight in persons with lower-limb amputation and its implication for their nutritonal assessment. *Am J Clin Nutr.* 2004;80(4):868-875.
85. Gunal A. How to determine 'dry weight'? *Kidney Int Suppl.* 2013;3(4):377-379.
86. Frankenfiled DC, Rowe WA, Cooney RN, Smith JS, Becker D. Limits of body mass index to detect obesity and predict body composition. *Nutrition.* 2001;17(1):26-30.
87. Flegal KM, Kit BK, Orpana H, Graubard BI. Association of all-cause mortality with overweight and obesity using standard body mass index categories. *JAMA.* 2013;309(1):71-82.
88. Zin T, Yusuff ASM, Myint T, Naing DKS, Htay K, Wynn AA. Body fat percentage, BMI and skinfold thickness among medical students in Sabah, Malaysia. *South East Asia J Public Health.* 2014;4(1):45-40.
89. Jensen TG, Dudrick SJ, Johnston DA. A comparison of triceps skinfold and upper arm circumference measurements taken in standard and supine positions. *JPEN J Parenter Enteral Nutr.* 1981;5(6):519-521.
90. Burden ST, Stoppard E, Shaffer J, Makin A, Todd C. Can we use mid upper arm anthropmetry to detect malnutrition in medical inpatients? A validation study. *J Hum Nutr Diet.* 2005;18(4):287-294.
91. Zuchinali P, Souza GC, Alves FD, et al. Triceps skinfold as a prognostic predictor in outpatient heart failure. *Arq Bras Cardiol.* 2013;101(5):434-441.
92. University of Colorado Denver. Waist circumference measurements in clinical research. http://www.ucdenver.edu/research/CCTSI/programs-services/ctrc/Nutrition/Documents/Waist%20Circumference%20Info%20for%20Web.pdf. Accessed March 14, 2017.
93. Jeyakumar A, Ghugre P, Gadhave S. Mid-upper-arm circumference (MUAC) as a simple measure to assess the nutritional status of adolescent girls as compared with BMI. *ICAN: Infant Child Adol Nutr.* 2013;5(1):22-25.
94. Cattermole GN, Graham CA, Rainer TH. Mid-arm circumference can be used to estimate weight of adult and adolescent patients. *Emerg Med J.* 2016;0:1-6.
95. Sultana T, Karim N, Ahmed T, Hossain I. Assessment of under nutrition of Bangladeshi adults using anthropometry: can body mass index be replaced by mid-upper-arm-circumference? *PLoS One.* 2015;10(4):1-8.
96. Powell NJ, Collier B. Nutrition and the open abdomen. *Nutr Clin Pract.* 2012;27(4):499-506.
97. Mei Z, Grummer-Strawn LM, de Onis M, Yip R. The development of a MUAC-for-height reference, including a comparison to other nutritional status screening indicators. *Bull World Health Organ.* 1997;75(4):333-341.
98. Powell-Tuck J, Hennessy EM. A comparison of mid upper arm circumference, body mass index and weight loss as indices of undernutrition in acutely hospitalized patients. *Clin Nutr.* 2003;22(3):307-312.
99. Tang AM, Dong K, Deitchler M, et al. Use of cutoffs for mid-upper arm circumference (MUAC) as indicator or predictor of nutritional and health-related outcomes in adolescents and adults: a systematic review. *Food and Nutrition Technical Assistance III Project (FANTA).* 2013;FHI 360/FANTA.
100. Hymers R. The use of mid upper arm circumference in the nutritional assessment of the critically ill patient. Scottish Intensive Care Society Web site. Scottish Intensive Care Society. http://www.scottishintensivecare.org.uk/uploads/2014-05-28-23-52-56-TheuseofMidUpperArmCircum-59986.pdf. Updated 2009. Accessed March 10, 2017.
101. Tartari RF, Ulbrich-Kulczynski JM, Filho AF. Measurement of mid-arm muscle circumference and prognosis in stage IV non-small cell lung cancer patients. *Oncol Lett.* 2013;5(3):1063-1067.
102. Wang J, Thornton JC, Bari S, et al. Comparisons of waist circumferences measured at 4 sites. *Am J Clin Nutr.* 2003;77(2):379-384.
103. de Koning L, Merchant AT, Pogue J, Anand SS. Waist circumference and waist-to-hip ratio as predictors of cardiovascular events: meta-regression analysis of prospective studies. *Eur Heart J.* 2007;28(7):850-856.
104. Janssen I, Katzmarzyk PT, Ross R. Waist circumference and not body mass index explains obesity-related health risk. *Am J Clin Nutr.* 2004;79(3):379-384.
105. Vazquez G, Duval S, Jacobs Jr. DR, Silventoinen K. Comparison of body mass index, waist circumference, and waist/hip ratio in predicting incident diabetes: a meta-analysis. *Epidemiol Rev.* 2007;29:115-128.
106. Ma W, Yang C, Shih S, et al. Measurement of waist circumference: midabdominal or iliac crest? *Diabetes Care.* 2013;36(6):1660-1666.
107. Mason C, Katzmarzyk PT. Variability in waist circumference measurements according to anatomic measurement site. *Obesity (Silver Spring).* 2009;17(9):1789-1795.
108. World Health Organization Expert Consultation. Waist circumference and waist-hip ratio. *Report of a WHO Expert Consultation.* http://www.who.int/nutrition/publications/obesity/WHO_report_waistcircumference_and_waisthip_ratio/en/ December,2008. Accessed October 29, 2017.
109. National Institutes of Health (NIH). According to waist circumference. Guidelines on Overweight and Obesity: Electronic Textbook Web site. https://www.nhlbi.nih.gov/health-pro/guidelines/current/obesity-guidelines/e_textbook/txgd/4142.htm Accessed March 14, 2017.
110. Cerhan JR, Moore SC, Jacobs EJ, et al. A pooled analysis of waist circumference and mortality in 650,000 adults. *Mayo Clin Proc.* 2014;89(3):335-345.
111. Britton KA, Massaro JM, Murabito JM, Kreger BE, Hoffmann U, Fox CS. Body fat distribution, incident cardiovascular disease, cancer, and all-cause mortality. *J Am Coll Cardiol.* 2013;62(10):921-925.
112. Price GM, Uauy R, Breeze E, Bulpitt CJ, Fletcher AE. Weight, shape, and mortality risk in older persons: Elevated waist-hip ratio, not high body mass index, is associated with a greater risk of death. *Am J Clin Nutr.* 2006;84(2):449-460.

113. Lear SA, James PT, Ko GT, Kumanyika S. Appropriateness of waist circumference and waist-to-hip ratio cutoffs for different ethnic groups. *Eur J Clin Nutr.* 2010;64:42-61.

114. Silver HJ, Welch EB, Avison MJ, Niswender KD. Imaging body composition in obesity and weight loss: challenges and opportunities. *Diabetes Metab Syndr Obes.* 2010;3:337-347.

115. Andreoli A, Scalzo G, Masala S, Tarantino U, Guglielmi G. Body composition assessment by dual-energy X-ray absorptiometry (DXA). *Radiol Med.* 2009;114:286-300.

116. Ross R, Goodpaster B, Kelley D, Boada F. Magnetic resonance imaging in human body composition research from quantitative to qualitative tissue measurement. *Ann N Y Acad Sci.* 2000;904:12-17.

117. Lee Y, Kwon O, Shin CS, Lee SM. Use of bioelectrical impedance analysis for the assessment of nutritional status in critically ill patients. *Clin Nutr Res.* 2015;4(1):32-40.

118. Kyle UG, Boseaus I, De Lorenzo AD, et al. Bioelectrical impedance analysis - part I: Review of principles and methods. Clin Nutr. 2004;23(5):1225-1243.

119. Kyle UG, Boseaus I, De Lorenzo AD, et al. Bioelectrical impedance analysis - part II: Utilization in clinical practice. *Clin Nutr.* 2004;23(5):1430-1453.

120. Walter-Kroker A, Kroker A, Mattiucci-Guehlke M, Glaab T. A practical guide to bioeletrical impedance analysis using the example of chronic obstructive pulmonary disease. *Nutr J.* 2011;10(35):1-8.

121. Savalle M, Gillaizeau F, Maruani G, et al. Assessment of body cell mass at bedside in critically ill patients. *Am J Physiol Endocrinol Metab.* 2012;303:E389-E396.

122. Chahar PS. Comparison of skinfold thickness measurement and bioelectrical impedance method for assessment of body fat. *World Appl Sci J.* 2013;28(8):1065-1069.

123. Andreoli A, Garaci F, Cafarelli FP, Guglielmi G. Body composition in clinical practice. *Eur J Radiol.* 2016;85(8):1461-1468.

124. Litchford M. Putting the nutrition focused physical assessment into practice in long-term care settings. *Ann Longterm Care.* 2013;21(11):38-41.

125. Radler DR, Lister T. Nutrient deficiencies associated with nutrition-focused physical findings of the oral cavity. *Nutr Clin Pract.* 2013;28(6):710-721.

126. Mordarski B. Nutrition-focused physical exam hands-on training workshop. *J Acad Nutr Diet.* 2016;116(5):868-869.

127. Fischer M, JeVenn A, Hipskind P. Evaluation of muscle and fat loss as diagnostic criteria for malnutrition. *Nutr Clin Pract.* 2015;30(2):239-248.

128. Esper DH. Utilization of nutrition-focused physical assessment in identifying micronutrient deficiencies. *Nutr Clin Pract.* 2015;30(2):194-202.

129. Russell MK. Functional assessment of nutrition status. *Nutr Clin Pract.* 2015;30(2):211-218.

130. Norman K, Stobäus N, Gonzalez MC, Schulzke J, Pirlich M. Hand grip strength: outcome predictor and marker of nutritional status. *Clin Nutr.* 2011;30(2):135-142.

131. Bohannon RW. Muscle strength: Clinical and prognostic value of hand-grip dynamometry. *Curr Opin Clin Nutr Metab Care.* 2015;18(5):465-470.

132. Wang AY, Sea MM, Ho ZS, Lui S, Li PK, Woo J. Evaluation of handgrip strength as a nutritional marker and prognostic indicator in peritoneal dialysis patients. *Am J Clin Nutr.* 2005;81(1):79-86.

133. Hillman TE, Nunes QM, Hornby ST, et al. A practical posture for hand grip dynanometry in the clinical setting. *Clin Nutr.* 2005;24(2): 224-228.

134. Matos LC, Tavares MM, Amaral TF. Handgrip strength as a hospital admission nutritional risk screening method. *Eur J Clin Nutr.* 2007;61(9):1128-1135.

135. Jakobsen LH, Rask IK, Kondrup J. Validation of handgrip strength and endurance as a measure of physical function and quality of life in healthy subjects and patients. *Nutrition.* 2010;25(5): 542-550.

136. Tufts University Nutrition Collaborative, Center for Drug Abuse and AIDS Research. Hand grip strength protocol. http://cdaar.tufts.edu/protocols/Handgrip.pdf. Updated September 2003. Accessed October 29, 2017.

137. Mendes J, Azevedo A, Amaral TF. Handgrip strength at admission and time to discharge in medical and surgical inpatients. *JPEN J Parenter Enteral Nutr.* 2014;38(4):481-488.

138. Flood A, Chung A, Parker H, Kearns V, O'Sullivan TA. The use of hand grip strength as a predictor of nutrition status in hospital patients. *Clin Nutr.* 2014;33(1):106-114.

139. Garcia MF, Meireles MS, Führ LM, Donini AB, Wazlawik E. Relationship between hand grip strength and nutritional assessment methods used of hospitalized patients. *Rev Nutr.* 2013;26(1):49-57.

140. Norman K, Stobäus N, Smoliner C, et al. Determinants of hand grip strength, knee extension strength and functional status in cancer patients. *Clin Nutr.* 2010;29(5):586-591.

141. Luna-Heredia E, Martín-Peña G, Ruiz-Galiana J. Handgrip dynamometry in healthy adults. *Clin Nutr.* 2005;24:250-258.

142. Jonnalagadda SS, Mitchell DC, Smiciklas-Wright H, et al. Accuracy of energy intake data estimated by a multiple-pass, 24-hour dietary recall technique. *J Am Diet Assoc.* 2000;100(3):303-308.

143. Kubena KS. Accuracy in dietary assessment: on the road to good science. *J Am Diet Assoc.* 2000;100(7):775-776.

144. Timon CM, van den Barg R, Blain RJ, et al. A review of the design and validation of web- and computer-based 24-h dietary recall tools. *Nutr Res Rev.* 2016;29(2):260-280.

145. Kirkpatrick SI, Collins CE. Assessment of nutrient intakes: introduction to the special issue. *Nutrients.* 2016;8(4):184-187.

146. Subar AF, Freedman LS, Tooze JA, et al. Addressing current criticism regarding the value of self-report dietary data. *J Nutr.* 2015;145(12):2639-2645.

147. Moshfegh AJ, Rhodes DG, Baer DJ, et al. The US Department of Agriculture automated multiple-pass method reduces bias in the collection of energy intakes. *Am J Clin Nutr.* 2008;88(2):324-332.

148. Blanton CA, Moshfegh AJ, Baer DJ, Kretsch MJ. The USDA automated multiple-pass method accurately estiamtes group total energy and nutrient intake. *J Nutr.* 2006;136(10):2594-2599.

149. Conway JM, Ingwersen LA, Moshfegh AJ. Accuracy of dietary recall using the USDA five-step multiple-pass method in men: an observational validation study. *J Am Diet Assoc.* 2004;104(4):595-603.

150. Chambers EI, McGuire B, Godwin S, McDowell M, Vecchio F. Quantifying portion sizes for selected snack foods and beverages in 24-hour dietary recalls. *Nutrition Research.* 2000;20(3):315-326.

151. Subar AF. Developing dietary assessment tools. *J Am Diet Assoc.* 2004;104(5):769-770.

152. National Cancer Institute. Usual dietary intakes: The NCI method. Epidemiology and Genomics Research Program Web site. https://epi.grants.cancer.gov/diet/usualintakes/method.html Updated July 17, 2015. Accessed October 29, 2017.

153. Sharp DB, Allman-Farinelli M. Feasibility and validity of mobile phones to assess dietary intake. *Nutrition.* 2014;30(11-12):1257-1266.

154. Bloomfield R, Steel E, MacLennan G, Noble DW. Accuracy of weight and height estimation in an intensive care unit: implications for clinical practice and research. *Crit Care Med.* 2006;34(8):2153-2157.

155. Heyland DK, Dhaliwal R, Jiang X, Day AG. Identifying critically ill patients who benefit the most from nutrition therapy: the

development and initial validation of a novel risk assessment tool. *Crit Care*. 2011;15(6):R268.

156. Rosa M, Heyland DK, Fernandes D, Rabito EL, Oliveira ML, Marcadenti A. Translation and adaptation of the NUTRIC score to identify critically ill patients who benefit the most from nutrition therapy. *Clin Nutr ESPEN*. 2016;14:31-36.
157. Kalaiselvan MS, Renuka MK, Arunkumar AS. Use of nutrition risk in critically ill (NUTRIC) score to assess nutritional risk in mechanically ventilated patients: a prospective observational study. *Indian J Crit Care Med*. 2017;21(5):253-256.
158. Rahman A, Hasan RM, Agarwala R, Martin C, Day AG, Heyland DK. Identifying critically-ill patients who will benefit most from nutritional therapy: further validation of the "modified NUTRIC" nutritional risk assessment tool. *Clin Nutr*. 2016;35(1):158-162.

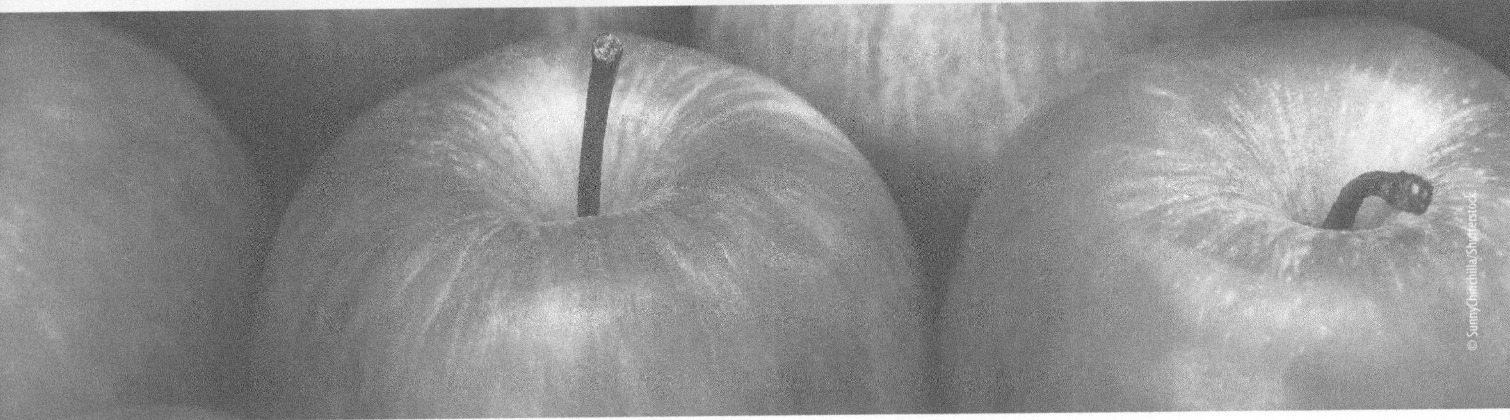

Clinical Assessment of Nutritional Status

Phyllis Famularo, DCN, RD, CSG, LDN, FAND

CHAPTER OUTLINE

- Introduction
- Nutritional Assessment
- Client History
- Food- and Nutrition-Related History
- Nutrition-Focused Physical Examination
- Malnutrition
- Estimating Energy Requirements
- Estimating Protein Requirements
- Estimating Fluid Requirements
- Nutritional Assessment and Management of Eating Disorders
- Nutritional Assessment and Management of the HIV Patient
- Mini Nutritional Assessment (MNA)
- Malnutrition Universal Screening Tool (MUST)
- Subjective Global Assessment (SGA)
- Chapter Summary

LEARNING OBJECTIVES

After reading this chapter, the learner will be able to:

1. Understand the components of a complete nutritional assessment.
2. Explain how the nutritional status assessment will vary based on the care setting, including acute care, long-term care, rehabilitation setting or community-dwelling patient or client.
3. Express the rationale for obtaining a client history when completing a nutritional assessment.
4. Identify and discuss the information collected in a client history.
5. Define the limitations of completing a food- and nutrition-related history.
6. Indicate how the findings from the nutrition-focused physical exam are used to define the nutritional status of the client.
7. Explain the differences between starvation-related malnutrition, chronic disease-related malnutrition, and acute disease- or injury-related malnutrition.
8. Determine energy requirements for healthy and unhealthy clients.
9. Describe the methods used for estimating protein requirements.
10. Calculate fluid needs for individuals as part of the nutrition-assessment process.
11. Create an awareness of the psychological and behavioral characteristics of an individual with eating disorders.
12. Discuss the impact of HIV on nutrition status.
13. Understand the process for completing the MNA, the MUST, and the SGA.

Introduction

A complete and thorough nutritional assessment is critical in determining the most appropriate nutritional plan of care for a patient, resident, or client. A nutritional assessment should have multiple components, including a **client history**, a food- and nutrition-related history, medication regimen, anthropometrics, laboratory and related medical tests, and nutrition-focused physical findings. The last component should include oral status and psychosocial aspects that can affect nutritional status. By using all of the available data, the clinician will be able to recommend and implement nutritional interventions that will lead to improved nutritional status or disease management. In addition to reviewing the components of a nutritional assessment, this chapter gives special consideration to the process for conducting a nutrition-focused physical examination and evaluating individuals for **malnutrition**. The chapter also presents information on the nutritional aspects and management of diseases such as human immunodeficiency virus and eating disorders, as well as the use of validated nutrition-screening and assessment tools.

Nutritional Assessment

Preview Adequate nutritional intake is essential to maintaining health, functional status, and overall quality of life. The burden of chronic disease can be ameliorated by consuming an appropriate combination of essential nutrients that incorporate a combination of carbohydrates, protein, fat, fluids, and micronutrients, including vitamins and minerals.

Nutritional status can be defined as "the health status of individuals or population groups as influenced by their intake and utilization of nutrients."[1] An individual's nutritional status can be determined by evaluating diet patterns and quality, the process of food and fluid intake, digestion, nutrient absorption, metabolism, and the excretion of waste products. Any factors that affect the intake and use of nutrients can affect nutritional status and health.

To determine if nutritional intake is meeting the individual's needs, a nutritional assessment should be completed. Differences in healthcare settings and target populations guides the process used to complete such an assessment. Its findings, however, will help define a nutrition prescription that will address the individual's nutritional needs and help promote maintenance or improvement of his or her nutritional status.

Nutrition Screening

Although a full nutritional assessment is the approach of choice in determining nutritional status, **nutrition screening** is the first-line process of identifying patients, clients, or groups that are at nutritional risk and will benefit from nutrition assessment and intervention by a nutrition professional.[2] Because of the limited nutrition resources in the community setting, a nutrition screen may be an acceptable approach for recognizing individuals at nutritional risk. In addition, the large number of admissions to acute-care facilities makes a nutritional screen highly recommended within the first 24 hours of admission so that nutritional risk can be identified and treatment implemented.[3] In the long-term care setting as well as rehabilitation centers that accept Medicare and Medicaid funds, a full nutrition assessment is required for all admissions as described in the regulations set forth by the Centers for Medicare and Medicaid (CMS).[4]

Many validated nutrition-screening tools have been developed and are available for members of the interprofessional team to use. The Academy of Nutrition and Dietetics (the Academy) has completed an evidence analysis to help define the sensitivity, specificity, and reliability of some of the available screens in identifying nutrition risks for different patient populations.[5] Sensitivity, specificity, and reliability can be defined as follows[6]:

- *Sensitivity.* How effective is the screening tool in detecting a disease or condition? The higher the sensitivity of a nutrition-screening tool, the fewer cases of nutrition risk that will go undetected.
- *Specificity.* How often does the screening tool give negative results in those who are free of the disease or condition? The higher the specificity of a nutrition-screening tool, the fewer well-nourished persons who are incorrectly labeled as at nutritional risk, and the fewer resources that are wasted on those who need no intervention.
- *Reliability.* Are results obtained by different investigators consistent when repeated with the same subjects?

A screening tool should be easy to administer and score, transferable from one care setting to another, effective in identifying the need for nutrition-assessment completion, and cost-effective. The use of screening tools facilitates early intervention for those at nutritional risk and includes relevant data on risk factors and the interpretation of data for intervention or treatment.[7] The **Mini Nutritional Assessment (MNA)** and the **Malnutrition Universal Screening Tool (MUST)** are two examples of validated instruments used to determine nutritional risk. These tools are discussed in detail later in this chapter.

Nutritional Assessment Purpose

The purpose of a nutritional assessment is to acquire, validate, and interpret data needed to identify nutrition-related problems, their root causes, and their relevance to overall health status. A **nutritional assessment** has been defined by the American Society of Enteral and Parenteral Nutrition (ASPEN) as "a comprehensive approach to diagnosing nutrition problems that uses a combination of the following: medical, nutrition, and medication histories; physical examination; anthropometric measurements; and laboratory data."[8] After completing the assessment, the nutrition professional identifies nutritional problems and develops a plan of care with specific interventions to maintain or improve nutritional outcomes. To facilitate nutrition care across health care settings, the Academy has developed the International Dietetics and Nutrition Terminology (IDNT), a standardized language for nutrition professionals. Using this language and evidence-based practice, registered dietitian nutritionists (RDNs) provide medical nutrition therapy (MNT) using nutrition assessment, nutrition diagnoses, interventions, and monitoring and evaluation standards across the continuum of health care.[9]

Components of Nutritional Assessment

Data collection for a nutritional assessment includes securing anthropometric and biochemical data; clinical assessment information, including client history, medical history, signs and symptoms, and medication use; and food and diet history. The mnemonic ABCD can be used to remember the four main components of the nutritional assessment:

A—Anthropometric
B—Biochemical
C—Clinical assessment
D—Dietary or food- and nutrition-related history

Anthropometry

Anthropometry is the study of the measurement of the human body in terms of the dimensions of bone, muscle, and adipose (fat) tissue. This includes the measurement of weight, height, weight changes, and body composition, including **body mass index (BMI)**, which is used to determine how the patient compares to reference standards. Results can indicate normal, undernutrition or malnutrition, or overnutrition (overweight and obese). Anthropometric measurements can be used to compare an individual to assess and monitor his or her nutritional status against standards for a population and relevant health studies. The anthropometric measurements most commonly used are height and weight, various circumference measurements, and skinfold thickness. More complex methods include bioelectrical impedance, dual-energy x-ray absorptiometry (DXA), body density, and total body water estimates that are not readily available in clinical settings.[10]

Weight Measurement

Body weight is one of the easiest and most routinely collected anthropometric measures. Weight is used to monitor the patient's or individual's nutritional status and is and is a rough estimate of energy stores.[11] Weight does not, however, provide information on actual body composition.[12] Because weight can be easily and non-invasively measured, it remains an important measurement in assessing nutritional status and determining energy requirements. Accurate weight measures are critical for the initial nutritional evaluation and subsequent assessments of the patient or individual. In addition, accurate weights are necessary to accurately dose chemotherapeutic agents, anesthetics, and other medications. A variety of conditions may make many patients unable to stand on a regular bathroom or upright beam scale. Also available are a variety of scales that allow an individual to stay seated or facilitates the weight to be obtained while the individual is in bed. Proper technique must be used because dangling limbs and improper zeroing can lead to wide fluctuations in weight measurements. It is important to weigh the patient in the same type of clothing, at the same time of the day, before eating and after voiding.[11] It is recommended that a patient who receives diuretic therapy or has varying edema be weighed in the morning shortly after rising; however, this may be not be possible for some patients or individuals, depending on the care setting. A scale-calibration schedule is critical, as is a battery-charging schedule for digital scales. Frequent training of staff that completes weight measurements is also essential.[13] Research conducted in acute-and long-term care settings has found that recorded weights can be inaccurate, and sometimes weights are not obtained at all.

Body weight measurements can be compared to reference standards published by the National

Center for Health Statistics, which provides data for infants, children, and adults using information from the National Health and Nutrition Examination Survey (NHANES).[14] Weight measurement data are divided into three-month increments for infants, one-year increments for children up to age 19 years, and 10-year increments for adults 20 years of age and older. It provides fifth percentile through 95th percentile data for weights of any given height. The final age grouping for adults is 80 years and older. Although these weight reference tables do not provide "ideal" weights for health, they represent the weight statuses of children and adults living in the United States today.

Weight Changes

Evaluation of weight changes is an important component when completing a nutrition assessment. Changes in weight, both losses and gains, have been shown to be predictive of negative health outcomes in adults. In a study of older adults, weight loss and weight cycling (alternating weight gain and weight loss) were noted to significantly affect mobility and mortality when compared to those with stable weights or weight gains.[15] Weight gain has also been identified as an indicator of mortality in the intensive care unit (ICU) or in patients with heart failure.[16,17] When assessing individuals with weight loss, the weight loss must be evaluated within the framework in which it occurred, such as in the context of acute illness or injury, chronic illness, and social or environmental circumstances. In acute illness or injury, a weight loss of more than 2% in one week, 5% in one month, and 7.5% in three months is considered severe. Weight loss is severe in chronic disease (organ failure, cancer, rheumatoid arthritis, etc.) and in the context of social or environmental circumstances (anorexia or starvation) if weight loss is more than 5% in one month, 7.5% in three months, 10% in 6 months, and 20% in one year. In long-term care communities (nursing homes) regulated by the CMS, significant weight loss is defined at 5% or more in one month and 10% or more in six months.

Because of the potential for poor outcomes in patients who have significant weight changes, weights should be taken at admission and monitored at routine intervals based on the clinical setting so that timely nutritional interventions can be put into place. When weight does change, it is important to investigate its root cause and determine the appropriate interventions.[18] For example, if a nursing home resident seems to have difficulty chewing and has experienced weight loss, then the appropriate intervention would be to provide softer foods and refer for a dental consult rather than provide a nutritional supplement between meals. The supplement may improve the caloric intake, but it will not address the chewing problem. For a patient with weight loss and difficulty chewing in an acute-care setting, a softer diet consistency and an oral nutritional supplement may be the appropriate intervention because of the significantly shorter length of stay. Quickly improving the patient's intake and weight status may help prevent readmission to the hospital.

Height Measurement

An accurate measurement of height is needed because many of the indicators of appropriate body weight require an individual's height.[11] Although the easiest method of obtaining height is a standing-height measurement using a stadiometer (standing scale), this may not always be feasible or accurate because of illness, kyphosis, and limited mobility. Several predictive methods can be used when an individual is unable to stand for a height measurement, and four methods have been reported for measuring height when an individual cannot be measured on a stadiometer: arm span (or a variation called *demispan*), knee height, forearm length (or ulnar length), and segmental measurement.

- *Arm span.* Arm span is correlated with height in both men and women (±10%).[19] This can be accomplished by having the patient extend both arms at the level of the shoulder with the back pressed against a flat surface for maximum accuracy. The measurement is taken from the longest fingertip on one hand to the longest fingertip on the other hand.[20] In the demispan, the distance is measured from the sternal notch to the tip of the longest fingertip and doubled to estimate stature. The demispan can be used for patients who cannot easily extend both arms, such as those who are contracted or have hemiplegia on one side of the body.[21]
- *Knee height.* While the patient is supine, both the knee and the ankle are held at 90-degree angles. One blade of a sliding broad-blade caliper is placed under the heel of the foot, and the other blade is placed on the anterior surface of the thigh. The shaft of the caliper is held parallel to the long axis of the lower leg, and pressure is applied to compress the tissue. Height (in cm) is then calculated as follows[21]:

  Females: Height in cm = 84.88 − (0.24 × age) + (1.83 × knee height)

HEIGHT (m)	Men (<65 years)	1.94	1.93	1.91	1.89	1.87	1.85	1.84	1.82	1.80	1.78	1.76	1.75	1.73	1.71
	Men (>65 years)	1.87	1.86	1.84	1.82	1.81	1.79	1.78	1.76	1.75	1.73	1.71	1.70	1.68	1.67
	Ulna length (cm)	32.0	31.5	31.0	30.5	30.0	29.5	29.0	28.5	28.0	27.5	27.0	26.5	26.0	25.5
HEIGHT (m)	Women (<65 years)	1.84	1.83	1.81	1.80	1.79	1.77	1.76	1.75	1.73	1.72	1.70	1.69	1.68	1.66
	Women (>65 years)	1.84	1.83	1.81	1.79	1.78	1.76	1.75	1.73	1.71	1.70	1.68	1.66	1.65	1.63

HEIGHT (m)	Men (<65 years)	1.69	1.67	1.66	1.64	1.62	1.60	1.58	1.57	1.55	1.53	1.51	1.49	1.48	1.46
	Men (>65 years)	1.65	1.63	1.62	1.60	1.59	1.57	1.56	1.54	1.52	1.51	1.49	1.48	1.46	1.45
	Ulna length (cm)	25.5	24.5	24.0	23.5	23.0	22.5	22.0	21.5	21.0	20.5	20.0	19.5	19.0	18.5
HEIGHT (m)	Women (<65 years)	1.65	1.63	1.62	1.61	1.59	1.58	1.56	1.55	1.54	1.52	1.51	1.50	1.48	1.47
	Women (>65 years)	1.61	1.60	1.58	1.56	1.55	1.53	1.52	1.50	1.48	1.47	1.45	1.44	1.42	1.40

FIGURE 1 Estimating height from ulna length.

Reproduced from Estimating height in bedridden patients. RxKinetics. http://www.rxkinetics.com/height_estimate.html. Date unknown. Accessed January 7, 2017.

Males: Height in cm = 64.19 – (0.04 × age) + (2.02 × knee height)

- *Forearm or ulnar length.* This method can also be used in patients who have osteoporosis, kyphosis, or arthritis. Forearm length can be measured from the tip of the acromial process of the scapula to the end of the styloid process of the ulna. Ulnar length must be converted to height (**FIGURE 1**).[22] A study using this method reported that although height decreases with age, arm measurements do not change to the same degree.[23]
- *Segmental measurement.* This method can be used for individuals who have severe neuromuscular deformities, as in cerebral palsy. Segment lengths should be measured between specific bony landmarks and as vertical distances between a flat surface and a bony landmark (heel to knee, knee to hip, hip to shoulder, and shoulder to top of head). The sectional measurements are then totaled to determine stature. Segments should not be measured from joint creases. This method has potential for error and there is only fair to poor agreement with actual height.[24]

Body Composition

Body Mass Index

Once accurate weight and height measurements have been obtained, BMI, a weight-to-height ratio, is calculated by dividing weight in kilograms by the square of a patient's height in meters. The result indicates whether the patient is overweight, normoweight, or underweight. A limitation of this measurement is that BMI does not measure body fat directly. However, research has shown that BMI is moderately correlated with more-direct measures of body fat, including skinfold thickness and bioelectrical impedance.[25,26] See **TABLE 1** for BMI calculations. The Centers for Disease Control and Prevention (CDC) has issued the BMI recommendations for adult 20 years of age and older for both men and women. Individuals with BMIs of less than 18.5 are classified as underweight. Those with BMIs between 18.5 and 24.9 are considered normal or at normal or healthy weights. A BMI of 30 or above is considered obese. Individuals who have BMIs of 30 or higher are at increased risk for developing diseases and health conditions such as:[27,28]

- All causes of death (increased mortality)
- Hypertension
- Dyslipidemia
- Type 2 diabetes
- Coronary heart disease
- Cardiovascular accident
- Gallbladder disease
- Osteoarthritis
- Sleep apnea and breathing problems
- Chronic inflammation and increased oxidative stress
- Some cancers (endometrial, breast, colon, kidney, gallbladder, and liver)
- Low quality of life
- Mental illness such as clinical depression, anxiety, and other mental disorders; and
- Body pain and difficulty with physical functioning

The prevalence of obesity in the United States was identified as 36.5% in 2011–2014. More than one-third of all adults in the United States have a BMI of 30 or greater. Although the rate of obesity has been increasing since the 1970s, this trend has leveled off

TABLE 1 Calculation of body mass index (BMI)

Measurement Units	Formula and Calculation
Kilograms and meters (or centimeters)	Formula: weight (kg) ÷ [height (m)]^2 With the metric system, the formula for BMI is weight in kilograms divided by height in meters squared. Because height is commonly measured in centimeters, divide height in centimeters by 100 to obtain height in meters. Example: Weight = 68 kg; height = 165 cm (1.65 m) Calculation: $68 \div (1.65)^2 = 24.98$
Pounds and inches	Formula: weight (lb) ÷ [height (in)]^2 × 703 Calculate BMI by dividing weight in pounds (lbs) by height in inches (in) squared and multiplying by a conversion factor of 703. Example: Weight = 150 lbs; height = 5'5" (65") Calculation: $[150 \div (65)^2] \times 703 = 24.96$

Modified from Centers for Disease Control and Prevention (CDC). Available at: https://www.cdc.gov/healthyweight/assessing/bmi/adult_bmi/index.html. Accessed January 19, 2017.

for all groups except women greater than 60 years of age.[29]

In recent years, BMI has been questioned as a significant factor in determining the nutrition status and mortality risk for older adults. The Nutrition Screening Initiative included the use of BMI and states that elderly persons with a BMI of more than 27 or less than 24 may be at increased risk for poor nutritional status. A meta-analysis of eight studies that included 370,416 subjects indicated that a BMI less than 22 was associated with a higher mortality risk in those ages 65 years and older. At higher ranges of BMI, mortality increased for younger adults at a BMI of 28.0 to 28.9, but did not tend to significantly increase in older adults.[30]

Skinfold and Circumference Measurements

BMI does not provide specific information about body composition, but skinfold and circumference measurements can be used to evaluate the actual composition of lean muscle tissue and adipose tissue. A nutritional assessment should include skinfold and circumference measurements, especially if malnutrition is suspected.

Skinfold Measures

These measurements are relatively easy to measure and noninvasive. Unlike body weight, they are also less affected by hydration status. Skinfold measurements generally correlate with more-complex body-composition measurements, including air-displacement plethysmography (ADP) and bioelectrical impedance (BIA).[31] Measurements are made using a skinfold caliper at the following body sites: triceps, biceps, subscapular, and suprailiac. Using the same side of the body for both skinfold and circumference measurements for an individual is recommended. Standardized methods have been developed to measure skinfold at each body site with trained clinicians conducting the measurements. For example, the triceps skinfold (TSF) is measured at a point midway between the lateral projection of the acromial process of the scapula and the inferior margin of the olecranon. With the individual's elbow flexed to 90 degrees, the midway point is determined using a tape measure on the posterior of the arm and then marked. If possible, the person should be standing; otherwise, he or she should be sitting upright in a chair. For the measurement, the skinfold is measured with the arm hanging loosely at the side. The triceps skinfold is picked up with the left thumb and index finger, approximately 1 cm from the marked location on the triceps. The skinfold is held for the duration of the measurement.[32] Standardized equations have been developed to predict body fat and calculate fat-free mass (FFM) using one or more skinfold measurements.[33] Skinfold measurements are thought to be comparable to more sophisticated techniques to assess for body fat, but recommendations also suggest that equations may need to be modified to address body-composition differences in obese subjects and various ethnic groups.[34]

Arm Circumference

Circumference measurements can be used alone or in combination with skinfold measurements or other circumferences to help evaluate nutritional status. The only tool required to measure arm circumference is a flexible tape measure in either metric or imperial measure. (If imperial measure is used, it will need to be converted to metric.) The mid–upper arm-circumference (MUAC) is measured at the same location used for the triceps skinfold. The measurement is taken with the elbow extended and the arm relaxed to the side of the body, with the palm facing the thigh.[11] MUAC data are available from the NHANES 2003–2006 for both adults and children by both age and gender in the United States and is expressed as means and percentiles. These data are collected to add to the knowledge about trends in child growth and development and trends in the distribution of body measurements in the American population.[35] The MUAC and the triceps skinfold measurements can be used to calculate the arm-muscle circumference (AMC) and the arm-muscle area (AMA), both of which estimate the amount of muscle or lean body mass (LBM) in the body. The following equation is used to calculate AMC and AMA and have been used to develop reference standards:

$$\text{AMC (cm)} = \text{MUAC (cm)} - [3.14 \times \text{TSF (mm)}]$$
$$\text{AMA (cm}^2) = \text{AMC}^2 \div 12.56$$

Calf Circumference

This circumference measurement is also monitored by the NHANES studies. The World Health Organization has recommended that calf circumference (CC) be used as a measure of nutritional status in older adults and is included as one of the anthropometric measurements used in the Mini Nutritional Status Assessment.[36,37] A study of 170 hospitalized older adult patients found a positive correlation between CC and BMI, AMC, TSF, MUAC, and AMA.[38] To measure CC, the subject should be sitting with the left leg hanging loosely or standing with his or her weight evenly distributed on both feet. Next, wrap the measuring tape around the calf at the widest part and note the measurement nearest to 0.1 cm. Take additional measurements above and below the point to ensure that the first measurement was the largest. For bed-bound patients, an alternate procedure is specified.[39] The person lies in a supine position with the left knee bent at a 90-degree angle. A CC of less than 31 cm is considered a risk factor for malnutrition. As with other circumference measurements, CC can be used alone or in combination with skinfold measurements to aid in evaluating nutritional status.

Waist Circumference and Waist-to-Hip Ratio

Although waist circumference and BMI are interrelated, waist circumference provides an independent risk predictor beyond BMI measurements. Waist circumference is particularly meaningful in individuals who are categorized as normal or overweight by BMI standards. At BMIs equal to or more than 35, waist circumference has little additional predictive power of disease risk beyond that of BMI, so it is not necessary to measure waist circumference in individuals with BMIs 35 and above. The waist circumference at which there is high risk of disease, including cardiovascular disease, type 2 diabetes, dyslipidemia, and hypertension, are as follows: men > 102 cm (> 40 inches) and women > 88 cm (> 35 inches).[40] Monitoring waist circumference over time, along with BMI, can provide an estimate of increased abdominal fat even without a change in BMI. In some ethnic groups, including Asian Americans, waist circumference is a better predictor of disease risk than BMI.[41] Waist circumference can be measured as follows with a flexible tape measure. Start at the top of the hip bone and bring the tape measure all the way around, level with the belly button. Ensure that the tape is straight around the waist and not tight. The breath should not be held while being measured. Waist-to-hip ratio (WTH) is also predictive of disease risk and is determined by measuring the waist and hip circumferences and then dividing the waist circumference by the hip circumference. For men, normal risk is a ratio of 0.90 or less; for women, 0.8 or less. For both men and women, a WTH ratio above 1.0 is considered at risk for cardiovascular and other chronic diseases. Studies show that waist circumference is more predictive of cardiovascular disease risk while others have reported that WTH ratio is a more sensitive indicator of disease risk.[42,43] Both measurements have been found to be predictive of cardiovascular events.[44] **TABLE 2** shows how disease risk is associated with overweight and underweight statuses.

Other Methods of Assessing Body Composition

More advanced techniques for measuring body composition are available. However, the equipment to complete the measurement, the time involved, and the requisite clinician training are factors that may limit the use of these techniques. These additional body-composition methods are used mainly in research studies and for specific conditions that require information regarding body composition.

Bioelectrical Impedance Analysis

BIA is a relatively quick, simple, and noninvasive method to measure body composition (lean body

TABLE 2 Overweight and obesity by BMI, waist circumference, and associated disease risk				
			Disease Risk* Relative to Normal Weight and Waist Circumference	
	BMI (kg/m²)	Obesity Class	Men ≤102 cm (≤40 in) Women ≤88 cm (≤35 in)	Men >102 cm (>40 in); Women >88 cm (>35 in)
Underweight	18.5	NA	Average	Average
Normal+	18.5–24.9	NA	Average	Average
Overweight	25.0–29.9	NA	Increased	High
Obesity	30.0–34.9 35.0–39.9	I II	High Very high	Very high Very high
Extreme Obesity	≥ 40	III	Extremely high	Extremely high

*Disease risk for type 2 diabetes, hypertension, and CVD.
+Increased waist circumference can also be a marker for increased risk even in persons of normal weight.

Adapted from Clinical guidelines on the identification, evaluation, and treatment of overweight and obesity in adults: the evidence report. National Heart Lung and Blood Institute in cooperation with The National Institute of Diabetes and Digestive and Kidney Diseases. NIH Publication No. 98-4083. September, 1998.

mass and fat mass). The technique determines body composition by measuring electrical conductivity under the premise that electric current flows at different rates through the body, depending on its composition. The body is composed mostly of water and ions by which electrical current can flow. Alternately, the body contains nonconducting materials (body fat) that provides resistance to the flow of electrical current. The principal of BIA is that electric current passes through the body at a differential rate, depending on body composition. Impedance is a drop in voltage when a small constant current with a fixed frequency passes between electrodes spanning the body. The procedure is as follows: Electrodes are placed on the hands and feet while an electrical current is passed through the body. Adequate hydration is necessary to ensure proper estimation of fat-free mass. Based on the measurements, predictive equations are used to measure total body water, FFM, and body cell mass (BCM) using gender, age, weight, height, and race. It has been suggested that alternative BIA equations be developed for diverse populations.[45]

Dual-Energy X-Ray Absorptiometry

DXA is used to measure body composition as well as bone-mineral density to assess the risk of osteoporosis. In 2008, the Center for Health Statistics released DXA data from an NHANES population-based sample using modern fan beam scanners. Reference values were provided for individuals from eight to 85 years old and separated for gender and ethnicity. The following data were provided: percent fat, fat mass/height^2, lean mass/height^2, appendicular lean mass/height^2, bone-mineral content, and bone-mineral density.[46] DXA tests are performed by a licensed radiologic technologist and involve passing two low-dose x-ray beams through the body that differentiate among fat-free tissue, fat tissue, and bone. The results provide a precise measurement of total body fat and its distribution. DXA is used to determine long-term alterations in body composition with aging and short-term changes as a result of interventions to modify body fat or LBM.[47,48]

Air-Displacement Plethysmography

Underwater weighing (or hydrostatic weighing) is considered the gold standard for obtaining body composition. A BOD POD is an ADP that uses whole-body densitometry to determine body composition (fat vs. lean body mass). Similar in principle to underwater weighing (air is used rather than water), the BOD POD measures body mass (weight) using a precise scale; volume is determined when a patient sits inside the BOD POD. Body density can then be calculated as mass/volume. Once the overall density of the body is determined, the relative proportions of body fat and lean body mass are calculated.[49] Results obtained using ADP (BOD POD) are similar to the underwater

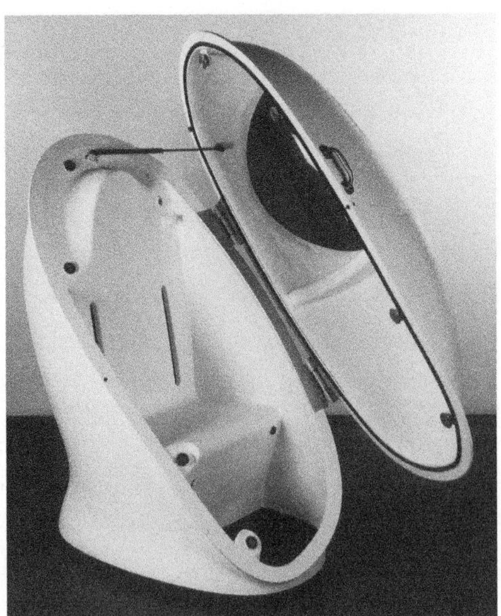

FIGURE 2 BOD POD (air-displacement plethysmography).

Courtesy of COSMED USA, Inc.

weighing technique.[50] The benefit of ADP is that it can be used throughout the life cycle from infants to adults, with excellent accuracy.[51] See **FIGURE 2**.

Biochemical Measures/Laboratory Data

In additional to anthropometric data, biochemical measures or laboratory data are necessary to complete a thorough nutritional assessment. Changes in biochemical data can be used to determine if nutrition interventions are effective, including adequacy of hydration, control of diabetes, and measures of nutritional adequacy or deficiency of specific micronutrients. Biochemical changes may be seen well before clinical signs of a nutrient deficiency occur. The nutrition professional should review the following laboratory tests: complete blood count (CBC); chemistry panel that includes electrolytes—sodium and potassium; glucose; blood urea nitrogen (BUN); creatinine; total protein; albumin; and blood lipids, including total cholesterol [high-density lipoproteins (HDLs) and low-density lipoproteins (LDLs) and triglycerides. Additional tests that may be useful to review are glycosylated hemoglobin (HbA1C); urinalysis; specific nutrient levels, including vitamin B_{12}; and iron, ferritin (storage iron), and folate.

Protein Status

Albumin and prealbumin (transthyretin) have been determined to be poor indicators of protein status, and low serum levels reflect inflammation in the body rather than inadequate protein status.[52,53] Although the clinician will take note that albumin or prealbumin levels are low as a sign of potential inflammation, conducting a **nutrition-focused physical examination (NFPE)** can provide a better indication of protein status.

Nutritional Anemias

The results obtained by a CBC exam are evaluated to determine the presence of anemia. There are many different forms of anemia. The manifestation of low hemoglobin (Hgb) and hematocrit and a high or low mean corpuscular volume (MCV) may indicate the presence of a nutritional anemia. The healthcare provider may determine that additional laboratory tests are required to determine if the anemia could be nutritional in nature. Laboratory results such as serum iron (Fe), total iron-binding capacity, and serum ferritin may be indicated to rule out iron-deficiency anemia in the presence of low MCV (small or microcytic red blood cells). Serum vitamin B_{12} and folate levels may be necessary if the MCV level is high (indicative of large or macrocytic red blood cells). The CBC can also indicate the presence of infection if the white blood cell count is elevated, which can correlate with a low albumin level and the presence of infection or inflammation.[54] Globally, iron deficiency is the most common nutrient deficiency. The CBC may also indicate a low total lymphocyte count (TLC), but many other factors can cause TLC to be low; therefore, its usefulness as an assessment of immune function and nutritional status is not reliable.[55]

Electrolytes, Blood Urea Nitrogen, and Creatinine

The nutrition professional will need to review laboratory results for electrolytes, BUN, and creatinine to evaluate hydration status and kidney function. Elevated serum sodium (hypernatremia) may indicate dehydration, and a low sodium level (hyponatremia) can indicate overhydration or impairment in adrenal function. Abnormal sodium levels can also be the result of medication effects such as diuretics and some types of antidepressants. In some instances, fluid intake may need to be limited to increase serum sodium levels to normal.[56] Elevated BUN can be a sign of impaired kidney function as well as dehydration or excessive protein intake. An elevated creatinine is a sign of kidney dysfunction. The best marker of kidney function, however, is glomerular filtration rate (GFR), which uses serum creatinine, age, gender, and race to determine the presence and stage of kidney disease.[57] The GFR equation is as follows:

$$\text{eGFR} = 186 \times \text{serum creatinine}^{-1.154} \times \text{age}^{-0.203} \times [1.210 \text{ if black}] \times [0.742 \text{ if female}]$$

Laboratory Values for Diabetes Mellitus

The clinician should also review fasting blood glucose (FBG). Although FBG has limited value regarding diabetes management, elevated blood glucose may indicate the need to check the glycosylated (or glycated) hemoglobin level. HbA1C is a test that measures the long-term control of blood glucose. Excess glucose in the blood is bound to hemoglobin (Hgb), and because a red blood cell has a life of approximately 120 days, the HbA1C test can indicate the average blood glucose over the past three to four months.[58] The amount of glucose bound to Hgb is expressed as a percentage with levels as follows:

- 4.9–5.2%—Normal
- 5.3–5.4%—Intermediate
- 5.5–6.5%—Prediabetic
- ≥ 6.6%—Diabetes Mellitus

The estimated average glucose (eAG) is another way to interpret glycosylated hemoglobin results. **TABLE 3** provides a list of estimated average glucose results based on the data reported by the A1C. For instance, a patient with an A1C of 8% has an eAG of 183 mg/dL. This information can be useful for the patient because it helps translate A1C tests into numbers that would more closely represent daily glucometer readings.

TABLE 3 Estimated average glucose

HbA1C (%)	eAG (mg/dL)
5	97
6	126
7	154
8	183
9	212
10	240
11	269
12	198

The relationship between A1C and eAG is described by the formula $28.7 \times A1C - 46.7 = eAG$.

Data from Nathan DM, Kuenen J, Borg R, Zheng H, Schoenfeld D, Heine RJ. Translating the A1C Assay Into Estimated Average Glucose Values. *Diabetes Care.* 2008;31(8):1-6.

Blood Lipid Levels

Serum cholesterol, lipoprotein levels, and triglycerides should be reviewed. Elevated serum cholesterol and elevated LDL cholesterol levels are risk factors for cardiovascular disease. A total cholesterol above 240 mg/dL and an LDL cholesterol level greater than 160 mg/dL indicate high risk.[59] Low cholesterol levels can be a sign of malnutrition and be predictive of mortality in older adults—unless the patient is taking cholesterol-lowering medications.[60,61] Elevated serum triglycerides (TGs) can be caused by obesity, poorly controlled diabetes, hypothyroidism, kidney disease, or excessive alcohol consumption. As with elevated total and LDL cholesterol, high TGs can increase the risk of heart disease.

Recap After anthropometric and laboratory data have been collected and reviewed, the nutrition professional will need to obtain additional information on the individual's food- and nutrition-related history to complete the data-collection process.

▸ Client History

Preview The client history is an important component of a complete nutritional assessment as it provides information regarding acute and chronic medical conditions that can have an impact on nutrition status. Based on the IDNT reference manual, client history includes the following: personal history; medical, health, and family history; treatments and complementary or alternative medicine use; and social history.[9]

Personal History

Personal history information pertinent to nutrition assessment includes age; gender; race or ethnicity; language spoken and written; literacy factors such as a language barrier or low literacy; educational level; physical disability, including impaired vision, hearing, or other; and mobility. These data are important to the nutritional assessment as the delivery of nutrition care and nutrition education and counseling may be affected by these factors. To express personal data or history, nutrition-assessment documentation may begin with, "Patient/client is a 65-year-old Spanish female with new-onset type 2 diabetes. Client speaks and reads English, 8th grade education level."

Medical, Health, and Family History

Medical, health, and family history includes current and past medical diagnoses, conditions, and illnesses that can have an effect on nutritional status. The new or current diagnoses should be listed first, including the patient's or client's chief nutritional complaint, which includes indicators such as poor appetite, weight gain, difficulty swallowing, and unstable blood glucose. In addition to primary nutrition complaints, medical history should include body system diagnoses including cardiovascular, endocrine or metabolism, excretory, gastrointestinal, gynecological, hematological or oncological, immune system issues such as food allergies, integumentary (skin), musculoskeletal, neurological, psychological, and respiratory. Family medical history should also be assessed if pertinent to the primary nutrition complaint. For example, if the patient has new-onset type-2 diabetes, it would be important to know which family members have diabetes; this would also be relevant for patients with new diagnoses of hyperlipidemia and other conditions. An example of documentation related to medical and health history is: "Patient with a history of hypertension and elevated blood lipids. Patient reports that both parents were prescribed medication for hypertension and high cholesterol."

Treatments

Treatments include both medical and surgical. Among the medical treatments are chemotherapy, dialysis, mechanical ventilation or oxygen therapy, ostomies, or current therapies such as occupational therapy, physical therapy, and speech therapy. Surgical treatments include coronary artery bypass, gastric bypass (type), intestinal resection, joint or orthopedic surgery or replacement, limb amputation, organ transplant, and total gastrectomy. In addition, palliative or end-of-life care is also considered under a treatment. A nutrition-assessment documentation might read, "Patient receiving dialysis three times weekly for end-stage kidney disease and experiencing decreased appetite due to fatigue and uremia."[9]

Social History

Social history is important to gather because nonmedical factors can affect nutrition intake and the retention of nutrition education as well. Social indicators include socioeconomic factors, living or housing situations, domestic issues, social and medical support systems, geographic location of the home, occupation, religion, history of recent crisis, and daily stress level. For a patient receiving home care services, documentation of social history in the nutritional assessment may note, "Patient lives in own home alone and receives one meal per day from Meals on Wheels. Patient's family lives over 100 miles away and is only able to visit and purchase groceries every other week."

The client history can be obtained through the patient or client and by family interview, from the medical record, or by reference from the healthcare provider or other involved agency. The nutrition clinician will need to review the subjective data, the information the patient or family member shares, and objective data, or what the clinician detects based on the client medical history to form an assessment of the patient's overall nutritional status.[62]

The detail of the client history needed to form a complete nutrition assessment varies on the primary nutrition-related complaint. For example, if a patient reports constipation, then the nutrition clinician will need to be aware of the patient's usual bowel pattern or frequency because this varies significantly within the patient population.[63,64] Other important client history information necessary to evaluate the root cause and treatment of constipation would include concurrent disease state(s), the current medication regimen, supplement use, activity level, and previous medical conditions or surgeries.[65] Once the client history is obtained, food and fluid intake will be reviewed with the patient. This is covered in the next section.

Recap The collection of the individuals' food- and nutrition-related history is an important component for the completion of a nutrition assessment. The patient's unique history can assist the nutrition professional in implementing nutrition interventions that will help the patient achieve nutritional goals.

Food- and Nutrition-Related History

Preview The **food- and nutrition-related history** is an important aspect of the nutrition assessment because it identifies current eating patterns and types and amounts of foods and beverages consumed. Previously called a diet history, the tool was developed in 1947 for use in food and nutrition research studies.[66]

Components of Food- and Nutrition-Related History

Components of the food- and nutrition-related history include information on a typical day's eating pattern, including meals, beverages, and snacks; occasional alternative foods consumed; usual portion sizes; past changes in eating patterns; food preferences and dislikes; food allergies, intolerances, or aversions; and ethnic, cultural, and religious practices and preferences. In addition, food security should be assessed as well as transportation availability, cooking facilities, and health-related dietary restrictions. Medication regimen, alcohol consumption, and nutritional and non-nutritional supplement use should be gathered to provide a complete picture of the client's intake patterns. The diet history can be taken for a three-day period with one weekend day or for one day if time is a limiting factor.

Common questions used when gathering a food history include the following.

- How many times do you eat each day?
- When you arise, do you consume any food or beverages?
- When do you eat next? Avoid using names for meal or snack periods.
- How many servings of fruits and vegetables do you eat in a day?
- Do you eat meat, poultry, and fish?
- Do you have an intolerance to milk, dairy products, or other foods?
- Are there any foods that you avoid?
- Do you follow a meal plan prescribed by a health practitioner such as a fat-restricted or salt-restricted diet?
- What medications do you take (prescription and over-the-counter)?
- How much alcohol do you drink in a day?
- In the past month, have you skipped meals for any of the following reasons:[65]
  - Not enough food or money to buy food
  - No transportation to grocery stores
  - No working appliances (stove or kitchen utensils) to prepare food
  - No place to store perishable foods (refrigerator or freezer)
  - No access to congregate meal programs
  - Inability to prepare meals because of physical or cognitive impairments
- How many meals did you skip in the past week?

Questions should be specific and not judgmental about food-intake behaviors to promote open and honest answers to the interviewer's questions. For example, do not ask, "What do you eat for breakfast?" but rather, "Do you eat any food or beverages when you wake in the morning?" To view videos of nutrition professionals conducting food histories, refer to the Internet links at the end of the chapter.

Food histories can be modified based on the presenting medical condition(s) of the client or patient in order to obtain additional information that aids in planning for nutritional care. For example, for a client with diabetes, asking about specific meal and snack times, readiness to change nutrition-related behaviors, travel frequency, typical macronutrient intake, usual physical activity, appetite and gastrointestinal issues, and so on will add important information to the diet history.[65] A standardized diet history tool has been developed to support the diagnosis of food allergies.[67] A version is available for both pediatrics and adults. See **TABLE 4** for the pediatric version.

Additional Methods to Determine Intake

Several other methods can be used to collect food-intake information if a food history is not completed because of time constraints, the individual is unable to provide the information, or data collection is required from multiple clients, as in epidemiological research. Direct observation of food and fluid intake, a 24-hour diet recall, a food-frequency questionnaire (FFQ), and diet checklists are additional options, depending on the setting and ability of individuals to participate. Observing meal intake can be useful in individuals who are not able to recall food intakes or provide a diet history. The nutrition professional or observer can witness for type and amount of foods consumed, intake of fluids, feeding ability, rate of eating, food preferences and dislikes, and ease of intake related to chewing and swallowing status.

The 24-Hour Recall

The 24-hour food recall is a structured interview that attempts to capture all foods and beverages consumed over the previous 24-hour period. The trained interviewer uses open-ended questions to capture the time of day and portion sizes of food and beverages consumed. Food models, pictures, and other visual aids may be used to improve the accuracy of the recall. Supplement intake may also be included, although the interviewer asks questions about food and beverage intake first. A 24-hour recall generally takes about 20 to 60 minutes to complete.[68] Automated 24-hour recall systems are available for collecting interviewer-administered 24-hour dietary recalls in person or by telephone. The US Department of Agriculture's (USDA)

TABLE 4 Pediatric diet history for food allergies

1	Feeding history: Breastfed; formula fed; N/A
2	If breastfed, review maternal diet; are there any foods being avoided or being consumed in excessive amounts?
3	a. What type of infant formula or milk substitute is the child taking? ☐ Standard infant cow's milk formula with or without prebiotics/probiotics (circle) ☐ Partially/extensively hydrolyzed casein/whey formula: Type ____________ ☐ Partially/extensively hydrolyzed rice formula: Type ____________ ☐ Amino acid formula: Type ____________ ☐ Infant soy formula: Type ____________ ☐ Nonfortified soy formula: Type ____________ ☐ Fortified soya milk: Type ____________ ☐ Other milk: Fortified? Yes/No (circle): Type ____________ b. How much formula is taken per 24 hours? ____________
4	Have complementary foods been introduced into the diet of the child? Yes No (circle)

5	Food	Age	Format—in what form was food given?	Any problems with weaning or with particular foods, e.g., colic or reflux?
	Fruits			
	Vegetables			
	Rice/corn			
	Meat/chicken			
	Fats/oils			
	Cow's milk			
	Egg			
	Wheat			
	Cod or other white fish			
	Salmon or other oily fish			
	Shellfish			
	Soy			
	Tree nuts (specify type)			
	Seeds			

(continues)

TABLE 4 (continued)		
6	Is the child refusing food/to feed? If YES, is the refusal associated with back arching or distress crying?	Yes No Yes No
7	Is the child experiencing early satiety or consuming only small portions?	Yes No
8	Have foods been eliminated previously? If YES, was this helpful?	Yes No Yes No
9	Are symptoms related to a specific food? If no, complete Question 10	Yes No Possibly
10	If no specific food identified, list the meals preceding the most recent reaction and two other reactions including the most severe (think of age-related foods and possible cross-reacting foods to inhalant allergens)	

Meal	Time of Onset of Symptoms (Minutes)	Symptom Type

Adapted from: Skypala, IJ. The development of a standardized diet history tool to support the diagnosis of food allergy. Clin Translational Allergy. 2015;5:7.

Automated Multiple-Pass Method is a research-based, multiple-pass approach that uses five steps designed to enhance complete and accurate food recall and reduce respondent burden.[69] Automated self-administered tools are available as well, including the National Cancer Institute's Automated Self-Administered 24-hour (ASA24) dietary assessment tool.[68]

Daily Food Checklist

A daily food checklist is another tool that can be used to gather and assess food and beverage intake. The tool provides a list of foods; over a one-day period, the respondent makes a check beside the food each time he or she eats it. The benefits of using a checklist are that the individual does not need to recall foods eaten the previous day and little effort is required to complete the list. The checklist can be used alone or in conjunction with another instrument such as the food-frequency questionnaire (FFQ) as the FFQ. The Observing Protein & Energy Nutrition (OPEN) study found that protein and energy intake estimates were closer to true intake when used in combination with an FFQ.[70] The National Institutes of Health have developed a seven-day automated checklist tool that can be completed online to facilitate data collection.[71]

Food-Frequency Questionnaire

The FFQ is a defined list of foods and beverages with response categories to indicate usual intake of food over a certain time period. To assess total intake, an individual is asked about approximately 80–120 foods and beverages and usual portion size consumed is typically requested for each item. The FFQ can also include questions regarding supplement intake to determine whether the individual is completing 100% of the recommended daily intake for micronutrients. Generally, the FFQ is self-administered and can be completed in 30–60 minutes. It should be able to capture total dietary intake if the individual is able to complete it accurately.[71] The FFQ is generally used for large population studies, and many types have been developed based on varied ethnic groups. It is age appropriate for children and older adults and those that query specific types of food intakes, including dietary fiber, vitamin D, flavonoid intake, and others.

The NHANES has developed an FFQ that does not ask information regarding portion size to reduce respondent burden.[72]

Recap From the information obtained from the client, the nutrition professional can determine both the qualitative and quantitative aspects of the individual's intake. Generally, the information collected from the diet history correlates with the client's nutritional status if the individual provides candid information. Diet histories do have some limitations; they can be time intensive and require a highly trained professional, preferably an RDN. In addition, the participant must be highly motivated to participate and be open and honest with the professional gathering the food-intake data. The client must also be able to remember the foods consumed in the past to provide an accurate assessment; individuals with acute illnesses or dementia may not be able to participate because of short-term memory loss.[73]

Nutrition-Focused Physical Examination

Preview The use of a nutrition-focused physical exam will help the nutrition professional validate and expand on the anthropometric and biochemical components, client history, and food- and nutrition-related histories.

Why Conduct a Nutrition-Focused Physical Examination?

An NFPE is a critical component of a complete nutritional assessment because it provides information that cannot be gleaned from the food- and nutrition-related history, client history, anthropometric measurements, biochemical data, and medical tests and procedures. An NFPE includes evaluation of physical appearance, muscle and fat wasting, swallowing function, appetite, and affect, which can help determine nutritional status, signs of malnutrition, and nutrient deficiencies.[9] First, the NFPE can provide objective data in which the examiner may find physical aspects that were not included in the food history but can also be used to relate to findings from other healthcare professionals. Second, the NFPE can be used to organize information and determine whether findings are associated with a nutrition problem. The NPFE helps identify two general categories for potential nutrient deficiencies: macronutrients (energy, protein, fluids) and micronutrients (vitamins and minerals).[74]

Historically, a physical examination conducted by a physician, advanced-practice nurse, or physician's assistant has been conducted on patients seeking medical care. The physical findings from the exam would be used to identify medical problems that could be appropriately treated through patient education, physical therapy, medications, surgery, or other medical procedures. Unlike the medical examination, the NFPE is specifically a tool that can be used by nutrition professionals to complement the other aspects of the nutritional assessment and be used to develop a nutrition diagnosis versus a medical diagnosis. It is common knowledge that serum albumin and prealbumin are not sensitive indicators of protein status. Serum albumin and prealbumin levels are affected by several factors, including the patient's total body water, liver function, and renal losses. Albumin also tends to be depressed in inflammatory states in the body, caused by acute injury or trauma, infections, and chronic disease states such as arthritis, heart disease, wounds, and cancers, to name a few.[52,75] An NFPE is a way to determine if protein intake is adequate based on physical manifestations such as muscle wasting and fluid retention, as well as other physical findings.

How to Conduct an NFPE

Physical characteristics that are pertinent when evaluating an individual's nutritional status include height and weight measurement and BMI, identification of edema and hydration status, identification of skin and mucosal changes, identification of fat loss, muscle wasting and loss of strength, identification of functional deficits, gastrointestinal factors that can affect the initiation of feedings, identification of nutritional neuropathies, and identification of psychological factors that can influence nutritional intake.[74]

The NFPE is a minimally invasive process. Techniques used in the NFPE include inspection, palpation and percussion. Inspection is the most commonly used technique. It involves observing various areas of the body with the unassisted eye and can include the use of a pen light to examine lesions or the oral cavity. Palpation is the process of using the hands to inspect the body. It can be used when examining subcutaneous fat loss in the triceps, muscle loss in the interosseous muscles in the hand, and skin turgor, and it can also be used to evaluate for pitting edema. Percussion is a method of tapping body parts with the fingers, hands, or a small instrument to assess for size, consistency, and borders of organs. Percussion can also assess the presence or absence of fluid in body areas.[76] This technique is when examining the abdomen, heart, and lungs.

Both the patient's external appearance and an evaluation of his or her skin, eyes, hair, oral cavity, abdomen, extremities, and nails can provide clues as to nutritional status and point toward nutritional deficiencies or factors that can affect nutritional intake.

An NFPE generally begins with a general observation of the body and skin, starting at the head and moving downward. Findings from overall appearance would include an observation of wasting or fat accumulation, as well as dermatitis, pigmentation changes, distended abdomen, liver enlargement, muscle wasting, presence of edema, and weakness of the extremities.[77] The initial inspection and observation will help the clinician determine areas that require additional examination.

Skin

The skin is the largest organ of the body, and nutrition-focused findings may be noted in a variety of areas and conditions. Examination of the skin is conducted using inspection and palpation. Skin should be inspected for color and uniform appearance, symmetry, hygiene, lesions, tears, bruising, edema, rashes, and flakiness. Light palpation can be used to assess for moisture, temperature, texture, turgor, and mobility. To assess for skin turgor, a small area on the forearm or sternal area is pinched between the thumb and forefinger. If the skin readily returns to place when released, hydration is estimated to be adequate. If the skin does not quickly return to place, then the patient may have inadequate fluid intake or have edema (fluid retention) in the area assessed. A variety of skin lesions can indicate nutritional deficiencies, and the clinician should document a lesion's color(s), shape, texture, elevation, or depression, as well as the presence and quality of any exudate, including color, volume, odor, consistency, and location on the body.[78] **TABLE 5** indicates the physical-exam findings with the potential association of nutrient deficiencies or insufficiencies.

Hair and Eyes

After completing the general observation of the patient and assessing skin status, the clinician should start looking at the patient from head to toe. Hair should be smooth and evenly distributed. Several signs of nutritional deficiencies and disease states can be determined from the hair. Coarse, dry, or brittle hair can be a sign of

TABLE 5 Nutrition-focused physical exam findings and associated nutritional deficiencies

	Physical Exam Finding	Potential Association with Nutrient Deficiency
Hair	Easily plucked without pain; dull; dry; lack of natural shine Corkscrew hair; unemerged coiled hairs Lanugo (very fine soft hair all over body) Color changes; depigmentation	Protein deficiency; malnutrition, essential fatty acid deficiency Vitamin C deficiency Calorie deficiency Protein-calorie malnutrition; manganese, selenium, copper deficiency
Eyes	Xanthelasma (small yellowish lumps around eyes) Angular blepharitis (inflammation of eyelids, "grittiness" under eyelids) Pale conjunctiva Night blindness, dry membranes, dull or soft cornea, infected/ulcerated eye Keratomalacia; Bitot's spots (white or gray spots on conjunctiva) Angular palpebritis (redness and fissures of eyelid corners) Red and inflamed conjunctiva, swollen and sticky eyelids	Hyperlipidemia Riboflavin, biotin, vitamin B_6, zinc deficiency Vitamin B_6, vitamin B_{12}; folate, iron, coper deficiency; anemias Vitamin A deficiency Niacin, riboflavin, iron, vitamin B_6 deficiency

TABLE 5 *(continued)*

	Physical Exam Finding	Potential Association with Nutrient Deficiency
Mouth, Gums, and Tongue	Soreness, burning Angular stomatitis or cheilitis (redness, scars, swelling or fissures at the corner of the mouth Gingivitis, swollen, spongy, bleeds easily, retracted gums Sore, swollen, scarlet, raw-beefy tongue Soreness, burning tongue, purplish/magenta colored Smooth, beefy-red tongue Glossitis (sore, swollen, red and smooth tongue)	Riboflavin deficiency Riboflavin, niacin, iron, vitamin B_6,vitamin B_{12} deficiency; vitamin A toxicity Vitamin C, niacin, folate, zinc deficiency; severe vitamin D deficiency; excessive vitamin A Folate, niacin deficiency Riboflavin deficiency Vitamin B_{12}, niacin deficiency Riboflavin, niacin, vitamin B_6, vitamin B_{12}, folate deficiency; severe iron deficiency
Neck	Thyroid gland enlargement; goiter	Iodine deficiency
Skin	Slow wound healing, pressure injury Acanthosis nigracans (velvety pigmentation in body folds, around neck, etc.) Eczema Follicular hyperkeratosis (goose flesh) Seborrheic dermatitis (scaliness, waxiness, oiliness, crusty plaques on the scalp, lips, nasolabial folds) Petechiae (purple or red spots due to bleeding under skin)	Zinc, vitamin C, protein deficiency; malnutrition; inadequate hydration Obesity; insulin resistance Riboflavin, zinc deficiency Vitamin A or C deficiency Biotin, vitamin B_6, zinc, riboflavin, essential fatty acid deficiency; vitamin A excess or deficiency Vitamin C or K deficiency
Skin	Xerosis (abnormal dryness) Pellegra (thick, dry, scaly, pigmented skin on sun-exposed areas) Pallor (pale skin) Poor skin turgor	Vitamin A, essential fatty acid deficiency Niacin, tryptophan, vitamin B_6 deficiency Iron, vitamin B_{12}, folate deficiency; anemia Dehydration
Nails	Beau's lines (transverse ridges, horizontal grooves on the nail) Muehrcke's lines (transverse white lines) Kolonychia (spoon-shaped, concave) Splinter hemorrhage Brittle, soft, dry, weak or thin; splits easily Central ridges	Severe zinc deficiency, protein deficiency, hypocalcemia Malnutrition; hypoalbuminemia Iron, protein deficiency; anemia Vitamin C deficiency Magnesium deficiency; severe malnutrition; vitamin A and selenium toxicity Iron, folate, protein deficiency
Skeletal and Muscular System	Demineralization of bone Epiphyseal enlargement of wrists, legs, and knees; bowed legs, rickets or osteomalacia, frontal bossing (prominent forehead) Bone tenderness/pain Calf tenderness, absent deep tendon reflexes; foot and wrist drop Peripheral neuropathy, tingling, "pins and needles" Muscle cramps	Calcium, phosphorous, vitamin D deficiency; excessive vitamin A Vitamin D deficiency Vitamin D deficiency Thiamin deficiency Folate, vitamin B_6, pantothenic acid, phosphate, thiamin, vitamin B_{12} deficiency; vitamin B_6 toxicity Chloride, sodium, potassium, magnesium, calcium, vitamin D deficiency; dehydration

Adapted from Mordarski, B, Wolff, J. *Nutrition Focused Physical Exam Pocket Guide*. Academy of Nutrition and Dietetics, 2015.

hypothyroidism. The presence of fine, silky hair is associated with hyperthyroidism. If a patient has fine, silky hair and has had recent weight loss, this could indicate that the thyroid is overactive and the patient may need to be evaluated by the physician for hyperthyroidism. Another abnormality would be hair that is sparse, thin, and easily plucked without pain, which could indicate a potential protein deficiency.[79]

Irregularities of the hair can also be seen on other areas of the body with hair. Lanugo—very fine soft hair all over the body—can indicate caloric deficiency and is seen in some patients with **anorexia nervosa (AN)**. Corkscrew hairs or unemerged coiled hairs can be seen with a vitamin C deficiency or with Menkes syndrome (a genetic syndrome that leads to copper deficiency, deterioration of the nervous system, and the presence of brittle, kinky hair).[79]

The eyes can also show indications of nutritional deficiencies and overall nutritional status. Eyes that appear "hollow" can indicate loss of subcutaneous fat as well as dehydration.[80] Vitamin deficiencies, especially vitamin A, can be observed in the eyes. Night blindness, dry membranes, dull or soft corneas, infection, or ulceration in the eyes can indicate a vitamin A deficiency, which can lead to keratomalacia. As a vitamin A deficiency advances, Bitot's spots may appear (foamy, silver-gray spots) on the membranes that cover the white of the eyes. Angular palpebritis (redness and fissures of the eyelid corners) can indicate niacin, riboflavin, iron, and vitamin B_6 deficiency. A condition called angular blepharitis (inflammation of eyelids or "grittiness" under the eyelids) can indicated riboflavin, biotin, vitamin B_6, or zinc deficiency. Angular blepharitis can also be caused by poor eye hygiene and must be ruled out if a vitamin deficiency is suspected. Pale conjunctiva may indicate that a vitamin B_6, vitamin B_{12}, folate, iron, or copper deficiency anemia may be present. Note that anemias are not always nutrition related, and the presence of non-nutritional anemia, as in the case of anemia of chronic disease, should be ruled out. The eye can also provide a window to the impaired lipid levels in the patient because xanthelasma (small, yellowish lumps around eyes) or white rings around the iris in both eyes can indicate hyperlipidemia.[79]

Oral Cavity: Mouth, Lips, and Tongue

Healthy oral status is critical in the maintenance of good nutritional status because the mouth is the entry point into the body for adequate nutrition and hydration. Abnormalities in the oral area can affect chewing or swallowing, which can contribute directly to malnutrition. Soreness and pale and burning lips and mouth can indicate riboflavin deficiency. Angular stomatitis or cheilitis (swelling or fissures at the corners of the mouth) can also indicate riboflavin deficiency as well as niacin, iron, vitamin B_6, and vitamin B_{12} deficiencies. Angular stomatitis can also be present in vitamin A toxicity. The tongue can also reflect the presence of nutrient deficiencies. A sore, swollen, beefy-red tongue can be caused by a folate or niacin deficiency. A burning, purplish, or magenta tongue may indicate lack of adequate riboflavin. Glossitis of the tongue (a sore, swollen, red, and smooth tongue) may reflect a deficiency of a number of B vitamins or iron. Gum health can also show signs and symptoms of vitamin deficiency. The presence of gingivitis and swollen, spongy, reddened gums can indicate a vitamin C, niacin, folate, zinc, or vitamin D deficiency.[79]

The oral exam should also evaluate the teeth. Missing teeth not only indicate generally poor nutrition but also inadequate dental care. Dental caries can indicate excessive sugar intake, a vitamin D or vitamin B_6 deficiency, or inadequate fluoride consumption. Excessive fluoride intake can present as gray-brown spots or mottling on the teeth. The patient or individual should be asked to open his or her mouth as wide as possible, and the opening should be the width of three fingers. This ensures that the patient can open his or her mouth wide enough to accommodate eating utensils and food intake. The presence of any lesions should be noted. An observation of the hard palate can be accomplished by asking the patient to tilt his or her head back. Look for any abnormal nodules, redness, or inflammation.[78] Does the patient have any clicking in the jaw? The presence of a temporal-mandibular joint problem can create soreness in this area and affect chewing.

Neck

The neck should be inspected for the presence of swollen or hard lymph nodes on either side of the neck, under the jaw, and behind the ears. Swollen lymph nodes can indicate recent infection, and hard and fixed lymph nodes can indicate a possible tumor. In the healthy state, lymph nodes should not be palpable. The thyroid also can be assessed for enlargement, which can indicate a goiter possibly caused by an iodine deficiency.[78]

Nails

The nails can indicate a variety of nutrient deficiencies and medical conditions. Beau's lines (transverse ridges, horizontal grooves on nails) can indicate a severe zinc or protein deficiency but can also be present after a severe illness such as a myocardial infarction or high fever. Muehrcke's lines (transverse white lines) may be present with malnutrition or hypoalbuminemia but also be present with chronic liver or renal disease. Spoon-shaped nails (koilonychia) may be present with iron or protein deficiency but can also be seen in patients with diabetes, systemic lupus, Raynaud's disease, and hypothyroidism.[79]

Abdomen

In general, a full abdominal evaluation is not completed for a routine NFPE, but it can be part of the exam if there is any indication of gastrointestinal abnormalities. The abdominal skin area should be observed first for color and surface characteristics. Color should be similar to the other areas of the body and show no signs of jaundice, cyanosis, redness, or bruising. A shiny and firm abdomen can indicate ascites caused by cirrhosis of the liver, heart failure, or malignancy. Symmetrical distention of the abdomen that is symmetrical may indicate obesity, enlarged organs, fluid retention, or gas. If the distention is not symmetrical, this could indicate a bowel obstruction, hernia, or cysts, among other conditions. Bowel sounds can be assessed by listening for clicks and gurgles with a stethoscope; a range of five to 35 per minute are noted to be normal. This should be completed for all four quadrants of the abdomen. Increased bowel sounds can indicate hunger, gastroenteritis, or early stages of intestinal obstruction. Decreased bowel sounds can occur with peritonitis and ileus.[75]

Bones and Muscles

Bone tenderness and pain may be related to a vitamin D deficiency, but medical causes such as fractures, arthritis, and cancer should be evaluated as possible sources of pain. Calf tenderness and foot and wrist drop may indicate a thiamine deficiency, and muscle twitching may be related to a magnesium or vitamin B_6 excess or deficiency, or a calcium or vitamin D deficiency.[75,79] If a medical examination has ruled out other causes of pain and tenderness in the bones and muscles, then nutrition could be reviewed for possible deficiencies or excesses.

Recap An NFPE is an important aspect of the nutritional assessment process to ensure that an accurate nutrition problem is identified. A nutrition-focused oral examination may provide important information as to the cause of inadequate intake, weight loss, or possible nutrient deficiencies. Remember to consider the population that is being examined because findings will vary based on age, gender, and medical conditions. Review YouTube videos for NFPEs; these offer more-thorough details about how to conduct an exam.

Malnutrition

Preview Simply defined, malnutrition is any nutritional imbalance.[81] Recent advances in the understanding of cytokine-driven inflammatory responses and greater knowledge about how inflammation can affect nutritional assessment and intervention has warranted further review of the criteria to define malnutrition syndromes.[82]

Nutrition and Inflammation

By itself, nutrition supplementation is not effective in preventing or reversing protein loss when the body is experiencing an active inflammatory state. Inflammation itself causes anorexia, and so further loss of LBM will occur. Adequate nutrition, however, can help limit additional protein losses and improve outcomes in the critically ill patient.[83] Acute inflammation also affects nutritional status by increasing the resting metabolic rate and energy requirements. Protein requirements are also greater because of inefficient protein utilization when compared to healthy adults. Expansion of the extracellular fluid compartment occurs as does the production of positive acute-phase reactants that are needed for the immune response and tissue repair. This prevents the production of albumin and skeletal muscle proteins.

Previous definitions of malnutrition were based on pediatric malnutrition syndromes in underdeveloped countries. Malnutrition that occurs in a critically ill adult in a developed nation, however, is often related to an inflammatory state and not inadequate intake initially. Use of serum albumin as a prognostic indicator of nutritional status has been challenged, and although albumin is low in hospitalized patients, it is caused by cytokine-mediated **inflammatory responses** caused by injury, inflammatory conditions, or infection.[52] Serum albumin can be drastically reduced by acute injury within 24 hours. Inflammation causes even greater changes in serum albumin than does protein-energy malnutrition (PEM). We use PED protein-energy deficiency in other chapters. does even when calorie and protein intakes are adequate. These factors all suggest that non-nutrition factors are more important determinants of serum albumin levels than either protein intake or nutrition status. Although it has a shorter half-life than albumin, prealbumin is also affected by inflammation, so its use in assessing nutritional status is also limited.[84]

Cachexia

Another malnutrition syndrome of some controversy among practitioners is the definition of cachexia. Many medical references define **cachexia** as wasting of both adipose tissue and skeletal muscle. The syndrome can be seen in a variety of conditions, including cancer and AIDS.[85] However, with the increased recognition of inflammation's impact on nutritional status, the European Society for Clinical Nutrition and Metabolism (ESPEN) has defined cachexia as a systemic proinflammatory condition with metabolic aberrations that include insulin resistance, increased lipolysis, increased lipid oxidation, increased protein turnover, and loss of both body fat and muscle.[86] Despite the mild to moderate intensity of cytokine-mediated inflammation, nutrition support alone is not effective without successfully treating the underlying condition. Modern medicine has been able to keep individuals alive in this proinflammatory state, although body cell mass erodes and muscle weakness increases.

Kwashiorkor

Kwashiorkor also has been defined as a pediatric PEM syndrome occurring in underdeveloped countries and is characterized by edema in underweight children who were thought to have inadequate protein intake but adequate caloric intake. Further review of the literature shows that some studies found no difference in the macronutrient intake of children who developed kwashiorkor compared to those who did not.[87] Edema reportedly resolved in these children before improvements in serum albumin and while they were still consuming a low-protein diet. Infection and other stressors may have contributed to the development of kwashiorkor syndrome in these children. Based on these factors, the diagnosis of kwashiorkor should not be routinely used for adult patients in developed countries because there appear to be additional factors responsible for pediatric kwashiorkor in underdeveloped nations. Malnutrition caused by inadequate protein intake is generally unusual in modern medicine because critically ill patients generally have inadequate intake of both protein and energy. Current nutrition-support interventions, when provided, contain balanced macronutrients, including protein, and adequate energy and essential micronutrients.[88]

Adult PEM, sometimes referred to as *marasmic kwashiorkor*, results from a systemic inflammatory response from infection, injury, or some other inflammatory condition that continues beyond several days. Although the classic Wellcome criteria for PEM in children is the presence or absence of edema and a body weight above or below 60% of the standard for that age, the weight limits are different for adults.[89] In adult PEM, weight at approximately 80% per standard weight for height is indicative of PEM. When albumin or prealbumin was considered a valid marker of protein status, patients were often given the PEM diagnosis; however, reduced protein levels are now known to be principal manifestations of systemic inflammatory responses and not of inadequate nutritional intake. Although patients with lowered albumin or prealbumin are at nutritional risk because of inflammation, they may not be malnourished. Malnutrition may ensue, as in a critically ill patient who has not had adequate intake for 10 to 14 days.[90] Early feeding in the most severe forms of systemic inflammation, including severe sepsis, multiple trauma, severe burns, and closed head injuries, can improve outcomes before PEM develops.[91,92,93]

Sarcopenia

Sarcopenia, another syndrome associated with malnutrition, may also be affected by inflammatory factors. Defined as a loss of skeletal muscle mass and strength with aging, sarcopenia includes a loss of α-motor neuron input, changes in anabolic hormones, decreased intake of dietary protein, and a decline in physical activity.[94] Loss of muscle mass can begin as early as the fourth decade of life, with evidence suggesting that skeletal muscle mass and skeletal muscle strength decline in a linear fashion, with as much as 50% of mass being lost by the eighth decade of life.[95] For diagnostic purposes, sarcopenia has been defined as appendicular skeletal muscle mass/height^2 ((m^2)) that is less than two standard deviations below the mean for young and healthy reference populations.[96] Research on sarcopenia has suggested that it is a "smoldering" inflammatory state propelled by both cytokines and oxidative stress.[53] Sarcopenia may be described as a condition of both cachexia and failure to thrive. Some evidence suggests that chronic disease triggers hormonal changes, and inadequate nutritional intake and declining activity levels may be multifactorial causes for sarcopenia.[97]

Although clinicians generally think of patients with sarcopenia as frail older adults, sarcopenia can occur in obese patients as well. Dubbed **sarcopenic obesity**, these patients also exhibit decreased muscle mass or strength and are characterized as having excess energy intake, limited physical activity, low-grade inflammation, insulin resistance, and changes in hormonal milieu. Muscle strength has been determined to be more important that muscle mass, so muscle "quality" is affected, which leads to a decrease in fiber size and number and a reduction in the contractility of the intact muscle fibers.[98] These manifestations can lead to functional limitations, increased morbidity, and a potential for increased mortality. In

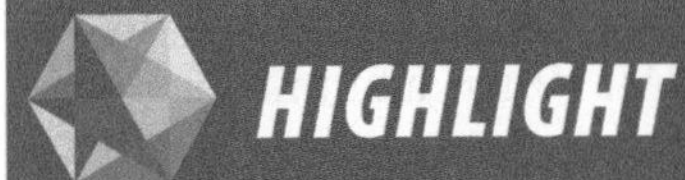

Sarcopenia

Because sarcopenia can have adverse outcomes such as immobility, falls, disability, and death in older adults, a rapid screen has been developed to increase the recognition and treatment of sarcopenia. Although the methodology to assess for sarcopenia can be ultrasound, BIA, computed tomography, or magnetic resonance imaging, a questionnaire has been validated to rapidly diagnose sarcopenia. The SARC-F was developed and found to have excellent specificity in identifying persons with sarcopenia. Evidence shows that sarcopenia can be alleviated by resistance exercise, leucine-enriched amino acids, and vitamin D. The screen takes less than 15 seconds to complete and is thus a cost-effective and quick evaluation to screen for sarcopenia. See **TABLE A**.

TABLE A

Component	Question	Scoring
Strength	How much difficulty do you have lifting and carrying 10 lbs?	None = 0 Some = 1 A lot or unable = 2
Assistance in walking	How much difficulty do you have walking across a room?	None = 0 Some = 1 A lot, uses aids, or unable = 2
Rise from a chair	How much difficulty do you have transferring from a chair or bed?	None = 0 Some = 1 A lot or unable without help = 2
Climb stairs	How much difficulty do you have climbing a flight of 10 stairs?	None = 0 Some = 1 A lot or unable = 2
Falls	How many times have you fallen in the last year?	None = 0 1–3 falls = 1 4 or more falls = 2

A SARC-F score of ≥ 4 indicates a high risk for sarcopenia.

Modified from Morley, JE, Cao, L. Rapid screening for sarcopenia. *J Cachexia Sarcopenia Muscle*. 2015;6:312-314. Malmstrom, TK, Miller, DK, Simonsick, EM, Ferruci, L, Morley, JE. SARC-F: a symptom score to predict persons with sarcopenia at risk for poor functional outcomes. *J Cachexia Sarcopenia Muscle*. 2016;7(1):28-36.

a study of 4,652 adults 60 years of age and older, the prevalence of sarcopenic obesity was 18.1% in women and 42.9% in men. Although sarcopenic obesity was higher in men, mortality risk was greater in women with sarcopenic obesity.[99]

The presence of inflammation helps to rule out nutrition intake as a causative factor of adult malnutrition. Once nutrition risk is identified due to compromised intake and/or loss of body mass (weight loss), the clinician determines whether inflammation is present. Inflammation is believed to be a causative factor for malnutrition if the individual has an active infection, presence of injury, the person has edema or low serum albumin, or altered C-reactive protein levels, among others. If inflammation is absent, starvation-related malnutrition (or malnutrition in the context of social or environmental circumstances including pure chronic starvation or anorexia nervosa) is suspected. If inflammation is of mild to moderate intensity and is sustained, this is suggestive of chronic disease-related malnutrition (as in organ failure, pancreatic cancer, rheumatoid arthritis, and sarcopenic obesity). If there is a marked inflammatory response, this is suggestive of acute disease or injury-related malnutrition (as in major infection, burns, trauma, and closed head injury).[88,100]

Adult Malnutrition

The Academy and ASPEN have developed a consensus statement for the identification and documentation of adult malnutrition (undernutrition).[101] This consensus statement will help determine the prevalence of malnutrition in various healthcare settings, especially in acute care where the Center for Medicare and Medicaid has voiced concerns about which malnutrition code is used and the wide variation in the prevalence and incidence within the same geographic area or populations with similar demographics.[102]

Diagnosis of Adult Malnutrition

The presence of malnutrition in the hospital setting was first portrayed in the 1974 article "The Skeleton in the Hospital Closet" in which the importance of adequate nutritional care could help reduce length of stay (LOS) and healthcare costs.[103] Current statistics on adult malnutrition range from 15% to 60%, depending on the patient population and the characteristics used to identify its occurrence.[104] Some medical conditions have higher rates of malnutrition than others, including pancreatic cancer (85%), lung cancer (13% to 50%), head and neck cancers (24% to 88%), gastrointestinal cancer (55% to 80%), cerebrovascular accident (16% to 49%), and chronic obstructive pulmonary disease (25%).[105] Nutrition deficits in hospital patients can lead to muscle loss and weakness, which can increase the risk for falls, pressure injuries, infections, delays in wound healing, and hospital readmission rates. Malnutrition as a comorbid condition can increase the LOS and time spent in rehabilitation.[106] As a result of all possible comorbidities and hospital LOS, identifying, diagnosing, and treating malnutrition in addition to the primary illness are critical processes.

Appropriate documentation and care of the malnourished hospitalized patient can lead to reimbursement for the additional care provided. With the transition to the 10th edition of the *International Classification of Disease* (ICD-10) in 2015, modifications have been made in coding. See **TABLE 6** for the ICD-9 and ICD-10 codes, which are available at www.cms.gov.icd10. Severe protein-calorie malnutrition can be considered a major complication or comorbidity (MCC) based on the primary diagnosis. Mild or moderate protein-calorie nutrition is considered a complication or comorbidity (CC).

Characteristics for the diagnosis of adult malnutrition have been defined so that the condition can be consistently detected and diagnosed. The Academy and ASPEN workgroups determined that the presence of two or more of the following characteristics are needed to further assess the individual for a diagnosis of malnutrition:[101]

- Insufficient energy intake
- Weight loss
- Loss of muscle mass
- Loss of subcutaneous fat
- Localized or generalized fluid accumulation that may sometimes mask weight loss and
- Diminished functional status as measured by handgrip strength

Patients should be assessed at admission and at frequent intervals throughout their stays based on screenings and assessment standards for various types of healthcare settings—acute, transitional, or long term. The clinician should share the data with all members of the healthcare team, including the physician, because the clinician is responsible for documenting a diagnosis of malnutrition.[100]

In addition to insufficient energy intake and weight loss, an NFPE specific to malnutrition can be conducted to assess for physical characteristics. Muscle mass loss can be assessed in the upper body because this area is more prone to muscle loss, independent of functional status. Assessment via inspection of the temporal area (depression at the temples), as well as the shoulders, clavicles, deltoids, pectoralis muscles, and interosseous muscles in the hands will reveal signs of muscle loss in the presence of malnutrition. Loss of subcutaneous fat can be best assessed in the orbital (eye), triceps (upper arm), and ribs and chest areas. The presence of pitting edema or fluid accumulation can be local (usually in the lower extremities) or generalized, and the clinician must consider other causes of fluid retention, including heart failure, liver and kidney disease, stomach cancer (ascites), lymphedema, and hyperthyroidism.[107] Muscle function reacts early to nutritional deprivation, and handgrip strength can be assessed using a dynamometer, a simple noninvasive marker of muscle strength in the upper extremities.[108] Clinical signs of inflammation may also be revealed with the NFPE, including fever or hypothermia as well as other nonspecific signs of systemic inflammatory response (e.g., tachycardia, and hyperglycemia).[100]

The diagnosis of malnutrition may not be appropriate for certain patients based on age or disease process. For example, a diagnosis of malnutrition should not be considered for the older adult who consistently consumes less than recommended calories but maintains a stable but lower than recommended weight and is able to function well in the

TABLE 6 ICD-9 and ICD-10 codes for malnutrition

ICD-9 Code	ICD-10 Code	ICD-9 Title	ICD-10 Title	Criteria/Description	MCC/CC
260	E40	Kwashiorkor should rarely be used in the United States.	Kwashiorkor should rarely be used in the United States.	Nutritional edema with dyspigmentation of skin and hair	MCC
260	E42	Kwashiorkor should rarely be used in the United States.	Marasmic kwashiorkor should rarely be used in the United States.		
261	E41	Nutritional marasmus should rarely be used in the United States.	Nutritional marasmus should rarely be used in the United States.	Nutritional atrophy; severe malnutrition otherwise stated; severe energy deficiency	MCC
262	E43	Other severe protein-calorie malnutrition	Unspecified severe protein-calorie malnutrition	Nutritional edema without mention of dyspigmentation of skin and hair	MCC
263	*E44	Malnutrition of moderate degree	Moderate protein-calorie malnutrition	No definition given (use criteria from the Academy or ASPEN)	CC
263.1	E44.1	Malnutrition of mild degree	Mild protein-calorie malnutrition	No definition given (use criteria from the Academy or ASPEN)	CC
263.2	E45	Arrested development following protein-calorie malnutrition	Retarded development following protein-calorie malnutrition		CC
263.8/9	E46	Other protein-calorie malnutrition	Unspecified protein-calorie malnutrition	A disorder caused by lack of proper nutrition or an inability to absorb nutrients from food. An imbalanced nutritional status resulting from insufficient intake of nutrients to meet normal physiological requirements.	CC
263.9	E64	Unspecified protein-calorie malnutrition	Sequelae of protein-calorie malnutrition		CC

MCC = major complications or comorbidities; CC = complications or comorbidities.

Adapted from: Phillips, W. Coding for malnutrition in the adult patient: what the physician needs to know. Practical Gastroenterol., September 2014. Retrieved January 2, 2017.

VIEWPOINT

Predatory Publishing

J. Scott Thomson, MS, MLIS, AHIP

It could happen to you!

- You receive an email inviting you to submit an article to an impressive-sounding journal and think, "That's strange. . . . I've never heard of this publisher."
- You receive an invitation to serve as editor or reviewer for a journal and think, "I've never heard of any of these people. How did they get my name?"
- Or you simply stumble onto a journal's website and something doesn't seem quite right.

If any of the above examples sound familiar, you may have had a brush with the less-reputable side of the scholarly publishing world: predatory publishing.

Predatory publishing is an emerging term used to describe any form of scholarly communication that exploits scholars or the peer-review system itself. The Internet has removed many of the traditional barriers to publishing, and this has led to a proliferation of new online publishers, many of whom use an open-access (OA) model of publication. Unlike traditional publications for which users have to pay to access content, OA publications are freely available online, and the costs associated with publication are recouped in other ways. One common method is to rely on the authors to pay the costs associated with publishing and editing their publications. Many OA publishers are legitimate, and some are even quite prestigious, but others have exploited the model, usually by creating predatory open-access journals.

Predatory OA journals are probably the most common form of predatory publishing encountered today. The exact details of how they work varies from instance to instance, but here's a typical example. An article is submitted to a journal and is quickly accepted for publication. Despite assurances of a traditional editorial and review process, the article receives little if any copy editing and is rushed into publication. The author never receives any notes, comments, or editing requests that would typically come from an established and scientific peer-review process. At some point in the process, the author may be presented with a substantial and often unexpected invoice for the costs associated with the publication and review of the paper.

Publishers of this type come in many shapes and sizes, and they use many different models to achieve their goals, which can make them difficult to spot. However, there is help. Many universities and organizations maintain guides with information to help you identify and avoid predatory publishers. Here are a few examples to help you get started.

- Rosalind Franklin University. Predatory Publishing. http://guides.rosalindfranklin.edu/predatorypublishing.
  This guide provides an overview of predatory publishing along with a list of red flags to look out for when evaluating a publisher.
- Think–Check–Submit. http://thinkchecksubmit.org/.
  This guide was created and maintained by a consortia of publishers and scholarly societies to help you pick the right journal for your research—and avoid the wrong ones!

Remember, this type of fraudulent activity isn't limited to journals. There are scams involving books and conferences, so when in doubt, check it out!

community environment. Other individuals for whom this criterion would not apply include patients with a muscle-loss condition related to a spinal cord injury but who consume adequate calories and protein, or terminally ill individuals for whom nutrition interventions would not be effective.[100]

A careful review of the patient's primary complaint, review of systems, medical, nutrition and psychosocial histories, physical exam results, laboratory markers of inflammation, anthropometric measures, food intake, and functional status should be reviewed to make the initial diagnosis of malnutrition. Based on the findings, a nutritional plan of care can be developed and should be reassessed frequently to ensure that the interventions put into place help to the patient to achieve optimal nutritional health.

Determining calorie, protein, and fluid needs for the individual is the next important step in the nutrition-assessment process and will be discussed in the next several sections.

Recap Most of the body's protein is contained in the skeletal muscle, which is the body compartment most affected by protein malnutrition. Cytokines have a significant effect on muscle regulation when inflammation is present, including promoting muscle catabolism, preventing protein synthesis and repair, affecting contractility and function, and triggering cell death. All of the effects of cytokines on muscle tissue contribute to the development of protein-energy undernutrition or malnutrition.[88]

▸ Estimating Energy Requirements

Preview The gold standard for measuring caloric needs is the use of indirect calorimetry. In the absence of the resources needed to conduct indirect calorimetry studies, predictive equations are used to define caloric needs.

Indirect Calorimetry

To complete a nutritional assessment and determine the effectiveness of planned nutrition interventions, an accurate determination of energy needs is required. Although the Academy's Evidence Analysis Library (EAL) has determined that the gold standard for determining energy needs or **resting metabolic rate (RMR)** is indirect calorimetry, this method is unrealistic for most clinical practice settings.[109] **Indirect calorimetry** is the measurement of pulmonary gas exchange; it measures the consumption of oxygen and the production of carbon dioxide. The amount and mixture of macronutrients (carbohydrate, fat, and protein) oxidized by the body produces a specific amount of heat and carbon dioxide and the consumption of a specific amount of oxygen. A ratio of carbon dioxide production to oxygen consumption, known as the *respiratory quotient* (RQ), is used to calculate metabolic rate.[110] The use of indirect calorimetry is costly because of equipment needs, requires more time to complete, and requires trained personnel to run the test. In addition, the condition of the patient must be considered; critically ill or cognitively impaired patients may not be able to participate in the measurement.[111] Portable indirect calorimeters, which measure gas exchange and RMR, have been around since the 1970s and are accurate to within 5%.[112] As a result of the challenges of using indirect calorimetry, several **predictive equations for estimating energy needs** have been developed to estimate energy requirements. These equations have been compared to indirect calorimetry, and the accuracy of each has been substantiated.[113] The equations recommended for assessing energy needs vary based on the type and health status of the individual being assessed. Intra-individual variations in energy needs of 7.5% to 17.9% also exist between individuals matched for age, gender, height, and weight.[114,115] Therefore, the determination of energy needs for an individual will be an estimate and may need to be adjusted based on changes in weight status and nutritional intake.

Predictive Equations for Estimating Energy Needs

In 2005, the EAL's Working Group determined the Mifflin–St. Jeor equation to be the most reliable equation for estimating resting energy requirement (REE). Equation results are within 10% in both nonobese and obese individuals when compared to other equations reviewed (Harris-Benedict, Owen, and the World Health Organization, Food and Agriculture Organization, and United Nations University, or WHO–FAO–UNO).[116,117,118,119] Estimates using the Mifflin–St. Jeor were found to be 82% accurate in the nonobese adult and 70% accurate in the obese adult (BMI >30). The Mifflin–St. Jeor in nonobese adults was noted to underestimate energy needs as much as 18% and overestimate needs by as much as 15% because of individual variability. In obese adults, errors in estimation tend to be underestimates, with maximal underestimation by 20% and maximal overestimation by 15%. For older adults, accuracy within 10% is not available because of limited research in this population group; the equation may underestimate needs by 18% in older men and 31% in older women.

The Harris-Benedict equation (HBE) was also evaluated by the EAL 2005 Working Group. Developed in 1919, this is the oldest tool for estimating energy needs.[120] This equation is only found to be 45% to 81% accurate in nonobese adults and tends to overestimate energy needs. Similarly, in obese individuals, only 38% to 64% of the estimates are accurate, with most errors tending to be overestimates. In older adults, accuracy within 10% is not possible and can both underestimate and overestimate needs in men and women because of individual variation. The Owen equation is, a lesser-known and seldom-used equation is 73% accurate in nonobese adults and 51% in obese adults.[121] As with the other equations, the data in older adults are limited and exist only for older white females with an underestimation of 27% and an overestimation of 12%. Accuracy of the WHO–FAO–UNO equation developed by Schofield is not reported for nonobese or obese adults in any of the evaluated studies. For older adults, the accuracy of this equation is unknown.[119,122]

Although the Mifflin–St. Jeor and Harris-Benedict equations for estimating energy needs are generally recommended for healthy adults, several equations have been developed specifically for critically ill patients. The Critical Illness Workgroup of the Academy's EAL

TABLE 7 Validated predictive equations for estimating energy needs

Healthy	Harris-Benedict (1919)	Men: Wt(13.75) + Ht(5) – age(6.8) + 66 Women: Wt(9.6) + Ht(1.8) – age(4.7) + 655
	Owen (1986, 1987)	Men: Wt(10.2) + 879 Women: Wt(7.2) + 795
	Mifflin–St. Jeor (1990)	Men: Wt(10) + Ht(6.25) – age(5) + 5 Women: Wt(10) + Ht(6.25) – age(5) – 161
	Livingston (2005)	Men: 293 × Wt(0.4430) – age(5.92) Women: 248 × Wt(0.4356) – age(5.09)
Critically ill	Swinanmer (1990)	BSA(941) – age(6.3) + T(104) + RR(24) + Vt(804) – 4243
	Ireton-Jones (1992)	Wt(5) – age(10) + Male(281) + Trauma(292) + Burns(851)
	Brandl (1999)	HBE(0.96) + HR(7) + Ve(32) + T(48) – 702
	Faisy (2003)	8(wt) + 14(ht) + 42(Ve) + 94(T) – 4834
	Penn State (1998, 2004, 2010)	Age ≥ 60 with BMI ≥ 30 kg/m^2: Mifflin(0.71) + Tmax(85) + Ve(64) – 3085 All others: Mifflin(0.96) + Tmax(167) + Ve(31) – 6212

Wt = weight (kg); Ht = height (cm); age in years; BMI = body mass index; BSA = body surface area in m^2; T = temperature in °C; RR = respiratory rate in breaths/min; Vt = tidal volume in L/breath; HBE = Harris-Benedict in kcal/day; HR = heart rate in beats/min; Tmax = maximum body temperature previous 24 hours in °C; Ve = minute ventilation in L/min.

Adapted from Frankenfield, DC, Ashcraft, CM. Estimating energy needs in nutrition support patients. Tutorial. *J Parenter Enteral Nutr.* 2011;35(5):564.

project evaluated the accuracy of the predictive equations for energy expenditure and concluded that the Ireton-Jones and Penn State equations were the most accurate in assessing critically ill obese patients.[119,123,124] Several other predictive equations have been developed for critically ill patients, including the Fick method and the HBE with stress factors.[125] The Critical Illness Workgroup concluded that these equations consistently underestimate patient needs and should not be used. The Swinamer equation was also evaluated in the critically ill, and it was determined that additional validation study is needed because there was insufficient evidence to reject this formula.[126]

The Ireton-Jones equation has been studied in both spontaneously breathing and ventilator-dependent patients.[123] The EAL Critical Illness Workgroup concluded that there was insufficient evidence to reject the equation and that further validation studies were needed to confirm its accuracy. The equation was revised in 1997 but did not perform as well as the 1992 version and is not recommended for use.[127] The Penn State equations are specific to ventilator-dependent patients.[124,128] The equations include the Harris-Benedict (HBE) equation and add max body temperature in the previous 24 hours, and ventilation in L/min. to determine estimated energy needs. Although only one study was evaluated by the EAL, both equations were unbiased and precise. The equation was accurate 79% of the time in nonobese patients and can be used for critically ill patients on ventilators. Additional validation was recommended because of the limited data available. **TABLE 7** lists equations that have been developed for both healthy and critically ill adult patients.

Recap The use of indirect calorimetry is costly because of equipment needs and both time and trained personnel requirements. In addition, a patient's condition must be considered critically ill, and cognitively impaired patients may not be able to participate in the measurement.[111] As a result of the challenges of using indirect calorimetry, several predictive equations have been developed to estimate energy requirements.

Estimating Protein Requirements

Preview Protein is needed for buildup and repair functions in the body. Protein is the only macronutrient that contains nitrogen.

Protein is the major building block in the body and is present in enzymes, membrane carriers, blood-transport molecules, the intracellular matrices, hair, fingernails, serum albumin, keratin, collagen, and hormones. Because of demand by every cell in the human body, a constant source of protein is needed to maintain the structural integrity and function of all cells. The major difference between proteins and the other macronutrients, (carbohydrates and fats) is that protein contains an amino or nitrogen group.[129]

Protein Requirements in Healthy Adults

Protein requirements are based on whether the body is in a healthy state or if disease status dictates that added or decreased protein is warranted by the medical condition. For healthy adults, the Recommended Daily Allowance (RDA) is 0.8 g/kg body weight per day of good-quality protein. The RDA for adult men is 56 g/day; for adult females, 46 g/day. At this level of intake, this amount of protein meets the needs of 97% to 98% of all healthy individuals in a group. Requirements for protein during pregnancy and lactation are higher because of fetal growth and the production of breast milk, with the Dietary Reference Intakes (DRIs) recommending 0.88 g/kg body weight during pregnancy and 1.05 g/kg during lactation; the RDA is set at 71 g protein for both pregnancy and lactation.[130]

Several studies have suggested that older adults may benefit from higher protein intakes to preserve bone and muscle mass. Osteoporosis and sarcopenia are morbidities frequently associated with aging. Evidence exists that the anabolic response of muscle to dietary protein is decreased in older adults. In addition, an increase in dietary protein increases circulating insulin growth factor, which has anabolic effects on both muscle and bone and increases calcium absorption, which is also beneficial to bone health.[131] Short-term studies in older individuals have reported positive outcomes on muscle mass at protein intakes of 1.6 to 1.8 g/kg per day; however, longer-duration studies are necessary to determine safety and efficacy.[132] It has been suggested that increasing the RDA for older individuals to 1.0 to 1.2 g/kg per day would be beneficial for bone and muscle health without compromising renal function, until long-term protein supplementation trials have been completed.[131]

Protein Needs in Critical Illness

Needs for dietary protein are increased for certain conditions in which catabolism is occurring in the body, such as in critical illnesses where the patient requires treatment in the intensive-care unit (ICU). These illnesses include sepsis and systemic inflammatory-response syndrome, trauma, neurological injuries such as traumatic brain injury or stroke, pancreatitis, respiratory failure, multiorgan failure, and surgery. There is limited evidence on defining the protein needs in patients who are critically ill. The 2007 Academy EAL work group on protein needs in critical illness concluded that there are not enough adequately powered studies to determine protein requirements in critically ill adults.[133] A study in which critically ill patients undergoing continuous renal-replacement therapy were provided with more than 2 g protein/kg/day reported that the probability of survival increased by 21% for every daily 1-g increase in nitrogen balance. After multivariate analyses controlled for age, gender, diagnosis, and Acute Physiology and Chronic Health Evaluation (APACHE) II score, no significant results connected protein intake with mortality.[134] Similarly, a review of protein needs in critically ill patients suggests that, although there are limited and poor-quality studies, 2.0 g to 2.5 g protein/kg normal body weight is safe and could be an optimal level for patients who are critically ill. In addition, it has been noted that most critically ill patients receive less than half of this level for the first week or longer in the ICU.[135] Patients who have sustained burns over at least 20% of total body surface area (TBSA) require 20% to 25% of energy intake in the form of protein, equivalent to 1.5 g/kg to 2.0 g/kg body weight.[136] For patients with burns covering of less than 10% of TBSA or obese patients, the recommendation for protein is 1.2g/kg body weight. Protein needs decrease as healing occurs, and adequacy of protein intake can be determined by wound healing of burns and donor sites, the adherence of skin grafts, and nitrogen-balance measurements.

The following is a summary of recommendations for protein needs in critical illness:[137]

- 20% to 25% of total calories for stressed patients, including those with burns
- 1.2 to 2.0 g/kg actual body weight if BMI is < 30 (may be higher in burn or trauma patients)
- 2.5 g/kg/day in early postop burn patients and as much as 4 g/kg/day during flow period

- 2.0 to 2.5 g/kg/day for continuous renal-replacement therapy
- ≥ 2.0 g/kg ideal body weight if BMI is 30 to 40 and hypocaloric feeding is used
- ≥ 2.5 g/kg ideal body weight if BMI is > 40 and hypocaloric is feeding used

Protein Needs for Pressure Injuries

Protein requirements are increased for patients with pressure injuries to promote healing. The National Pressure Ulcer Advisory Panel, the European Pressure Ulcer Advisory Panel, and the Pan Pacific Pressure Injury Alliance joined together to develop the most current guidelines for the prevention and treatment of pressure injuries, including nutrition recommendations.[138] The seven recommendations regarding protein requirements are as follow:

1. Provide adequate protein for positive nitrogen balance for adults assessed to be at risk of a pressure injury.
2. Offer 1.25 g to 1.5 g protein/kg body weight daily for adults at risk of a pressure injury who are assessed to be at risk of malnutrition, when compatible with goals of care; reassess as conditions change.
3. Provide adequate protein for positive nitrogen balance for adults with pressure injuries.
4. Offer 1.25 grams to 1.5 grams protein/kg body weight daily for adults with current pressure injuries who are assessed to be at risk of malnutrition, when compatible with goals of care; reassess as conditions change.
5. Offer high-calorie, high-protein nutritional supplements in addition to the usual diet to adults with nutritional risk and pressure-injury risk if nutritional requirements cannot be achieved by dietary intake.
6. Assess renal function to ensure that high levels of protein are appropriate for the individual. (Clinical judgment is needed to determine the level of protein required for each individual based on the number of pressure injuries present, current overall nutritional status, comorbidities, and tolerance to nutritional interventions.)
7. Supplement with high protein, arginine, and micronutrients for adults with pressure injuries at stage III or IV or multiple pressure ulcers when nutritional requirements cannot be met with traditional high-calorie and protein supplements.[138]

Protein Needs for Chronic Kidney Disease

Adjustments in protein intake are necessary for patients with chronic kidney disease (CKD), depending on the stage of renal disease and whether the patient is receiving dialysis. Dietary intake of protein for individuals not receiving dialysis with a glomerular filtration rate of <25 mL/min (stage IV CKD) are advised to consume a diet providing 0.60 g protein/kg body weight/day, which will limit toxic nitrogenous metabolites, the development of uremic symptoms, and the occurrence of other metabolic consequences. Evidence-based guidelines support that a low-protein diet may slow the progression of renal failure and delay the need for dialysis. Approximately 50% of the protein should be of high biological value.[139] For individuals already receiving dialysis therapy, protein intake depends on the type of dialysis, maintenance hemodialysis (MHD), or chronic peritoneal dialysis (CPD), requiring 1.2 g protein/kg body weight/day and 1.2 g to 1.3 g protein/kg body weight/day, respectively. For both MHD and CPD, 50% of protein should be of high biological value. For patients in the earlier stages (I to II) of CKD, protein intake at the DRI level is recommended with 12% to 15% of calories from protein (0.8 g protein/kg body weight/day) to slow the progression of the disease. At stage III CKD, reducing protein intake to 10% of calories is recommended.[140] The nutrition professional should consider the overall nutritional status of the patient when estimating protein needs to prevent excessive or inadequate protein intakes. If a patient with CKD has a pressure injury as a comorbidity, protein needs may need to be adjusted to meet healing requirements as well as address the current stage of CKD.

Recap Protein requirements are based on whether the body is in a healthy state or if disease status dictates added or decreased protein. For healthy adults, the RDA is 0.8 g/kg body weight per day of good-quality protein. Needs for dietary protein are increased for certain conditions in which catabolism is occurring in the body.

Estimating Fluid Requirements

Preview Adequate fluid intake is needed to sustain life because the amount of water in the average adult's body is must be from 50% to 65%, depending on gender and age. Fluids are needed for almost all body functions, including digestion, and metabolism, excretion of waste products, as a medium for biochemical reactions, as a regulator of body temperature, as a conductor of electrical messages to muscles and nerves, and to lubricate joints.

Equations for Estimating Fluid Needs

For adults, several equations are used to calculate fluid needs as part of a nutritional assessment. The body surface area (BSA) method allows for 1,500 mL/m^2 × BSA = mL fluid required daily. This method is not routinely used to estimate fluid needs.[141] The Adolph method, which is also known as the Recommended Dietary Allowance method, uses 1 ml of fluid per calorie of intake. The fluid-balance method is urine output + 500 ml per day, and the Holiday-Segar method is based on body weight with 100 mL/kg for the first 10 kg body weight, + 50 mL/kg for the second 10 kg body weight + 20 mL/kg for the remaining kg body weight (< 50 years of age), or + 15mL for remaining kg body weight (> 50 years of age).[142,143,144] Generally, most nutrition clinicians use the single-calculation equations for estimating fluid needs for normal-weight adults as follows: 25 mL/kg for patients with congestive heart disease or renal failure; 30 mL/kg for average adults; and 35 mL/kg for patients with infection or draining wounds.[145,146] For obese adults, the following equation has been suggested:[145]

$$[(\text{kg body weight} - 20) \times 15] + 1500$$

Despite the different methods available to calculate fluid needs, the Academy's EAL concluded that there is no evidence supporting either clinical or biochemical measurements as a gold standard for addressing hydration status in individuals.[147]

Factors That Can Impact Fluid Needs

The nutrition professional must be aware of factors that can alter fluid requirements so that adjustments to the assessment can be made. If a patient is exhibiting conditions such as anabolism, burns, constipation, dehydration, diarrhea, emesis, fever, fistulas or drains, hemorrhage, hot or dry environments, hyperventilation, hypotension, medications, nasogastric suctioning, and polyuria, the individual's fluid intake must reflect increased needs. Fluid needs are also estimated to show a 7% increase for each degree Fahrenheit above normal body temperature in individuals with increased body temperature. Polyuria can results from poor glucose control, excess alcohol, excess caffeine, and osmotic diuresis. The following conditions may decrease fluid requirements: cardiac disease (especially heart failure), edema, fluid overload, hepatic failure with ascites, medications, renal failure, syndrome of antidiuretic hormone, significant hypertension, and "third spacing" of fluids.[148]

Recap Despite the importance of fluid in the body, the Academy's EAL concluded there is no evidence, either clinical or biochemical measurements, that are available to best assess hydration status in individuals, although several methods have been described.

Nutritional Assessment and Management of Eating Disorders

Preview Conditions such as eating disorders require special nutrition considerations. Eating disorders (EDs) encompass many different conditions, including anorexia nervosa, bulimia nervosa, and binge eating.[149]

The *Diagnostic and Statistics Manual of Mental Disorders*, 5th edition (DSM-V), defines anorexia nervosa as a restriction of energy intake relative to required needs that leads to a significantly low body weight in the context of age, developmental trajectory, and physical health.[150] **Bulimia nervosa (BN)** is characterized by episodes of binge eating, or consuming a large amount of food quickly followed by vomiting or purging. **Binge-eating disorder (BED)** is described as recurrent eating of large quantities of food to the point of feeling uncomfortably full and not regularly vomiting or purging the excess intake. In addition to the three main eating disorders, a category of other feeding and eating disorders or eating disorders not otherwise specified includes the following:

- Atypical anorexia nervosa (weight is not below normal)
- Bulimia nervosa (with less-frequent behaviors)
- Binge-eating disorder (with less-frequent occurrences)
- Purging disorder (purging without binge eating)
- Night eating syndrome (excessive nighttime food consumption)
- Avoidant–restrictive food-intake disorder (failure to consume adequate amounts of food, with serious nutritional consequences but without the psychological features of anorexia nervosa)
- Pica (eating things that are not food and do not provide nutritional value) and
- Rumination disorder (regurgitation of food that has already been swallowed; the regurgitated food is often reswallowed or spit out)

Prevalence of Eating Disorders

In a study of the prevalence of eating disorders in a nationally representative sample of 10,123 adolescents aged 13 to 18 years, the current rates of five eating disorders were similar to previous studies: AN 0.3%, BN 0.9%, BED 1.6%, subthreshold anorexia nervosa 0.8%, and subthreshold binge-eating disorder 2.5%.[151] Additional findings indicated there was no female preponderance for AN or BN and only 3% to 28% had specifically discussed eating or weight problems with a healthcare professional.

Because of the complex psychodynamics of EDs, treatment is a collaborative effort that involves medical, psychiatric, psychosocial, and nutritional interventions. Nutrition professionals who work with patients with EDs should receive initial and ongoing training on the management of psychiatric disorders as well as in working with specific population groups such as adolescents, athletes, and obese patients who exhibit BEDs.[152] The nutrition professional may be the first person to recognize an individual's symptoms of an ED, or this professional may be the initial health practitioner who is consulted by the patient for his or her condition.

Management of Eating Disorders

Despite the prevalence of EDs, evidence-based practice guidelines on nutrition management are lacking. A review of nutrition practice management of EDs concluded that few studies have addressed the effectiveness of the nutrition interventions prescribed for this category of disease.[153] The guidance supports the importance of nutrition and establishes that the goals of initial treatment for anorexia nervosa are to restore weight, improve nutrition status, and aim for a return to normal eating. However, limited information exists on how to achieve these goals.[154,155,156,157,158] It has been suggested that nutrition interventions are at times neglected as effective behavioral therapy will restore normal eating behaviors. One study noted that nutritional professionals who work with EDs have the best nutritional knowledge when compared to other healthcare professionals who work with these patients, so it is important to have an RDN on the healthcare team in the management of EDs.[159] One key missing factor in the nutrition treatment of these individuals is a working definition of what "normal eating patterns" actually encompass.[153]

Nutrition Guidelines for Eating Disorders

The American Psychiatric Association's nutritional rehabilitation guidelines for AN include goals such as restoring weight, normalizing eating patterns, achieving normal perceptions of hunger and satiety, and correct biological and psychological sequelae of malnutrition. Starting calorie needs should be estimated at 30–40 kcals/kg per day or approximately 1,000–1,600 kcals/day. During the weight-gain phase, intake amounts are increased to as high as 70-100 kcals/kg per day as some male patients require a large number of calories to gain weight. Established expected rates of controlled weight gain are 2–3 lb/week for hospitalized patients and 0.5–1 lb/week for outpatients. Patients gaining excessive amounts of weight should be monitored for refeeding syndrome and fluid retention, especially for those weighing < 70% of healthy body weight. In addition to increased calorie intake, patients may benefit from vitamin and mineral supplementation. Serum potassium should be monitored in patients who are persistently vomiting.[157]

Goals for individuals with BN are to help the patient develop a structured meal pattern that helps reduce the episodes of dietary restriction and the urge to binge and purge. Adequate caloric intake can help prevent craving and promote satiety. Nutrition restoration is not a central focus of treatment, because most BN patients are of normal weight. Note that although these individuals maintain a normal weight, this does not equate to a healthy nutritional status.[157]

Although the American Psychiatric Association provides treatment regimens and goals for EDs, specific nutrition interventions have been recommended for the nutrition professional based on review of 41 topic papers, studies, and guidelines on EDs.[153] See **TABLE 8** for a list of nutrition interventions.

Eating Disorders in Special Populations

The nutrition professional should be aware of eating disorders in special population groups, including athletes and adolescents. Athletes may initially diet to reduce body weight for enhanced performance, but this behavior can lead to true eating disorders. These disorders are more prevalent in sports that promote LBM, including running, wrestling, gymnastics, and dance.[160] Female athletes who do not consume adequate caloric intake may experience changes in bone-mineral density typical of osteoporosis and amenorrhea in addition to low body weight. Healthcare professionals who work with adolescents should be aware that this age period has increased vulnerability to EDs because of peer pressure and biological changes in the body that are specific to that age group. A developing trend in EDs includes adolescents with type 1 diabetes mellitus who omit taking insulin as a means of controlling their weight. This has been referred to as *diabulimia*.[152]

TABLE 8 Nutrition interventions recommended by the American Psychiatric Association	
Topic	**Intervention**
Provide education on meal planning	Focus on "when" rather than "what" the patient eats and aid with the establishment of a regular pattern of meals and snacks. Plan the introduction of a variety of foods including "binge foods "and "forbidden foods." Use food exchange lists, food models, and portion-controlled foods to ensure a variety of food choices. Make changes in steps rather than at one time. Include fats from dressings, butter, nuts, seeds, avocado, and olive oil. Provide an outline of several model intake days based on calorie needs. Have patients help develop eating plans that will give them confidence to succeed. Help families develop healthy guidelines for family meals.
Provide accurate nutrition information to patient including on the following topics	Metabolism, energy requirements, determinants of body weight Nutrition myths and misinformation Normal calorie and fat intake Dental health and gut function Calcium intake and osteoporosis Fluid intake Reading nutrition labels
Provide advice on normal eating	Eat for enjoyment and health and aim for flexible and spontaneous eating behaviors. Focus on what others eat and what normal eating really means rather than aiming for a perfect diet. Restrict eating to one room in the house. Sit down when eating and do not engage in other activities while eating. Develop sensitivity to cues for eating: presence of appetite, time of day, social situation, and visual appeal. Use appropriate utensils and eat at a moderate pace. Avoid measuring food. Eat with others when possible.
Review psychological education topics.	Biological and psychological effects of starvation. List consequences of binge eating and purging. Help overcome guilt associated with eating fattening or high calorically dense foods. Provide education on disadvantages of avoiding food and food groups and encourage increasing food choices and food experiences.
Provide advice on stopping weight-loss behaviors.	Help patient refrain from restrictive dieting, break the binge–purge cycle in BN, and restore a healthy weight in AN. Avoid excessive exercise. Comment on stability of weight even when eating behaviors have improved. Support patients to accept and maintain a healthy body weight.
Develop rapport and therapeutic alliance when providing nutrition counseling.	Engage client: show genuine concern; aim for trusting and open relationship, which will help patients share fears and abnormal eating behaviors. This promotes trust in the nutrition professional and increases openness to change. Establish supportive rather than confrontational relationship. Remain nonjudgmental with nonadherence and manipulative behaviors. Show empathy; acknowledge how difficult it is to make changes in food behaviors. Collaborate with the patient by involving patient in food planning and decision making.

(continues)

TABLE 8 (continued)	
Topic	**Intervention**
	Use motivational strategies; discuss barriers to change and examine pros and cons of change. Use goal setting by having patient leave each session with a goal he or she can accomplish. Identify how the goal will benefit the person. Demonstrate skills, including maintaining a sense of humor, being firm and consistent, remaining calm, refraining from power struggles, being persuasive and curious, establishing credibility, and being warm, open, patient, and encouraging.
Use behavioral strategies.	Avoiding weighing between sessions. Develop a hierarchy of food and eating situations and start with the easiest to change. Explain self-monitoring to identify links between emotions and food. To reduce binge eating: limit access to food that encourages binge eating; after episode of binge eating, encourage person to return to usual eating pattern for the next scheduled meal; limit the amount of food available at the meal and discard leftovers; avoid missing snacks or meals; avoid eating from large packages and containers; teach healthy coping behaviors to promote self-control.
Promote practical and social eating skills.	Practice going to a restaurant and eating in a group and for special occasions. Provide advice on shopping, meal preparation, cooking, and meal plans. Discuss the relationship between food and culture to explain eating in social context.
Discuss appetite regulation.	Encourage increased attention to normal hunger and satiety cues. Explain how appetite generally reflects biological needs.
Dietary guidelines during inpatient treatment	Promote a food environment that is planned and secure for consistency and control. Place limitations on foods that patients may refuse to eat; allow three to five dislikes. Discourage the use of caffeinated beverages. Encourage the consumption of a varied diet that includes energy-dense foods; avoid energy-dilute foods and chewing gum.
Refeeding	Introduce food gradually with small frequent feedings to reduce sensations of bloating. Reduce the use of raw fruits and vegetables because of their filling effects. These foods are not calorically dense and delay gastric emptying. Use whole grains and bran to aid in constipation. Advise patients that they will have feelings on being overly full for 2–3 weeks as the body adjusts to food and encourage eating regardless of fullness. Yogurt may help improve immunological markers independently of weight gain. Avoid excessive sodium to reduce the risk of fluid and electrolyte overexpansion. Provide a structured, low-stress environment with support and encouragement.
Meal supervision	Patients should be supervised for one hour after each meal. Set expectations about the amount of food that should be eaten in a set time period. The reintroduction of food can be facilitated by therapist modeling and clinicians' own healthy attitudes about eating and weight. Encouragement from other patients and staff members can help overcome initial resistance to eating. Provide both empathy and understanding of patient's struggle while encouraging consumption of food.

Modified from American Psychiatric Association. American Psychiatric Association; treatment of patients with eating disorders, 3rd ed. *Am J Psychiatry*. 2006;163(7):1-54. Hart, S, Russell, J, Abraham, S. Nutrition and dietetic practice in eating disorder management. *J Hum Nutr Diet*. 2011;24:144-153.

Recap Nutrition assessment and management are integral components of treatment for the ED patient. Specialized training, collaboration with the interdisciplinary team, and communication skills are needed to ensure that the nutrition practitioner is well versed not only in the nutritional care of the ED patient but also in the behavioral aspects of treatment so that nutrition interventions and nutrition counseling can be delivered effectively. There continues to be a need for evidence-based nutrition and behavior therapies for EDs to improve treatment outcomes.

Nutritional Assessment and Management of the HIV Patient

Preview HIV is a retrovirus, an RNA retrovirus that inserts a DNA copy of its genome into host cells, particularly immune cells, to replicate. As a result, the immune cells (known as CD4 or T-cells) become dysfunctional, which leads to cell destruction. Other cells such as disease-fighting macrophages are also rendered dysfunctional. The condition makes it difficult for the body to fight off infections and some other diseases; these **opportunistic infections** take advantage of a weak immune system and signal that the person is suffering from acquired immunodeficiency syndrome (AIDS). As a result, the disease process itself leads to malnutrition and wasting. The infection causes an inflammatory response and can decrease lean body mass.

Prevalence of Human Immunodeficiency Virus

The **human immunodeficiency virus (HIV)** can be passed to others via direct contact with bodily fluids. Transmission to others can occur through unprotected sex, needle sharing, or exposure to HIV-infected blood. A mother with HIV can infect her child during pregnancy, delivery, or breastfeeding.[161,162] Nearly 34 million people in the world today live with HIV infections. Although the global occurrence of AIDS has plateaued, it remains one of the leading causes of death around the world, especially in Africa.[163] In the United States, an estimated 1.1 million people over the age of 13 years live with HIV or AIDS, and infection rates are highest in groups that are the most subject to health disparities.[164] The prevalence of this disease points to the large number of individuals who could benefit from improved medical care for HIV and AIDS, including nutrition care.

Importance of Nutrition in HIV

Nutrition is an essential component in promoting the health and quality of life of individuals living with HIV. Anorexia and inadequate intake are not the only contributors to the development of malnutrition seen in HIV and AIDS patients. Gastrointestinal disorders, including nausea, vomiting, and malabsorption; altered nutrient and metabolite use; increased energy requirements; and side effects of medications used to treat the disease are among the many causes of the impaired nutritional status seen in these individuals.[165] The nutritional complications of the disease may be caused by the HIV infection itself, opportunistic infections, or the medication regimens prescribed for disease management.[166] Nutritional assessment of the HIV patient should include evaluation of anthropometry (including estimation of body cell mass and fat distribution of lipodystrophy), biochemical tests, medication-related side effects, client history, food history, and physical examination, which would include NFPE findings that may influence nutritional status.[167,168,169,170]

Weight Loss in HIV

Weight loss is one sign of disease progression in HIV infection and is indicative of malnutrition.[171] As little as 5% weight loss is associated with increased mortality risk.[172] Typically, weight loss in HIV infection has a disproportionately higher loss of LBM in men and a higher loss of fat in women early in the disease, and increasing LBM loss as the disease progresses.[173] The AIDS wasting syndrome, defined in 1987 by the CDC, is the unintentional weight loss of more than 10% of premorbid body weight.[174]

Medication treatments such as the use of protease inhibitors and highly active antiretroviral therapy (HAART) promote weight increase in these individuals. The weight increase promoted by medication use does not translate into LBM repletion. Medication administration has been associated with a pathologic redistribution of body fat in peripheral areas, fat atrophy, and visceral adiposity known as **lipodystrophy**.[175] This makes the anthropometric assessment of height, body weight, lean body mass, and fat distribution an important component of the nutritional assessment for individuals with HIV. In assessing weight loss, the criteria specified by the Academy and ASPEN can be used to determine whether the weight loss indicates moderate or severe malnutrition.[100] An NPFE should be used to assess for muscle wasting and fat loss, gain, or lipodystrophy, depending on the treatment regimen of the patient.[100]

Biochemical Measurements in HIV

Biochemical measurements are also important parts of the nutritional assessment of HIV patients. **TABLE 9** lists the recommended biochemical measurements for baseline assessment.[165] Metabolic abnormalities associated with the disease can lead to altered use, storage, and excretion of nutrients. These include impaired immune function, side effects of medications (including antiretroviral therapies), infections, and changes in hormonal status. A fasting lipid profile can provide information on lipid metabolism and can be compared to physical assessment in patients who have fat redistribution. Individuals with HIV and evidence of lipodystrophy are known to have increased LDL cholesterol, increased triglycerides, and decreased HDL cholesterol levels. This lipid profile can increase the risk for developing cardiovascular disease.[176] Individuals with a diagnosis of HIV are also known to suffer from altered insulin sensitivity, mitochondrial toxicity, and lactic acidosis.[177,178] Abnormal plasma proteins, micronutrients, and other nutrition-related laboratory values have been associated with an increased mortality risk.[179–181] Laboratory values specifically affected by this disease include albumin, transthyretin, glucose, vitamin B_{12}, C-reactive protein, zinc, and serum iron, to name a few. Abnormal laboratory results are often related to the systemic inflammatory response rather than to true nutritional deficiencies. Anemia of chronic disease is often present in these individuals.[182]

Food- and Nutrition-Related History in HIV

Client and food histories are also a vital component of an accurate nutrition assessment. The following information should be obtained when assessing a patient with HIV:[165,182]

- Current diagnoses including opportunistic infections and chronic illnesses
- Use of alcohol, tobacco, and recreational drugs (some recreational drugs may influence appetite)
- Past surgeries that may affect nutritional status (e.g., gastrointestinal surgeries)
- Current medications, medication management, and medication compliance
- Bowel habits
- Exercise level
- Weight history and changes in weight status
- Food history
- Issues that would affect nutritional intake, including difficulty chewing or swallowing, mouth pain, changes in taste, anorexia, or satiety issues
- Food allergies, intolerances, or aversions
- Vitamin or mineral supplements or herbal therapies
- Social and financial issues that affect food security, including living situation and family and friend support
- Food-preparation abilities and facilities, including food-safety techniques
- Ethnic and religious beliefs

Food–Drug Interactions in HIV

There are many drug–nutrient interactions and medication side effects that the nutrition professional should be cognizant of when conducting a nutrition assessment. **TABLE 10** shows a list of medications and specific directions regarding whether the medication should be taken with or without food.[183] A component of the nutrition assessment

TABLE 9 Recommended biochemical measures for baseline assessment in HIV

Biochemical Parameter
Albumin, prealbumin
Complete blood count with differential
Fasting lipid profile (total cholesterol, HDL cholesterol, LDL cholesterol, TG)
Fasting blood glucose
Renal panel (creatinine, BUN, total calcium, phosphorous, chloride, potassium, CO_2, and sodium)
Liver panel (total protein, alanine aminotransferase, aspartate aminotransferase, alkaline phosphatase, bilirubin, gamma-glutamyl transferase, lactate dehydrogenase, and prothrombin time)
CD4, CD8, and viral load
Serum testosterone
Serum zinc and selenium
Serum vitamin A, folate, and vitamin B_{12}

Adapted from: Earthman, et. Al. Evaluation of nutrition assessment parameters in the presence of human immunodeficiency virus infection. *Nutr Clin Prac.* 2004;19:330-339.

TABLE 10 HIV drugs and food interactions	
Medication	**Food Requirements**
Nucleoside/Nucleotide Reverse Transcriptase Inhibitors	
Abacavir (*Ziagen*)	May be taken with or without food
Emtricitabine (*Emtriva*)	May be taken with or without food
Lamivudine (*Epivir*)	May be taken with or without food
Tenofovir disproxil (*Viread*)	Take with food
Zidovudine (*Retrovir*)	May be taken with or without food, although taking with food may reduce nausea.
Combination Pills	
Atripla (efavirenz, emtricitabine, & tenfovir disoproxil combined)	Take on empty stomach (preferably at bedtime) to reduce incidence of side effects. Avoid taking soon after a high fat meal at this increases risk of side effects.
Lamivudine and zidovudine (sometimes called Cobivir)	May be taken with or without food, although taking with food may reduce nausea
Descovy (tenofovir alafenamide and embtricitabine combined)	Take with or without food
Eviplera (rilpivirine, emtricitabine and tenofovir disproxil combined)	Take with food
Kivexa (lamivudine and abacavir combined	May be taken with or without food
Stribild (elvitegravir, emtricitabine, tenofovir and cobicistat, a boosting agent)	Take with food
Triumeq (dolutegravir, abacavir and lamivudine combined)	May be taken with or without food
Trizivir (zidovudine, lamivudine and abacavir combined)	May be taken with or without food
Truvada (Tenofovir disproxil and emtricitabine combined)	Take with or after food
Non-Nucleoside Reverse Transcriptase Inhibitors	
Efavirenz (*Sustiva*)	Take on empty stomach (preferably at bedtime) to reduce incidence of side effects. Avoid taking soon after a high fat meal at this increases risk of side effects.
Etravirine (*Intelence*)	Take with or after food (within two hours after a main meal or within ½ hour after a snack).
Nevirapine (*Viramune and Viramune prolonged-release*)	Take with or without food.
Rilpivirine (*Edurant*)	

TABLE 10 *(continued)*

Protease Inhibitors	
Atazanavir (*Reyataz*) (taken with a booster dose of ritonavir or cobcistat)	Take with or after food (within two hours after a main meal or within ½ hour after a snack).
Darunavir (Prezista) (always taken with a booster dose of ritonavir or cobicistat	Taken with or after food (within ½ hour after a meal).
Fosamprenavir (*Telzir*) (usually taken with ritonavir)	May be taken with or without food.
Lopinavir/ritonavir (*Kaletra*)	Take with or without food
Ritonavir (*Norvir*)	May be taken with or without food, but taken with fatty meal minimizes risk of nausea.
Tipranavir (*Aptivus*) (must be taken with ritonavir)	Take with or after food to reduce the side effects.
Fusion and Entry Inhibitors	
Maraviroc (Celsnetri)	May be taken with or without food.
Enfuvirtide (*Fuzeon*)	Administered by injection. No food restrictions
Integrase Inhibitors	
Dolutegravir (*Tivicay*)	May be taken with or without foods. If patient has some resistance to integrase inhibitors, it should be taken with food.
Raltegravir (*Isentress*)	May be taken with or without food; do not chew, crush, or split tablets.

Modified from: Interactions between drugs and food. AIDSMAP. Available at: http://www.aidsmap.com/Interactions-between-drugs-and-food/page/3080183/#item3080185nd food., Updated August 2016. Retrieved November 12, 2016.

should include a discussion on current medications and timing of medications (in relation to meals and dosing) in efforts to assist the patient in assessing the need for changes to promote medication efficacy. For instance, some medications for HIV should be taken with food; if the patient skips a meal, the medication may cause nausea, which can further interfere with promoting an optimum nutrition status and affect nutrition status. In addition, if the patient is taking medications such as isoniazid (an antitubercular medication) for opportunistic infections, this increases the requirement for pyridoxine, folate, niacin, and magnesium. For optimum effectiveness, these medications should be taken with food.

A clinical evaluation of gastrointestinal (GI) function is recommended in patients with HIV. In a study of 671 HIV-infected patients, 88% exhibited at least one abnormality of GI function.[184] Diarrhea was present in 38.9%, a history of liver disease was present in 40.3%, and 12.2% had at least one stool pathogen. Other GI complications of the disease include malabsorption, nausea and vomiting, stomatitis or odynophagia, dysgeusia, and oral or esophageal candidiasis (thrush). Many of the symptoms occur as a result of opportunistic infections or medication side effects. A summary of GI concerns in HIV patients is depicted in **TABLE 11**. An NFPE is useful in assessing the HIV patient for malnutrition as well as for signs of vitamin and mineral deficiencies. HIV patients may exhibit iron-deficiency anemia. This can occur as a side effect of some of the medications used to treat the disease. An NFPE may help identify pale conjunctiva and koilonychias.

TABLE 11 Problems observed in HIV-infected individuals

Problem	Possible Causes and/or Implications
Anorexia	Opportunistic infections and medications
Diarrhea	Opportunistic infections, including foodborne infections including *Salmonella*, *Campylobacter*, and *Cryptosporidium*; medications; or HIV-associated enteropathy (no enteric pathogen identified)
Malabsorption	Opportunistic infections (e.g., *Mycobacterium*, avium complex, *Cytomegalovirus*); HIV-associated enteropathy; symptoms may include steatorrhea, bloating, or diarrhea
Nausea and vomiting	Non-Hodgkin's and Burkett's lymphomas; medications; food-borne opportunistic infections
Stomatitis	Oral ulcers, oral or esophageal candidiasis can cause sore mouth or painful swallowing or both
Dysgeusia	Altered taste caused by medications or zinc deficiency
Oral or esophageal problem	Yeast infection association with sore mouth and oral or esophageal ulcers, candidiasis (thrush), pain with eating or swallowing.

Adapted from Earthman, et. Al. Evaluation of nutrition assessment parameters in the presence of human immunodeficiency virus infection. *Nutr Clin Prac*. 2004;19:330-339.

Importance of Food Safety in HIV

Because the HIV patient's immune function is depressed, food safety is a critical topic to review during the food- and nutrition-related history and MNT. The US Food and Drug Administration has developed online material to reduce the risk of foodborne illness. This tool describes foods that can potentially be a greater risk in persons with HIV or AIDS.[185] All foods—meats, poultry, shellfish, and eggs—should not be consumed raw, and raw milk should be avoided. Raw sprouts should be cooked; hot dogs and deli meats should be reheated to 165 °F. Soft cheeses should be avoided, and hard cheeses and processed cheeses should be chosen. All raw vegetables should be thoroughly washed or cooked. Assurance of a safe water supply is also critical in preventing opportunistic infections.

Nutritional Management of HIV

Since the success of HAART in 1996 to treat HIV, the nutritional management of the disease has changed. In the early years of HIV treatment, the major nutritional concern was wasting or "slim disease," but with effective medical therapy, new complications of medical progress have surfaced, including insulin resistance, fat redistribution, dyslipidemia, lactic acidosis, food safety, and bone abnormalities. Even though modern HIV management requires significant expertise in dealing with these nutrition issues, there have not yet been guidelines issued that specifically target the nutritional care of HIV patients.[186] Despite the use of HAART, undernutrition or wasting continues to be a concern, especially in developing countries that do not have access to medical treatments. MNT is indicated when significant weight loss (> 5% in three months) or a significant loss of BCM (> 5% in three months) has occurred. MNT should be considered when BMI is below 18.5 kg/m^2. The combination of oral food and enteral nutrition is appropriate. However, if oral intake is possible, nutrition intervention should be implemented in the following steps: nutrition counseling, calorie-dense, high-protein food choices, and oral nutritional supplements. Enteral or parenteral nutrition should be used if adequate intake cannot be achieved orally. Protein intake should achieve 1.2 g/kg per day and may be increased to 1.5 g/kg per day in acute illness. Goals of nutritional support include an improved nutritional status, decreased functional impairment from undernutrition (muscular fatigue), improved tolerance to antiretroviral treatment, alleviated GI symptoms (nausea, diarrhea, bloating), and improved quality of life.[187] The nutritional management of conditions related to HAART and prolonged survival of the HIV patient, including dyslipidemia and bone abnormalities, should be based on current guidelines for these disorders.

Nutrition assessment and management of the HIV patient is critical to survival. Nutrition counseling and nutrition counseling with oral nutrition supplements have shown to positively influence health outcomes in HIV.[188,189,190]

Recap The nutrition professional is an important part of the interprofessional team who not only addresses undernutrition but also implements nutrition interventions that address the secondary complications related to medication management and the increased survival rate of patients with HIV.

Mini Nutritional Assessment

Preview Although nutrition screens do not provide the entire clinical picture, they do help identify those at nutritional risk so that MNT can be initiated.

Development of the Mini Nutritional Assessment

The development of the Mini Nutritional Assessment started in 1989 when researchers in geriatric practice identified the need for a nutrition screening and assessment tool to identify institutionalized, frail, and older adults. Nutrition assessments were not then routinely performed in clinical practice outside the United States. The goal was to develop a nutrition-assessment tool that would be analogous to the Mini-Mental Status Exam, a tool used to assess cognitive function. The ideal nutrition-assessment tool needed to be reliable, inexpensive, and quick to perform.[191] The MNA was initially validated in 1990–1991 and further validated in the New Mexico Aging Process Study, a longitudinal survey on nutrition and aging in 2001 by the Nestlé Research Centre in Switzerland. In 2001, an MNA short form (MNA-SF) was developed and validated.[192] Since 1994, the MNA has been translated into 24 languages. Many studies continue to evaluate the sensitivity, specificity, and reliability of the tool in different settings and different countries. In both medical practice and clinical research, the MNA is the most widely used tool for nutritional screening and assessment in older adults.

Completing the MNA

The MNA helps categorize older adults as well nourished, at risk of malnutrition, or malnourished. Its 18 self-reported questions were derived from the four parameters of assessment: anthropometric, general, diet and food history, and self-assessment. The screen is performed as a two-step process. **FIGURE 3** depicts a full MNA tool. The MNA-SF can be completed as a first-step screening tool to determine if further evaluation is needed. The first six items on the MNA makes up the MNA-SF (Part 1, Screening), which can help detect a decline in intake or appetite over the preceding three months, chewing or swallowing problems, digestive issues, weight loss in the previous three months, current mobility impairment, an acute illness or major stress in the previous three months, a neuropsychological problem (dementia or depression), and a decrease in BMI.

If the MNA-SF shows the individual to be at nutritional risk, then the full MNA (Part 2, Assessment) can be completed. The second part of the MNA assesses living arrangements, the presence of polypharmacy, pressure injuries, the number of complete meals eaten daily, the amount and frequency of specific foods and fluids, and the mode of feeding. The individual reports nutrition and health status, and the screener measures height and weight (to calculate BMI), midarm circumference, and calf circumference.[191,193] The MNA-SF takes only a few minutes to complete; if nutrition risk is noted, then completing the assessment section of the MNA takes an additional 10–15 minutes. Scores from both parts are added to determine risk of malnutrition. If cognitive impairment is present, caregiver or healthcare staff may provide the information on meal intakes and weight changes.

The MNA in Various Clinical Settings

The MNA has been evaluated in older adults in different clinical settings, including community, home care, outpatients, hospital, and long-term care patients with good acceptability and validity. When different settings are compared for the prevalence of malnutrition, there are extremely large differences per settings. The presence of malnutrition in the community has been reported as 1%–2%;

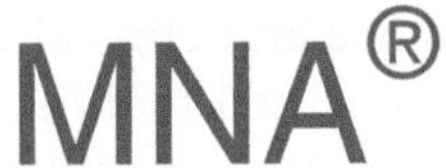

Nestlé
NutritionInstitute

Last name: First name:

Sex: Age: Weight, kg: Height, cm: Date:

Complete the screen by filling in the boxes with the appropriate numbers. Total the numbers for the final screening score.

Screening

A Has food intake declined over the past 3 months due to loss of appetite, digestive problems, chewing or swallowing difficulties?
0 = severe decrease in food intake
1 = moderate decrease in food intake
2 = no decrease in food intake ☐

B Weight loss during the last 3 months
0 = weight loss greater than 3 kg (6.6 lbs)
1 = does not know
2 = weight loss between 1 and 3 kg (2.2 and 6.6 lbs)
3 = no weight loss ☐

C Mobility
0 = bed or chair bound
1 = able to get out of bed / chair but does not go out
2 = goes out ☐

D Has suffered psychological stress or acute disease in the past 3 months?
0 = yes 2 = no ☐

E Neuropsychological problems
0 = severe dementia or depression
1 = mild dementia
2 = no psychological problems ☐

F1 Body Mass Index (BMI) (weight in kg) / (height in m)^2
0 = BMI less than 19
1 = BMI 19 to less than 21
2 = BMI 21 to less than 23
3 = BMI 23 or greater ☐

IF BMI IS NOT AVAILABLE, REPLACE QUESTION F1 WITH QUESTION F2.
DO NOT ANSWER QUESTION F2 IF QUESTION F1 IS ALREADY COMPLETED.

F2 Calf circumference (CC) in cm
0 = CC less than 31
3 = CC 31 or greater ☐

Screening score
(max. 14 points) ☐☐

12-14 points: ☐ Normal nutritional status
8-11 points: ☐ At risk of malnutrition
0-7 points: ☐ Malnourished

FIGURE 3 Mini-Nutrition Assessment.

Reproduced from Mini Nutritional Assessment (MNA). Nestlé Nutrition institute. https://www.mna-elderly.com/forms/mini/mna_mini_english.pdf. Retrieved July 1, 2017.

in home care 4%–9%; in outpatients 9%; in hospitalized patients 20%–23%; and in long-term care patients 21%–37%.[194,195] In 11 studies that evaluated cognitively impaired individuals, the prevalence of malnutrition was 15% (range of 0%–62%), and the risk of malnutrition was 44% (range of 19%–87%).[191] **FIGURE 4** indicates how the scoring on the MNA can be used to guide nutrition interventions.

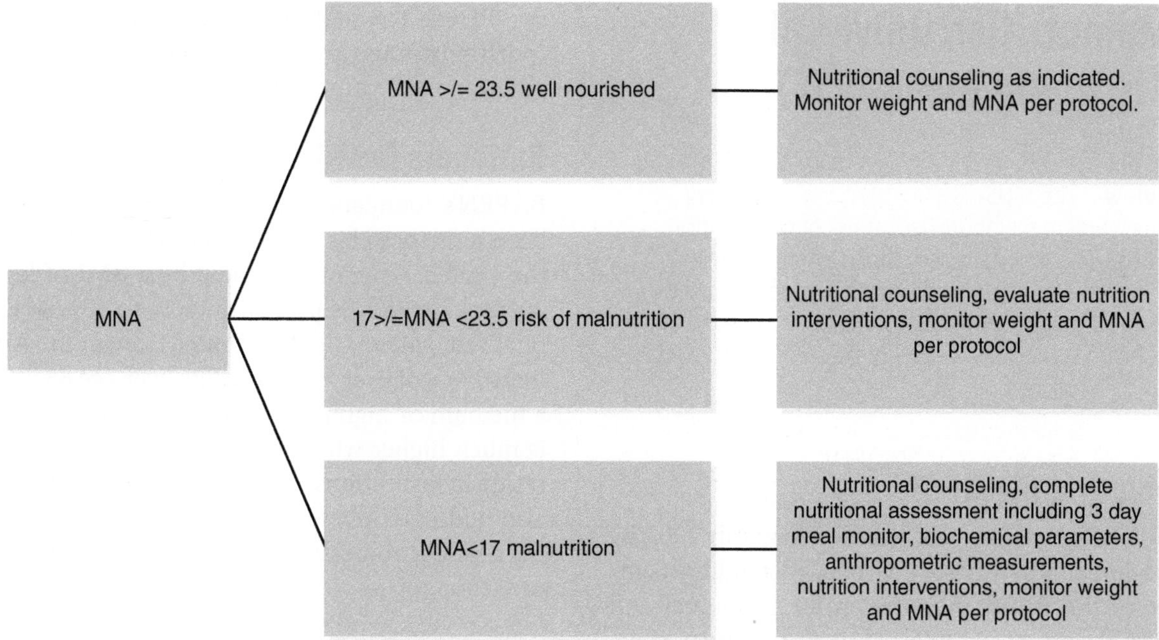

FIGURE 4 The MNA diagnostic tool for malnutrition and a guide for nutritional intervention.

Data from Lim, SL, et al. *J Parenter Enteral Nutr*. 2016;40(7):966-972.

The MNA in Nutrition Research Studies

More than 200 studies have been published that used the MNA in clinical research. The International Association of Gerontology and International Academy of Nutrition and Aging Task Force recommends the use of the MNA for nutrition studies in older adults.[191] Intervention studies have noted associations with improvements in MNA scores. Both the MNA and MNA-SF have been found to be sensitive, specific, and accurate in identifying nutritional risk in older adults.[195] The MNA is widely used in nutrition research studies focusing on older adults. Christner reported that both the MNA and the MNA-SF were useful for evaluating malnutrition risk in older hospitalized patients when compared to the Nutrition Risk Screening 2002 (NRS-2002) tool.[196] Agreement between the MNA and MNA-SF was highly significant for malnutrition and for patients at risk of malnutrition ($p < 0.001$), whereas no agreement was found between the MNA-SF and the NRS 2002. The MNA indicated that 91.1% of the older hospitalized patients were either malnourished or at risk of malnutrition; the MNA-SF indicated that 93.4% were malnourished or at risk. The NRS 2002, however, revealed that only 66.0% of patients fell into the malnourished or at-risk category, which was significantly different from the MNA and MNA-SF results.

An iteration of the MNA-SF has been developed for patients undergoing hemodialysis, because the short form was found to underestimate the risk of malnutrition. However, research comparing the results obtained using the full MNA and the subjective global assessment (SGA) tools yielded comparable outcomes. The modification to increase accuracy in identifying malnutrition in individuals receiving hemodialysis treatment is an example of a disease-specific MNA-SF nutritional screen. Dubbed the MNA-T1, this screen switched the self-reported nutritional status questions with neuropsychological problems.[197] Other derivations of the MNA and MNA-SF will probably be developed to address specific conditions and diseases.

Limitations of the MNA

Although no specific limitations of the MNA-SF nutritional screen and the MNA nutritional assessment have been noted, the MNA is specific to older adults and is not as reliable in predicting malnutrition and risks as the MUST is for younger adults (20 to 64 years of age).[198]

Recap The MNA and the MNA-SF are useful and ready-to-use tools for older adults.

Malnutrition Universal Screening Tool (MUST)

Preview The MUST is a five-step tool to identify adults who are malnourished, at risk of malnutrition, or obese. This tool includes management guidelines that can be used to initiate nutrition interventions or care plans to address risk factors. It can be used in all healthcare settings as well as in the community, and by all care workers.

Completing the MUST

The MUST screening tool was developed in 2003 by the Malnutrition Advisory Group, a standing committee of the British Association for Parenteral and Enteral Nutrition (BAPEN).[199] It is the most commonly used nutrition-screening tool in the United Kingdom and is also used in other countries. In addition to the standard screening tool, a MUST calculator, a Malnutrition Self-Screening Tool, and a mobile application are available to clinicians. The MUST is available in six languages, including English.

To use the tool, go to http://www.bapen.org.uk/pdfs/must/must_full.pdf. To complete the MUST, the clinician must complete the steps listed in **TABLE 12**.

Rationale for MUST Development

BAPEN's foundation for developing the MUST has been influenced by the overall level of malnutrition in the United Kingdom. Defined by a BMI of less than 20, malnutrition is present in 10% to 40% of all hospitalized patients in the United Kingdom. An estimated one of every seven adults over age 65 years has a medium or high risk for malnutrition. This statistic is much higher when the number of individuals that reside in institutions is taken into account. The MUST also addresses obesity (BMI >30). Obesity increases the risk of chronic disease prevalence as well as healthcare costs.

Validity of the MUST

The MUST has been validated in hospital inpatients and has been shown to predict clinical outcomes, including length of hospital stay, discharge destination from the hospital, rate of admission to the hospital, number of physician visits, and overall mortality. Patients with

TABLE 12 Steps to complete the MUST screen

Step Number	Description
Step 1	Measure height and weight to get a BMI score using chart provided. If unable to measure height, use recently documented or self-reported height; or use other method of determining height—demispan, ulna, or knee height. If height or weight cannot be obtained, use subjective criteria to assist in judgment of nutritional risk.
Step 2	Note percentage unplanned weight loss and score using tables provided.
Step 3	Establish acute disease effect and score.
Step 4	Add scores from steps 1, 2, and 3 to obtain overall risk of malnutrition.
Step 5	Use management guidelines or local policy to develop care plan.
Calculating screen score	Scoring for the tool rates items as 0, 1, or 2 as follows: ■ BMI 20.0 kg/m² = 0 points; 18.5–20.0 kg/m² = 1 point; < 18.5 kg/m² = 2 points ■ Weight loss within the last 3 to 6 months less than 5% = 0 points; 5%–10% = 1 point; > 10% = 2 points ■ Presence of acute disease: add 2 points in the case of acutely ill patients with no nutritional intake or likelihood of no nutritional intake for more than 5 days. ■ A cumulative score of 0 indicates low risk of malnutrition; a score of 1 point indicates a moderate risk of malnutrition; a score of ≥ 2 points strongly suggests increased risk of malnutrition.

Modified from Stratton RJ, Hackston A, Longmore D, et al. Malnutrition in hospital outpatients and inpatients: Prevalence, concurrent validity and ease of use of the Malnutrition Universal Screening Tool (MUST) for adults. *Br J Nutr*. 2004;92:799-808.

higher MUST scores have up to two to four longer LOS in high- than low-risk patients in elderly medical hospital wards.[200] In the community, the MUST is a predictor of rate of hospital admissions and physician visits. It has also contributed to the body of literature that supports nutrition interventions that improve patient outcomes. In a study of 150 hospital admissions for people ages 85 ± 5.5 years, the MUST screen identified 58% of patients are at nutrition risk. Although only 56% of the patients could be weighed, the authors indicated that all the patients could be screened with the MUST by using the subjective criteria for weight (see MUST tool under "Online Resources"). Those patients with no measured or reported weight had a greater risk of malnutrition and poorer clinical outcomes than those who could be weighed. Researchers concluded that the MUST screen could be used to determine nutrition risk for all patients, even those who cannot be weighed.[201]

Evaluation of the MUST

Since the introduction of the MUST, many studies have been conducted in a variety of healthcare settings and geographic locations, and with different patient types and medical diagnoses. A study of nursing home residents attempted to determine the agreement between the MNA, the MNA-SF, the Nutrition Risk Screening (NRS-2002), and the MUST.[202] Predictive value and survival analysis were performed to compare the nutrition risk classifications measured from the different tools. The MNA was considered the reference tool in the study. Results identified 22.6% of women and 17% of men as malnourished. In addition, 56.7% of females and 61% of males were at risk of malnutrition. Agreement between the MNA, NRS-2002, and the MUST was considered to be "fair." All of the screening tools point toward a significant association between malnutrition and mortality. Since the MUST and the NRS-2002 do not assess the functional, psychological and cognitive elements that are important risk factors in older adults residing in institutions, the MNA has been identified as the most appropriate tool in this care setting.

A study focusing on nursing home residents compared the use of the MNA, the NRS-2002, and the MUST. The concluded that the MNA was the most appropriate tool for these individuals. Both the NRS-2002 and MUST identified malnutrition in 8.6% of the 200 nursing home residents, whereas the MNA identified malnutrition in 15.4% of the sample.[203] Based on these results, the MNA may be more sensitive at capturing the risk of elderly patients who may be at marginal risk of malnutrition and could benefit from nutrition interventions.

In a comparison study of the MUST and the MNA-SF in 149 older hospitalized patients (65–99 years of age), findings indicated a moderate agreement between the MUST and the MNA-SF. Both screens predicted mortality, but the LOS increased progressively as risk level increased in the MNA-SF; this was not reported with the MUST. Patients with normal risk on the MNA-SF had an average LOS of six days, those "at risk" had an average LOS of nine days, and the malnourished individuals had an average LOS of 12 days. The MNA-SF was also noted to be superior to the MUST in predicting hospital readmission rates.[204]

Disease- or condition-specific studies have been conducted comparing nutrition-screening tools, including the MUST. One study compared the adequacy of the MNA-SF, NRS-2002, and MUST nutritional screening tools in 215 post–hip repair surgical patients (71.6% female; mean age 83.5 ± 6.09 years). For this sample, the MNA identified 95 individuals at risk of malnutrition and 25 malnourished. The MUST results were different, identifying 31 individuals at low risk for malnutrition and 13 at high risk. The NRS-2002 identified 70 individuals at medium risk and 11 at high risk for malnutrition. No differences in LOS and complications were noted between the patients' nutritional statuses of each screening tool, but only the MNA-SF predicted that well-nourished patients would have lower rates of readmission over a six-month follow-up period. The MNA-SF was the most accurate tool at predicting mortality 36 months after surgery.[205]

Malnutrition Self-Screening Tool

A Malnutrition Self-Screening Tool has been developed by BAPEN that is based on the MUST. An electronic version of this tool can be viewed at http://www.malnutritionselfscreening.org/self-screening.html. The validity of the Malnutrition Self-Screening Tool was determined in a study involving outpatient individuals with irritable bowel disease (IBD). Malnutrition is a common comorbidity affecting clinical outcomes in patients with IBD.[206] This was a prospective validation study with a total sample of 154 individuals suffering from IBD. The self-administered tool was completed by the patients and followed by a MUST screen conducted by healthcare professionals. All patients were able to complete the screen independently. There was a high level of agreement between the MUST conducted by healthcare staff and the self-assessment completed by the IBD individuals. Ninety-six percent of the patients reported that the Malnutrition

Self-Screening Tool was easy to understand and complete. Use of self-screening nutritional-risk tools can help identify patients who need additional nutrition support without increasing time for staff to conduct the evaluation. Self-screening tools are appropriate for community-living adults who are able to complete the tool with no or limited assistance. This format can help clinicians and researchers identify a greater number of patients at nutritional risk for malnutrition.[207]

Limitations of the MUST

Although it has been determined that the MUST is a valid screening tool for the identification of malnutrition in adults, its use has several limitations. The tool requires a height and weight to determine BMI. If the height and weight cannot be obtained, then the subjective criteria outlined by the tool can be used to determine nutrition risk and the parameter that affects the final score. Several studies, especially the ones using older adults as their sample, have reported that the MNA or the MNA-SF is a more accurate indicator of nutritional risk and predictor of LOS, hospital admission, and mortality. A positive aspect of the tool is that training time for the healthcare professional is less than one hour and the self-screening tool is easy for community-living adults to complete without assistance.[200]

Recap To prevent malnutrition and identify individuals at risk, nutrition screening should be conducted for community-dwelling adults. Any of the validated nutritional screening tools discussed thus far can be used to help identify malnutrition and the chance of reducing the incidence of comorbid conditions that are exacerbated by inadequate nutritional status.

Subjective Global Assessment

Preview Although the MNA and the MUST are nutrition-screening tools, the **subjective global assessment (SGA)** is a validated nutritional assessment tool that involves evaluating five components of a patient's medical history (weight status and dietary-intake changes, gastrointestinal symptoms, functional capacity, and metabolic stress from disease) and three components of physical examination (muscle wasting, fat depletion, and nutrition-related edema).[208–210]

Subjective Global Assessment Seven-Point Scale

The SGA consists of a subjective summation of the eight components that classifies patients into one of three categories: A = well nourished, B = moderately malnourished, and C = severely malnourished.[208] **FIGURE 5** shows the conventional SGA tool. The SGA has been researched in different patient types and has been determined to be a valid assessment tool in older adults, clinical and surgical hospital patients, rehabilitation center patients, critical-care patients, and children.[211,212,213,214]

Developed almost 30 years ago, the SGA is not an efficient tool for detecting small changes in nutrition status during follow-up assessments.[215,216] To make the SGA more sensitive in detecting small changes in nutrition status, the tool was expanded to a seven-point scale. The seven-point SGA scale was tested in a study with a patient sample consisting of 680 peritoneal dialysis patients. Ratings for nutrition status range from one to seven, with ratings of one to two denoting severe malnutrition, three to five indicating moderate malnutrition, and six to seven indicating a well-nourished individual. The revisions accomplished the goal of making the tool more sensitive to detect small changes without sacrificing the original ratings of the conventional SGA.[217] The sensitivity of the seven-point SGA was further confirmed in a study of 67 adult inpatients assessed as malnourished (per the SGA) and then reassessed using both the conventional SGA and the seven-point SGA at one, three, and five months after the baseline assessment. It took a significantly shorter time to note a one-point change using the seven-point SGA than the conventional SGA tool. This tool can be used to help identify individuals needing nutrition interventions.[218] See **FIGURE 6** for the seven-point SGA tool.

Patient-Generated Subjective Global Assessment

Another iteration of the SGA is the **patient-generated subjective global assessment (PG-SGA)**. This tool has been specifically developed for patients with cancer.[219] When compared to the conventional SGA, the PG-SGA includes additional questions regarding nutritional symptoms and short-term weight loss. The PG-SGA was designed so that patients could complete their medical histories using checkboxes. The physical exam is then completed by the healthcare professional, physician,

A. History
1. Weight Change
Maximum weight _____ Wt. 1 year ago _____ Wt. 6 months ago _____ Current Wt. _____
Overall loss in past 6 months: Amount = _________ lbs; % loss _________.
Change in past 2 weeks: _____ increase;
_____ no change;
_____ decrease.
Other history: (Change in clothing size, loose fitting clothes, etc.)
A = No significant change; B = 5-10% weight loss; C = 10% or more sustained weight loss
2. Dietary-intake change (relative to normal)
(Have eating patterns changed over last several weeks or months? Has amount of food eaten changes? Are certain foods they used to eat that they no longer eat? What happens if they try to eat more? How does typical breakfast, lunch, dinner compare with 6 to 12 months ago?
A = No significant change; B = poor but improving or borderline but declining; C = starvation, unable to eat.
3. Gastrointestinal symptoms (that persisted for > 2 weeks)
_____ None (A); _____ Some symptoms (B) (nausea, vomiting, diarrhea); _____ Many symptoms (C)
4. Functional capacity
_____ No dysfunction (e. g. full capacity) (A)
_____ Dysfunction: Mild (B); _____ Severe (C) _____ Duration = # _____ weeks.
5. Disease and its relation to nutritional requirements
Metabolic demand (stress): _____ No stress (A); _____ Low—moderate stress (B); _____ High stress (C)

B. Physical (for each trait specify: A = normal, B = mild-moderate, C = severe)
__________ loss of subcutaneous fat (triceps, chest)
__________ muscle wasting (quadriceps, deltoids)
__________ ankle edema
__________ sacral edema
__________ ascites

C. SGA rating (select one)
__________ A = Well-nourished
__________ B = Moderately (or suspected of being) malnourished
__________ C = Severely malnourished

FIGURE 5 Subjective global assessment.

Adapted from: Subjective Global Assessment. Covinsky, KE, Martin, GE, Beyth, RJ, et al. The relationship between clinical assessments of nutritional status and adverse outcomes in older hospitalized medical patients. *J Am Geriatr Soc.* 1999;47:532-538.

nurse, or RDN. The Scored PG-SGA is an advanced version of the PG-SGA. This version allows for a numerical score to be generated that indicates whether a patient is well nourished, moderately nourished, or severely malnourished. For each component of the Scored PG-SGA, points from zero to four are assigned to each criterion, depending on the effect of the symptom on nutritional status. The total points are calculated, and the score is used to guide the level of nutrition intervention appropriate for the risk level.[220] The Scored PG-SGA was also evaluated as an assessment tool to identify malnutrition in older adults admitted to rehabilitation centers, in efforts to address the strong evidence showing malnutrition is both underrecognized and underdiagnosed in rehabilitation settings.[221] Fifty-seven older adults admitted to a rehabilitation center were assessed for malnutrition using the Scored PG-SGA, the MNA, or the *International Statistical Classification of Diseases and Health Related Problems*, 10th revision, *Australian Modification* (ICD10-AM) to determine the validity of the tools and the prevalence of malnutrition.[211,222] The incidence of malnutrition varied, with the nutrition assessment tool used with 28% of patients noted to be malnourished with the MNA, 46% with the ICD10-AM, and 53% with the Scored PG-SGA. The Scored PG-SGA showed strong concurrent validity, whereas the MNA indicated moderate concurrent validity. The Scored PG-SGA nutrition assessment tool was determined to be suitable for nutrition assessment in the older adult population, although caution must be taken with the MNA to identify all patients at risk of malnutrition.

Point SGA tool

Assessment criteria

Weight	Rating	7	6	5	4	3	2	1
Weight loss		0%	<3%	3-<5%	5-<7%	7-<10%	10-<15%	>/=15 %
Weight increase trend	Add one point							
Weight loss trend- in one month	Deduct 1 point							
Intake (in the last 2 weeks)		100%	>75%-100%	50-75%- but increasing	50-75%-- no change or decreasing	<50% but increasing	<50%-no change or decreasing	<25%
Gastrointestinal symptoms (present for > 2 weeks): nausea, vomiting, diarrhea		No symptoms	Very few intermittent symptoms (once/ day)	Some symptoms (2-3 times/ week) improving	Some symptoms (2-3 times/ week) No change	Some symptoms (2-3 times/ week) getting worse	Some or all symptoms >3 times/ day	
Functional status (nutrition related)		Full functional capacity		Mid to moderate loss of stamina			Severe loss of functional ability (bedridden)	
Disease affecting nutritional needs		No increase in metabolic demands		Mild to moderate increase in metabolic demands			Drastic increase in metabolic demands	
Muscle waste (at least 3 areas)		No depletion		Mild to moderate depletion			Severe depletion	
Fat stores		No depletion		Mild to moderate depletion			Severe depletion	
Edema (nutrition related)		No edema		Mild to moderate edema			Severe edema	
Nutritional status		Well nourished		Mild to moderately malnourished			Severely malnourished	
Overall SGA rating (select one)		**7**	**6**	**5**	**4**	**3**	**2**	**1**

FIGURE 6 Seven-point SGA tool.

Data from Lim SL, Lin XH, Daniels L. Seven-Point Subjective Global Assessment Is More Time Sensitive Than Conventional Subjective Global Assessment in Detecting Nutrition Changes. *J Parenter Enteral Nutr*. 2016;40(7):966-972.

Evaluation of the Subjective Global Assessment Tool

In a systematic literature view, Fink et al. reported that several nutrition screening tools are more sensitive than the SGA in identifying nutrition risk in patients. Based on their analysis, the NRS 2002 was a better predictor of postoperative complications and the Mini Nutrition Assessment screening tool was reported to be the best suited for elderly hospitalized patients.[223] Note that this review was only based only on the conventional SGA and does not reflect the iterations of the SGA that may be more sensitive to changes in nutrition status—namely, the seven-point SGA, the PG-SGA, and the Scored PG-SGA.

Recap When the conventional SGA was developed in the late 1980s, the physical examination for fat loss, muscle wasting, and edema was typically performed by a physician or advanced-practice nurse; however, with the training of other healthcare professionals on nutrition-focused physical examination, however, by training other healthcare professionals to perform NFPEs, the SGA can be completed by any trained healthcare professional. RDNs trained to complete an NFPE are able to conduct an SGA and use other nutritional assessment tools to assess for malnutrition and promptly implement nutrition interventions.

▸ Chapter Summary

A complete and thorough nutrition assessment is based on gathering all factors that can affect nutritional status. Anthropometric and biochemical data as well as medical and food- and nutrition-related history must be assembled. This data can be used to confirm or refute nutrition-focused physical findings to determine the presence of nutritional problem(s).

Adult malnutrition has been defined by the Academy and ASPEN collaboration in recent years, and parameters have been established that will help the clinician determine the incidence of malnutrition in different healthcare settings. In addition, evidence-based formulas have been developed and validated to determine energy, protein, and fluid needs in various conditions and disease states.

Two specific nutrition-related conditions have been reviewed—HIV infection and eating disorders. Many other conditions and diseases, however, require specialized nutrition interventions, including diabetes, kidney disease, and heart disease, among others. Anthropometric, biochemical, client, and food- and nutrition-related history as well as nutrition-focused physical findings are all important aspects to consider when completing a nutritional assessment for these and other conditions or disease states.

Several nutrition screening and assessment tools have been developed to aid clinicians in determining nutritional risk, and these tools help identify and intervene early to prevent the development of severe malnutrition. These tools have been validated in various healthcare settings to help not only nutrition professionals but also all healthcare professionals in identifying nutritional risk and promote referral to RDNs for prompt nutrition interventions.

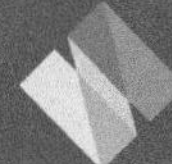

CASE STUDY

Anorexia Nervosa

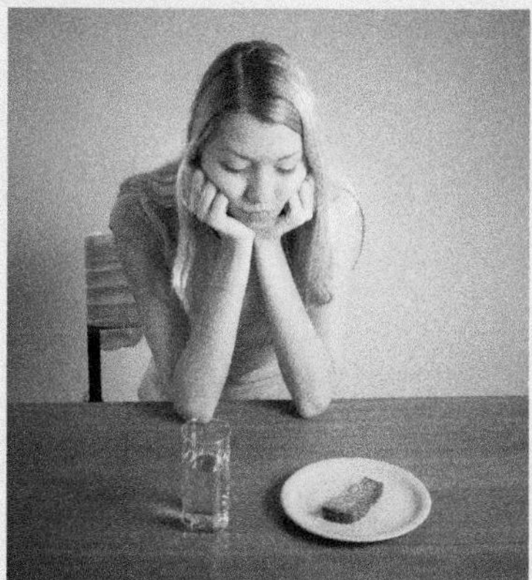

Dawna, a 26-year-old woman, was admitted to the hospital with a diagnosis of anorexia nervosa and long-standing history of restrictive-eating behavior with purging. She had lost one-third of her body weight over 6 months. On admission, Dawna was 5'6" tall and weighed 82 lbs, with a BMI of 13.2. Her resting heart rate was 50 beats per minute. She was afebrile. Laboratory values included C-reactive protein (0.7 mg/dL), white blood cell count (6,200 mm^3), prealbumin (25 mg/dL), and fasting blood glucose (75 mg/dL). Dawna exhibited generalized loss of muscle and subcutaneous fat. Other findings included lanugo hairs. Markedly underweight status was evident, with weight loss of 42 lbs over 6 months. Midarm muscle circumference measurement was below the fifth percentile.

Questions:

1. What malnutrition syndrome would you anticipate in a patient who presents with anorexia nervosa? How would you confirm this?
   a. Severe malnutrition in the context of chronic illness
   b. Severe malnutrition in the context of environmental or social circumstances
   c. Severe malnutrition in the context of acute injury
   d. Mild or moderate malnutrition in the context of chronic illness
2. What factors indicate the type of malnutrition diagnosed?
3. Consider Dawna's history and clinical diagnosis, clinical signs and results from a physical examination, anthropometric data, laboratory indicators, dietary intake, and functional outcomes. Would you suspect reduced handgrip? Why?

Use **TABLES A** and **B**, which describe the clinical characteristics to be used to identify, document, and support a diagnosis of malnutrition.

TABLE A Characteristics to support a diagnosis of malnutrition						
	Malnutrition in Acute Illness or Injury		**Malnutrition in Chronic Illness**		**Malnutrition in Social or Environmental Circumstances**	
Clinical Characteristics	Nonsevere or moderate malnutrition	Severe malnutrition	Nonsevere or moderate malnutrition	Severe malnutrition	Nonsevere or moderate malnutrition	Severe malnutrition
Intake	<75% of estimated energy needs for >7 days	≤50% of estimated energy needs for ≥5 days	<75% of estimated energy needs for ≥1 month	<75% of estimated energy needs for ≥1 month	<75% of estimated energy needs for ≥3 month	<50% of estimated energy needs for ≥1 month
Weight Loss	1–2% in one week 5% in one month 7.5% in three months	>2% in one week >5% in one month >7.5% in three months	5% in one month 7.5% in three months 10% in six months 20% in 12 months	>5% in one month >7.5% in three months >10% in six months >20% in 12 months	5% in one month 7.5% in three months 10% in six months 20% in 12 months	>5% in one month >7.5% in three months >10% in six months >20% in 12 months
Body Fat	Mild	Moderate	Mild	Moderate	Mild	Moderate
Muscle Mass	Mild		Mild		Mild	
Fluid Accumulation/ Edema	Mild	Moderate to severe	Mild	Severe	Mild	Severe
Reduced Handgrip	Not applicable	Measurably reduced	Not applicable	Measurably reduced	Not applicable	Measurably reduced

Note: A minimum of two of the six clinical characteristics should be present for diagnosis of either severe or nonsevere malnutrition.

1. White JV, Guenter P, Jensen G, et al. Consensus Statement: Academy of Nutrition and Dietetics and American Society for Parenteral and Enteral Nutrition: Characteristics Recommended for the Identification and Documentation of Adult Malnutrition (Undernutrition). *Journal of Parenteral and Enteral Nutrition*. 2012;36(3):275-283.
2. Kondrup J. Can food intake in hospitals be improved? *Clin Nutr*. 2001;20:153-160.
3. Blackburn GL, Bistrian BR, Maini BS, Schlamm HT, Smith MF. Nutritional and metabolic assessment of the hospitalized patient JPEN J Parenter Enteral Nutr. 1977;1:11-22.
4. Klein S, Kinney J, Jeejeebhoy K, et al. Nutrition support in clinical practice: review of published data and recommendations for future research directions. National Institutes of Health, American Society for Parenteral and Enteral Nutrition, and American Society for Clinical Nutrition. *JPEN J Parenter Enteral Nutr*. 1977;21:133-156.
5. Rosenbaum K, Wang J, Pierson RN, Kotler DP. Time-dependent variation in weight and body composition in healthy adults. *J Parenter Enteral Nutr*. 2000;24:52-55.
6. Keys A. Chronic undernutrition and starvation with notes on protein deficiency. JAMA. 1948;138:500-511.
7. Sacks GS, Dearman K, Replogle WH, Cora VL, Meeks M, Canada T. Use of subjective global assessment to identify nutritionassociated complications and death in long-term care facility residents. J Am Coll Nutr. 2000;19:570-577.
8. Norman K, Stobaus N, Gonzalez MC, Schulzke J-D, Pirlich M. Hand grip strength: outcome predictor and marker of nutritional status. *Clin Nutr*. 2011;30:135-142.
9. Hagan JC. Acute and chronic diseases. In: Mulner RM, ed. Encyclopedia of Health Services Research. Vol 1. Thousand Oaks, CA Sage; 2009:25.
10. American Dietetic Association Evidence Analysis Library. Does serum prealbumin correlate with weight loss in four models of prolonged protein-energy restriction: anorexia nervosa, non-malabsorptive gastric partitioning bariatric surgery, calorie-restricted diets or starvation. http://www.adaevidencelibrary.com/conclusion.cfm?conclusion_statement_id=251313&highlight=prealbumin& home=1. Accessed July 5, 2017.
11. American Dietetic Association Evidence Analysis Library. Does serum prealbumin correlate with nitrogen balance? http://www.adaevidencelibrary.com/conclusion.cfm?conclusion_statement_id=251315&highlight=prealbumin&home=1. Accessed July 5, 2017.
12. American Dietetic Association Evidence Analysis Library. Does serum albumin correlate with weight loss in four models of prolonged protein-energy restriction: anorexia nervosa, non-malabsorptive gastric partitioning bariatric surgery, calorie-restricted diets or starvation. http://www.adaevidencelibrary.com/conclusion.cfm?conclusion_statement_id=251263&highlight=albumin&home=1. Accessed July 5, 2017.
13. American Dietetic Association Evidence Analysis Library. Does serum albumin correlate with nitrogen balance? http://www.adaevidencelibrary.com/conclusion.cfm?conclusion_statement_id=251265&highlight=albumin&home=1. Accessed July 5, 2017.

TABLE B

	Intake	Weight Loss	Nutrition Focused Physical Exam	Body Fat	Muscle Mass	Fluid Accumulation/ Edema	Reduced Handgrip
Description of clinical Characteristics	Malnutrition occurs due to insufficient food and nutrient intake or malabsorption. Recent nutrient consumption compared against estimated nutritional needs is a primary standard for defining malnutrition. The clinician should conduct or review the food and fluid intake history, calculate optimal energy needs, compare them with calculated energy consumed, and report insufficient intake as a percentage of calculated energy needs over time.	The clinician should evaluate current weight considering other clinical findings, together with the presence of under- or overhydration. Weigh change is assessed over time and reported as a percent of weight loss from the previous weight.	Malnutrition normally manifests in the form of physical changes that can be identified via a nutrition focused physical exam. Weigh, body fat, muscle mass, fluid accumulation, and handgrip changes should be documented as part of conducting and documenting a nutrition focused physical exam.	Loss of subcutaneous fat (as seen in orbital cavity, triceps, and fat covering the ribcage)	Muscle loss as seen in wasting of the temples, clavicles, shoulders, interosseous muscles, scapula, thigh, and calf	Evaluate the individual for generalized or localized fluid accumulation. This is usually seen in the extremities (especially the lower extremities), genital edema, or ascites. Weight loss is often disguised by generalized edema. Unplanned, unexplained weight increase can be seen in the presence of fluid accumulation.	Compare measurements to measurement standards provided by the dynamometer manufacturer.

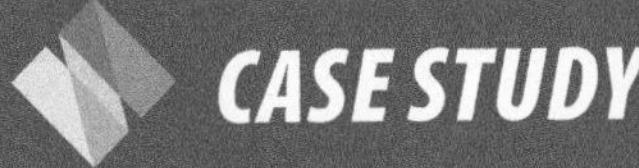

CASE STUDY

Cirrhosis with Portal Hypertension and Ascites

Steven, a 52-year-old man, sees you for a follow-up clinical appointment. He has an established history of cirrhosis and portal hypertension in the setting of long-term ethanol abuse. Steven had gained 10 lbs over the prior 2 weeks and exhibits massive ascites. Additional findings included mild encephalopathy with poor concentration, asterixis, and sclera icterus. A family member reports that Steven's food intake had been severely compromised for weeks. At presentation, the patient is 5'8" tall and weighs 161 lbs (usual weight ~150 lbs). He is afebrile. Laboratories included total bilirubin (3.8 mg/dL), aspartate aminotransferase (96 IU/L) alanine aminotransferase (111 U/L), alkaline phosphatase (162 IU/L), serum albumin (1.7 g/dL), prothrombin time (18 seconds), white blood cells (3700 mm^3), C-reactive protein (27 mg/L), prealbumin (6.8 mg/dL), hemoglobin (8 g/dL), hematocrit (32%), and fasting glucose (107 mg/dL). Physical findings are notable for ascites and extensive loss of muscle and subcutaneous fat.

Questions:

1. What nutrition syndrome would you anticipate in a patient who presents with cirrhosis with portal hypertension and ascites, and how would you confirm this?
   a. Severe malnutrition in the context of chronic illness
   b. Severe malnutrition in the context of environmental or social circumstances
   c. Severe malnutrition in the context of acute injury
   d. Mild or moderate malnutrition in the context of chronic illness
2. What factors indicate the type of malnutrition diagnosed?

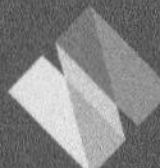

CASE STUDY

Multiple-Trauma Victim

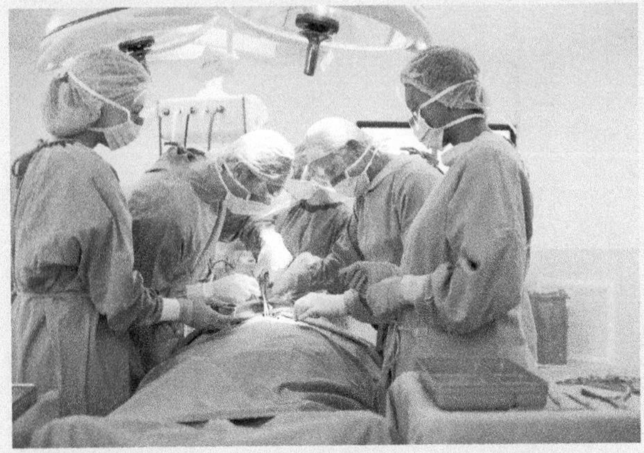

Stuart, a 38-year-old man, is suffering from multiple traumas secondary to a motor vehicle accident. His injuries include a ruptured spleen, grade III liver laceration, left femur fracture, and bilateral pulmonary contusions. His status was post damage control celiotomy, splenectonmy, and packing of the liver. He was transferred to the trauma intensive-care unit on a ventilator, where he continued to be resuscitated. Postsurgery day two of admission, Stuart had a temperature (102°F), heart rate (98 beats per minute), respiratory rate (26 breaths per minute), white blood cell count (25K/mm^3), and pCO_2 (28 mm Hg). He was markedly edematous, with a weight gain of 15 lbs above his usual body weight. His open abdomen was dressed. Additional laboratory data: C-reactive protein (45 mg/dL), serum albumin (2.6 g/dL), prealbumin (11.0 mg/dL) and glucose (220 mg/dL). He has an increased metabolic rate by indirect calorimetry (REE of 3,000 kcal). Dietary intake is anticipated to be compromised for a week or more. He is reported to have been well nourished with suitable dietary intake before his injury.

Questions:

1. What malnutrition syndrome would you anticipate in a multiple-trauma victim early in his course? How would you confirm this?
   a. Severe malnutrition in the context of chronic illness
   b. Severe malnutrition in the context of environmental or social circumstances
   c. Severe malnutrition in the context of acute injury
   d. Mild or moderate malnutrition in the context of chronic illness
2. What factors indicate the type of malnutrition diagnosed?

Learning Portfolio

Key Terms

Anorexia nervosa (AN)
Anthropometry
Binge-eating disorder (BED)
Body mass index (BMI)
Bulimia nervosa (BN)
Cachexia
Client history
Food- and nutrition-related history
Human immunodeficiency virus (HIV)
Indirect calorimetry
Inflammatory response
Kwashiorkor
Lipodystrophy
Malnutrition
Malnutrition Universal Screening Tool (MUST)
Mini Nutrition Assessment (MNA)
Nutritional assessment
Nutritional status
Nutrition-focused physical examination (NFPE)
Nutrition screening
Opportunistic infection
Patient-generated subjective global assessment (PG-SGA)
Predictive equations for estimating energy needs
Resting metabolic rate (RMR)
Sarcopenia
Sarcopenic obesity
Subjective global assessment (SGA)

Study Questions

1. The height of a patient with severe muscular deformities or multiple contractures can best be measured by:
   a. Standing height.
   b. Segmental measurement.
   c. Arm span.
   d. Bioelectrical impedance analysis.
2. Effective medications for managing HIV have resulted in other metabolic abnormalities that require nutrition management. Which of the following occurs?
   a. Lipodystrophy
   b. Nutritional anemias
   c. Low blood glucose levels
   d. Elevated HDL cholesterol levels
3. What characteristic is not included in the diagnosis of adult malnutrition?
   a. Loss of subcutaneous fat
   b. Insufficient protein intake
   c. Diminished functional status
   d. Insufficient energy intake
4. Bone tenderness and pain may be present with a __________ deficiency.
   a. Vitamin A
   b. Vitamin C
   c. Vitamin D
   d. Vitamin K
5. ____________ is a method of determining body composition that is generally equivalent to underwater weighing.
   a. Air-displacement plethysmography
   b. Bioelectrical impedance analysis
   c. Waist-to-hip ratio
   d. Dual-energy x-ray absorptiometry
6. Which component is generally *not* part of a client history?
   a. Medical history
   b. Surgeries
   c. Treatments
   d. Dietary supplement use
7. A major limitation of a food- and nutrition-related history may be:
   a. Interviewer questions that are too specific.
   b. Too many interview questions to answer.
   c. Clients with impaired cognition may not be able to provide accurate information.
   d. Information given by the caregiver is not the same as the client would provide.
8. The most commonly used technique for a nutrition-focused physical exam is:
   a. Inspection.
   b. Palpation.
   c. Percussion.
   d. Manipulation.

9. A limitation of the Malnutrition Universal Screening Tool is that:
   a. It requires a current height and weight to determine BMI.
   b. It can only be completed by advanced healthcare practitioners.
   c. It takes a significant amount of time to complete.
   d. It should only be used for hospitalized patients.

10. Bitot's spots may be present in which deficiency?
    a. Iron
    b. Folate
    c. Vitamin A
    d. Vitamin D

11. The prevalence of obesity in American adults is:
    a. 15.3%.
    b. 26.7%.
    c. 36.5%.
    d. 41.2%.

12. A predictive resting energy equation noted to be specific for ventilator-dependent patients is the:
    a. Mifflin–St. Jeor.
    b. Penn State.
    c. Harris-Benedict.
    d. Owen.

13. The extent to which a nutritional screen gives negative results in those who are free of the disease or condition is called:
    a. Sensitivity.
    b. Reliability.
    c. Accuracy.
    d. Specificity.

14. Spoon-shaped nails can be present in a:
    a. Vitamin A or vitamin D excess.
    b. Vitamin C deficiency.
    c. Protein or iron deficiency.
    d. Riboflavin deficiency.

15. Gray-brown spots or mottling on teeth can indicate:
    a. A vitamin C deficiency.
    b. Excessive sugar intake.
    c. A high acid intake.
    d. Excess fluoride intake.

16. Adult malnutrition is similar to pediatric:
    a. Kwashiorkor.
    b. Marasmus.
    c. Marasmic kwashiorkor.
    d. Cachexia.

17. Sarcopenia is characterized by the loss of:
    a. Lean muscle mass and body fat.
    b. Body fat.
    c. Muscle mass.
    d. Body weight.

18. Appropriate interventions for weight change or weight loss in patients are determined by:
    a. Starting with an oral nutrition supplement first.
    b. Altering the diet consistency.
    c. Liberalizing the diet.
    d. Investigating the root cause of the weight loss.

19. Malnutrition in the context of social or environmental circumstances may be present in patients with:
    a. Major infection.
    b. Cancer.
    c. Rheumatoid arthritis.
    d. Anorexia nervosa.

20. A patient with a hemoglobin A1C of 7.9% has an estimate average glucose (eAG) of approximately:
    a. 212 mg/dL.
    b. 80 mg/dL.
    c. 183 mg/dL.
    d. 97 mg/dL.

21. Muscle mass loss is *not* assessed in which one of the following areas of the body?
    a. Ribs or chest area
    b. Temporal area
    c. Clavicle area
    d. Interosseous area of the hand

22. The equation found most reliable in predicting resting energy requirements is the ______________ equation.
    a. Harris-Benedict
    b. Ireton-Jones
    c. Penn State
    d. Mifflin–St. Jeor

23. Recommended protein intakes for patients at risk of malnutrition or with existing pressure injuries who are assessed to be at risk of malnutrition is:
    a. 1.0–1.2 g/kg body weight.
    b. 1.25–1.5 g/kg body weight.
    c. 1.5–1.7 g/kg body weight.
    d. ≥ 2.0 g/kg body weight.

24. A diet history tool that asks the client to recall food and beverage intake from the previous day is called a:
    a. Food-frequency questionnaire.
    b. Daily food checklist.
    c. 24-hour food recall.
    d. Direct meal observation.

25. Recommendations for protein in a patient who is in stage III CKD are:
    a. 10% of calorie intake from protein.
    b. 15% of calorie intake from protein.
    c. 0.8 g/kg body weight.
    d. 1.0 g/kg body weight.
26. Weight gain goals for hospitalized patients with anorexia nervosa are:
    a. Preventing further weight loss while in hospital.
    b. 0.5 – 1.0 lb/week
    c. 1 – 2 lb/week
    d. 2 – 3 lb/week
27. Which of the nutrition-screening and assessment tools contains both a nutrition-screening tool and a nutritional assessment?
    a. Nutrition risk screening
    b. Malnutrition Universal Screening Tool
    c. ubjective global assessment
    d. Mini Nutritional Assessment
28. The best indicator of kidney function is:
    a. Glomerular filtration rate.
    b. Serum creatinine.
    c. Blood urea nitrogen.
    d. Serum sodium level.
29. The subjective global assessment does not review which of the following?
    a. Change in body weight
    b. Gastrointestinal symptoms
    c. Biochemical measures
    d. Functional capacity
30. Coarse, dry, brittle hair can indicate:
    a. Hyperthyroidism.
    b. Hypothyroidism.
    c. Hyperparathyroidism.
    d. Protein deficiency.

Discussion Questions

1. Discuss the difference between a nutrition screen and a nutrition assessment.
2. Compare and contrast the diagnosis of adult malnutrition in the following contexts: acute injury or illness, chronic illness, and social or environmental circumstances.
3. Discuss the positive aspects and the limitations of the MUST.

Activities

1. Conduct a food- and nutrition-related history interview with one of your friends or family members. Use the list of questions in the section on food history to conduct the interview.
2. Review the history of a patient or client. What details of the client history are important in completing a nutritional assessment?
3. Contact a local senior center and ask the director if you can conduct a Mini Nutritional Assessment and a Malnutrition Universal Screening Tool at the center. Determine whether any individuals are at nutritional risk. Tell any individuals who are at nutritional risk to follow up with their physicians.
4. Calculate your estimated energy needs using three of the predictive equations. What were the differences in the results?
5. Calculate the protein and fluid needs for an older adult female who is 62 inches and 130 lbs with a current pressure injury who is assessed to be at risk of malnutrition.
6. Measure the height of a peer using the methods described in the chapter.
7. Once the height and weight are obtained, calculate the BMI. What does the BMI tell you about your peer?
8. View the Nestlé Nutrition Institute videos under "Online Resources" section that follows. Conduct a basic NFPE with one of your peers.
    a. What nutrient deficiency were you able to identify in your peer? What physical signs were used to determine the identified deficiency?
    b. If no nutrition deficiency was identified, what physical characteristics did you use to reach that conclusion?

Online Resources

Snapshot—NCP Step 1: Nutrition Assessment

https://www.andeal.org/vault/2440/web/files/20140602-NA%20Snapshot.pdf

Academy of Nutrition and Dietetics Critical Thinking Skills in Nutrition Assessment and Diagnosis

http://www.eatrightpro.org/~/media/eatrightpro%20files/practice/position%20and%20practice%20papers/practice%20papers/practice%20papers/practice%20paper%20critical%20thinking%20skills%20in%20nutrition%20assessment.ashx

Skinfold measurement technique video

https://youtu.be/XMpifYMxHVo

Diet History Part 1

https://www.youtube.com/watch?v=76OfeSesBw0

Diet History Interview

https://www.youtube.com/watch?v=CruhCMRTpnQ

Patient-Generated Subjective Global Assessment

http://pt-global.org

The Minnesota Semistarvation Experiment

http://www.epi.umn.edu/cvdepi/video/the-minnesota-semistarvation-experiment/

Alliance to Advance Patient Nutrition

http://malnutrition.com

Nutrition Focused Physical Assessment Part 1: Setting the Stage for Success

https://www.nestlenutrition-institute.org/Resources/Online-Conferences/Pages/NutritionFocusedPhysicalAssessmentPart1SettingtheStageforSuccess.aspx

Nutrition Focused Physical Assessment Part 2: Creating Your Malnutrition Toolbox

https://www.nestlenutrition-institute.org/Resources/online-conferences/Pages/NutritionFocusedPhysicalAssessmentPart2CreatingYourMalnutritionToolbox.aspx

Nutrition Focused Physical Assessment Part 3: Micronutrient Deficiencies

https://www.nestlenutrition-institute.org/Resources/online-conferences/Pages/NutritionFocusedPhysicalAssessmentPart3MicronutrientDeficiencies.aspx

Mini Nutrition Assessment Resources: Nestlé Nutrition institute

http://www.mna-elderly.com/

Malnutrition Universal Screening Tool (MUST)

http://www.bapen.org.uk/pdfs/must/must_full.pdf

Malnutrition Self-Screening Tool

http://www.malnutritionselfscreening.org/self-screening.html

References

1. Mann J, Truswell S. *Essentials of Human Nutrition*. 4th ed. New York, NY: Oxford University Press; 2012.
2. Ferguson M. Nutrition Screening Evidence Analysis Project presentation; 2009; February 10. https://www.andeal.org/topic.cfm?key=2193&cat=3853.
3. American Society of Parenteral Enteral Nutrition (ASPEN). Malnutrition Screening for Hospital Patients Widespread but Hospitals Fall Short on Nutrition Care Plans. https://www.nutritioncare.org/Press_Room/2014/Malnutrition_Screening_for_Hospital_Patients_Widespread_but_Hospitals_Fall_Short_on_Nutrition_Care_Plans/.
4. Department of Health and Human Services, Centers for Medicare & Medicaid Services. Revisions to Appendix PP: Interpretive Guidelines for Long-Term Care Facilities; 2008. https://www.cms.gov/Regulations-and-Guidance/Guidance/Transmittals/downloads/R36SOMA.pdf.
5. Academy of Nutrition and Dietetics. Nutrition Screening (NSCR) Systematic Review (2009–2010). http://www.andeal.org/topic.cfm?menu=3584.
6. Nestlé Nutrition Institute. Validity in Screening Tools. MNA Mini Nutrition Assessment. http://www.mna-elderly.com/validity_in_screening_tools.html.
7. American Dietetic Association. ADA's definitions for nutrition screening and nutrition assessment: Identifying patients at risk. *J Am Diet Assoc*. 1994; 94(8):838-839.
8. ASPEN. Board of Directors and Clinical Practice Committee. Definition of terms, style, and conventions used in ASPEN Board of Directors–approved documents; 2015. https://www.researchgate.net/publication/7557179_Definition_of_Terms_Style_and_Conventions_Used_in_ASPEN_Guidelines_and_Standards.

9. Academy of Nutrition and Dietetics. *International Dietetics and Nutrition Terminology (IDNT) Reference Manual: Standardized Language for the Nutrition Care Process.* 4th ed. Chicago, IL: Academy of Nutrition and Dietetics; 2013.
10. Duren DL, Sherwood BJ, Czerwinski SA, et al. Body composition comparisons and interpretation. *J Diab Sci Technol.* 2008; 2(6):1139–1146.
11. Chernoff R. *Geriatric Nutrition: The Health Professional's Handbook.* 4th ed. Burlington, MA: Jones & Bartlett Learning; 2014; 443.
12. Roche AF. Anthropometric variables: effectiveness and limitations. In: *Assessing the Nutritional Status of the Elderly: State of the Art Report of the Third Ross Roundtable on Medical Issues.* Columbus, OH: Ross Laboratories; 1982.
13. Collins N. Measuring height and weight. *Adv Skin Wound Care.* 2002; 15(2):91–92.
14. Centers for Disease Control and Prevention (CDC). *Anthropometric Reference Data for Children and Adults: United States, 2007–2010.* https://www.cdc.gov/nchs/data/series/sr_11/sr11_252.pdf.
15. Murphy RA, Patel KV, Kritchevsky SB. Weight change, body composition, and risk of mobility disability and mortality in older adults: A population-based cohort study. *J Am Geriatr Soc.* 2014; 62:1476–1483.
16. You JW, Seung JL, Kim YE, et al. Association between weight change and clinical outcomes in critically ill patients. *J Crit Care.* 2013;28(6):923–927.
17. Nakagawa T, Toyazaki T, Chiba N, et al. Prognostic value of body mass index and change in body weight in postoperative outcomes of lung cancer surgery. *Interact Cardiovasc Thorac Surg.* 2016; 23(4):560–566.
18. American Medical Directors Association. *Clinical Practice Guideline: Altered Nutritional Status in the Long-Term Care Setting.* Columbia, MD: American Medical Directors Association; 2010.
19. Rossman I. The anatomy of aging. In: Rossman I, ed. *Clinical Geriatrics.* Philadelphia, PA: Lippincott; 1979.
20. Mitchell MK. *Nutrition Across the Life Span.* Philadelphia, PA: WB Saunders Company; 1997: 479.
21. Estimating height in bedridden patients. http://www.rxkinetics.com/height_estimate.html.
22. Pribram V. *Nutrition and HIV.* Appendix 10. Equations to Calculate Height and Estimation of Height from Ulna Length; 2013. http://onlinelibrary.wiley.com/doi/10.1002/9781118786529.app10/pdf.
23. Auyeung TW, Lee JS, Kwok T, et al. Estimation of stature by measuring fibula and ulna bone length in 2443 older adults. *J Nutr Health Aging.* 2009; 13(10):931–936.
24. Haapala H, Peterson MD, Daunter A, Hurvitz EA. Agreement between actual height and estimated height using segmental limb lengths for individuals with cerebral palsy. *Am J Phys Med Rehabil.* 2015; 94(7): 539–546.
25. Freedman DS, Horlick M, Berenson GS. A comparison of the Slaughter skinfold-thickness equations and BMI in predicting body fatness and cardiovascular disease risk factor levels in children. *Am J Clin Nutr.* 2013; 98(6):1417–1424.
26. Wohlfahrt-Veje C, Tinggaard J, Winther K, et al. Body fat throughout childhood in 2647 healthy Danish children: Agreement of BMI, waist circumference, skinfolds with dual x-ray absorptiometry. *Eur J Clin Nutr.* 2014; 68(6):664–670.
27. National Heart Lung and Blood Institute (NHLBI). *Managing Overweight and Obesity in Adults: Systematic Evidence Review from the Obesity Expert Panel.* Washington, DC: NHLBI; 2013.
28. Bhaskaran K, Douglas I, Forbes H, dos-Santos-Silva I, Leon DA, Smeeth L. Body-mass index and risk of 22 specific cancers: A population-based cohort study of 5.24 million UK adults. *Lancet.* 2014;384(9945):755–765.
29. NCHS Data Brief No. 219. Prevalence of obesity among adults and youth: United States, 2011–2014; 2015. https://www.cdc.gov/nchs/data/databriefs/db219.pdf.
30. Winter JE, MacInnis RJ, Nowson CA. The influence of age on the BMI and all-cause mortality association: A meta-analysis. *J Nutr Health Aging*; 2016; 7:1–5.
31. Hillier SE, Beck L, Petropoulou BA, Clegg ME. A comparison of body composition measurement techniques. *J Hum Nutr Dietet.* 2014; 27:626–631.
32. Harrison GG, Buskirk ER, Carter JEL, et al. Skinfold thickness and measurement technique. In: Lohman TG, Roche AF, Martorell R, eds., *Anthropometric Standardization Reference Manual.* Champaign, IL: Human Kinetics; 1988.
33. Durnin JV, Womersley S. Body fat assessed from total body density and its estimation from skinfold thickness: Measurements of 481 men and women aged from 16-72 years. *Br J Nutr.* 1974; 32:77–79.
34. Chambers AJ, Parise E, McCrory JL, Cham R. A comparison of prediction equations for the estimation of body fat percentage in non-obese and obese older Caucasian adults in the United States. *J Nutr Health Aging.* 2014; 18(6):586–590.
35. CDC. *Anthropometric Reference Data for Children and Adults: United States, 2003–2006*; 2008. http://www.cdc.gov/nchs/data/nhsr/nhsr010.pdf.
36. de Oms M, Habicht JP. Anthropometric reference data for international use: Recommendations from a World Health Organization Expert Committee. *Am J Clin Nutr.* 1996; 64:650–658.
37. Guigoz Y, Bruno V, Garry PL. Assessing the nutritional status of the elderly: The Mini Nutritional Assessment as part of the geriatric evaluation. *Nutr Rev.* 1996; 54:S59–S65.
38. Portero-McClellan KC, Staudt C, Silva FR, et al. The use of calf circumference measurement as an anthropometric tool to monitor nutritional status in elderly inpatients. *J Nutr Health Aging.* 2010; 14(4):266–270.
39. Nutrition screening as easy as MNA. A guide to completing the Mini Nutrition Assessment (MNA). Nestle Nutrition Institute. http://www.mna-elderly.com/forms/mna_guide_english.pdf.
40. Chan JM, Rimm EB, Colditz GA, Stampfer MJ, Willett WC. Obesity, fat distribution, and weight gain as risk factors for clinical diabetes in men. *Diabetes Care.* 1994; 17:961–969.
41. Potts J, Simmons D. Sex and ethnic group differences in fat distribution in young United Kingdom South Asians and Europids. *J Clin Epidemiol.* 1994; 47:837–841.
42. Dobbelsteyn CJ, Joffres MR, MacLean DR, Flowerdew G. A comparative evaluation of waist circumference, waist-to-hip ratio and body mass index as indicators of cardiovascular risk factors. The Canadian Heart Health Surveys. *Intern J Obesity.* 2001; 25(5):652–661.
43. Czemichow S, Kengne AP, Huxley RR, et al. Comparison of waist-to-hip ratio and other obesity indices as predictors of cardiovascular disease risk in people with type 2 diabetes: A prospective cohort study from ADVANCE. *Eur J Cardiovasc Prev Rehabil.* 2011; 18(2):312–319.
44. de Koning L, Merchant AT, Pogue J, Anand SS. Waist circumference and waist-to-hip ratio as predictors of cardiovascular events: Meta-regression analysis of prospective studies. *Eur Heart J.* 2007; 28(7):850–856.

45. Dehghan M, Merchant AT. Is bioelectrical impedance accurate for use in large epidemiological studies? *Nutr J.* 2008; 7:26.
46. Kelly TL, Wilson KE, Heymsfield SB. Dual energy x-ray absorptiometry body composition reference values from NHANES, 2009. *PLoS One.* 2009; 4(9):e7038. http://journals.plos.org/plosone/article/citation?id=10.1371/journal.pone.0007038.
47. Houtkooper LB, Going SB, Sproul J, et al. Comparison of methods for assessing body composition over 1 y in postmenopausal women. *Am J Clin Nutr.* 2000; 72:401–406.
48. Gallagher D, Kovera AJ, Clay-Williams G, et al. Weight loss in postmenopausal obesity: No adverse alterations in body composition and protein metabolism. *Am J Physiol Endocrinol Metab.* 2000; 279:E124–E131.
49. How Does the BOD POD Work? http://ybefit.byu.edu/Portals/88/Documents/How%20Does%20The%20BOD%20POD%20Work.pdf.
50. Maddalozzo GF, Cardinal BJ, Snow CA. Concurrent validity of the BOD POD and dual energy x-ray absorptiometry techniques for assessing body composition in young women. *J Am Diet Assoc.* 2002; 102(11):1677–1679.
51. Fields DA, Gunatilake R, Kalaitzoglou E. Air displacement plethysmography: Cradle to grave. *Nutr Clin Prac.* 2015; 30(2):219–226.
52. Banh L. Serum proteins as markers of nutrition: What are we treating? Nutrition Issues in Gastroenterology. Series No. 43. *Prac Gastroenterol.* 2006; 30(10):46–64.
53. Jensen GL. Inflammation roles in aging and sarcopenia. *J Parenter Enteral Nutr.* 2008; 32(6):656–659.
54. Chan LN, Mike LA. The science and practice of micronutrient supplementations in nutritional anemia: An evidence-based review. *J Parenter Enteral Nutr.* 2014; 38(6):656–672.
55. Kuzuya M, Kanda S, Koike T, et al. Lack of correlation between total lymphocyte count and nutritional status in the elderly. *Clin Nutr.* 2005; 24(3):427–432.
56. Morley JE. Dehydration, hypernatremia, and hyponatremia. *Clin Geriatr Med.* 2015; 31(3):389–399.
57. National Kidney Foundation. Glomerular filtration rate (GFR). https://www.kidney.org/kidneydisease/siemens_hcp_gfr.
58. Foreback, C. Glycated hemoglobin in the diabetic patient. *Med Lab Observer.* 2015; 47(6):14–20.
59. NHLBI. What is cholesterol? https://www.nhlbi.nih.gov/health/health-topics/topics/hbc/.
60. Zarny LA, Berstein LH. Serum cholesterol: an indicator of malnutrition. *J Am Dietet Assoc.* 1995; 95(9):A25.
61. Hamada S, Gulliford MC. Mortality in individuals aged 80 and older with type 2 diabetes mellitus in relation to glycosylated hemoglobin, blood pressure, and total cholesterol. *J Am Geriatr Soc.* 2016; 64:1425-1431.
62. Bickley LS. *Bates' Guide to Physical Examination and History Taking.* 11th ed. Chapter 1, Overview: Physical Examination and History Taking. Philadelphia, PA: Wolters Kluwer Health/Lippincott Williams & Wilkins; 2013: 4–6.
63. Ternent CA, Bastawrous AL, Morin NA, Ellis CN, Hyman NH, Buie WD. Standards Practice Task Force of the American Society of Colon and Rectal Surgeons. Practice parameters for the evaluation and management of constipation. *Dis Colon Rec.* 2007; 50:2013–2022.
64. Müller-Lissner S, Kamm M, Scarpignato C, Wald A. Myths and misconceptions about chronic constipation. *Am J Gastroenterol.* 2005; 100:124–129.
65. Academy of Nutrition and Dietetics. Nutrition Care Manual. Client History Gastrointestinal Disease, Constipation. https://www.nutritioncaremanual.org/topic.cfm?ncm_toc_id=268232.
66. Burke BS. The diet history as a tool in research. *J Am Diet Assoc.* 1943; 23:1041–1046.
67. Skypala IJ, Venter C, Meyer R, et al. The development of a standardized diet history tool to support the diagnosis of food allergy. *Clin Transl Allergy.* 2015; 5(7). http://ctajournal.biomedcentral.com/articles/10.1186/s13601-015-0050-2#Abs1.
68. National Cancer Institute (NCI). 24-hour dietary recall (24HR) at a glance. https://dietassessmentprimer.cancer.gov/profiles/recall/.
69. US Department of Agriculture. Automated multiple-pass method. https://www.ars.usda.gov/northeast-area/beltsville-md/beltsville-human-nutrition-research-center/food-surveys-research-group/docs/ampm-usda-automated-multiple-pass-method/.
70. NCI. Observing protein & energy nutrition (OPEN) study. http://epi.grants.cancer.gov/past-initiatives/open/.
71. NCI. Food frequency questionnaire at a glance. https://dietassessmentprimer.cancer.gov/profiles/questionnaire/.
72. NCI. Usual Dietary Intakes: NHANES Food Frequency Questionnaire (FFQ). http://epi.grants.cancer.gov/diet/usualintakes/ffq.html?&url=/diet/usualintakes/ffq.html.
73. Bernstein M, Munoz N. Chapter 7: Nutritional Assessment for the Older Adult. In: *Nutrition for the Older Adult.* 2nd ed. Burlington, MA: Jones and Bartlett Learning; 2016:179.
74. Scollard T. Malnutrition and nutrition-focused physical assessment. Power Point presentation at Utah Academy of Nutrition and Dietetics annual meeting, March 27, 2015. http://www.eatrightutah.org/docs/AM15-Speaker2-01c.pdf.
75. Collins N, Harris C. The physical assessment revisited: Inclusion of the nutrition-focused physical exam. *Ostomy Wound Manag.* 2010. http://www.o-wm.com/files/owm/pdfs/Nutrition411_Layout%201.pdf.
76. MedlinePlus. Percussion. https://medlineplus.gov/ency/article/002281.htm.
77. Bistrain BR. Clinical nutritional assessment. In: Goldman L, Ausiello D, eds. *Cecil Medicine.* 23rd ed. Philadelphia, PA: Saunders Elsevier; 2008.
78. Seidel HM, Stewart RW, Ball JW, Dains JE, Flynn JA, Solomon BS. *Mosby's Guide to Physical Examination.* 7th ed. St. Louis, MO: Mosby; 2011.
79. Mordarski B, Wolff J. *Nutrition Focused Physical Exam Pocket Guide.* Chicago, IL: Academy of Nutrition and Dietetics; 2015.
80. Gross CR, Lindquist RD, Wooley AC, Granieri R, Allard K, Webster B. Clinical indicators of dehydration severity in elderly patients. *J Emerg Med.* 1992; 10(3):267–274.
81. *Dorland's Illustrated Medical Dictionary.* 32nd ed. New York, NY: Elsevier Health Sciences Division; 2011.
82. Jensen GL. Inflammation as the key interface of the medical and nutrition universes: A provocative examination of the future of clinical nutrition and medicine. *J Parenter Enteral Nutr.* 2006; 30:453–463.
83. Simpson F, Doig GS. Parenteral vs. enteral nutrition in the critically ill patient: A meta-analysis of trials using the intention to treat principle. *Intensive Care Med.* 2005; 31(1):12–23.
84. Lopez-Hellin J, Baena-Fustegueras JA, Schwartz-Riera S, Garcia-Arumi E. Usefulness of short-lived protein as nutritional indicators in surgical patients. *Clin Nutr.* 2002; 21:119–125.
85. Chabner BA, Thompson EC. Cachexia in cancer. Merck Manual (professional version). http://www.merckmanuals.com/professional/hematology-and-oncology/principles-of-cancer-therapy/cachexia-in-cancer.

86. Arends J, Bodoky G, Bozzetti F, et al. ESPEN guidelines on enteral nutrition: Non-surgical oncology. *Clin Nutr.* 2006; 25:245–259.
87. Lin CA, Boslaugh S, Ciliberto HM, et al. A prospective assessment of food and nutrient intake in a population of Malawian children at risk for kwashiorkor. *J Pediatr Gastroenterol Nutr.* 2007; 44(4):487–493.
88. Jensen GL, Bistrain B, Roubenoff R. Heimburger DC. Malnutrition syndromes: A conundrum vs continuum. *J Parenter Enteral Nutr.* 2009; 33(6):710–716.
89. Wellcome Trust Working Party. Classification of infantile malnutrition. *Lancet.* 1970; 2:302–303.
90. Plank LD, Connolly AB, Hill GL. Sequential changes in the metabolic response in severely septic patients during the first 23 days after the onset of peritonitis. *Ann Surg.* 1998; 228(2):146–158.
91. Lewis SJ, Egger M, Sylvester PA, Thomas S. Early enteral feeding versus "nil by mouth" after gastrointestinal surgery: Systematic review and meta-analysis of controlled trials. *Br Med J.* 2001; 323:1–5
92. Artinian V, Krayem H, DiGiovine B. Effects of early enteral feeding on the outcome of critically ill mechanically ventilated medical patients. *Chest.* 2006; 129:960–967.
93. Perel P, Yanagawa T, Bunn F, et al. Nutritional support for head-injured patients. *Cochrane Database Sys Rev.* 2006; 4:CD001530.
94. Morley JE, Baumgartner RN, Roubenoff R, et al. Sarcopenia. *J Lab Clin Med.* 2001; 137:231–243.
95. Metter EJ, Conwit R, Tobin J, Fozard JL. Age-associated loss of power and strength in the upper extremities in women and men. *J Gerontol A Biol Sci Med Sci.* 1997; 52:B267–B276.
96. Iannuzzi-Sucich M, Prestwood KM, Kenny AM. Prevalence of sarcopenia and predictors of skeletal muscle mass in healthy older men and women. *J Gerontol A Biol Sci Med Sci.* 2002; 57(12): M772–M777.
97. Walston JD. Sarcopenia in older adults. *Curr Opin Rheumatol.* 2012; 24(6): 623–627.
98. Stenholm S, Harris TB, Rantanen T, et al. Sarcopenic obesity: Definition, etiology, and consequences. *Curr Opin Clin Nutr Metab Care.* 2008; 11(6):693–700.
99. Batsus JA, Mackenzie TA, Barre LK, et al. Sarcopenia, sarcopenic obesity, and mortality in older adults: Results from the National Health and Nutrition Examination Survey III. *Euro J Clin Nutr.* 2014; 68:1001–1007.
100. White JV, Guenter P, Jensen G, et al. Consensus statement of the Academy of Nutrition and Dietetics/American Society for Parenteral and Enteral Nutrition: Characteristics recommended for the identification and documentation of adult malnutrition (undernutrition). *J Acad Nutr Diet.* 2012; 112:730–738.
101. White JV, Guenter P, Jensen G, et al. Consensus statement of the Academy of Nutrition and Dietetics/American Society for Parenteral and Enteral Nutrition: characteristics recommended for the identification and documentation of adult malnutrition (undernutrition). *J Parenter Enteral Nutr.* 2012; 36(3):275–283.
102. Bentley DV. Diagnosis coding confusion discussed at ICD-9-CM Coordination and Maintenance Meeting. Just Coding. March 29, 2011. www.justcoding.com.
103. Butterworth CE. The skeleton in the hospital closet. *Nutr Today.* 1974; 9:4–7.
104. Mueller C, Compher C, Druyan ME, et al. Nutrition screening, assessment, and intervention. *J Parenter Enteral Nutr.* 2011; 35(1):16–24.
105. National Alliance for Infusion Therapy and the American Society for Parenteral and Enteral Nutrition Public Policy Committee and Board of Directors. Disease-related malnutrition and enteral nutrition therapy: A significant problem with a cost-effective solution. *Nutr Clin Pract.* 2010; 25(5):548–554.
106. National Heart, Lung, and Blood Institute Acute Respiratory Distress Syndrome (ARDS) Clinical Trials Network, Rice TW, Wheeler AP, et al. Initial trophic vs. full enteral feeding in patients with acute lung injury: The EDEN randomized trial. *JAMA.* 2012; 307(8)795–803.
107. Dennett C. Nutrition-focused physical exam. *Todays Dietitian.* 2016; 18(2):36.
108. Norman K, Stobäus N, Gonzalez MC, Schulzke JD, Pirlich M. Hand grip strength: Outcome predictor and marker of nutritional status. *Clin Nutr.* 2011; 30:135–142.
109. Compher CW, Frankenfield DC, Roth-Yoursey L. Evidence Analysis Working Group. Best practice methods to apply to measurement of resting metabolic rate in adults: A systematic review. *J Am Diet Assoc.* 2006; 106:881–903.
110. Frankenfield DC, Ashcraft LM. Estimating energy needs in the nutrition support patient. *J Parenter Enteral Nutr.* 2011; 35(5):563–570.
111. Foltz MB, Schiller MR, Ryan AS. Nutrition screening and assessment: Current practices and dietitians' leadership roles. *J Am Diet Assoc.* 1993; 93:1388–1395.
112. Phang PT, Rich T, Ronco J. A validation and comparison study of two metabolic monitors. *J Parenter Enteral Nutr.* 1990; 14:259–264.
113. Academy of Nutrition and Dietetics. Nutrition Care Manual. Predictive equations: validation of prediction equations. https://www.nutritioncaremanual.org/topic.cfm?ncm_toc_id=144908.
114. Shetty PS, Henry CJ, Black AE, Prentice AM. Energy requirements of adults: an update on basal metabolic rates (BMRs) and physical activity levels (PALs). *Eur J Clin Nutr.* 1996; 50:S11–S23.
115. Shetty P. Energy requirements of adults. *Public Health Nutr.* 2005; 8(7A):994–1009.
116. Heymsfield SB, Harp JB, Rowell PN, Nguyen AM, Pietrobelli A. How much may I eat? Calories estimates based upon energy expenditure prediction equations. *Obes Rev.* 2006; 7:361–370.
117. Frankenfield DC, Smith JS, Cooney RN, Blosser SA, Sarson GY. Relative association of fever and injury with hypermetabolism in critically ill patients. *Injury.* 1997; 28:617–621.
118. Frankenfield D, Roth-Yousey L, Compher C. Comparison of predictive equations for resting metabolic rate in nonobese and obese adults: A systematic review. *J Am Diet Assoc.* 2005; 105(5):775–789.
119. EAL Working Group—Energy Needs. Academy of Nutrition and Dietetics Evidence Analysis Library. EE: Evidence analysis: Estimating RMR with prediction equations (2006). https://www.andeal.org/topic.cfm?menu=5299&cat=2694.
120. Harris JA, Benedict FG. A biometric study of human basal metabolism. *Proc Natl Acad Sci USA.* 1918; 4(12):370–373.
121. Owen OE, Holup JL, D'Alessio DA, et al. A reappraisal of the caloric requirements of men. *Am J Clin Nutr.* 1987; 46(6):875–885.
122. Schofield WN. Predicting basal metabolic rate, new standards and review of previous work. *Hum Nutr Clin Nutr.* 1985; 39(Suppl 1): 5–41.

123. Ireton-Jones CS, Turner WW Jr, Liepa GU, Baxter CR. Equations for the estimation of energy expenditures in patients with burns with special reference to ventilatory status. *J Burn Care Rehabil.* 1992; 13(3):330–333.
124. Frankenfield DC. Energy Dynamics. In: Matarese LE, Gottschlich MM, eds. *Contemporary Nutrition Support Practice: A Clinical Guide.* Philadelphia, PA: WB Saunders; 1998:79–98.
125. Frankenfield D, Hise M, Malone A, Russell M, Gradwell E, Compher C. Evidence Analysis Working Group. Prediction of resting metabolic rate in critically ill adult patients: Results of a systematic review of the evidence. *J Am Diet Assoc.* 2007; 107(9):1552–1561.
126. Swinamer DL, Grace MG, Hamilton SM, Jones R, Roberts P, King EG. Predictive equation for assessing energy expenditure in mechanically ventilated critically ill patients. *Crit Care Med.* 1990; 18:657–661.
127. Ireton-Jones CS, Jones JD. Why use predictive equations for energy expenditure assessment? *J Am Diet Assoc.* 1997; 97:A44.
128. Frankenfield D, Smith S, Cooney RN. Validation of 2 approaches to predicting resting metabolic rate in critically ill patients. *J Parenter Enteral Nutr.* 2004; 28(4):259–264.
129. National Academies of Science, Engineering, and Medicine. Chapter 10: Protein and Amino Acids. In: *Dietary Reference Intakes for Energy, Carbohydrate, Fiber, Fat, Fatty Acids, Cholesterol, Protein, and Amino Acids (Macronutrients).* Washington, DC: National Academies Press; 2005. https://www.nap.edu/read/10490/chapter/12.
130. Dietary Reference Intakes (DRIs): Recommended Dietary Allowances and Adequate Intakes, Total Water and Macronutrients. https://fnic.nal.usda.gov/sites/fnic.nal.usda.gov/files/uploads/DRI_RDAs_Adequate_Intakes_Total_Water_Macronutrients.pdf.
131. Gaffney-Stomberg E, Insogna KL, Rodriguez NR, Kerstetter JE. Increasing dietary protein requirements in elderly people for optimal muscle and bone health. *J Am Geriatr Soc.* 2009; 57:1073–1079.
132. Wolfe RR. The underappreciated role of muscle in health and disease. *Am J Clin Nutr.* 2006; 84:475–482.
133. Academy of Nutrition and Dietetics Evidence Analysis Library. Critical Illness (2006-2007): Protein needs. "What level of protein intake or what protein delivery is associated with improvements in mortality?" http://www.andeal.org/topic.cfm?menu=3369&cat=3369.
134. Scheinkestel CD, Kar L, Marshall K, et al. Prospective randomized trial to assess caloric and protein needs of critically ill, anuric, ventilated patients requiring continuous renal replacement therapy. *Nutrition.* 2003; 19(11-12):909-916.
135. Hoffer LJ, Bistrian BR. Appropriate protein provision in critical illness: A systematic and narrative review. *Am J Clin Nutr.* 2012; 96:591–600.
136. Mayes T, Gottschlich MM. Burns. In: Matarese LE, Gottschlich MM, eds. *Contemporary Nutrition Support Practice.* 2nd ed. Philadelphia, PA: WB Saunders Co; 2003: 595–615.
137. Academy of Nutrition and Dietetics. Nutrition Care Manual. Critical illness: Comparative standards. https://www.nutritioncaremanual.org/topic.cfm?ncm_toc_id=269153.
138. National Pressure Ulcer Advisory Panel, European Pressure Ulcer Advisory Panel, and Pan Pacific Pressure Injury Alliance. *Prevention and Treatment of Pressure Ulcers: Quick Reference Guide.* 2nd ed.; 2014. http://www.npuap.org/wp-content/uploads/2014/08/Quick-Reference-Guide-DIGITAL-NPUAP-EPUAP-PPPIA-Jan2016.pdf.
139. National Kidney Foundation Kidney Disease Outcomes Quality Initiative (KDOQI). KDOQI Clinical Practice Guidelines for Nutrition in Chronic Renal Failure. http://www2.kidney.org/professionals/KDOQI/guidelines_nutrition/doqi_nut.html.
140. Stall S. Protein recommendations for individuals with CKD stages 1–4. *Nephrol Nurs J.* 2008; 35(3):279–282.
141. Snively WD. Body surface area as a dosage criterion in fluid therapy: Theory and application. *Metabolism.* 1957; 6(1):70–87.
142. Adolph EF. The metabolism and distribution of water in body and tissues. *Physiol Rev.* 1933; 13(3):336–371.
143. American Dietetic Association. Chapter 1, Nutrition Assessment of Adults. In: *Manual of Clinical Dietetics.* 6th ed. Chicago, IL: American Dietetic Association; 2000: 33.
144. Holliday MA, Segar WE. The maintenance need for water in parenteral fluid therapy. *Pediatrics.* 1957; 19(5):823–832.
145. Brummit P. Clinical Dietitians in Healthcare Facilities. *Dietary Documentation Pocket Guide.* 2nd ed. Chicago, IL: American Dietetic Association; 2002.
146. Kobriger AM. *Hydration: Maintenance: Dehydration, Laboratory Values, and Clinical Alterations.* Chilton, WI: Kobriger Presents; 2005.
147. Academy of Nutrition and Dietetics. Evidence Analysis Library. *Hydration: Estimating Fluid Needs*; 2007. http://www.andeal.org/topic.cfm?menu=2820&cat=3217.
148. Dietetics in Health Care Communities. *Pocket Resource for Nutrition Assessment.* 8th ed. Chicago, IL: Academy of Nutrition and Dietetics; 2013.
149. National Eating Disorder Association. Types and Symptoms of Eating Disorders. http://www.nationaleatingdisorders.org/general-information.
150. The Center for Eating Disorders at Sheppard Pratt. *Anorexia Nervosa.* http://www.eatingdisorder.org/eating-disorder-information/anorexia-nervosa/.
151. Swanson S, Crow S, Le Grange D, Swendsen J, Merikangas K. Prevalence and correlates of eating disorders in adolescents. Results from the National Comorbidity Survey Replication Adolescent Supplement. *Arch Gen Psychiatr.* 2011; 68(7):714–723.
152. American Dietetic Association: Standards of Practice and Standards of Professional Performance for registered dietitians (competent, proficient, and expert) in disordered eating and eating disorders (DE and ED). *J Am Diet Assoc.* 2011; 111:1242-1249.e37.
153. Hart S, Russell J, Abraham S. Nutrition and dietetic practice in eating disorder management. *J Hum Nutr Diet.* 2011; 24:144-153.
154. Gowers S, Pilling S, Treasure J, et al. Eating disorders. In: *Core Interventions in the Treatment and Management of Anorexia Nervosa and Related Eating Disorders.* London: National Institute for Clinical Excellence; 2004: 1–261.
155. Winston AP, Gowers S, Jackson AA, et al. *Guidelines for the Nutritional Management of Anorexia Nervosa.* London: Royal College of Psychiatrists; 2005: 42.
156. Ozier AD, Henry BW. Position of the American Dietetic Association: Nutrition intervention in the treatment of eating disorders. *J Am Diet Assoc.* 2011; 111:1236–1241.
157. American Psychiatric Association. American Psychiatric Association; treatment of patients with eating disorders, 3rd ed. *Am J Psychiatry.* 2006; 163(7):1–54.

158. Wakefield A, Williams H. *Practice Recommendations for the Nutritional Management of Anorexia Nervosa in Adults*; 2009: 1-45. http://cedd.org.au/wordpress/wp-content/uploads/2014/09/Practice-Recommendations-for-the-Nutritional-Assessment-of-Anorexia-Nervosa-in-Adults.pdf.
159. Cordery H, Waller G. Nutritional knowledge of health care professionals working in the eating disorders. *Eur Eat Disord Rev.* 2006; 14:462–467.
160. Rosen DS. Identification and management of eating disorders in children and adolescents. *Pediatrics.* 2010; 126:1240–1253.
161. Meyer RR, Alder R. Human immunodeficiency virus (HIV). *Magill's Medical Guide* (online edition); 2016. http://www.cengage.com/search/productOverview.do?N=197+4294891683&Ntk=P_EPI&Ntt=20284504821069771651498819252478625389&Ntx=mode%2Bmatchallpartial.
162. HIV in the United States: At a Glance. http://www.cdc.gov/hiv/pdf/statistics_basics_factsheet.pdf.
163. UNAIDS. *Global Report: UNAIDS Report on the Global AIDS Epidemic*; 2013. http://files.unaids.org/en/media/unaids/contentassets/documents/epidemiology/2013/gr2013/UNAIDS_Global_Report_2013_en.pdf.
164. CDC. About HIV/AIDS. http://www.cdc.gov/hiv/basics/whatishiv.html.
165. Earthman CP. Evaluation of nutrition assessment parameters in the presence of human immunodeficiency virus infection. *Nutr Clin Prac.* 2004; 19:330–339.
166. Nerad J, Romeyn M, Silverman E, et al. General nutrition management in patients infected with human immunodeficiency virus. *Clin Infect Dis.* 2003; 36(Suppl):S52–S62.
167. Grinspoon S, Mulligan K. Weight loss and wasting in patients with human immunodeficiency virus. *Clin Infect Dis.* 2003; 36(Suppl):S69–S78.
168. American Dietetic Association and Dietitians of Canada. Position of the American Dietetic Association and Dietitians of Canada: Nutrition intervention in the care of persons with human immunodeficiency virus infection. *J Am Diet Assoc.* 2000; 100:708–717.
169. Shevitz AH, Knox TA. Nutrition in the era of highly active antiretroviral therapy. *Clin Infect Dis.* 2001; 32:1769–1775.
170. Polsky B, Kotler D, Steinhart C. HIV-associated wasting in the HAART era: Guidelines for assessment, diagnosis, and treatment. *AIDS Patient Care STD.* 2001;15:411–423.
171. Palenicek JP, Graham NM, He YD, et al. Multicenter AIDS Cohort Study Investigators: weight loss prior to clinical AIDS as a predictor of survival. *J Acquir Immune Defic Sydr.* 1995; 10:366–373.
172. Tang A, Forrester J, Spiegelman D, Knox TA, Tchetgen E, Gorbach SL. Weight loss and survival in HIV positive patients in the era of highly active antiretroviral therapy. *J Acquir Immune Defic Syndr.* 2002; 31(2):230–236.
173. Kotler DP. Nutritional alterations associated with HIV infection. *J Acquir Immune Defic Syndr.* 2000; 25(Suppl):S81–S87.
174. Council of State and Territorial Epidemiologists, AIDS Program, Center for Infectious Diseases. Revision of the CDC surveillance case definition for acquired immunodeficiency syndrome. *Morb Mortal Wkly Rep.* 1987; 36(Suppl 1):1S-15S.
175. McDermott AY, Shevitz A, Knox T, Moen K, Johansen D, Paton N. Effect of highly active antiretroviral therapy on fat, lean, and bone mass in HIV-seropositive men and women. *Am J Clin Nutr.* 2001; 74:679–686.
176. Hadigan C, Meigs JB, Corcoran C, et al. Metabolic abnormalities and cardiovascular disease risk factors in adults with human immunodeficiency virus infection and lipodystrophy. *Clin Infect Dis.* 2001; 32:130–139.
177. Nolan D, Hammond E, Martin A, et al. Mitochondrial DNA depletion and morphologic changes in adipocytes associated with nucleoside reverse transcriptase inhibitor therapy. *AIDS.* 2003; 17:1329–1338.
178. Gelato MC. Insulin and carbohydrate dys-regulation. *Clin Infect Dis.* 2003; 36(suppl 2):91–95.
179. Jones CY, Tang AM, Forrester JE, et al. Micronutrient levels and HIV disease status in HIV-infected patients on highly active antiretroviral therapy in the Nutrition for Healthy Living cohort. *J Acquir Immune Defic Syndr.* 2006; 43:475–482.
180. Papathakis PC, Rollins NC, Chantry CJ, Bennish ML, Brown KH. Micronutrient status during lactation in HIV-infected and HIV-uninfected South African women during the first 6 months after delivery. *Am J Clin Nutr.* 2007; 85:182–192.
181. Drain PK, Baeten JM, Overbaugh J, et al. Low serum albumin and the acute phase response predict low serum selenium in HIV-1 infected women. *BMC Infect Dis.* 2006; 6:85.
182. Fields-Gardner C, Campa A. Position of the American Dietetic Association: Nutrition intervention and human immunodeficiency virus infection. *J Am Diet Assoc.* 2010; 110:1105–1119.
183. NAM AIDSMAP. Interactions Between Drugs and Food. http://www.aidsmap.com/Interactions-between-drugs-and-food/page/3080183/#item3080185nd food.
184. Knox T, Speiegelman D, Skinner SG, Gorbach S. Diarrhea and abnormalities of gastrointestinal function in a cohort of men and women with HIV infection. *Am J Gastroenterol.* 2000; 95:3482–3489.
185. US Food and Drug Administration. Food Safety for People with HIV/AIDS. http://www.fda.gov/Food/FoodborneIllnessContaminants/PeopleAtRisk/ucm312669.htm#Transport.
186. Bartlett JG. Integrating nutrition therapy into medical management of human immunodeficiency virus. *Clin Infect Dis.* 2003; 36(Suppl 2):551.
187. Ockengaa J, Grimbleb R, Jonkers-Schuitemac C, et al. ESPEN guidelines on enteral nutrition: Wasting in HIV and other chronic infectious diseases. *Clin Nutr.* 2006; 25:319–329.
188. Rabeneck L, Palmer A, Knowles JB, et al. A randomized controlled trial evaluating nutrition counseling with and without oral supplementations in malnourished HIV-infected patients. *J Am Diet Assoc.* 1998; 98:434–438.
189. Burger B, Schwenk A, Junger H, et al. Oral supplements in HIV infected patients with chronic wasting: A prospective trial. *Med Klin.* 1994; 89:579–581, 633.
190. Berneis K, Battegay M, Bassetti R, et al. Nutritional supplements combined with dietary counseling diminish whole body protein catabolism in HIV-infected patients. *Eur J Clin Invest.* 2000; 30:87–94.
191. Secher M, Soto ME, Villars H, Abellan van Kan G, Vellas B. The Mini Nutritional Assessment (MNA) after 20 years of research and clinical practice. *Rev in Clin Gerontol.* 2007; 17:293–310.
192. Rubenstein LZ, Harker JO, Salvá A, Guigoz Y, Vellas B. Screening for undernutrition in geriatric practice: Developing the short-form mini-nutritional assessment (MNA-SF). *J Gerontol A Biol Med Sci.* 2001; 56:366-372.
193. Nestlé Nutrition Institute. MNA Mini Nutritional Assessment. http://www.mna-elderly.com/default.html.

194. Guigoz Y, Laque S, Vellas B. Identifying the elderly at risk for malnutrition: The Mini Nutritional Assessment. *Clin Geriatr Med.* 2002; 18:737–757.
195. Guigoz Y. The Mini Nutritional Assessment (MNA) review of the literature. What does it tell us? *J Nutr Health Aging.* 2006; 10:466–486.
196. Christner S, Ritt M, Volkert D, et al. Evaluation of the nutritional status of older hospitalized geriatric patients: A comparative analysis of a Mini Nutritional Assessment (MNA) version and the Nutritional Risk Screening (NRS 2002). *J Human Nutr Diet.* 2016; 29(6):704–713.
197. Tsai AC, Chang TL, Chang MZ. An alternative short-form Mini-Nutritional Assessment for rating the risk of malnutrition in persons on hemodialysis. *J Clin Nurs.* 2013; 22:2830–2837.
198. van Bokhorst-de van der Schueren MA, Guaitoli PR, Jansma EP, de Vet HC. Nutrition screening tools: Does one size fit all? A systematic review of screening tools for the hospital setting. *Clin Nutr.* 2014; 33(1):39–58.
199. British Association of Parenteral and Enteral Nutrition (BAPEN). Malnutrition Universal Screening Tool (MUST). http://www.bapen.org.uk/pdfs/must/must_full.pdf.
200. Elia M. The "MUST" report; nutritional screening of adults—A multidisciplinary responsibility: Development and use of the "Malnutrition Universal Screening Tool" ("MUST") for adults. Redditch: BAPEN; 2003.
201. Stratton RJ, King CL, Stroud MA, Jackson AA, Elia M. "Malnutrition Universal Screening Tool" predicts mortality and length of hospital stay in acutely ill elderly. *Br J Nutr.* 2006; 95:325–330.
202. Donini LM, Poggiogalle E, Molfino A, et al. Mini-Nutritional Assessment, Malnutrition Universal Screening Tool, and Nutrition Risk Screening tool for the nutritional evaluation of older nursing home residents. *J Am Med Direc Assoc.* 2016; 17:959.e11–959.e18.
203. Diekmann R, Winning K, Uter W, et al. Screening for malnutrition among nursing home residents—a comparative analysis of the Mini Nutritional Assessment, the nutritional risk screening, and the Malnutrition Universal Screening Tool. *J Nutr Health Aging.* 2013; 17(4):326–331.
204. Rasheed S, Woods RT. Predictive validity of "Malnutrition Universal Screening Tool" ("MUST") and short form Mini Nutrition Assessment (MNA-SF) in terms of survival and length of hospital stay. *e-ESPEN Journal.* 2013; 8:e44–e50.
205. Koren-Hakin T, Weiss A, Hershkovitz A, et al. Comparing the adequacy of the MNA-SF, NRS-2002 and MUST nutritional tools in assessing malnutrition in hip fracture operated elderly patients. *Clin Nutr.* 2016; 35:1053–1058.
206. Valentini L, Schulzke J. Mundane, yet challenging: The assessment of malnutrition in inflammatory bowel disease. *Eur J Intern Med.* 2011; 22(1):13–15.
207. Sandhu A, Mosli M, Yan B, et al. Self-screening for malnutrition risk in outpatient inflammatory bowel disease patients using the Malnutrition Universal Screening Tool (MUST). *J Parenter Enteral Nutr.* 2015; 40(4):507–510.
208. Detsky AS, McLaughlin JR, Baker JP, et al. What is subjective global assessment of nutritional status? *J Parenter Enteral Nutr.* 1987; 11:8–13.
209. Baker JP, Detsky AS, Wesson DE, et al. Nutritional assessment; a comparison of clinical judgment and objective measurements. *N Engl J Med.* 1982; 306:969–972.
210. Hirsch S, Obaldia N, Petermann M, et al. Subjective global assessment of nutritional status: Further validation. *Nutrition.* 1991; 7:35–37.
211. Marshall S, Young A, Bauer J, Isenring E. Malnutrition in geriatric rehabilitation: Prevalence, patient outcomes, and criterion validity of the scored Patient-Generated Subjective Global Assessment and the Mini Nutritional Assessment. *J Acad Nutr Diet.* 2016; 116:785–794.
212. Raslan M, Gonzalez MC, Torrinhas RS, Ravacci GR, Pereira JC, Waitzberg DL. Complementarity of subjective global assessment (SGA) and nutritional risk screening 2002 (NRS 2002) for predicting poor clinical outcomes in hospitalized patients. *Clin Nutr.* 2011; 30(1):49–53.
213. Bector S, Vagianos K, Suh M, Duerksen DR. Does the Subjective Global Assessment predict outcomes in critically ill medical patients? *J Intens Care Med.* 2016; 31(7): 485–489.
214. Secker DJ, Jeejeebhoy KN. Subjective Global Nutrition Assessment for children. *Am J Clin Nutr.* 2007; 85(4): 1083–1089.
215. Visser R, Dekker FW, Boeschoten EW, Stevens P, Krediet RT. Reliability of the 7-point subjective global assessment scale in assessing nutritional status of dialysis patients. *Adv Perit Dial.* 1999; 15:222–225.
216. Kalantar-Zadeh K, Kleiner M, Dunne E, Lee G, Luft F. A modified quantitative subjective global assessment of nutrition for dialysis patients. *Nephrol Dial Transplant.* 1999; 14(7):1732–1738.
217. Churchill DN, Taylor DW, Keshaviah PR. Adequacy of dialysis and nutrition in continuous peritoneal dialysis: association with clinical outcomes. Canada-USA (CANUSA) Peritoneal Dialysis Study Group. *J Am Soc Nephrol.* 1996; 7:198–207.
218. Lim SL, Lin XH, Daniels L. Seven-point Subjective Global Assessment is more time sensitive than conventional Subjective Global Assessment in detecting nutrition changes. *J Parenter Enteral Nutr.*2016; 40:966–972.
219. Ottery FD. Rethinking nutritional support of the cancer patient: The new field of nutritional oncology. *Sem Oncol.* 1994; 21:770–778.
220. Ottery FD. Patient-Generated Subjective Global Assessment. In: McCallum PD, Polisena CG, eds. *The Clinical Guide to Oncology Nutrition*, Chicago, IL: American Dietetic Association; 2000: 11–23.
221. Watterson C, Fraser A, Banks M, et al. Evidence based practice guidelines for the nutritional management of malnutrition in patients across the continuum of care. *Nutr Diet.* 2009; 66(Suppl 3):S1–S34.
222. National Centre for Classification in Health. Australian Coding Standards for I.C.D.-10-AM. Sydney, Australia: National Centre for Classification in Health; 2008.
223. Da Silva Fink J, Daniel de Mello P, Daniel de Mello E. Subjective global assessment: A systematic review of the literature. *Clin Nutr.* 2015; 34:785–792.

Chart Review

A thorough nutrition assessment begins with a review of the patient's medical chart. The medical chart provides information on the patient's medical history, diagnosis or diagnoses, physical assessment, treatment, laboratory data, medications, social history, and response to treatment. This chapter reviews the various systems, their nutritional implications, and intervention.

The Nutrition Care Process according to the American Dietetic Association involves four steps:

1. *Nutrition assessment*: The nutrition assessment is a systematic approach used to collect, record, and interpret relevant data from patients, clients, family members, caregivers, and other individuals and groups. It takes into consideration anthropometric data, diet/medical history, biochemical data, and social history.
2. *Nutrition diagnosis*: The nutrition diagnosis is the diagnosis of nutrition-related problems based on signs and symptoms from the assessment data.

3. *Nutrition intervention*: The nutrition intervention is a plan designed to address the nutrition diagnosis for which goals are developed with the patient/client and reviewed for modification as needed.
4. *Nutrition monitoring and evaluation:* This step identifies the progress made on the plan of care and measures outcomes.

In reviewing the patient's medical record, it is important you have a clear understanding of the medical diagnosis(es) and its impact on nutritional status, food–drug interaction, and laboratory values. These topics are covered in detail in this chapter.

MEDICAL DIAGNOSIS

Medical diagnosis varies from one patient to another, and some patients present with multiple diagnoses. In assessing the patient's nutritional status, you often can find that for some patients one diagnosis takes precedence over another. The diagnosis is pivotal to your assessment. For example, you review the chart of a patient who has a diagnosis of hypertension, but also has poor oral intake. As a dietitian, your primary focus is to ensure adequate caloric intake, and in this case, that might mean offering a regular diet instead of a sodium-restricted diet so as to encourage good oral intake.

Let's say JB is admitted to your facility with a history of hepatic encephalopathy and has severe depletion of albumin with wasting syndrome. Instead of reducing protein intake because of the hepatic encephalopathy, your focus now shifts to the low albumin and wasting syndrome. The goal, therefore, is to provide adequate protein and calories to improve nutritional status. Lactulose/neomycin is usually administered to decrease the ammonia level and subsequently improve hepatic encephalopathy.

I remember some years ago during my internship, I encountered a patient who was diagnosed with cancer, but who also had diabetes. I went into his room because I had received a nutrition consult for diabetes management. I put all my instruction sheets together and was ready to show off my counseling skills.

His wife was with him as I entered the room. I introduced myself and began sharing my expertise in diabetes management when his wife said, "We are not worried about his diabetes; that is the least of our concerns.

My husband has cancer." I realized then that the diagnosis that concerned her most was cancer, and therefore the couple was not prepared to receive counseling on managing diabetes. It is important to listen to your patient to determine learning readiness.

You can never be familiar with all the diagnoses that exist, but when in doubt, "check it out." Make use of the physicians on your team and get a better understanding of the diagnoses because in almost all cases, nutrition plays a vital role in the recovery process. Whatever the diagnosis, the aim is to provide adequate nutrition to reduce the risk of malnutrition because malnutrition slows recovery time for patients. Sometimes it becomes necessary to focus on the diagnosis with the greatest impact on the patient's medical and nutritional health.

SURGICAL REVIEW AND HISTORY

Some, if not all, surgical procedures have a direct impact on patients' nutritional status and outcome. Surgery is almost always accompanied by weight loss resulting from fasting before the procedure and decreased oral intake immediately following the procedure. It is not unusual for a patient's hemoglobin, hematocrit, and albumin levels to fall significantly following surgery. This section highlights some common surgical procedures and their nutritional implications.

Gastric Bypass Surgery

In an effort to manage weight, many obese individuals turn to surgical procedures. In recent years, the number of gastric bypass surgeries being performed yearly has increased. According to the Centers for Disease Control and Prevention (CDC), more than 60% of Americans are overweight, and about 3 in 10 are obese. Gastric bypass involves reducing the size of the stomach by applying rows of stainless steel staples across the top of the stomach so that only a small opening into the distal stomach is left open. This is then connected to the small intestine by means of an intestinal loop (Mahan & Escott-Stump, 2008).

Nutritional Implications and Intervention

Gastric bypass surgery patients take in less food and absorb less of what they ingest, putting them at risk for developing nutritional deficiencies.

Bloating, nausea, and vomiting are common in these patients. The goal of nutrition therapy is to maximize nutritional intake in small quantities and prevent "dumping syndrome," which occurs when food passes too quickly from the stomach to the small intestine. Symptoms of dumping syndrome may include feelings of nausea, feelings of fullness, stomach cramping, diarrhea, weakness, sweating, and a fast heart rate.

Another complication of gastric bypass surgery is the formation of gallstones, which frequently leads to the need for gallbladder surgery. Most surgeons remove the gallbladder during the gastric bypass surgery to prevent this from happening. Patients should be monitored for potential anemia and deficiencies of potassium, magnesium, folate, and vitamin B_{12}. Vitamin and mineral supplements are necessary for life following surgery.

Short Bowel Syndrome

Short bowel syndrome is often the result of extensive intestinal resection and is characterized by diarrhea, malabsorption, and malnutrition related to a shortened intestinal remnant. "Patients who are at the greatest nutritional and dehydration risk generally have < 115 cm of residual small intestine in the absence of colon in continuity or < 60 cm of residual small intestine with colon in continuity" (Buchman, 2004).

Hydration and nutritional status are difficult to maintain without nutrition support when more than 75% of the small intestine has been resected. To assess the nutritional status of patients with short bowel syndrome effectively, you need to know the extent of the resection, whether the ileocecal valve was removed, which segment of the small bowel remains, and the adaptation potential of the remaining gut. "An intact colon may absorb up to 1200 cal/day" (Buchman, 2004).

Nutritional Implications and Intervention

With extensive ileal resections, the proximal gut does not gain the capacity to absorb bile salts or vitamin B_{12}, and the ileal "brake" on upper gut transit is lost [illegible] cal valve may lead to bacterial overgrowth. As a co[illegible], progressive dehydration, hypovolemia [illegible] malabsorption of fat, fat-soluble vitamins (A, D, E, and K), vitamin B_{12} and divalent cations (calcium, magnesium, zinc, and copper) may develop (Bernard, 1993).

Anemia resulting from vitamin B_{12} deficiency in patients with short bowel syndrome (SBS) is believed to be linked to *Lactobacillus* overgrowth; lactobacilli require vitamin B_{12}, for growth (Hojo Bando, Itoh, Taketomo, & Ishii, 2008).

One of the major complications of short bowel syndrome is chronic diarrhea resulting from malabsorption. After massive small bowel resection, increased gastrointestinal losses can often cause dehydration, hyponatremia, hypokalemia, hypomagnesemia, hypocalcemia, and metabolic acidosis. Most patients require total parenteral nutrition (TPN) for 7 to 10 days following the resection. Energy requirements are generally 25–35 cal/kg/day, and protein requirements are 1.0–1.5g/kg/day.

Patients may also experience steatorrhea, and MCT oil is usually recommended to enhance absorption of nutrients. MCT oil, however, lacks linoleic acid, an essential fatty acid. Plant oils, for example, safflower and sunflower, are good sources of linoleic acid. Reducing fat intake helps to decrease steatorrhea.

Fluid requirements are modified to prevent dehydration. You must, however, monitor fluid status daily for clinical signs of fluid overload or dehydration. Oral rehydration solutions (ORSs) are recommended to reduce sodium loss.

The goal of nutrition therapy for the patient with short bowel syndrome is to ensure adequate fluid and electrolyte replacement, stabilize diarrhea, prevent loss of or replace water-soluble and fat-soluble vitamins, and prevent vitamin B_{12} deficiency. Vitamin K deficiency may occur in patients who do not have a colon because colonic bacteria synthesize 60% of daily vitamin K requirements.

Patients with short bowel syndrome who do not receive TPN are generally in negative calcium balance, and you should prescribe a supplement (800–1500 mg/day) (Buchman, 2004).

If the colon is intact, the patient is at increased risk of developing calcium oxalate renal stones. Patients presenting with calcium oxalate kidney stones should restrict dietary oxalate. Foods high in oxalate include tea, cola drinks, chocolate, nuts, green leafy vegetables, celery, strawberries, blueberries, and tangerines. Frequent meals consisting of complex carbohydrate and soluble fiber are strongly encouraged in the patient with an intact colon.

Missing Body Parts

From time to time, a patient will present to your facility with missing body parts, whether it be an arm, a leg, or even a breast. Because breast size varies from one woman to another and body weight differs among patients, it is important to ascertain the patient's body weight prior to mastectomy and after mastectomy when the patient resumes a normal eating pattern because weight loss immediately after surgery might be a combination of breast tissue loss as well as blood and fluid loss.

Amputations

You can calculate the patient's approximate body weight loss following an amputation by using this list as a guide:

Hand represents	0.7% loss	Foot represents	1.5% loss
Forearm with hand represents	2.3% loss	Lower leg and foot represents	6.0% loss
Entire arm represents	5.0% loss	Entire leg represents	16.0% loss

Nutritional Implications and Intervention

Missing body parts affect the estimated caloric and protein needs of the patient. To determine the ideal body weight (IBW) of the patient with a missing body part, first establish the IBW prior to amputation, and then subtract the percentage of the missing body part as well as the weight of any prostheses.

Coronary Artery Bypass Grafting Surgery

When a coronary artery becomes narrowed or clogged, the section of the heart that it supplies suffers. Coronary artery bypass grafting surgery (CABG) is a way to treat the blocked artery by creating new passages for blood to flow to the heart muscles. It works by taking arteries or veins from other parts of the body, called grafts, and using them to reroute blood around the clogged artery. Coronary artery bypass grafting surgery, however, does not cure atherosclerosis because the new grafts are susceptible to atherogenesis, the formation of plaques in the inner lining of the arteries (Mahan & Escott-Stump, 2008).

This surgical procedure is increasingly performed in older adults who are vulnerable to undernutrition. Among the risk factors associated with adverse outcomes are low serum albumin and body mass index (BMI). Rich et al. retrospectively analyzed the effect of hypoalbuminemia (serum albumin level < 3.5 g/dL) on postoperative complications in 92 patients (> 75 years of age) undergoing cardiac surgery over a 2-year period. Fourteen percent were hypoalbuminemic, and hypoalbuminemia was the most significant predictor of postoperative renal dysfunction and a contributor to postoperative length of stay. Patients classified as having hypoalbuminemia, hypoalbuminemia and liver insufficiency, or hypoalbuminemia and congestive heart failure had an increased likelihood of postoperative organ dysfunction, gastrointestinal bleeding, nosocomial infections, extended length of intensive care unit stay, prolonged duration of mechanical ventilation, and hospital death.

"In another series of 886 Swedish cardiac surgery patients (63% were ≥ 65 years of age), a low preoperative serum albumin level was also associated with an increased rate of postoperative infection, and a low preoperative BMI increased the risk for death. Engleman et al. also demonstrated that low preoperative serum albumin level (< 2.5 g/dL) and low BMI (< 20 kg/m^2) independently predicted mortality after cardiac surgery" (DiMaria-Ghalili, 2008).

> DiMaria-Ghalili systematically examined the relationship between nutrition markers (BMI, serum albumin, and transferrin levels) before surgery and again at 4–5 days post-surgery and 4–6 weeks post-discharge, as well as biomedical and general health outcomes, in 91 elderly patients undergoing elective CABG surgery. Although older patients undergoing elective CABG had a normal preoperative nutrition status, weight loss during the later phases of the surgical stress response was problematic. Older patients undergoing elective CABG lost an average of 5.2% ± 4.3% of their weight from pre-surgery to 6 weeks post-discharge. The more weight lost during this period, the lower their level of self-reported physical health and the greater their chances of being readmitted to the hospital. Thus, older CABG patients who lose weight in the postoperative period may increase their vulnerability to adverse health outcomes, including hospital readmission." (DiMaria-Ghalili, 2008, Oct–Nov; *23* (5), 498)

Nutritional Implications and Intervention

To reduce the risk of mortality following cardiac surgery it is important that you conduct a thorough nutrition evaluation on the patient. Decreased dietary intake can lead to weight loss and subsequent malnutrition.

Depression is associated with decreased oral intake, decreased appetite, and weight loss. Weight loss especially in older adults correlates with increased mortality. Postoperative weight loss is also common in the CABG patient.

Like other postsurgical procedures, the postoperative CABG patient is put on a liquid diet that is low in fat and cholesterol until the individual is able to tolerate regular consistency. Patients are advised to follow a low-fat, low-cholesterol diet after discharge; however, because of the metabolic demands of CABG surgery, some surgeons advise patients not to make dietary changes until their appetite has returned to normal to ensure that adequate calories and proteins are consumed to promote recovery. This recommendation is appropriate because CABG patients frequently report decreased appetite and a change in the taste of food in the early weeks after discharge (DiMaria-Ghalili, 2008).

Pancreatectomy

The pancreas is the central organ for digestion and for control of glucose homeostasis. Whenever a patient experiences complications of chronic or acute pancreatitis or pancreatic malignancies, pancreatic surgery may be necessary. According to the National Cancer Institute, one of the following types of surgery may be used to remove tumors in the patient with pancreatic cancer:

- *Whipple procedure:* The head of the pancreas, the gallbladder, part of the stomach, part of the small intestine, and the bile duct are removed. Enough of the pancreas is left to produce digestive juices and insulin.
- *Total pancreatectomy:* The whole pancreas, part of the stomach, part of the small intestine, the common bile duct, the gallbladder, the spleen, and nearby lymph nodes are removed.
- *Distal pancreatectomy:* The body and the tail of the pancreas and usually the spleen are removed.

Nutritional Implications and Intervention

Most patients develop diabetes mellitus following pancreatectomy, requiring them to have insulin substitution. Hypoglycemia is the most difficult clinical problem to handle following pancreatectomy, and therefore carbohydrate intake must be adequate while monitoring blood glucose.

Alterations in glucagon regulation is considered a potential side effect of partial pancreatectomies (Schrader et al., 2009). Glucagon injection is administered when blood sugar drops significantly low.

Improvements in postoperative management include auto-islet cell transplantation, advances in insulin formulations, and the use of glucagon rescue therapy, which allow much tighter control of blood glucose than previously possible. This markedly lessens the risk of life-threatening hypoglycemia and decreases the risk of long-term complications, resulting in improved quality of life for these patients (Heidt, Burant, & Simeone, 2007).

The main clinical manifestations of exocrine pancreatic insufficiency are fat malabsorption, which is called steatorrhea and which consists of fecal excretion of more than 6 g per day of fat; weight loss; abdominal pain; and abdominal swelling sensation (Bini, 2007). There is also malabsorption of carbohydrates and protein, but fat malabsorption is more severe.

The presence of weight loss requires an increased energy intake. Dietary protein and carbohydrates should be high. Medium chain triglycerides (MCTs) are recommended for patients with steatorrhea because these fatty acids are hydrolyzed more rapidly.

The extent of malabsorption depends on the original disease process and the type and extent of surgical resection. Pancreatectomy interferes with the production of pancreatic enzymes necessary to digest nutrients, so to reduce the risk of malnutrition, pancreatic enzyme supplements (extracts) are given. The medical therapy target is to correct fat, protein, and carbohydrate malabsorption with pancreatic extracts, and secondary diabetes mellitus with insulin. Pancreatic extracts must be given with meals for good effect.

Ileostomy/Colostomy

An ostomy may be required when part of the urinary tract or bowel does not work and an alternate route must be created for the flow of waste. In the procedure, an opening called a stoma is surgically created between the body surface and the intestinal tract, allowing defecation from the intact portion of the intestine.

When the entire colon, rectum, and anus have to be removed following severe colitis, Crohn's disease, colon cancer, or intestinal trauma, an **ileostomy** or opening into the ileum is performed. If only the rectum and anus are removed, a **colostomy** can provide entrance to the colon.

The consistency of the stool from an ileostomy is liquid, whereas that from a colostomy ranges from mushy to fairy well formed. Odor is a major concern for the patient with an ileostomy or colostomy.

Nutritional Implications and Intervention

Foods that tend to cause odor from a colostomy are corn, dried beans, onions, cabbage, highly spiced foods, and fish. Fibrous vegetables should be avoided, and patients must chew foods well to prevent food getting caught at the point where the ileum narrows as it enters the abdominal wall, causing a food blockage.

Symptoms of blockage include the following:

- Objectionable odor
- Change in discharge from a semisolid to a thin liquid
- Increase in volume of output
- Cramping
- Distended abdomen
- Vomiting
- No ileostomy output, which usually occurs when there is complete blockage

Because of excessive losses of salt and water in patients with ileostomy, it is important that the diet be adequate in sodium and water. Electrolytes should be monitored closely. Gas-forming foods such as Brussels sprouts, peas, spinach, corn, cabbage, broccoli, string beans, dried beans, beer, cucumbers, carbonated beverages, and mushrooms should be limited.

If diarrhea occurs, the patient should follow a low-residue diet. Strained banana, applesauce, boiled rice, and tapioca are some foods that may help alleviate diarrhea.

WEIGHT HISTORY

The patient's weight is pivotal to the nutrition assessment. When a patient is first admitted to the hospital or nursing home, his or her ideal body weight is not the main concern because that patient might be overweight but still malnourished because of poor oral intake prior to admission. It is, therefore, important to ascertain the patient's usual body weight and compare that weight to the current weight to determine severity of weight loss, if any. Patients should be weighed on admission. If you are unable to obtain weight from the patient's chart, utilize family members to obtain an estimated weight until the accurate weight measurement is available. Should you decide to use an estimated weight based on visual assessment, or as reported by the patient or family members, you should document the term *estimated weight* or *reported weight* in the nutrition assessment. Make an effort to obtain the patient's correct weight as soon as possible after admission. Patients can be malnourished, yet present with normal weight because of fluid overload. Therefore, use the patient's ideal body weight to determine caloric and protein needs.

Height is important in determining ideal body weight. Ideally, the patient should be measured to obtain an accurate height; if you are unable to do so, using the height reported by the patient is acceptable. You can also obtain height information from the patient's driver's license. If you must estimate height then document it as *estimated height.*

Determining Ideal Body Weight

You can determine the ideal body weight by following these guides:

Male: Allow 106 pounds for the first 5 ft and 6 pounds for each additional inch.

Female: Allow 100 pounds for the first 5 ft and 5 pounds for each additional inch. If the patient is less than 5 ft, subtract 5 pounds for each inch shorter than 5 ft.

Always create a weight range, which is usually 10% below and 10% above ideal body weight. For example, a woman who is 5ft 5 in. tall would have a weight range of 113–138 pounds.

Determining Adjusted Body Weight

Adjusted body weight is used for patients whose current weight is greater than or equal to 125% of their ideal body weight. Today body mass index (BMI) is most commonly used to determine overweight and obesity status.

Formula:

$$(\text{Actual weight} - \text{Ideal body weight}) \times 25\% + \text{Ideal weight} = \text{Adjusted body weight}$$

Example: For a male 5 ft 8 in. tall who weighs 250 pounds, the calculation for adjusted body weight is as follows:

$$\text{Actual weight (250 pounds)} - \text{Ideal body weight (154 pounds)} = 96 \text{ pounds}$$

$$96 \times .25 = 24 \text{ pounds}$$

$$24 + 154 = 178 \text{ pounds}$$

$$\text{Adjusted body weight} = 178 \text{ pounds}$$

Determining Weight Change

Here are the formulas for calculating weight changes:

- % Ideal body weight = Current weight ÷ Ideal body weight × 100
- % Usual body weight = Current weight ÷ usual body weight × 100
- % of Weight change = (Usual body weight − Current weight ÷ Usual body weight × 100)

UBW refers to previous weight at a specific point in time, for example, 1 month ago, or 6 months ago. **Table 1-1** shows guidelines on how to interpret weight changes.

Nutritional Implications and Intervention

Based on weight history and severity of weight loss, if any, the focus should be on maximizing oral intake or providing alternate feeding as soon as possible if oral intake is not feasible or is unachievable. Malnutrition is quite common in patients in hospitals and nursing homes.

Approximately 70–80% of malnourished patients currently enter and leave the hospital without healthcare practitioners acting to treat their malnutrition and without the diagnosis appearing on their discharge summary (Lean, 2008).

Factors attributed to malnutrition include anorexia, adjusting to hospitalization, dysphagia, metabolic disorder (e.g., cachexia secondary to cancer), AIDS, malabsorption, gastrointestinal distress, and a delayed response to poor caloric and protein intake.

Research studies indicate that up to 55% of older adults admitted to hospitals suffer from malnutrition. The challenge, therefore, is to prevent weight loss because unplanned severe weight loss correlates with poor nutrition outcome and increases length of stay in the hospital.

Table 1–1 Interpretation of Percentage Weight Change

Interpretation

Weight loss/gain of 1% to 2% in 1 week is significant. Weight loss/gain of > 2% in 1 week is severe.

Time	Significant Weight Loss (%)	Severe Weight Loss (%)
1 week	1–2	> 2
1 month	5	> 5
3 months	7.5	> 7.5
6 months	10	> 10

SKIN INTEGRITY

A pressure ulcer or pressure sore is a localized injury to the skin and/or underlying tissue, usually over a bony prominence, as a result of pressure. Pressure ulcers usually result from an inadequate supply of oxygen and nutrients to the skin's epithelial and supportive tissues. Pressure ulcers are staged to classify the degree of tissue damage observed. (See **Table 1–2**.)

The number of hospital patients with pressure sores, also called decubitus ulcers or bed sores, rose from 280,000 cases in 1993 to 455,000 cases in 2003—a 63% increase—according to data from the Department of Health and Human Services Agency for Healthcare Research and Quality (AHRQ) (Russo & Elixhauser, 2006).

Usually, nurses assess the skin integrity of the patient/resident using the Braden Scale and document it in the medical chart. However, because nutrition plays such a vital role in the healing process, the dietitian must be involved and must address matters relating to wound healing.

The Centers for Medicare and Medicaid Services (CMS) guidelines released on November 12, 2004, stipulate that facilities need to concentrate on residents' risk factors for and prevention of pressure sores, not just the Braden Scale (Beckrich & Aronovitch, 1999).

Risk Factors Associated With Delayed Wound Healing

Immobility and inactivity are primary risk factors for developing pressure ulcers. Malnutrition characterized by protein-calorie deficiency, anemia,

Table 1–2 Stages of Pressure Ulcers

Stages of Pressure Ulcers	Description	Nutrition Consideration
Stage I	Skin is warm to touch. Usually a persistent area of redness in lightly pigmented skin. In darker skin tones, the ulcer may appear with persistent red, blue, or purple hues.	• Ensure adequate caloric and fluid intake. • Recommend 30–35 cal/kg and 0.8–1.1 g protein per kg, more for patients who are malnourished or who have an albumin level < 3.5 mg/dL. • Add MVI to regimen.
Stage II	Partial thickness skin loss involving epidermis, dermis, or both. The ulcer is superficial and presents clinically as an abrasion, blister, or a shallow open ulcer.	• Ensure adequate caloric and fluid intake. • Recommend 30–35 cal/kg. • Recommend 1.1–1.3 g protein/kg, more for patients who are malnourished or who have an albumin level < 3.5 mg/dL. • Add MVI once a day and vitamin C 500 mg once a day to regimen.
Stage III	Full thickness skin loss involving damage to, necrosis of subcutaneous tissue that may extend down to, but not through underlying fascia.	• Ensure adequate caloric and fluid intake. • Recommend 35 cal/kg and 1.3–1.5 g protein/kg. • Add MVI once a day and vitamin C 500 mg per day.
Stage IV	Full thickness skin loss with extensive destruction, tissue necrosis, or damage to muscle, bone, or supporting structures (e.g., tendon, joint capsule).	• Ensure adequate caloric and fluid intake. • Recommend 35 cal/kg. Increase calories if patient is underweight or has had weight loss. • Recommend 1.5–2.0 g protein/kg body weight. • Add MVI once a day, vitamin C 500 mg twice a day. (Zinc is recommended only if there is evidence of zinc deficiency.)

vitamin deficiency, and dehydration is also a major risk factor. Malnutrition impedes healing for both chronic and acute wounds. Dehydration can result in an increase in blood glucose, which slows the healing process. Steroids and anticoagulants can also delay wound healing. Impaired wound healing may occur in patients taking glucocorticoids because these drugs suppress inflammatory cells and collagen synthesis (Ayello & Cuddington, 2004). The use of anticoagulants such as heparin/warfarin has a negative impact on the earliest stage of wound healing.

Patients who are immunocompromised such as older adults, those with cancer, and those with HIV/AIDS have reduced or delayed inflammatory response and may be at risk for infection or wound compromise. It is important that you assess for adequate calorie, protein, and fluid intake to aid wound healing.

Several randomized controlled trials have concluded that vitamin C, zinc, and arginine improve the rate of pressure ulcer healing (Desneves, Todorovic, Cassar, & Crowe, 2005). Clinical trials have demonstrated an improvement in healing rates with enhanced enteral formulas containing zinc, arginine, and vitamin C. Zinc is especially useful when there is a decrease in serum albumin.

Preventing Pressure Ulcers

The goal for pressure ulcers should be zero occurrences. Pressure ulcer prevention strategies should include the following six key elements:

- Conduct a pressure ulcer admission assessment for all patients.
- Reassess risk for all patients daily.
- Inspect skin daily.
- Manage moisture.
- Optimize nutrition and hydration.
- Minimize pressure. (Duncan, 2007)

Pressure ulcers are costly and painful and can be fatal if not treated aggressively. Preventing pressure ulcers help to save healthcare dollars.

GASTROINTESTINAL REVIEW

The gastrointestinal review looks at all factors involving the gastrointestinal (GI) tract and its impact on nutritional status.

Nausea and Vomiting

Nausea is an uneasiness of the stomach that often accompanies the urge to vomit, but doesn't always lead to vomiting. Vomiting, or emesis, can be caused by gastroparesis, as in uncontrolled diabetes, chemotherapy in cancer patients, food allergies, viral infection, or medications.

Investigate the nature of the emesis. Does the emesis consist of partially or fully digested food? Is it coffee ground in color, or is there blood? Coffee-ground emesis is indicative of gastrointestinal bleeding, which could cause a decrease in hemoglobin and hematocrit. It results from blood that has been in the stomach for a period of time, which indicates a slow bleed. An active GI bleed is indicated by bloody emesis.

It is also important to know when the vomiting occurs. Is it after meals? If so, how long after the meal does it occur? After which foods are consumed does the vomiting occur? This information is crucial to the nutrition intervention. Food elimination may be necessary if vomiting occurs consistently with some foods. Also consider that gastric tumor may cause emesis of undigested food. Emesis that is yellow or green may suggest the presence of bile, which could indicate gallbladder disease.

Nutritional Implications and Intervention

Persistent nausea and vomiting have the potential for anorexia with subsequent weight loss and dehydration. Bloody emesis can cause anemia, causing weakness and dizziness with increased risk for falls, especially in older adults. Vomiting decreases potassium and sodium levels as well. It is not unusual for a patient to report "being afraid to eat" lest he starts vomiting. Fluids should be encouraged and high-potassium foods given to prevent electrolyte imbalance. You must investigate the cause of the vomiting and address it. The diet should be low in fiber and fat. A promotility drug or other antiemetic medication is usually given to increase gastric emptying.

Stools and Diarrhea

Diarrhea is defined as the frequent passage of liquid stools greater than three per day for two consecutive days that may or may not be associated with a pathologic state. Some patients experience diarrhea with the use of antibiotics, and this may last for the duration of the antibiotic therapy. Diarrhea can also be caused by viral gastroenteritis; food poisoning;

malabsorption syndrome, which includes lactose intolerance, gluten malabsorption, inflammatory bowel disease—Crohn's disease, ulcerative colitis, and irritable bowel syndrome. Chemotherapy and laxatives containing magnesium are also associated with diarrhea.

Upper gastrointestinal (GI) bleed may cause dark, tarry stools. Iron supplements, however, may cause the stool to be dark as well, so a guaiac test is usually performed to determine the presence of blood. Stool sample is smeared on a card to test for blood in the stool. A dark red to black tarry appearance of the stool is indicative of a loss of 0.5 mL to 0.75 mL of blood from the upper gastrointestinal tract. Inflammatory bowel disease, stomach ulcers, colitis, and hemorrhoids may cause GI bleed.

Meat consumption prior to a stool test can give a false-positive test because of the presence of hemoglobin and myoglobin in the meat. Aspirin, alcohol, and excess vitamin C in amounts greater than 500 mg/day may cause a false-negative test (Fischbach, 2003).

Lower gastrointestinal bleed tends to cause frank bleeding, that is, obvious bleeding such as vomiting blood or seeing actual blood in the stools. Clay-colored stools may be indicative of jaundice.

Nutritional Implications and Intervention

You must investigate the cause of the diarrhea. If diarrhea is caused by the presence of *Clostridium difficile* (c-diff), antibiotic therapy is usually initiated.

It is wise to avoid lactose products and apple juice because these can exacerbate diarrhea. If persistent diarrhea is not caused by antibiotics, then antidiarrheal medications should be considered to improve diarrhea to prevent weight loss and ensure nutrient adequacy. Whatever the cause of the diarrhea, adequate fluids and electrolytes must be maintained to prevent dehydration and electrolyte imbalance. Oral rehydration solutions are used frequently to ensure electrolyte balance.

A variety of studies have found probiotic consumption to be useful in the treatment of many types of diarrhea, including antibiotic-induced diarrhea in adults. In Finland, the efficacy of *Lactobacillus* GG yogurt in preventing erythromycin-associated diarrhea was studied. Sixteen healthy volunteers were given erythromycin acistrate 400 mg t.i.d. for a week. The volunteers were randomly assigned to one of two groups taking twice daily 125 mL of either *Lactobacillus* GG fermented yogurt or pasteurized regular yogurt as placebo during the drug treatment. Subjects receiving *Lactobacillus*

GG yogurt with erythromycin had less diarrhea than those taking pasteurized yogurt. Other side effects of erythromycin, such as abdominal distress, stomach pain, and flatulence, were less common in the GG yogurt group than in the placebo yogurt group (Siitonen et al., 1990).

Teitelbaum (2005) reports in the *Pediatric Infectious Disease Journal* that probiotics were beneficial in treating infectious diarrhea when co-administered with a variety of antibiotics. The study of 16 healthy volunteers taking erythromycin for 1 week found that co-administration of *Lactobacillus* GG yogurt not only reduced the number of days with diarrhea from 8 to 2 but also decreased associated side effects such as abdominal pain from 39% to 23% (Teitelbaum, 2005).

Stools with a positive guaiac warrant further investigation of the underlying problem, and it should be addressed immediately. Diet should be rich in iron and protein to prevent hypoalbuminemia and anemia.

Constipation and Fecal Impaction

Constipation is the passage of small amounts of hard, dry stools, usually fewer than three times a week. Symptoms of constipation include feeling bloated, uncomfortable, and sluggish. Sudden watery diarrhea in someone who has chronic constipation is usually an indication of a fecal impaction. A fecal impaction is a large mass of dry, hard stool that can develop in the rectum as a result of chronic constipation. This mass may be so hard that it cannot be excreted, so the patient has to be disimpacted. In severe cases, the patient may require hospitalization. Fecal impaction can be fatal.

Contributory Factors

Specific factors contribute to constipation and fecal impaction:

- *Specific diseases/disorders*: Several disorders can cause constipation. These include neurologic disorders such as multiple sclerosis, Parkinson's disease, stroke, and spinal injuries. Metabolic and endocrine conditions including diabetes, underactive or overactive thyroid glands, and hypercalcemia also contribute to constipation.
- *Medications*: Medications that can cause constipation include pain medications (especially narcotics), antacids that contain aluminum and calcium, blood pressure medications (calcium channel blockers), anti-Parkinson drugs, antispasmodics, antidepressants, iron supplements, diuretics, and anticonvulsants.

- *Lack of physical activity*: Lack of physical activity can lead to constipation. Bedridden patients with stroke, dementia, or cerebral palsy are at high risk. The frequent use of laxatives for elimination over time can lead to loss of bowel function, causing chronic constipation.
- *Caffeine and alcohol*: Alcohol and liquids containing caffeine, such as coffee and cola drinks, have a diuretic effect and can increase the risk for dehydration and subsequent constipation.

Nutritional Implications and Intervention

Constipation causes bloating and discomfort and affects the patient's appetite. The risk of constipation can be reduced by encouraging the patient to increase fluid intake, gradually introduce fiber in the diet, and avoid excessive intake of banana, which can promote constipation. Encourage patients to limit intake of caffeine-containing beverages and increase physical activity, including range of motion for those who are bedridden.

The Prevalence of Enteral/Parenteral Nutrition (Nutrition Support)

Enteral Nutrition

If a patient's oral intake is suboptimal, proper documentation such as calorie count and/or food record of oral intake with percentages consumed should be in place to support the need for alternate feeding. If the patient is unable to make decisions about alternate feeding, contact the family to make the decision. In the absence of family involvement, the matter should be referred to the ethics committee of the facility for a decision to be made.

Enteral nutrition is administered into the gastrointestinal tract via percutaneous endoscopic gastrostomy (PEG), a nasogastric tube (NGT), percutaneous endoscopic jejunostomy (PEJ), or a orogastric tube (OGT).

Indications for early enteral nutrition include the following:

- Major head injuries, torso or abdominal trauma
- Major upper GI surgery that precludes oral intake for > 5 days
- Second- or third-degree burns over more than 20% of the body
- Chronical malnourishment in patients anticipated to be without oral intake for > 5 days

Enteral nutrition support is contraindicated in the following situations:

- When aggressive therapy is not warranted—poor prognosis
- When there is intractable vomiting or diarrhea
- Intestinal obstruction, peritonitis, short bowel syndrome with 75% or more resection of the small intestine and ileus
- When there is high output proximal fistula
- When a patient has severe acute pancreatitis

The caloric and protein needs of the patient are based on his or her medical condition. Formulas are designed to meet specific needs, for example, formula containing reduced carbohydrate for patients with diabetes, branched chain amino acids for patients with liver failure, and reduced water for patients with pulmonary conditions. Specialized formulas containing extra protein and calories, glutamine, arginine, and zinc are used for the critically ill patient. Adequate calories should be provided so that protein is not used for energy.

A patient new to tube feeding should start feeding at a lower rate, for example, 20–40 mL/hour. Calorically dense formulas such as those offering 1.5–2.0 cal/mL should start at a much lower rate of 10–15 mL/hr. Feeding should be gradually advanced in small increments every 8–12 hours until actual caloric needs are met in those patients who are hemodynamically stable. Feeding for the unstable patients should be advanced as can be tolerated.

Complications of Enteral Nutrition Following are the common complications of enteral nutrition:

- *Diarrhea*: Diarrhea and vomiting are associated with too rapid an infusion rate during feeding. Diarrhea can also be the result of intestinal atrophy; medications such as antibiotics, laxatives, or sorbitol-containing meds; or the presence of *Clostridium difficile* bacteria. Poor handling of formula can introduce bacteria as well. A hypertonic formula and hypoalbuminemia are also associated with diarrhea.
- *Constipation*: Constipation while on enteral nutrition can be attributed to lack of activity, inadequate fluids and fiber, and use of pain medications and narcotics.
- *Refeeding syndrome*: Refeeding syndrome can occur if the malnourished patient is fed too aggressively. Refeeding syndrome is charac-

terized by acute drops in the plasma levels of phosphorus, potassium, and magnesium. It may involve anemia, respiratory distress, tetany, and severe or fatal cardiac arrythmias. Monitoring of electrolytes, fluid input/output, glucose, and daily weights is important in preventing refeeding syndrome.

- *Aspiration*: A misplaced tube can cause aspiration. Patients receiving tube feeding may experience apirations evidenced by repeated pneumonia with an increase in temperature. A jejunostomy tube may be considered as an alternate route for feeding, though there is never an absolute lack of risk of aspiration. Other contributory factors to aspiration include decreased intestinal motility and gastric emptying. It is important that the head of the bed be elevated at a 45° angle during feeding to prevent aspiration.
- *Dehydration*: Dehydration in patients receiving enteral nutrition is associated with a hypertonic formula without sufficient free water. Excessive protein intake and hyperglycemia also can cause dehydration. Fluid needs are estimated at 1 mL/cal. You must calculate the water content of the formula and the water used for medications, and then determine free water flushes to meet the fluid needs of the patient. If there is evidence of constipation, increase fluids; however, be sure to monitor electrolytes to ensure that there is no hypervolemia (fluid overload).
- *Overhydration*: Overhydration of patients receiving enteral nutrition can lead to hyponatremia, or low serum sodium. Symptoms of hyponatremia include fatigue, lethargy, confusion, seizures, decreased consciousness, or coma. Reducing fluid intake can correct the sodium level.
- *High gastric residual volume*: Gastric residual volume is used as an indicator of the patient's tolerance for enteral feeding. Residuals should be less than 200 mL. If there is a high residual volume in the patient who is tube fed, take the following actions:
    1. Switch to a low-fat, low-fiber formula or diet if the patient is being fed orally as well.
    2. Administer the solution at room temperature.
    3. Consider adding Reglan (metoclopramide) for increased gastric emptying.
    4. Reduce tube feeding rate.

5. Consider a proton pump inhibitor to improve the integrity of the gastrointestinal tract; examples include Protonix (pantoprazole), Prevacid (lansoprozole), Prilosec (omeprazole), Nexium (esomeprazole magnesium).
6. Tighten glycemic control in the diabetic patient to glucose < 200 mg/dL.
7. Do not stop feeding, but repeat residuals in 4 hours.
8. If no improvement occurs, consider total parenteral nutrition (TPN).

Monitor patients who are receiving enteral nutrition carefully for electrolyte balance. Dilantin (phenytoin), an anticonvulsant, should be given 2 hours before or after tube feeding to increase bioavailability of the drug.

Parenteral Nutrition

Parenteral nutrition is usually administered into the veins. Peripheral parenteral nutrition (PPN) is administered into the veins of the arm, whereas total parenteral nutrition (TPN) is administered into the superior or inferior vena cava or the jugular vein. TPN is also called IVH, intravenous hyperalimentation.

Medicare guidelines stipulate that daily TPN be considered reasonable and necessary for a patient with severe pathology of the alimentary tract that does not allow absorption of sufficient nutrients to maintain weight and strength commensurate with the patient's general condition.

Qualifications for Parenteral Nutrition Conditions that qualify for parenteral nutrition include the following:

- A condition involving the small intestine and/or its exocrine glands that significantly impairs the absorption of nutrients.
- Disease of the stomach and/or intestine which is a motility disorder and impairs the ability of nutrients to be absorbed through the GI system The gut does not work.
- Need for nothing by mouth (NPO) status longer than 7 days, or few days if the patient presents with high nutrition risk.
- Nutritional needs that are greater than the amount of nutrients that can be delivered enterally.

Contraindications for Parenteral Nutrition Parenteral nutrition should not be used in the following situations:

- When there is a functioning GI tract
- When prognosis is poor
- In mild to moderate nutrition risk patients with short-term NPO status

Factors to consider for parenteral nutrition are caloric, fluid, protein, carbohydrate, fat, vitamin, mineral, and electrolyte needs of the patient.

Components of Parenteral Nutrition

- *Carbohydrate:* In the form of dextrose. Dextrose concentrations vary from 10% to 70%. Dextrose is calculated at 3.4 cal/g.
- *Protein:* Amino acids (AA) are available in 3% to 10% solutions. AA is calculated at 4 cal/g.
- *Lipids:* Available in 10–20% solutions. Ten percent lipids are calculated at 1.1 cal/mL and, 20% lipids at 2 cal/mL.
- *Electrolytes:* Provided as part of the general solutions to meet requirements. Amounts vary according to individual patient needs.
- *Vitamins and minerals:* Daily maintenance dosage given in standard solutions. May be adjusted to meet patient needs.
- *Trace elements:* Maintenance dosage provided in standard solutions.
- *Medications:* Insulin may be added to the solution for blood glucose control.

Calculating Parenteral Nutrition Formulas

1. *Calculate caloric needs.* Using the sample patient described in the preceding table, the caloric requirement is 1860 cal /day (30 cal/kg; $30 \times 62 = 1860$ calories).
2. *Determine protein needs.* Assuming that the patient is moderately ill, provide 1.2 g/kg to 1.5 g/kg. Protein needs would therefore be 74–93 g/day.
3. *Determine if the solution meets the needs of the patient.* First, find the volume of solution provided to the patient. Infusion for this patient begins at 18:00 hours (6 pm) and runs until 10:00 hours (10 am) at 84 mL/hr providing 1344 mL of solution over 16 hours. At 10:10 am the rate was reduced to 63 mL/hr to run for 8 hours providing 504 mL.

Sample Parenteral Nutrition Description

Patient: Jane Doe

Age: 64 years

Sex: Female

Height: 64.0 inches

Weight: 62 kg

Medication Description

Large Volumes	Dose	Dose Quantity	Rate Frequency	Next Time
Dextrose 40%	400 g	1 ea	84 mL/hr IV	10/31/08 18:00 hrs
Freamine III 10% 1000 mL	100 g	1 ea		
Sodium chloride 23.4% 30 mL	154 mEq	1.2833 ea	63 mL/hr Administer at 10 am daily and infuse over 8 hours	11/1/08 10:00 hrs
Potassium acetate 40 mEq/20 mL INJ	38 mEq	0.95 ea		
Calcium gluconate 10% 10 mL INJ	18.6047 mEq	4 ea		
Magnesium sulfate 50% 2 mL INJ	12.8 mEq	1.58 ea		
Multi trace elements 5 1 mL	1 mL	1 ea		
MVI12 10 mL INJ	10 mL	1 ea		
Potassium phosphate 3 mmo/mL 5mL	44 mEq	2 ea		
Potassium chloride 40 mEq/20 mL INJ	60 mEq	1.5 ea		
Insulin human reg 100 U/mL (LVP)	30 U	0.3 mL		
Lipid 10% 500 mL	500 mL	1 ea		

Also contains phosphate 20 mEq, sodium 10 mEq, and acetate 89 mEq

Total run time is 24 hours providing 1848 mL of solution. Note well that the constituents of the solution indicated on the TPN description are per 1000 mL (1 liter) of solution.

Calculate:

$$\text{Calories from dextrose: } 1.848 \text{ L} \times 400 \times 3.4 = 2513 \text{ cal}$$

$$\text{Calories from fat: } 1.848 \text{ L} \times 500 \times 1.1 = 1016 \text{ cal}$$

$$\text{Total non-protein cal} = 3529 \text{ cal}$$

$$\text{Total protein } 1.848 \text{ L} \times 100 = 185 \text{ g}$$

$$\text{Calories from protein (freamine) } 1.848 \text{ L} \times 100 \times 4 = 739 \text{ cal}$$

The solution above provides calories and protein in excess of required amounts. Unlike enteral nutrition formula, TPN usually begins at a high rate and decreases gradually. Monitor patient for weight gain. Insulin is provided to reduce the risk of hyperglycemia.

Nutritional Implications and Intervention Careful documentation must be in place to support the need for parenteral nutrition (PN). Review such documentation periodically for possible weaning and transitioning to oral or enteral nutrition.

A patient who is placed on PN who has been without nutrition for some time is at risk for **refeeding syndrome**. To minimize the risk of refeeding syndrome in PN patients, administer PN at one half the total calories and increase nutritional intake gradually to estimated nutritional requirements.

The National Institute for Clinical Excellence (NICE) recently recommended that parenteral nutrition should be limited to a maximum of 50% of the calculated requirements for the first 48 hours after initiation.

Hyperglycemia is associated with the initiation of PN and sometimes requires the use of insulin to control high blood glucose especially in patients who have diabetes or who experience sepsis. Blood glucose should be monitored frequently.

There is an increased risk for sepsis in patients receiving PN because the gut is not being used. There is also the risk of overfeeding critically ill patients, consequences of which can be fatal. Excessive carbohydrate infusion can result in hypercapnia, which increases the work of the lungs and potentially prolongs the need for mechanical ventilation. Overfeeding can also lead to hyperglycemia and an accumulation of fat in the liver. Severe hyperglycemia results in profound dehydration.

Excessive protein can lead to azotemia, hypertonic dehydration, and metabolic acidosis if the kidneys are unable to properly adjust urea excretion or acid–base balance. Hypertriglyceridemia and fat overload can occur as a result of excessive fat infusion. Monitor blood triglycerides closely. Respiratory distress, coagulopathies, and abnormal liver function tests are the primary manifestations of fat overload (Klein, Stanek, & Wiles 1998). The energy goal is based on the patient's actual weight and 25–30 cal/kg is recommended. The protein recommendation ranges from 1.5–2.0 g/kg body weight depending on the severity of illness. Use the ideal body weight to determine caloric and protein requirements in obese patients.

CARDIOVASCULAR REVIEW

The cardiovascular review takes into consideration the presence of a cerebral vascular accident (CVA) or stroke, congestive heart failure (CHF) or pleural effusion, angina, myocardial infarction (heart attack), hypertension, and obesity. If the patient presents with diabetes, the risk of coronary artery disease is increased. Diabetes causes an increase in triglycerides and a decrease in high-density lipoprotein (HDL). In most cases, once blood glucose is controlled and weight is decreased, triglycerides improve drastically even without medication.

Cerebral Vascular Accident

Cerebral vascular accidents (CVAs), commonly known as stroke, usually occur as a result of uncontrolled hypertension. In most cases, CVAs affect the patient's swallowing ability, speech, and ability to feed himself or herself. Patients experience an overall decline in activities of daily living (ADLs). The stroke patient is at increased risk for weight loss resulting from decline in swallowing and feeding skills. Encourage patients to use adaptive feeding devices to attain some level of independent feeding. Proper positioning is extremely important. The patient should be positioned at or close to a 90° angle as much as possible. The speech therapist determines the consistency of fluids and solids because most patients who have suffered a stroke are dysphagic.

If a patient is on a modified consistency, for example, a pureed diet, consult the speech pathologist before advancing the diet, even if the patient shows improvement in chewing and/or swallowing skills.

A diet low in sodium is usually recommended to help control hypertension. Other complications with CVA include pressure sores and contractures resulting from immobility.

Congestive Heart Failure

Congestive heart failure (CHF) occurs when the heart loses its ability to act as a pump. Some precipitating causes are pulmonary embolism, infection, anemia, myocarditis, arrythmias, and myocardial infarction.

Some symptoms of heart failure are shortness of breath; fatigue or weakness; persistent coughing or wheezing; swelling of the legs, ankles, and feet; third spacing fluid accumulation in the abdomen; lack of appetite; confused thinking; and increased or irregular heartbeat.

Angina and Myocardial Infarction

Heart disease remains the number one killer in the United States. Angina or chest pain occurs when the supply of oxygen to the heart becomes low. Angina is usually a precipitating factor of a heart attack, though not all chest pains are related to a heart condition. If blood flow to the heart is reduced as a result of buildup of plaque, primarily cholesterol along the artery (atherosclerosis), heart cells can die, resulting in a heart attack.

Patients who have diabetes or HIV/AIDS are at increased risk for heart disease. Most patients with type 2 diabetes present with increased triglycerides and decreased HDL. Medications such as Kaletra (lopinavir, ritovavir) used to treat HIV/AIDS patients may cause an increase in triglycerides. Increased triglycerides alone are not a risk factor for heart disease, but suggests to the clinician that there is an increased intake of carbohydrates, especially simple carbohydrates. Increased alcohol intake can also cause an increase in triglycerides. Risk factors for coronary heart disease include age, hereditary factors, overweight, smoking, high blood pressure, and sedentary lifestyle.

Increased homocysteine, an amino acid, in the blood is also associated with coronary heart disease. Folic acid and vitamin B_{12} are usually given to reduce homocysteine levels, but no studies prove that an individual can reduce his or her risk of coronary heart disease by taking these supplements (National Institutes of Health, 2005).

The lipid profile of the patient is the most important blood test for risk assessment. C-reactive protein (CRP), a substance produced in the liver, when elevated has been shown to be associated with an increased risk of heart disease. However, most physicians will not order this test unless the lipids associated with heart disease are also elevated, such as low-density lipoprotein (LDL), total cholesterol, and triglycerides, and also if high-density lipoprotein (HDL) is reduced. CRP levels less than 1 mg/L are considered low risk for a cardiovascular event in the next 10 years. Depending on medical history and other factors, a person having a CRP of 1–3 mg/L could have up to a 20% risk of having a heart attack in the next decade. Those with CRP levels of 3 mg/L or more per liter have the highest risk (National Institutes of Health, 2005).

Lowering high blood pressure and other lifestyle changes can help reduce CRP and improve overall cardiovascular health.

Hypertension

Hypertension is defined as blood pressure greater than 140/90 mmHg. Smoking, high cholesterol, obesity, and diabetes increase the risk of hypertension. The incidence of high blood pressure increases with age, but is today seen in children and adolescents, especially those who are overweight. Uncontrolled hypertension can affect the blood vessels, causing them to become thicker and less elastic, and blood clots can form and stick to the vessel walls. If a clot becomes dislodged, it can enter the bloodstream and do serious damage to various organs.

Prolonged high blood pressure can cause poor blood flow to the heart muscle, so the muscle cannot get the oxygen it needs, thereby causing ischemia. Over time, the heart grows larger; heart enlargement is one of the causes of cardiovascular disease. Besides affecting the heart and blood vessels, prolonged high blood pressure can affect the brain, as in stroke; the kidneys, reducing blood flow and weakening them; and can cause blood vessel constriction, tiny bleeding, and deposits of fat in the eyes. These changes in the eye result in worsening vision and loss of sight.

Obesity

There is a direct association between abdominal obesity and the risk of coronary heart disease. The Framingham Heart Study confirms that obesity is strongly predictive of CHD. Risk for CVD is particularly raised when abdominal obesity is present. Abdominal obesity is defined by a waist circumference greater than 102 cm (40 inches), in men, or 88 cm (35 inches) in women (National Cholesterol Education Program, Third Report, 2009). Encourage the individuals to make lifestyle changes to reduce weight and subsequent risk of heart disease.

Medications Used to Treat Heart Failure

Several types of drugs have been used and are proven useful in the treatment of heart failure. These include angiotensin-converting enzyme (ACE) inhibitors such as Vasotec (enalapril), lisinopril, and captopril; and angiotensin II receptor blockers (ARBs), which include losartan and Diovan (valsartan). These drugs decrease the workload of the heart. Digoxin, also referred to as digitalis, increases the strength of the heart muscle contractions and tends to slow the heartbeat. Beta blockers such as Coreg (carvedilol), Lopressor (metoprolol tartrate) and Zebeta (bisoprolol fumarate) also slow the heart rate.

Diuretics, for example, Furosemide (Lasix) and Spironolactone (Aldactone), are used to reduce fluid retention in patients with congestive heart failure. Lasix is potassium wasting, causing a decrease in serum potassium. Unlike Lasix, Aldactone is primarily potassium sparing. Aldactone prevents salt retention because it inhibits the production of aldosterone known to increase blood pressure.

Nutritional Implications and Intervention

Because of altered fluid status in the patient with congestive heart failure, weight must be interpreted with caution. The patient's oral intake, diet, and weight history provide needed information to determine caloric needs.

Fluid and electrolyte status must be monitored closely. Lasix can cause an increase in blood glucose (Pronsky, 1997). Renal function and potassium levels should be monitored regularly. Potassium supplements are usually given when potassium level drops significantly low. Spironolactone (Aldactone), on the other hand, can raise the level of potassium in the blood to dangerous levels, at which time a potassium-lowering drug such as Kayexalate (sodium polystyrene) may be given to improve hyperkalemia. High potassium can affect heart function. Diarrhea usually occurs with Kayexalate; fluids should therefore be monitored to prevent dehydration.

It is not unusual for a patient with CHF to develop cardiac cachexia, characterized by a marked loss of adipose tissue and lean body mass. Anorexia, depression, nausea and vomiting, and difficulty breathing because of pulmonary edema are some of the precipitating factors in the development of cardiac cachexia.

Restricted activity and a diet low in sodium are usually recommended for the patient with CHF. Fluid restriction may be necessary to help control retention of fluid.

The initial intervention for the patient who presents with the risk factors of coronary heart disease is lifestyle changes—weight loss for overweight patients, smoking cessation, a diet low in fat and cholesterol, reduced intake of simple carbohydrates to control hypertriglyceridemia, good glucose control for patients with diabetes, and increased physical activity. These all help to reduce low-density lipoprotein (LDL) and increase high-density lipoprotein (HDL). A low-sodium diet is also recommended to help control hypertension. The goal is to achieve and maintain a blood pressure of less than 130/80 mmHg. Medications, such as those used for patients with congestive heart failure, are also used to control high blood pressure.

Soluble fiber found in oats, legumes, fruits, and psyllium helps to lower cholesterol and LDL. Niacin is also used with good effect but can cause increased bleeding when used in combination with anticoagulants. Niacin should not be used in patients with kidney problems.

Aspirin or other anticoagulants such as Coumadin (warfarin) are added to prevent blood clots. Monitor the patient's platelets and International Normalized Ratio (INR) regularly when on anticoagulants to ensure that there is no bleeding.

For patients with diabetes, check their lipid profile one to two times a year. It is also important that there be pre-prandial and postprandial readings to determine efficacy of medication and diet regimen. Check hemoglobin AIC two to four times a year as part of the patient's scheduled medical visit (Joslin Diabetes Center, 2009).

PSYCHIATRIC REVIEW

The psychiatric review of the patient takes into consideration the patient's mental status including his level of consciousness; orientation to place, person, and time; impaired or unimpaired memory; decision-making skills; communication skills; presence of hallucination and illusion; and psychomotor behavior. Psychomotor behavior looks at whether the patient resists care, medication, or food; exhibits inappropriate or disruptive behavior such as smearing or throwing feces; is self-abusive; or displays sexual behavior, screaming, disrobing in public, noisiness, or disruptive sounds.

Some patients might not display disruptive behavior but may have mood issues. They may be sad or worried most of the time; may have reduced social interaction, self-depreciation, repetitive physical movements, repetitive physical complaints, fearfulness, paranoia, insomnia, persistent anger with others; and others cry a lot. Diagnoses that suggest psychosis include anxiety disorder, depression, and bipolar disorder.

Nutritional Implications and Intervention

All of the psychiatric situations mentioned have some impact on the patient's nutritional status. Medications used for psychosis and their interaction with nutrition are discussed later in this chapter. Some antidepressants such as Prozac (fluoxetine) and Luvox (fluvoxamine meleate) may cause constipation, thereby increasing the patient's need for extra fluids. Patients who take lithium to treat manic depressive disorder should maintain a consistent intake of sodium to stabilize the drug level because low sodium intake can cause delay in the excretion of lithium from the body, which might result in lithium toxicity. Other conditions that can lower sodium and cause a buildup of lithium include heavy sweating, fever, vomiting, diarrhea, and use of diuretics. Patients taking lithium should have adequate fluid intake to reduce toxicity of the drug.

Abilify (aripiprazole) used to treat schizophrenia and acute manic bipolar disorder has been associated with increased blood sugar.

Those patients with dementia including Alzheimer's disease tend to wander a lot and hardly ever sit to eat a meal. They are usually agitated and restless. Frequent wandering may increase energy needs as much as 1600 calories or more/day. Patient may make inappropriate food choices, forget to eat, or have problem recalling if they have eaten. These patients are at risk for weight loss and should be closely monitored. Offer small frequent meals one plate at a time—finger foods are best.

Some patients are paranoid, thinking that someone is trying to kill them by poisoning their food, so they refuse to eat. They do better with packaged and canned foods, which should be opened in their presence. Encouragement and support are always needed to ensure desirable outcomes for psychotic patients. A thorough review of the patient's mental status is important so that you can plan appropriately for the interview and intervention.

INFECTIOUS DISEASES

Infectious diseases include hepatitis A, B, and C; HIV/AIDS; tuberculosis, malaria, food-borne illnesses, bacterial meningitis, bacterial pneumonia, gastroenteritis, urinary tract infection, typhoid fever, dysentery, and cholera to name a few.

This section focuses on some of the more common infectious diseases seen in acute and long-term care, namely, hepatitis A, B, and C; HIV/AIDS; urinary tract infection; tuberculosis; bacterial pneumonia; and meningitis.

Hepatitis A

Hepatitis A is a liver disease caused by the hepatitis A virus. Hepatitis A is transmitted by the fecal-oral route and is contracted through contaminated drinking water, food, and sewage. Symptoms include anorexia, nausea, vomiting, abdominal pain, dark urine, and jaundice. Serious complications can occur in patients whose immune system is compromised such as older adults and very young children.

In 2007, 2,979 acute symptomatic cases of hepatitis A were reported. The estimated number of new infections was 25,000 (Centers for Disease Control and Prevention, 2009a).

Hepatitis B

Hepatitis B is a serious disease caused by a virus that attacks the liver. The virus, which is called hepatitis B virus (HBV), can cause lifelong infection, cirrhosis (scarring) of the liver, liver cancer, liver failure, and death.

During the past 10 years, an estimated 60,000–110,000 persons were infected with HBV annually, and 5,000 died from HBV-related disease in the United States (Finelli & Bell, 2008). More than 350 million people worldwide are infected with the hepatitis B virus. An estimated 620,000 persons worldwide die from hepatitis B virus-related liver disease each year (Centers for Disease Control and Prevention, 2009b).

Hepatitis B is a blood-borne disease and is transmitted via intravenous (IV) drug use, sex, and childbirth. Hepatitis B infection is common among healthcare workers.

Signs and symptoms of hepatitis B infection are similar to those of hepatitis A—jaundice, fatigue, abdominal pain, loss of appetite, nausea, vomiting, and joint pain.

According the Centers for Disease Control and Prevention (2009), about 30% of persons have no signs or symptoms.

Hepatitis C

Hepatitis C is a disease of the liver caused by the hepatitis C virus (HCV). It is one of the most common causes of chronic liver disease in the United States today, affecting more than 4 million Americans. At least 80% of patients with acute hepatitis C ultimately develop chronic liver infection, and 20% to 30% develop cirrhosis. Between 1% and 5% of patients may develop liver cancer. Hepatitis C is now the number-one cause for liver transplantation in the United States (National Institutes of Health, 2002).

Symptoms of hepatitis C infection include jaundice, abdominal pain (right upper abdomen), fatigue, loss of appetite, nausea and vomiting, low-grade fever, pale or clay-colored stools, dark urine, generalized itching, and bleeding varices (dilated veins throughout the gastrointestinal tract).

Nutritional Implications and Intervention

The liver is the largest and one of the most versatile organs in the body. Its functions include the following:

- *Carbohydrate metabolism*: The liver stores glucose as glycogen, breaks down glycogen to supply glucose when levels become low,

and produces glucose from noncarbohydrate sources such as lactic acid and amino acids.
- *Conversion of amino acids to glucose and the synthesis of non-essential amino acids.*
- *Detoxification of ammonia*: The liver converts ammonia to urea for excretion by the kidneys.
- *Storage of fat-soluble vitamins and some minerals as well as vitamin* B_{12}.
- *Synthesis of triglycerides, phospholipids, cholesterol, and bile salts.* Bile is essential for the absorption of the fat-soluble vitamins A, D, E, and K.
- *Removal of bacteria, alcohol, and toxic substances from the blood:* The liver converts toxins to substances that can be excreted from the body.
- *Synthesis of drugs and medications.*

When the liver is damaged its functioning is impaired.

Malnutrition is quite common in patients with chronic liver disease. Factors that contribute to malnutrition include a severely restricted diet, altered taste, portal hypertension, weakness, fatigue, early satiety in the presence of ascites, and malabsorption leading to inadequate intake of calories and protein. Protein-calorie malnutrition (PCM)—a condition of body wasting related to dietary deficiency of calories and protein—is found in 65–90% of patients with advanced liver disease and in almost 100% of candidates for liver transplantation (Henkel & Buchman, 2006).

Patients with hepatitis accompanied by ascites and varices should receive a sodium-restricted diet. In the absence of hepatic encephalopathy, protein should be increased greater than or equal to 1.5 g/kg of body weight. If the patient is experiencing hepatic encephalopathy evidenced by neurologic changes and an increase in ammonia level, a diet providing 0.8–1.0 g/kg is considered adequate because severe restriction of protein may cause further malnutrition.

A high ammonia level in the absence of neurologic changes is not considered hepatic encephalopathy. Most physicians will prescribe lactulose and/or neomycin to treat patients with hepatic encephalopathy. Lactulose causes diarrhea, and therefore fluid and electrolytes should be replenished to avoid dehydration. Branch chain amino acids (BCAA) supplementation may improve hepatic encephalopathy.

Patients with liver disease should be encouraged to avoid substances that are toxic to the liver, including alcohol. Even moderate amounts of alcohol speed up the progression of hepatitis C, and alcohol reduces the effectiveness of treatment.

Liver damage can cause bile to back up in the liver so that it is not available to the small intestine for the digestion of fats. When fat is not absorbed, it is excreted in large amounts in the feces, resulting in steatorrhea. Medium-chain triglycerides (MCTs) can help alleviate this condition.

A low serum albumin level is associated with liver disease because the damaged liver cannot synthesize protein and is therefore not a reliable marker for determining nutritional status. Because of fluid shift as in the presence of edema and ascites, you also cannot use weight to determine caloric needs.

In determining nutritional status in the patient with end-stage liver disease (ESLD), Henkel and Buchman (2006) suggest the use of anthropometry, subjective global assessment (SGA), which looks at weight loss during the previous 6 months, changes in dietary intake, gastrointestinal symptoms, functional capacity, metabolic demands, signs of muscle wasting, and the presence of presacral or pedal edema, and also the use of indirect calorimetry. Hand-grip strength was also considered to be a good predictor of complications in patients with advanced liver disease.

The diet should provide adequate calories and protein to prevent or reduce the risk of protein-calorie malnutrition (PCM). Small frequent meals are advised with a late evening snack to reduce protein breakdown. If oral intake is suboptimal, enteral nutrition should be initiated.

HIV/AIDS

HIV (human immunodeficiency virus) is a virus that attacks the body's immune system. The immune system protects the body from infections and diseases.

The Centers for Disease Control and Prevention now estimates that 1.1 million adults and adolescents (prevalence rate: 447.8 per 100,000 population) were living with diagnosed or undiagnosed HIV infection in the United States at the end of 2006. The majority of those living with

HIV were nonwhite (65.4%), and nearly half (48.1%) were men who have sex with men (MSM). The HIV prevalence rates for blacks (1,715.1 per 100,000) and Hispanics (585.3 per 100,000) were, respectively, 7.6 and 2.6 times the rate for whites (224.3 per 100,000; Morbidity and Morality Weekly Report, 2008). An estimated 55,000–58,500 new HIV infections occur in the United States each year (CDC, 2008).

AIDS is the late stage of the HIV infection in which the patient's CD4 cell count falls below 200 or the patient develops serious AIDS-defining diseases including but not limited to wasting syndrome, toxoplasmosis, recurrent pneumonia, esophageal candidiasis, Kaposi's sarcoma, *Mycobacterium avium* complex (MAC), tuberculosis, herpetic ulcers, and progressive multifocal leukoencephalopathy.

A patient may have HIV for a number of years before being diagnosed. Patients may present with flu-like symptoms, headache, cough, diarrhea, swollen glands, lack of energy, loss of appetite, weight loss, fever, sweats, repeated yeast infections, skin rashes, pelvic and abdominal cramps, sores in the mouth or on certain parts of the body, or short-term memory and/or vision loss.

Urinary Tract Infection

Urinary tract infection can occur anywhere along the urinary tract and is usually caused by bacteria from the anus entering the urethra and then the bladder, which leads to inflammation and infection in the lower urinary tract.

Symptoms of a urinary tract infection include pressure in the lower pelvis, pain or burning with urination, frequent or urgent need to urinate, cloudy urine, bloody urine, and foul or strong urine odor.

Pulmonary Tuberculosis

Pulmonary tuberculosis (TB) is a contagious bacterial infection caused by Mycobacterium tuberculosis (M. tuberculosis). The lungs are primarily involved, but the infection can spread to other organs.

Individuals with immune system damage caused by AIDS have a higher risk of developing active tuberculosis—either from new exposure to TB or reactivation of dormant mycobacteria. Symptoms include cough, mild fever, fatigue, unintentional weight loss, hemoptysis, night sweats, and phlegm-producing cough.

Treatment for TB includes rifampin, which can cause a significant increase in uric acid. An increase in uric acid can lead to gouty arthritis.

Pneumonia

Pneumonia is a common illness that affects millions of people each year in the United States. Pneumonia is an inflammation of the lungs caused by an infection. Bacterial pneumonias tend to be the most serious and the most common cause of pneumonia in adults. The most common pneumonia-causing bacterium in adults is Streptococcus pneumoniae (pneumococcus). The main symptoms of pneumonia are cough with greenish or yellow mucus, bloody sputum, fever, sharp or stabbing chest pain worsened by deep breathing or coughing, rapid shallow breathing, and shortness of breath. Other symptoms include headache, loss of appetite, excessive fatigue, and confusion in older people.

Nutritional Implications and Intervention

Most infectious diseases are accompanied by weight loss, increased temperature, anorexia, increased sweat, fatigue, increased risk for dehydration, and shortness of breath as in the case of pneumonia.

Antibiotics are usually administered to treat many infectious diseases, which oftentimes increase the need for more fluids and electrolytes because the patient may experience diarrhea with fluid and electrolyte imbalance.

Pay special attention to adequate nutrition and fluid intake in patients with infectious diseases. High-potassium foods such as fruit juices and banana are recommended for electrolyte replacement. Weight loss is common; therefore the diet should be adequate to meet calorie and protein needs. Small frequent meals are recommended to correct anorexia and fatigue. The patient may also require a nutritional supplement to meet dietary needs if meal intake is inadequate.

Patients treated with highly active antiretroviral therapy (HAART) for the management of HIV/AIDS should be carefully monitored for risk factors of CHD caused by some medications; for example, Kaletra (lopinavir, ritonavir) is known to cause hyperlipidemia. Other medications induce hepatotoxicity, osteopenia/osteoporosis/osteonecrosis, insulin resistance, and hypertension. Anemia is common in patients with HIV/AIDS; Procrit (epoetin alfa) and ferrous sulphate are usually given to improve this condition.

If the patient presents with oral thrush, modify the diet to allow for easy swallowing.

MUSCULOSKELETAL REVIEW

The musculoskeletal review looks at the body's network of tissues and muscles that are responsible for both voluntary and involuntary movements. Symptoms of decline in the functions of the musculoskeletal system include loss of subcutaneous fat, muscle wasting, edema, painful or swollen joints, and progressive weakness of the muscles. Bow legs, knock knees, and pigeon chest may be a result of protein-energy deficiency and poor intake of vitamins D and C and calcium.

Muscular dystrophy is a disorder of the musculoskeletal system. According to the National Institute of Neurological Disorder and Stroke (2009), muscular dystrophy is characterized by progressive weakness and degeneration of the skeletal muscles that control movement. Medical treatment for muscular dystrophy includes corticosteroids to slow muscle degeneration, anticonvulsants to control seizure and some muscle activity, immunosuppressants to delay dying of muscle cells, and antibiotics to fight respiratory infections. Occupational therapy, physical therapy, and assistive technology are also used in the care of patients with muscular dystrophy.

Nutritional Implications and Intervention

Because the patient's physical movement is compromised, there is an increased risk for overweight, blood clots, calcium deficiency, constipation, and increased blood sugar secondary to use of steroids in patients predisposed to diabetes. Anticonvulsant medications can also contribute to constipation.

The diet should provide adequate calories to maintain normal weight and should also be high in calcium and vitamin D for bone health. In cases where blood thinners are administered to prevent blood clots, monitor the patient for any signs or symptoms of gastrointestinal bleed. Adequate fluids and fiber should be provided to prevent or aid in relieving constipation.

PSYCHOSOCIAL REVIEW

Psychosocial data give information regarding the patient's economic status, occupation, education level, and mental status. This information proves helpful in formulating questions for the interview process. For example, a patient who is undomiciled (homeless) cannot follow a strict diet order; diet teaching must therefore be short and simple with no more than two objectives.

It is important to ascertain patients' food security, which is access to sufficient food at all times for an active and healthy lifestyle; and food insecurity, which is limited or uncertain availability of nutritionally adequate and safe food. Living and shopping arrangements, and availability of a cooking range, refrigerator, and food storage area are critical components that must be included in the psychosocial review of the patient. If the patient has limited access to food, refer the patient to a social worker, who can assist the patient in accessing community resources.

Determining the patient's education level is crucial for the interview. Never assume a patient who has a bachelor's or master's degree is knowledgeable in the area of nutrition and dietetics. As the expert in nutrition, you must ask all the relevant questions needed to complete the assessment thoroughly. Questions may include asking the patient about his or her medical condition and which foods may exacerbate or help improve the outcome. See Chapter 2 for more details.

PULMONARY REVIEW

Gas exchange is the major function of the pulmonary system. The lungs enable the body to obtain oxygen to meet its cellular and metabolic demands and remove the carbon dioxide produced by these processes (Mahan & Escott-Stump, 2008).

There is a strong correlation between malnutrition and pulmonary disease. Malnutrition may impair lung function. Low protein levels resulting from malnutrition contribute to the development of pulmonary edema. When hemoglobin levels are low because of anemia, less oxygen is carried by the blood, resulting in weakness, fatigue, and possibly death. The malnourished patient with lung disease is at risk for developing respiratory infections.

Asthma, bronchitis, and emphysema are collectively known as nonspecific lung diseases. Chronic obstructive pulmonary disease (COPD) is a slowly progressive disease of the airways characterized by a gradual loss of lung function resulting from chronic bronchitis, emphysema, or both. Cigarette smoking is the most important risk factor.

Nutrition Implications and Intervention

Epidemiologic studies indicate that malnourished patients with COPD have a worse prognosis than those who are well nourished. Weight loss in the patient with COPD is caused by the increased work of breathing, frequent recurrent respiratory infections, chronic sputum production, and frequent coughing. Shortness of breath and fatigue can interfere with the patient's ability to prepare and consume meals.

Breathing requires more energy for people with chronic obstructive pulmonary disease (COPD). The muscles used in breathing might require 10 times more calories than those of a person without COPD; hence, the diet must provide adequate calories to meet the increased caloric needs: 30–35 cal/kg is usually recommended for maintenance and 45 cal/kg for anabolism or maintenance during catabolic state.

It is important to monitor biochemical data for any signs of anemia and hypoalbuminemia because these factors can affect the nutritional outcome of the patient with COPD. In the presence of pulmonary edema, sodium should be restricted. Anemia, if present, should be treated aggressively with medication and/or injections such as Aranesp (darbepoetin alfa) or Procrit (epoetin alfa) to enhance good nutritional outcome. The diet should be balanced to provide adequate protein of high biological value and other iron-rich foods. For patients who are on a mechanical ventilator, take care not to overfeed them because this will impede weaning as a result of increased respiratory quotient (RQ—the ratio of carbon dioxide produced to oxygen consumed) and excessive carbon dioxide.

BIOCHEMICAL DATA REVIEW

This section looks at the biochemical data you can use to further assess the patient's medical and nutritional status. Most physicians tend to use the following format for recording lab values:

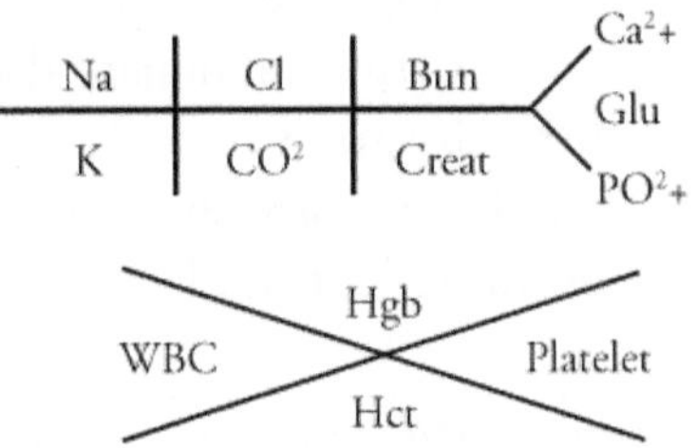

Key:

Na	Sodium	$Ca^{2}+$	Calcium
K	Potassium	Glu	Glucose
Cl	Chloride	$PO^{2}+$	Phosphorus
CO^{2}	Carbon oxide	WBC	White blood cells
BUN	Blood urea nitrogen	Hgb	Hemoglobin
Crea	Creatinine	Hct	Hematocrit

See **Table 1-3** for a more detailed description of these items.

REVIEW OF MEDICATIONS

Review of medications and potential food–drug interaction is important in assessing a patient's nutritional status. This section examines the categories of drugs with emphasis on their nutritional implications. The nutritional implications listed are by no means exhaustive, and you should consult food–medication interaction texts for more details; for example, Zaneta M. Pronsky, *Food–Medication Interactions*, 15th ed. (Pronsky, Z. M., 2008).

Because most drugs are metabolized in the liver, patients with a history of liver disease should have liver function tests done regularly.

See **Table 1-4** for detailed explanations of the nutritional implications of classes of drugs.

(text continues on page 54)

Table 1–3 Biochemical Data

Lab Test	Reference Range	Comments
Albumin	3.5–5.0 g/dL	Albumin values should be interpreted with caution because values can be increased with dehydration and steroid use. Values are usually low with edema/ascites, cancer, liver and kidney disease, and malnutrition. Decreases with prolonged hospital stay and immobility. Because of its 21-day half-life, albumin does not give acute changes in nutritional status.
Prealbumin	16–40 mg/dL	Because of its short half-life of about 2 days, prealbumin is more sensitive to acute changes in nutritional status; it is, however, affected by inflammation. Prealbumin level is usually checked whenever a patient is started on enteral/parenteral nutrition.
Blood urea nitrogen (BUN)	8–23 mg/dL	End product of protein metabolism. Increases with dehydration, renal dysfunction, high protein intake, protein catabolism, gastrointestinal hemorrhage, and diabetes. BUN decreases with overhydration, malnutrition, and liver disease.
Calcium	8.5–10.8 mg/dL	50% of calcium is bound to albumin; the rest is ionized calcium. A low calcium level may be caused by poor protein intake. It also decreases with elevated phosphorus and disorders of vitamin D metabolism. Excessive use of intravenous fluids will decrease albumin and thus decrease serum calcium. Calcium increases with cancer and hyperparathyroidism. Carbohydrates increase the intestinal absorption of calcium. For the patient with chronic kidney disease, corrected calcium is equal to (4.0 – Albumin) × 0.8 + Calcium.
Creatinine	0.7–1.5 mg/dL	Creatinine increases with kidney disease, dehydration, excessive exercise, starvation, hyperthyroidism, diabetic acidosis, muscular dystrophy, obstruction of the urinary tract, and high protein intake.
Sodium	136–145 mEq/L	Decreased sodium level, or hyponatremia, usually is indicative of fluid overload rather than low serum sodium. It is associated with severe burns, diarrhea, vomiting, excessive IV fluids, diuretics, SIADH, edema, diabetic acidosis, and severe nephritis. Sodium level increases with dehydration, primary aldosteronism, Cushing's disease, and diabetes insipidus.

Lab Test	Reference Range	Comments
Chloride	95–103 mEq/L	Alteration in serum chloride is hardly a primary problem. It is, however, significant in monitoring acid-base balance and water balance. Chloride levels decrease with severe vomiting, diarrhea, ulcerative colitis, severe burns, diabetic acidosis, overhydration, fever, infections, and use of drugs such as diuretics. It is increased with dehydration, anemia, and cardiac decompensation.
Potassium	3.5–5.0 mEq/L	Potassium controls the rate and force of contraction of the heart muscles. Most frequent causes of potassium deficiency/depletion are gastrointestinal loss and IV fluid administration without adequate potassium supplements. Other factors associated with hypokalemia are potassium-depleting diuretics, steroid and estrogen use, malnutrition, renal disease, liver disease with ascites, chronic stress, and fever. Hyperkalemia (increased levels of > 5.5) is frequently caused by renal failure. Cell damage as in burns, accidents, surgery, and chemotherapy causes a release of potassium into the blood, thereby causing hyperkalemia. Other factors include acidosis, internal hemorrhage, uncontrolled DM, and overuse of potassium supplements.
Ammonia (NH^3)	30–70 ug/dL	Ammonia is an end product of protein metabolism and is converted to urea by the liver. Increased ammonia in the blood affects brain function. Increased ammonia levels occur in liver disease, azotemia, severe heart failure, pulmonary disease, and Reye's syndrome. A high-protein diet and vigorous exercise also can cause an increase in ammonia level.
Phosphorus	2.6–4.5 mg/dL	Phosphorus is regulated by the kidneys, and elevated levels are associated with kidney dysfunction and uremia. Other factors associated with hyperphosphatemia (increased phosphorus level) include hypoparathyroidism, excessive intake of vitamin D, hypocalcemia, and Addison's disease. Low phosphorus level is associated with hyperparathyroidism, rickets or osteomalacia, diabetic coma, hyperinsulinism, and overuse of phosphate binders. Whenever phosphorus level is decreased, calcium is increased, and whenever calcium is decreased, phosphorus is increased.

(continues)

Table 1-3 Biochemical Data (continued)

Lab Test	Reference Range	Comments
Hemoglobin (hgb)	F: 12-16 g/dL M: 13.5-17.5 g/dL	Hemoglobin transports oxygen and carbon dioxide. Anemia occurs when hemoglobin, hematocrit, and/or red blood cell count numbers are low. Low hemoglobin levels are associated with cirrhosis of the liver, severe hemorrhage, hyperthyroidism, severe burns, systemic diseases such as Hodgkin's disease, leukemia, and systemic lupus erythematosus. Some HIV medications are associated with anemia. Increased levels of hemoglobin are associated with polycythemia (an increased production of red blood cells), dehydration, COPD, and congestive heart failure.
Hematocrit (hct)	F: 35-45% M: 39-49%	A decreased hematocrit value indicates anemia. Like hemoglobin, low levels are also associated with cirrhosis of the liver, hyperthyroidism, leukemia, severe burns, prosthetic heart valves, and acute massive blood loss. Levels are elevated with polycythemia and severe dehydration.
Red blood cells (RBC)	F: 3.5-5.5 M/mm^3 M: 4.3-5.9 M/mm^3	Red blood cells are found in the red bone marrow and transport oxygen and carbon dioxide. Anemia results when RBCs are low in conjunction with low hemoglobin (hgb) and hematocrit (hct) levels. The conditions that are associated with low hgb/hct are the same for low RBCs. There is a normal decrease in RBC during pregnancy due to an increase in body fluids. Levels are elevated with polycythemia and severe dehydration.
Ferritin	F: 12-150 ng/mL M: 15-200 ng/mL	Ferritin is the primary storage form of iron in the body. Decreased ferritin value is associated with Iron (Fe) deficiency anemia. Values increase with iron overload, inflammatory diseases, chronic renal failure, malignancy, and hepatitis.
Mean corpuscular hemoglobin (MCH)	26-34 pg/RBC	The MCH is an expression of the average weight of the hemoglobin in the red blood cell. An increase in MCH is associated with macrocytic anemia. Hyperlipidemia will cause a false increase in MCH. A decrease in MCH is associated with microcytic anemia.

Lab Test	Reference Range	Comments
Mean corpuscular hemoglobin concentration (MCHC)	32–37 g/dL	The MCHC is an expression of the average concentration of hemoglobin in the red blood cell. Decreased values are associated with iron deficiency, macrocytic anemia, and thalassemia, an inherited blood disorder characterized by abnormal hemoglobin. Hypochromic anemia is characterized by an MCHC of 30 or less (Fischbach, 2003). An increase in MCHC usually indicates spherocytosis, an inherited disorder of red blood cells where the red cells are smaller, rounder, and more fragile than normal. They tend to get trapped in the spleen, where they break down. MCHC is not increased in pernicious anemia.
Mean corpuscular volume (MCV)	87–103 um³/RBC	The MCV indicates whether the red blood cell appears normocytic, microcytic, or macrocytic, which is used to classify anemias. If the MCV is greater than 103 mm³, the red cells are macrocytic; if they are within normal range, the red blood cells are considered normocytic. Increased MCV values are associated with vitamin B_{12} and folate deficiency.
Total iron binding capacity (Transferrin Test)	240–450 ug/dL 200–400 mg/dL	Transferrin regulates iron absorption and transport in the body. Total iron binding capacity (TIBC) reflects the transferrin content of the blood. An increased TIBC reflects iron-deficiency anemia, whereas a decrease in TIBC reflects iron overload as in chronic inflammatory disease, pernicious anemia, sickle cell anemia, chronic infection, hepatic disease, nephrotic syndrome, cancer, and malnutrition.
Magnesium (Mg)	1.3–2.1 mEq/L	Magnesium deficiency is rare in a normal diet. Mg is important in the absorption of calcium and calcium metabolism. Low levels of Mg occur in the patient with a history of malnutrition, chronic diarrhea, alcoholism, ulcerative colitis, hepatic cirrhosis, hyperthyroidism, and hypoparathyroidism. Increased levels may be seen in dehydration, use of antacids containing Mg such as milk of magnesia, diabetic acidosis, Addison's disease, and hypothyroidism.

(continues)

Table 1-3 Biochemical Data (continued)

Lab Test	Reference Range	Comments
Glycosylated hemoglobin (HgbA1c)	Nondiabetic: 4.0–6.0% Diabetic: < 7.0% A1c Avg Glu 4.0–6.0 60–120 6.1–7.0 121–150 7.1–8.0 151–180 8.1–10.0 181–240 10.1–12.0 241–300 12.1–13.0 301–330	This test provides information on the efficacy of treatment for blood glucose. The more glucose the red blood cell is exposed to, the higher the percentage of glycosylated hemoglobin. Splenectomy decreases life span of red blood cells, so may give a falsely increased level. Hemolysis, on the other hand, gives a falsely decreased level.
Glucose	• 70–110 g/dL Fasting (normal) • 110–125 g/dL Fasting (defined by the American Diabetes Association to be prediabetic) • > 126 g/dL Fasting (on 2 occasions, defined by ADA as diabetes)	Blood glucose is regulated by *glucagon*, which causes an increase in glucose, and *insulin*, which causes a decrease in glucose levels. Increased blood sugar (*hyperglycemia*) usually indicates diabetes but is also associated with other conditions such as acute stress (myocardial infarction, meningitis, and encephalitis), Cushing's disease, hyperthyroidism, pancreatitis, adenoma of the pancreas, brain damage, use of steroids, diuretics, and chronic malnutrition. Low blood sugar (*hypoglycemia*) is associated with overuse of insulin, bacterial sepsis, Islet carcinoma of the pancreas, hepatic necrosis, glycogen storage disease, and hypothyroidism.
High-density lipoprotein (HDL)	**Desirable** F: > 40 mg/dL M: > 50 mg/dL	HDL is referred to as "good" cholesterol because it is believed that HDL serves as carriers that remove cholesterol from the peripheral tissues and transport it back to the liver for catabolism and excretion. A high level of HDL is an indication of a healthy metabolic system. HDL is increased with exercise. Decreased values are associated with an increased risk for CHD. Cigarette smoking, end-stage liver disease, diabetes, obesity, hyperthyroidism, and increased triglyceride are also associated with decreased HDL values.

Lab Test	Reference Range	Comments
Low-density lipoprotein (LDL)	**Desirable:** < 130 mg/dL < 100 mg/dL for DM < 70 mg/dL with an occurrence of coronary artery disease (CAD)	Increased LDL levels are caused by a family history of hyperlipidemia, a diet high in cholesterol and saturated fat, nephrotic syndrome, multiple myeloma, diabetes, hepatic disease, and pregnancy. High LDL, referred to as "bad cholesterol," is associated with coronary artery disease.
Triglycerides	< 150 mg/dL	Triglycerides account for about 95% of the fat stored in tissues. Increased triglyceride by itself does not indicate a risk factor for cardiovascular disease (CVD). Levels are increased in pancreatitis, poorly controlled diabetes, myocardial infarction, nephrotic syndrome, liver disease, and hypothyroidism. Levels are decreased with malnutrition, malabsorption, and hyperthyroidism.
Chol/HDL Ratio	**Male** **Female** < 4.2 < 3.9 4.2–7.3 3.9–5.7 7.4–11.5 5.8–9.0 > 11.5 > 9.0	Level of Risk Low average risk Average risk Increased average risk High average risk
Cholesterol, total	**Desirable:** 120–199 mg/dL	High levels of cholesterol are associated with atherosclerosis, a risk of coronary artery disease. Hypothyroidism, uncontrolled diabetes, nephrotic syndrome, and obesity are conditions associated with high cholesterol. Cholesterol levels are decreased when there is malabsorption, liver disease, hyperthyroidism, anemia, sepsis, stress, use of antibiotics, malnutrition, terminal stages of diseases such as cancer, severe infections, and pernicious anemia.

Note: Please note that reference values vary slightly from one lab to another. ADA = American Diabetes Association; Avg Glu = average glucose; CHD = coronary heart disease; COPD = chronic obstructive pulmonary disease; DM = diabetes mellitus; F = female; M = male; SIADH = syndrome of inappropriate antidiuretic hormone secretion

Table 1–4 Nutrition Implications of Certain Classes of Medications

Medications	Nutritional Implications
Analgesics Examples include MS Contin, Percocet, Nonsteroidal anti-inflammatory drugs (NSAIDs)	Monitor for constipation especially with Oxycontin and Percocet. Take with food to decrease gastrointestinal effect.
Antacids Examples include Maalox, Mylanta, Amphojel	Aluminum-containing antacids should not be used by older persons with bone problems or with Alzheimer's disease. The aluminum may cause their condition to worsen. Take Fe++ separately by 2 hours. Increased fluids are required to prevent constipation.
Antianemic Examples include ferrous sulfate, ferrous gluconate, Epogen, Aranesp	Ferrous sulfate contributes to constipation. Increased fluid is required and a stool softener is usually added to the regimen to alleviate constipation. Ferrous sulfate should be given in conjunction with Epogen for good effect. Frequent iron studies are essential. Monitor for hemachromatosis (iron overload).
Antibiotics Examples include cephlosporins, penicillin, aminoglycosides	The most common side effects of antibiotics are GI distress and diarrhea. Increased intake of fluids and electrolytes is encouraged.
Anticoagulants Examples include Coumadin	Increased risk of GI bleeding evidenced by black tarry stools, bleeding gums, blood in urine/stools, blotches under the skin, shortness of breath, and sudden weakness. Anticoagulants decrease platelets.
Anticonvulsants Examples include Tegretol, phenobarbital, Neurontin, Dilantin, Depakene, Depakote	Drugs such as phenobarbital and Dilantin interfere with intestinal absorption of calcium by increasing vitamin D metabolism in the liver. Long-term use of these drugs may lead to osteomalacia or rickets in children. Tube feeding decreases the bioavailability of Dilantin. Tube feeding should be stopped 2 hours before and after administering the drug.
Antidepressants Examples include Prozac, Zoloft, Luvox Paxil, Celexa, Wellbutrin	May cause dry mouth, blurred vision, constipation, fatigue, loss of appetite, and weight loss.
Antidiarrheals Examples include Kaopectate, Lomotil, Imodium	Diarrhea may increase fluid and electrolyte needs. May cause constipation, dry mouth, nausea, vomiting.

Medications	Nutritional Implications
Antiemetics Examples include Reglan, Compazine, Phenergan	May cause dry mouth, constipation, or diarrhea. May alter insulin requirements in people with diabetes.
Anti-GERD/proton pump inhibitors Examples include, Prevacid, Protonix	Proton pump inhibitors (PPIs) reduce gastric acid production. It is best for patients to take them before meals. PPIs may decrease absorption of iron and vitamin B_{12}.
Antigouts Examples include Zyloprim	Zyloprim is used to treat gouty arthritis, which occurs as a result of too much uric acid in the blood. Alcohol increases uric acid production and therefore should be limited or avoided. Excess amounts of vitamin C increase the risk of kidney stone formation while on Zyloprim. Lots of fluids are encouraged for adequate urine output.
Antihyperlipidemics These include: 1. Statins—for example, Lipitor, Pravachol 2. Fibrates—for example, Lopid, Tricor 3. Niacin—for example, Niacor, Niaspan 4. Resin—for example, cholestyramine (L-cholest, Questran)	Used to improve abnormal lipid values. Side effects include but not are limited to diarrhea, constipation, vomiting, joint and muscle pain, gas, headache, unusual bleeding or bruising, and loss of appetite. Medication is used in combination with a low-fat, low-cholesterol diet.
Antihypertensives/Diuretics Examples include Aldactone, Lasix, calcium channel blockers, ACE inhibitors	Aldactone is potassium sparing, while Lasix is potassium wasting. Potassium levels should be monitored frequently.
Antimanics Examples include lithium	Side effects of lithium include weakness, nausea, fatigue, increased thirst and urination. Consistent sodium intake is required to stabilize the drug level. Extra fluids are required, approximately 2–3 L/day.
Antineoplastics Examples include Thiotepa, Chlorambucil, etoposide phosphate	Common side effects include decrease in the number of blood cells in the bone marrow, nausea, vomiting, constipation, diarrhea, and quite often a change in taste. Loss of appetite and weakness also occur. Increased fluid intake is necessary. Unusual bleeding and/or bruising may occur.

(continues)

Table 1-4 Nutrition Implications of Certain Classes of Medications (continued)

Medications	Nutritional Implications
Antipsychotics Examples include Risperdal, Zyprexa, Seroquel, Haldol	May cause weight gain. Diet and exercise are important to manage weight. Dry mouth, increased salivation, and constipation are also some other side effects.
Antiretrovirals Examples include protease inhibitors (PIs), non-nucleoside reverse transcriptase inhibitors (NNRTIs), and nucleoside reverse transcriptase inhibitors (NRTIs)	Common side effects to antiretroviral therapy include lipodystrophy, insulin resistance, lactic acidosis, hyperlipidemia, osteoporosis/osteopenia, and hepatotoxicity. Loss of appetite, diarrhea, and subsequent weight loss may also occur.
Antirheumatics Examples include methotrexate	Methotrexate is used to treat rheumatoid arthritis and some neoplastic disease. Its side effects include decreased appetite, diarrhea, nausea/vomiting, mouth sores, and possibly unusual bruising/bleeding. It should not be taken with pain medication because this increases the effect of the drug. Alcohol intake with methotrexate can cause very serious liver damage. Methotrexate blocks folic acid synthesis. Folinic acid is used to reduce this side effect associated with use of the drug. Increased fluid intake is encouraged to increase urine output.
Antituberculosis Examples include Rifampin, pyrazinamide (PZA), isoniazid (INH)	May increase glucose in patients taking sulfonylureas for diabetes. Increased uric acid occurs with Rifampin and pyrazinamide. Isoniazid affects vitamin D metabolism, thereby causing a decrease in calcium and phosphorus. High-tyramine foods should be avoided. Isoniazid may also cause liver damage, especially in patients older than 50 years of age.
H^1-Antagonists (antihistamines) Examples include Claritin, Benadryl, Allegra, Zyrtec	Antihistamines are used to relieve allergy symptoms. Side effects may include dry mouth/throat, confusion, headache or tachycardia, blurred vision. Should not be used in combination with Periactin also an antihistamine used to improve appetite.

Medications	Nutritional Implications
Hypnotics/Sedatives Examples include Klonopin, Xanax, Valium, Ativan, BuSpar	May cause bradycardia, heart palpitation, hypotension, nausea/vomiting, dry mouth, constipation, dizziness in coordination, and confusion.
Laxatives Examples include Senna, Dulcolax, Lactulose	Electrolyte imbalance may occur with excessive use. Increased fluid intake is needed with lactulose to prevent constipation. Monitor electrolytes with long-term use.
Muscle Relaxants Examples include Lioresal, Robaxin	May cause epigastric distress. Patients should take these with food to decrease gastrointestinal distress.
Nonsteroidal anti-inflammatory drugs (NSAID) Examples include aspirin, Ecotrin, Bufferin, Motrin	May exacerbate ulcer disease, gastritis, and gastroesophageal reflux disease. Aspirin may cause bleeding, especially in those patients using anticoagulants.
Oral hypoglycemics *Sulfonylureas*—Glucotrol, Glyburide *Biguanide*—Glucophage *Meglitinides*—Prandin *Thiazolidinediones* (*TZD*)—Actos, Avandia (insulin sensitizers) *Alpha-glucosidase inhibitors*—Precose, Glyset	Glucophage reduces hepatic glucose production. It causes weight loss and an increase in creatinine levels. Patients should avoid alcohol with oral hypoglycemic medication because it can cause a drop in blood sugar. Precose, Glyset decrease the absorption of complex carbohydrates in the upper GI tract, thereby reducing postprandial hyperglycemia. Recent studies indicate that there is a potential risk for developing heart-related conditions with the use of Avandia.
Steroids Examples include systemic steroids such as prednisone, and inhaled steroids	May increase blood sugar in the patient who is predisposed to diabetes. May also cause GI bleeding/perforation. Osteoporosis may occur with long-term use.
Thyroid preparations Examples include Synthroid	May cause weight gain. Iron decreases absorption—patients must take it separately by 4 hours.

Note: GI = gastrointestinal.

SUMMARY

Reviewing the patient's medical chart and taking an in-depth look at the nutritional implications of the disease/medical condition and food–drug interactions and having a clear understanding of the laboratory data provides you with the tools necessary to formulate a proper plan of care for the patient. The chart review also helps you to prepare for the patient interview and educate the patient accordingly.

REVIEW QUESTIONS

1. A 32-year-old woman with below knee amputation (BKA) is admitted to your facility. She weighs 204 pounds and reported her height was 5 ft 9 in. Calculate her adjusted IBW.
2. Patient HS is an 82-year-old woman who is a resident in a nursing home. She does not ambulate, uses a geri-chair, and has a history of constipation. Her height is 62 inches and actual weight is 180 pounds. Patient is fed via G-tube. Formula provides 1200 cal, 54 g protein, and 780 cc water.

Biochemical data: Alb 3.0 BUN 24 Na 134 Ca 7.7 Ammonia 68
Modular: Promod 2 scoops via GT TID
Fluids: 100 cc water flushes administered before and after feeding, 200 cc q shift and 25 cc automatic water flush every hour × 13 hr/day

Patient was noted with a 5% weight gain in 1 month. Evaluate the patient's nutritional status and provide a recommendation for the MD.

REFERENCES

Ayello, E. A., & Cuddington, J. (2004, March). Conquer chronic wounds with wound bed preparation. *Nurse Practitioner: The American Journal of Primary Health Care, 29*(3), 8–25.

Bartlett J. G., & Gallant, J. E. (2005). *Medical management of HIV infection.* Baltimore: Johns Hopkins University Press.

Beckrich, K., & Aronovitch, S. A. (1999). Hospital-acquired pressure ulcers: A comparison of costs in medical vs surgical patients. *Nursing Economics, 17,* 263–271.

Bernard, D. K., & Shaw, M. J. (1993, August). Principles of nutrition therapy for short bowel syndrome. *Nutrition in Clinical Practice,* 8, 153–162.

Bini, L., Fantini, L., Pezzilli, R., Campana, D., Tomassetti, P., Casadei, R., Calculli, L., & Corinaldesi, R. (2007). Medical therapy of malabsorption in patients with head pancreatic resection. *Journal of the Pancreas, 8*(2), 151–155.

Buchman, A. (2004). The medical and surgical management of short bowel syndrome. *Medscape General Medicine, 6*(2), 12.

Burkhead G., Maki, G., AIDS Institute. (2001, March). *Mental health care for people with HIV infection: HIV clinical guidelines for the primary care practitioner.* New York: New York State Department of Health.

Centers for Disease Control and Prevention. (2009). *HIV/AIDS Today.* Retrieved October 1, 2009, from http://www.cdcnpin.org/scripts/hiv/hiv.asp

Centers for Disease Control and Prevention. (2009a). *FAQs for Health Professionals: Hepatitis A.* Retrieved October 1, 2009, from http://www.cdc.gov/hepatitis/HAV/HAVfaq.htm#general

Centers for Disease Control and Prevention. (2009b). *FAQs for Health Professionals: Hepatitis B.* Retrieved October 1, 2009, from http://www.cdc.gov/hepatitis/HBV/HBVfaq.htm#overview

Centers for Disease Control and Prevention. (2008). *HIV Incidence.* Retrieved August 15, 2008, from www.cdc.gov/hiv/topics/surveillance/incidence.htm

Desneves, K. J., Todorovic, B. E., Cassar, A., & Crowe, T. C. (2005, December). *Treatment with supplementary arginine, vitamin C and zinc in patients with pressure ulcers: A randomized controlled trial. Clinical Nutrition, 24*(6),979–987.

DiMaria-Ghalili, R. A. (2008). Nutrition risk factors in older coronary artery bypass graft patients. *Nutrition in Clinical Practice, 23*(5), 494–500.

Duncan, K. D. (2007). Preventing pressure ulcers: the goal is zero. Joint Commission Journal on Quality and Patient Safety, *33*(10), 605–610.

Finelli, L., & Bell, B. P. (2008). *Manual for the surveillance of vaccine-preventable diseases* (4th ed.), chapt 4: Hepatitis B.

Fischbach, F. (2003). *Manual of laboratory and diagnostic tests* (7th ed.) New York: Lippincott, Williams & Wilkins.

Heidt, D.G., Burant, C., & Simeone, D. M. (2007, February). Total pancreatectomy: Indications, operative technique, and postoperative sequelae. *Journal of Gastrointestinal Surgery, 11*(2), 209–216.

Henkel, A. S., & Buchman, A. L. (2006). Nutritional support in patients with chronic liver disease. *Nature Clinical Practice: Gastroenterology and Hepatology, 3*(4), 202–209.

Hojo, K., Bando, Y., Itoh, Y., Taketomo, N., & Ishii, M. (2008, March). Abnormal fecal *Lactobacillus* flora and vitamin B_{12} deficiency in a patient with short bowel syndrome. *Journal of Pediatric Gastroenterology and Nutrition, 46*(3), 342–345.

Joslin Diabetes Center and Joslin Clinic. (2009). *Clinical Guideline for adults with diabetes.* Retrieved October 1, 2009, from http://www.joslin.org/Files/Adult_guidelines_041109_grade_updating.pdf

Klein, C., Stanek, G. S., & Wiles, C. E. (1998). Overfeeding macronutrients to critically ill adults: Metabolic complications. *Journal of American Dietetic Association, 98,* 795–806.

Kopp-Hoolihan, L. (2001). Nutrition and therapeutic effects of probiotics. *Journal of American Dietetic Association, 101*, 229–238, 241.

Lean, M. (2008). Malnutrition in hospitals. *British Medical Journal, 336*, 290.

Mahan, K. L. & Escott-Stump, S. (2008). *Krause's food and nutrition therapy* (12th ed.). St. Louis, MO: Saunders.

Morbidity and Mortality Weekly Report (MMWR). (October 3, 2008). *HIV/AIDS in the United States, 57*(39), 1073–1076.

National Center for Immunization and Respiratory Diseases, Centers for Disease Control and Prevention. (2009, May). *Hepatitis B and hepatitis B vaccine [slideshow]*. Retrieved September 15, 2009, from http://www.cdc.gov/vaccines/pubs/pinkbook/downloads/Slides/HepB11.ppt

National Cholesterol Education Program. (2001, May). *Third report of the National Cholesterol Education Program (NCEP) Expert Panel on detection, evaluation, and treatment of high blood cholesterol in adults (Adult Treatment Panel III) executive summary*. Washington, DC: National Heart, Lung, and Blood Institute, National Institutes of Health. NIH Publication No. 01-3670. Retrieved October 1, 2009, from http://www.nhlbi.nih.gov/guidelines/cholesterol/atp_iii.htm

National Institutes of Health, National Institute on Aging. (2005, April). *Aging hearts and arteries: A scientific quest*. NIH Publication No. 05-3738. Bethesda, MD: Office of Communications and Public Liaison.

National Institutes of Health. (2002). *Management of hepatitis C: 2002*. Consensus Conference Statement, June 10–12. Retrieved September 15, 2009, from http://consensus.nih.gov/2002/2002HepatitisC2002116html.htm

National Institute for Health and Clinical Excellence. (February 22, 2006). Nutritional support in adults: Oral nutrition support, enteral, tube feeding and parenteral nutrition. Retrieved October 1, 2009, from http://www.nice.org.uk/guidance/CG32

National Institute of Neurological Disorders and Stroke. (October 19, 2009). Retrieved October 1, 2009, from http://www.ninds.nih.gov/disorders/md/md.htm

Pronsky, Z. M. (1997). *Food–medication interactions* (10th ed.). Birchunville, PA: Food Medication Interactions.

Rich, M. W., Keller, A. J., Schechtman, K. B., Marshall, W. G. Jr., & Kouchoukos, N. T. (1989, March). Increased complications and prolonged hospital stay in elderly cardiac surgical patients with low serum albumin. *American Journal of Cardiology, 63*(11), 714–718.

Russo, C., & Elixhauser, A. (2006). *Hospitalizations related to pressure sores, 2003*. Retrieved October 1, 2009, from http://www.ahrq.gov/news/enews/enews197.htm

Schrader, H., Menge, B. A., Breuer, T. G. K., Ritter, P. R., Uhl, W., & Schmidt, W. E., et al. (2009). Impaired glucose-induced glucagon suppression after partial pancreatectomy. *Journal of Clinical Endocrinology and Metabolism, 94*(8), 2857–2863.

Siitonen, S., Vapaatalo, H., Salminen, S., Gordin, A., Saxelin, M., & Wikberg, R., et al. (1990). Effect of *Lactobacillus* GG yoghurt in prevention of antibiotic diarrhoea. *Annuals of Medicine, 22*(1), 57–9.

Spratto, G., & Woods, A. L. (2007). 2008 PDR nurse's drug handbook. Clifton Park, NY: Thomson Delmar Learning.

Teitelbaum, J. E. (2005). Probiotics and the treatment of infectious diarrhea. *Pediatric Infectious Disease Journal, 24*(3), 267–268.

ADDITIONAL RESOURCES

National Cancer Institute: www.cancer.gov

National Institutes of Heath (NIH): www.nih.gov

Centers for Disease Control and Prevention: www.cdc.gov

Doenges, M., Moorhouse, M. F., & Murr, A. (2008). *Nursing Diagnosis Manual: Planning, Individualizing and Documenting Client Care* (2nd ed.). Philadelphia, PA: F. A. Davis Company.

The Interview

The interview is part of the first step in the Nutrition Care Process. It provides additional information that is not found in the chart, and as such, you need to pose open-ended questions and not be judgmental, but be a good listener. Listening carefully shows that you care. The aim is to obtain as much information as possible to conduct a complete and thorough nutrition assessment. Speak clearly and slowly. Questions should be concise and specific without room for ambiguity.

Use the patient's primary language during the interview and make use of the language bank in your facility. If you use a translator for the interview, always introduce yourself and the translator. It is very important that when you use a translator you speak directly to the patient rather than asking the translator to ask the questions. The translator should listen for your cue to translate the questions as they are asked. Avoid body language that may be offensive to the patient.

This chapter covers some very important components of the interview, including obtaining weight history, diet history, bowel movement information, eating patterns, race and diseases, culture and dietary practices, religion and dietary practices, and the use of herbal supplements. With this information, you can conduct a thorough assessment of the patient and provide intervention that meets his or her dietary needs.

OBTAINING DIET HISTORY

Following are sample open-ended questions you can use to obtain information on the patient's diet:

Instead of: Did you have breakfast this morning?

Ask: What did you have for breakfast this morning?

Instead of: How is your appetite?

Ask: How much of your meals do you usually consume? Half or more? Or, How many times during the day do you have something to eat?

Instead of: Do you drink?

Ask: What do you normally drink with your meals? What do you drink between meals?

Instead of: Do you drink water?

Ask: What time of the day do you normally drink water?

Instead of: Do you drink alcohol?

Ask: How many times do you have beer, whiskey, or other alcoholic beverages during a given week, if any?

Instead of: Do you have problem chewing or swallowing?

Ask: Does it hurt when you swallow? Do you find yourself coughing a lot while eating or drinking? Do you have difficulty chewing some foods?

Instead of: How are your bowel movements?

Ask: Do you move your bowels every day, every other day, or every three days?

Follow-up questions might be:

How would you describe your bowel movement—hard, soft, watery, or pebbly? Do you find yourself having to strain to move your bowels?

Instead of: Are you on a special diet?

Ask: What foods were you told to avoid?

Other open-ended questions that are useful in obtaining diet history may include the following:

- Who prepares the food at home?
- Who does the shopping?
- Do you obtain food from any other source such as soup kitchen, food pantry?
- What is a typical breakfast, lunch, dinner, or snack for you?
- What time do you normally have breakfast, lunch, dinner, or a snack?
- How often do you eat outside the home? For example, do you eat at a cafeteria at school/work, fast food, restaurants, homes of friends and family? What do you usually order when you eat out? (Charney & Ainsley, 2009)

OBTAINING WEIGHT HISTORY

Weight history is a sensitive issue, especially for the obese patient. *Never* tell a patient he or she is obese.

Sample questions for obtaining weight history for the obese patient might be the following:

"I noticed that your weight is 276 pounds. Is this your usual weight?"
"Are you comfortable with this weight?"
"Have you gained or lost weight recently?"
"How long have you been at this weight?"
"Have you tried losing weight in the past? If yes, what did you do?"
"Was it effective?"
"Are you interested in losing weight?"

As you interview the patient for weight history, always compare current weight with usual body weight and also determine weight loss or gain over a specific period of time. Provide suitable prompts for the patient to give you the time period.

Sample questions might include these:

"Your current weight is 101 pounds. Have you lost weight recently?"
"How much did you weigh before you started losing weight?"
"How long ago was that—a month ago, three months ago, six months ago, a year or more?"

24-HOUR RECALL

The 24-hour recall is not the most reliable tool for collecting information for a complete assessment because patients quite often tell clinicians what they want to hear. It is not a useful tool for interviewing young children and or older adults because of its reliance on memory (Gibson, 2005).

Accuracy in recalling what they ate in the last 24 hours can be a challenge for many people. Most patients have difficulty determining actual portion sizes. Always have on hand actual portion size examples, such as bowls, cups, spoons, plates, or pictures of these items. Food models are great for portion size demonstrations.

To achieve some level of accuracy with 24-hour recalls, it is best to start with the last meal eaten and work your way back to the first meal of the day. It is important to ask the patient about method of food preparation and about any additives, such as salad dressing, whipped cream, sour cream, and so forth. Answers will enable you to achieve a good estimate of caloric intake. Always ask the patient if this intake is typical of a regular day or whether he or she eats differently on the weekends and when dining out.

FOOD FREQUENCY QUESTIONNAIRE

Food frequency questionnaires (FFQ) are most useful when you assess the nutritional status of a large group of people, as was done in the National Health and Nutritional Examination Survey (NHANES) studies. But they are sometimes used for individual assessments, too. An FFQ asks the participant the number of times he or she eats a particular food over a period of time. FFQs provide you with information on the patient's usual intake and enable you to modify the diet to include choices from all the food groups.

THE RELATIONSHIP BETWEEN RACE/ ETHNICITY AND DISEASES

As you proceed with the interview, it is important to bear in mind that some chronic medical conditions are more prevalent among certain ethnic groups and races. *Race*, as defined by Webster's, is "a distinct group of people who share certain inherited physical characteristics." Some of the most common diseases affecting various ethnic groups are discussed in this section.

Hypertension and diabetes are said to be more prevalent among African Americans than their white counterparts. African Americans, Hispanic Americans, Asian Americans, and Native Americans all have an increased genetic predisposition for **diabetes**. Blindness caused by diabetes and kidney failure rank high among African Americans. The reason for this health disparity could be that patients seek treatment too late in the disease process, receive substandard care from their primary care physician, fail to engage in adequate physical activity; food practices and culture could also be contributors.

Asian Americans have the highest rate of **hepatitis B** in the United States. The rate of prevalence among Chinese Americans is five times higher than that in Caucasian Americans (American Liver Foundation, 2006).

Cystic fibrosis is an inherited disease that affects sodium channels in the body and causes respiratory and digestive problems. It is the most common fatal hereditary disorder affecting Caucasians in the United States. It affects about 1 in 2500 Caucasians and 1 in 25 is a carrier of the defective gene. Risk factors include a family history of cystic fibrosis or unexplained infant death.

Hereditary hemochromatosis (HHC), caused by the body absorbing too much iron, is another common genetic disease affecting Caucasians. One out of every 200 to 400 people is thought to carry a genetic mutation that causes HHC.

Systemic lupus erythematosus (**SLE** or **lupus**), a chronic autoimmune disease that is potentially debilitating and sometimes fatal, is three times more common in African American women than in Caucasian women. It is also more common in women of Hispanic, Asian, and Native American descent than in Caucasians.

Sickle cell anemia is an inherited disease of the red blood cells, which can cause attacks of pain and damage to vital organs and can lead to early death. It is more common among African Americans and Hispanics of Caribbean ancestry. Sickle cell anemia also affects people of Arabian, Greek, Maltese, Italian, Sardinian, Turkish, and Indian ancestry.

Thalassemia is a group of inherited diseases of the blood that causes red blood cell deficiencies. The most severe form, **alpha thalassemia**, results in fetal or newborn death and affects mainly individuals of Southeast Asian, Chinese, and Filipino ancestry.

Tay-Sachs disease is a fatal inherited disease of the central nervous system. Affected babies lack the necessary protein for breaking down certain fatty substances in the brain and nerve cells. These substances build up and gradually destroy brain and nerve cells to the point when the entire central nervous system shuts down, causing the child to go blind, be paralyzed, and die by age 5. Tay-Sachs occurs most frequently in descendants of central and eastern European Jews (Fertility Treatment Center, 2009).

Gaucher's disease is the most frequent hereditary lysosomal deposit storage disorder. It is characterized by a deficiency of the enzyme glucocerebrosidase that leads to an accumulation of substrate in the interior of the macrophage lysosomes. It is a multisystemic disease. In the majority of patients, there is hepatosplenomegaly, anemia, and thrombocytopenia. Skeletal involvement is also important and is frequently the most disabling manifestation (Campo, Calabuig, Aquilar, & Estelles, 2004). This disease is commonly found among Jewish people of eastern European ancestry.

UNDERSTANDING CULTURE AND DIETARY PRACTICES

Culture refers to the perspective, practices, and products of a social group. In conducting an interview with the patient, it is important for you to understand the patient's cultural practices.

In the *Journal of Continuing Education in Nursing*, Cuellar, Cahill, Ford, and Aycock (2003) report that by the year 2080, an estimated 51.1% of the population will be Hispanics, followed by African Americans and Asians.

Obtaining information about the patient's beliefs and cultural practices is as important as reviewing his or her medical condition. Cultural practices can significantly affect medical and nutritional outcomes.

In her article, "Best Culturally Competent Communication Tool," Loreno Drago, (2008) suggests using the following open-ended questions, part of which she refers to as the ETHNIC model:

> "What do you think may be the reason you have these symptoms?"
> "Do you know anyone else who has this condition, and how is it treated?"
> "What kinds of medicines, home remedies, or other treatments have you tried for this illness?"
> "Is there anything you eat, drink, or do (or avoid) on a regular basis to stay healthy?"
> "Are there any foods you eat to treat this condition?"
> "How do you prepare these foods and how often do you eat them?"
> "Have you sought advice from alternative/folk healers, friends, or other people who are not doctors?" (Drago, 2008)

Most culturally accepted foods are high in sodium and fat and low in calcium from diary products. There is an increased use of coconut milk and meat consumption in the Hispanic community. Coconut milk is high in saturated fat. Other popular food items include rice and beans, boiled or fried plantains, Spanish cheese, yucca (cassava), and sweet beans, that is, beans with condensed milk.

In Caribbean cultures, natural substances are used for healing, including herbs. Ginger tea, for example, is used for stomach pain, garlic for high blood pressure, and sour orange for respiratory congestion, to name a few. Homemade soups such as cow foot and fish tea are thought to give strength and are common items on the weekly menu. Salads are served mainly on Sundays and hardly during the week. Goat meat, oxtail, and codfish are frequently consumed. Most foods are fried or prepared with a lot of oil.

Prayer is another important component of Caribbean cultures. When sick, people of Caribbean cultures pray to God for help before seeking medical attention. They have a strong belief in faith healing.

Rice is a staple food in Asian cuisine, and foods are usually heavily spiced. There is also an increased consumption of pork among people from the Philippines.

Nutritional Implications and Intervention

Because of the high fat, high sodium content of most culturally accepted foods, it is not uncommon for you to see obesity, hyperlipidemia, hypertension, and diabetes among patients from diverse cultures.

Be cautious when counseling different ethnic groups so as not to make too many drastic changes that will lead to noncompliance. Make an effort to find out the ingredients used in cooking so as to better understand the impact that a particular food has on the patient's nutritional status. Listen carefully to patient's fears and concerns to determine their readiness to change. If a patient is on a restricted diet, changes should be timely and gradual.

RELIGION AND FOOD PRACTICES

Religion is a major influence on the foods most people eat. The role of food in cultural and religious practices is complex and varies among individuals and communities. You must be aware of the religious practices of the patient so as to ensure the patient can comply on some level with a therapeutic diet. Diets provided while patients are confined to a facility should meet the patients' religious mandates.

Buddhism

Some Buddhists include fish in their diet, but most are vegetarians. Most do not eat meat and do abstain from all beef products. The birth, enlightenment, and death of the Buddha are the three most commonly recognized festivals for feasting, resting from work, or fasting. Buddhist monks fast completely on certain days of the moon, and they routinely avoid eating any solid foods after the noon hour.

Hinduism

The cow is sacred to Hindus. Some do eat meat, but not beef. Pork, fowl, ducks, snails, and crabs are also avoided. Most Hindus are strict vegetarians. Although the eating of beef is prohibited, milk, yogurt, and butter are allowed. Many devout Hindus fast on the 18 major Hindu holidays, as well as on numerous personal days, such as birthdays and anniversaries of deaths and marriages. They also fast on Sundays and on days associated with various positions of the moon and planets.

Islam

The term *haram* in the Muslim religion refers to those foods that are prohibited such as pork, alcohol, foods that contain emulsifiers (because emulsifiers may be made from animal fats), tinned vegetables that include emulsifiers, frozen vegetables with sauce, particular margarines, and bread or bread products that contain dried yeast. Gelatine can be made from pig and, because pork is *haram*, products containing gelatine are forbidden. Caffeinated drinks such as coffee and tea are sometimes considered *haram*.

Fasting is practiced regularly on Mondays and Thursdays, and more often for six days during Shawwal (the 10th month of the Islamic year) and for the entire month of Ramadan (the ninth month). Fasting on these occasions includes abstention from all food and drink from sunrise to sunset. The fast is broken in the evening by a meal called the *iftar*, which traditionally includes dates and water or sweet drinks, and is resumed again at sunrise.

Judaism

The term *kosher* refers to the methods of processing foods according to the Jewish laws. Meat and dairy products are never consumed at the same meal; in fact, separate cooking utensils are used during the preparation. Kosher and nonkosher foods cannot come into contact with the same plates. Jewish laws dictate the slaughter and removal of blood from meat before it can be eaten. Animals such as pigs and rabbits and creatures of the sea, such as lobster, shrimp, and clams, are prohibited.

Mormonism

Mormonism promotes abstinence from tobacco, alcohol, coffee, tea, chocolate, and illegal drugs. Products from the land, such as grains, fruits, vegetables, and nuts, are to take the place of meats. Meats, sugar, cheeses, and spices are to be avoided. Reason and self-control in eating are expected in order to stay healthy.

Rastafarianism

People who are devoted to Rastafarianism are completely vegetarians. Some Rastafarians eat fish that are no longer than 12 inches. Pork and shellfish are strictly prohibited. The true Rastas eat only **I-tal** food, which is cooked but served in the rawest form possible, without salts, preservatives, or condiments. *I-tal* food is unique food because it never touches chemicals and is completely natural. Drinking preferences are for anything that is herbal, such as tea. Liquor, milk, coffee, and soft drinks are viewed as unnatural. Marijuana is used during religious observances and is considered to have medicinal properties.

Roman Catholicism

The dietary practices of devout Catholics center around the restriction of meat and fasting behaviors on specified holy days. On designated days, Catholics may abstain from all food, or they may restrict meat and meat products. Water or nonstimulant liquids are usually allowed during the fast.

Seventh-Day Adventists

The Seventh-Day Adventist Church promotes a lacto-ovo vegetarian diet. Pork and shellfish are strictly prohibited. Meat, fish, coffee, tea, and alcohol are avoided (Waibel, 2004).

Nutritional Implications and Intervention

The practice of fasting is almost universal across religious groups, and most religions regard it as a mechanism to discipline followers in a humbling way for spiritual growth. Fasting in the absence of water can lead to dehydration. Some religions emphasize strict adherence to a vegetarian diet (vegan), which puts the growing child and older adults at risk for vitamin B_{12} deficiency. Vitamin B_{12} is found only in animal products and is responsible for the formation of DNA and red blood cell count development. In the absence of animal products, vitamin B_{12} supplementation becomes necessary.

During fasting, people with diabetes may experience a drop in blood glucose. Fasting is not recommended for people with diabetes; however, if a patient insists on fasting, explain the nutritional implications of the fast to him or her and give the option to consume some form of carbohydrate to prevent hypoglycemia. It is advisable for the patient to contact his or her physician prior to the fast for possible adjustment of the diabetes medication or insulin for the duration of the fast.

THE USE OF HERBAL SUPPLEMENTS

In the United States, approximately 38% of adults (about 4 in 10) and approximately 12% of children (about 1 in 9) use some form of complementary and alternative medicine (CAM). The most common types of CAM are herbs, vitamins, chiropractic care, relaxation techniques, spirituality, massage, acupuncture, naturopathy, Chinese medicine, guided imagery, Ayurveda, and chelation. The use of herbal/dietary supplements is the mostly commonly used CAM therapy among adults and is greatest among women and those with higher levels of education and higher incomes.

The sale of dietary supplements today is a $30 billion a year business, and older adults are the main target market. Some dietary supplements interfere with conventional medicines and as such, patients should be advised of the risk of serious complications.

In conducting a thorough nutrition assessment, ask about the use of herbal/dietary supplements. Some patients do not consider this important information or realize that it can be potentially dangerous, so do not volunteer this information. The American Dietetic Association suggests using the following four-step process for evaluating dietary supplement use: Ask, Evaluate, Educate, and Document. **Table 2–1** provides a fuller description of the process.

Table 2–1 Evaluating Dietary Supplement Use

ASK:
• What dietary supplements are you taking? (Type—vitamin, mineral, botanical, amino acid, fiber.) • What antacids or other over-the-counter medications or food products are being consumed that provide supplemental nutrients, herbals, fiber, etc.? • Why are you taking the dietary supplement(s)? Include review of patient's diagnosis/symptoms for which they may take supplements (e.g., osteoarthritis, heart disease, high blood pressure, night sweats, loss of memory, fatigue). • How long have you been taking the dietary supplement(s)? • What dose? How much? (For each, include chemical form; review and photocopy labels.) • What frequency? How often? (For each.) • Sources of supplements—over-the-counter or prescribed, Internet, health care provider, etc. • Manufacturer • Is it touted as being preventive or to have treatment effects? What does the label claim? Supplemental brochures/materials? • Who recommended the supplement—media, physician, nurse, dietetics professional, alternative medicine practitioner, friend, family?
EVALUATE:
• Dietary intake (including intake of fortified food or beverages) • Health status/health history (include lifestyle habits such as smoking, alcohol, exercise) • Biochemical profile • Prescribed and over-the-counter medications • Clinical response • Adverse events, symptoms
EDUCATE:
• Scientific evidence of benefit and/or effectiveness • Potential interaction with foods, nutrients, and/or medications or other dietary supplements • Appropriate dose, brand, and chemical form; duration of supplementation; appropriate follow-up • Quality of products, manufacturers, good manufacturing practices (United States Pharmacopoeia, Consumer Labs) • Mechanism of action of the primary active ingredient • Duration of use • How to store the dietary supplement • Administration instructions: with or without food?, potential food-supplement interactions • Awareness and reporting of any side effects/adverse events, symptoms • Recommend concurrent dietary changes • Remember a supplement should *supplement* the diet

DOCUMENTATION:

- List specific supplements and brand name of each supplement being taken
- Record batch number from bottle in case of an adverse event
- Patient perception, expected level of compliance
- Monitor efficacy and safety including health outcomes and adverse effects
- Medication-supplement or supplement-supplement interactions
- Timeline for follow-up

Source: © 2005 Elsevier, Inc. Practice Paper of the American Dietetic Association: Dietary Supplements Journal of the American Dietetic Association, 15 (Vol. 105, Issue 3), 460–470.

Interactions Between Frequently Used Supplements and Conventional Medicines

Blood thinning agents, such as **warfarin/Coumadin** and **Heparin** are prescribed to prevent occurrence or reoccurrence of heart attack in patients who are at risk for heart disease. However, when these medications are used in combination with some dietary supplements, they can cause prolonged bleeding, which can be fatal if left untreated.

St. John's wort, for example, which is used by many people to treat depression, when taken in combination with warfarin can cause prolonged bleeding and has also been reported to reduce the effects of some antihypertensive medications. St. John's wort may also be responsible for reducing the effectiveness of digoxin, used to treat congestive heart failure.

Feverfew, **ginseng**, **garlic**, **ginkgo biloba**, and **ginger** are also examples of supplements that can cause unusual bleeding or bruising when used in combination with warfarin. Ginkgo biloba has been associated with brain hemorrhage and blood clot. Vitamin E is also known to have blood-thinning effects. Garlic, when used with certain medications to treat HIV/AIDS, may decrease the effectiveness of these medications. One such medication is Saquinavir. Use of garlic caplets lead to a significant decline in plasma concentration of Saquinavir (Piscitelli, Burnstein, Welden, Gallicano, Falloon, 2002).

Omega-3 fatty acids found in fish oils are primarily used to reduce the risk of cardiovascular disease and treat immune disorders, but when used in combination with warfarin can cause unusual bleeding and bruising.

Glucosamine, which is promoted to decrease pain and stiffness in osteoarthritis, may worsen insulin resistance in people with diabetes. This may result in the need to increase doses of diabetes medications or possibly add insulin to the regimen (Shane-McWhorter, 2002).

The Consumer Advisory of the U.S. Food and Drug Administration (FDA) in March 2002 warned that **kava**-containing dietary supplements may be associated with liver-related injuries, including hepatitis, cirrhosis, and liver failure (FDA, 2002). Supplements containing kava are promoted to aid in relaxation (e.g., to relieve stress, anxiety, and tension), sleeplessness, menopausal symptoms, and other uses.

FDA warns consumers to avoid red yeast rice products promoted on the Internet as treatment for high cholesterol. FDA testing revealed that the products contain lovastatin, a cholesterol-lowering drug. It further states that red yeast rice products are a threat to health because the possibility exists that lovastatin can cause severe muscle problems leading to kidney impairment. This risk is greater in patients who take higher doses of lovastatin or who take lovastatin and other medicines that increase the risk of muscle adverse reactions. These medicines include the antidepressant nefazodone, certain antibiotics, drugs used to treat fungal infections and HIV infections, and other cholesterol-lowering medications (FDA, 2007).

Liqiang 4 dietary supplement, promoted as being useful for the control of diabetes, is shown to contain glyburide, a drug that could have serious, life-threatening consequences in some people. The FDA warns that people who have low blood sugar or diabetes can receive dangerously high amounts of glyburide by consuming Liqiang 4 (FDA, 2005).

Dietary/Herbal Treatments and Diabetes Type 2

The National Center for Complementary and Alternative Medicine (2008) reports on the safety and effectiveness of six dietary supplements used to treat diabetes. The supplements are alpha-lipoic acid, chromium, coenzyme 10, garlic, magnesium, and omega-3 fatty acids.

The research findings are as follows:

- *Alpha-lipoic acid (ALA)*: A few studies indicate glucose uptake in muscle, insulin sensitivity, and/or weight loss in patients who take

ALA. ALA may significantly lower blood glucose in patients with diabetes, and therefore close monitoring of blood glucose is necessary. ALA may lower blood levels of iron and may interact with some medications such as antacids and decrease the effectiveness of some anticancer drugs.

- *Chromium*: There is not enough evidence to show that chromium is beneficial in the management of diabetes. Chromium can add to insulin in its effect on blood glucose, which can cause the blood glucose level to drop low. The development of kidney problems can be a serious side effect of chromium supplementation in people with diabetes. Other possible side effects include vomiting, diarrhea, and gastrointestinal bleeding.
- *Coenzyme Q10*: There is not enough scientific evidence to support the effectiveness of Coenzyme Q10 (CoQ10) in treating diabetes. It may interact with other medications such as warfarin and some medications used for high blood pressure treatment and cancer chemotherapy.
- *Garlic*: No evidence-based study supports the benefit of garlic in treating type 2 diabetes.
- *Magnesium*: The relationship between diabetes and magnesium is not fully understood, though low levels of magnesium are commonly found in people with diabetes. Some studies have suggested that low magnesium levels may make glucose control worse in type 2 diabetes, but additional studies are needed to establish whether magnesium supplementation is beneficial in treating diabetes.
- *Omega-3 fatty acids (fish oils)*: Randomized clinical trials have found that omega-3 fatty acids lower triglycerides, but have no significant effect on fasting blood glucose, HbA1c, total cholesterol, or HDL cholesterol. Fish oil in high doses can interact with blood-thinning and hypertensive medications.

Nutritional Implications and Intervention

Certain supplements can boost blood levels of certain drugs to dangerous levels. You must ask patients which herbal supplements they are taking and be nonjudgmental when commenting on these products.

By understanding the side effects of these commonly used herbal/dietary supplements, you can educate your patients to make informed choices. Encourage patients to discuss their use of supplements with their physician and pharmacist (Shane-McWhorter, 2002).

FOOD ALLERGY AND INTOLERANCE

Food allergy and intolerance are more commonly seen in children but can also be present in adults. Obtaining information on any food allergy, adverse reaction, and/or food intolerance is extremely important, especially in an in-patient setting. Food allergy can be fatal if medical intervention is delayed.

Here are some sample questions to ask the patient to help you determine food allergy or intolerance:

"Are there any foods that make you sick after eating them?"
"What symptoms do you experience after eating these foods?"
"What do you do to relieve these symptoms?"
"What foods do you eat in lieu of the foods to which you are allergic?"

Definitions

- *Adverse food reaction*: Generic term referring to any undesirable reaction following the ingestion of food
- *Food allergy*: An abnormal response to food triggered by the body's immune system (National Institute of Allergy and Infectious Diseases, 2009)
- *Food intolerance:* Result of nonimmunologic mechanism as in lactase deficiency, bacterial food poisoning, and pancreatic insufficiency

Symptoms of food allergy include itching in the throat, difficulty swallowing or breathing, diarrhea, vomiting, nausea, abdominal pain, gastrointestinal bleeding, itching of the skin, flushing, eczema, asthma, and hives (urticaria). In severe cases, anaphylaxis may occur, where, in addition to some or all of the preceding symptoms, there is a sudden drop in blood pressure, tightening of the throat, chest pain, cyanosis, shock, and eventual death if not treated in time. A symptom occurring more than 3 or 4 hours after ingesting food is not food allergy.

Major Food Allergens

- Soy
- Wheat
- Cow's milk
- Egg
- Fish
- Shellfish
- Peanuts and tree nuts

A study reported in the *Journal of the American Dietetic Association* found that children with two or more food allergies were shorter based on height-for-age percentiles than those with one food allergy (Christie, Hine, Parker, & Burks, 2002).

Nutritional Implications and Intervention

Most common food allergens are inconspicuously hidden in foods, but when consumed can have very serious, life-strengthening effects. You must alert patients to these hidden allergens and provide alternate foods that will meet their nutritional needs. The Food Allergy and Anaphylaxis Network is an excellent resource for information on food allergy. See **Figure 2–1** below for foods that may contain food allergens as listed on food labels.

The growing child needs calcium, as do adults and older adults. If a patient presents with allergy to cow's milk, then discuss alternate choices to ensure the person receives adequate intake of calcium. Alternate choices include but are not limited to calcium-fortified rice or soy milk, fortified orange juice, tofu, calcium-fortified bread and cereal, fish eaten with bones in, and green vegetables except spinach. (The calcium in spinach is not bioavailable because of the presence of oxalate, which binds with calcium and makes it unavailable to the body.)

Patients should be advised to always have an EpiPen Auto-Injector or Benadryl (diphenhydramine) in immediate reach at home or when eating out because there is a high probability of cross contact in the preparation of some foods. It is best to avoid processed foods to reduce the risk of cross contact with food allergens.

How to Read a Label for a Milk-Free Diet

All FDA-regulated manufactured food products that contain milk as an ingredient are required by U.S. law to list the word "milk" on the product label.

Avoid foods that contain milk or any of these ingredients:

- butter, butter fat, butter oil, butter acid, butter ester(s)
- buttermilk
- casein
- casein hydrolysate
- caseinates *(in all forms)*
- cheese
- cottage cheese
- cream
- curds
- custard
- diacetyl
- ghee
- half-and-half
- lactalbumin, lactalbumin phosphate
- lactoferrin
- lactose
- lactulose
- milk *(in all forms, including condensed, derivative, dry, evaporated, goat's milk and milk from other animals, low-fat, malted, milkfat, nonfat, powder, protein, skimmed, solids, whole)*
- milk protein hydrolysate
- pudding
- Recaldent®
- rennet casein
- sour cream, sour cream solids
- sour milk solids
- tagatose
- whey *(in all forms)*
- whey protein hydrolysate
- yogurt

Milk is sometimes found in the following:

- artificial butter flavor
- baked goods
- caramel candies
- chocolate
- lactic acid starter culture and other bacterial cultures
- luncheon meat, hot dogs, sausages
- margarine
- nisin
- nondairy products
- nougat

The Food Allergy & Anaphylaxis Network

11781 Lee Jackson Hwy.
Suite 160
Fairfax, VA 22033-3309
Phone: 703-691-3179
Fax: 703-691-2713
www.foodallergy.org
faan@foodallergy.org

How to Read a Label for a Soy-Free Diet

All FDA-regulated manufactured food products that contain soy as an ingredient are required by U.S. law to list the word "soy" on the product label.

Avoid foods that contain soy or any of these ingredients:

- edamame
- miso
- natto
- shoyu
- soy *(soy albumin, soy cheese, soy fiber, soy flour, soy grits, soy ice cream, soy milk, soy nuts, soy sprouts, soy yogurt)*
- soya
- soybean *(curd, granules)*
- soy protein *(concentrate, hydrolyzed, isolate)*
- soy sauce
- tamari
- tempeh
- textured vegetable protein *(TVP)*
- tofu

Soy is sometimes found in the following:

- Asian cuisine
- vegetable broth
- vegetable gum
- vegetable starch

Keep the following in mind:

- **The FDA exempts highly refined soybean oil from being labeled as an allergen.** Studies show most allergic individuals can safely eat soy oil that has been highly refined (***not*** cold pressed, expeller pressed, or extruded soybean oil).
- Most individuals allergic to soy can safely eat soy lecithin.
- Follow your doctor's advice regarding these ingredients.

How to Read a Label for a Peanut-Free Diet

All FDA-regulated manufactured food products that contain peanut as an ingredient are required by U.S. law to list the word "peanut" on the product label.

Avoid foods that contain peanuts or any of these ingredients:

- artificial nuts
- beer nuts
- cold pressed, expeller pressed, or extruded peanut oil
- goobers
- ground nuts
- mixed nuts
- monkey nuts
- nut pieces
- nutmeat
- peanut butter
- peanut flour
- peanut protein hydrolysate

Peanut is sometimes found in the following:

- African, Asian *(especially Chinese, Indian, Indonesian, Thai, and Vietnamese)*, and Mexican dishes
- baked goods *(e.g., pastries, cookies)*
- candy *(including chocolate candy)*
- chili
- egg rolls
- enchilada sauce
- marzipan
- mole sauce
- nougat

Keep the following in mind:

- Mandelonas are peanuts soaked in almond flavoring.
- **The FDA exempts highly refined peanut oil from being labeled as an allergen.** Studies show that most allergic individuals can safely eat peanut oil that has been highly refined (not cold pressed, expeller pressed, or extruded peanut oil). Follow your doctor's advice.
- A study showed that unlike other legumes, there is a strong possibility of cross-reaction between peanuts and lupine.
- Arachis oil is peanut oil.
- Many experts advise patients allergic to peanuts to avoid tree nuts as well.
- Sunflower seeds are often produced on equipment shared with peanuts.

Figure 2–1 How to Identify Food Allergens from Food Labels

How to Read a Label for a Wheat-Free Diet

All FDA-regulated manufactured food products that contain wheat as an ingredient are required by U.S. law to list the word "wheat" on the product label. The law defines any species in the genus Triticum as wheat.

Avoid foods that contain wheat or any of these ingredients:

bread crumbs
bulgur
cereal extract
club wheat
couscous
cracker meal
durum
einkorn
emmer
farina
flour *(all purpose, bread, cake, durum, enriched, graham, high gluten, high protein, instant, pastry, self-rising, soft wheat, steel ground, stone ground, whole wheat)*
hydrolyzed wheat protein
Kamut
matzoh, matzoh meal *(also spelled as matzo, matzah, or matza)*
pasta
seitan
semolina
spelt
sprouted wheat
triticale
vital wheat gluten
wheat *(bran, durum, germ, gluten, grass, malt, sprouts, starch)*
wheat bran hydrolysate
wheat germ oil
wheat grass
wheat protein isolate
whole wheat berries

Wheat is sometimes found in the following:

glucose syrup
soy sauce
starch *(gelatinized starch, modified starch, modified food starch, vegetable starch)*
surimi

How to Read a Label for an Egg-Free Diet

All FDA-regulated manufactured food products that contain egg as an ingredient are required by U.S. law to list the word "egg" on the product label.

Avoid foods that contain eggs or any of these ingredients:

albumin *(also spelled albumen)*
egg *(dried, powdered, solids, white, yolk)*
eggnog
lysozyme
mayonnaise
meringue *(meringue powder)*
ovalbumin
surimi

Egg is sometimes found in the following:

baked goods
egg substitutes
lecithin
macaroni
Marzipan
marshmallows
nougat
pasta

Keep the following in mind:

- Individuals with egg allergy should also avoid eggs from duck, turkey, goose, quail, etc., as these are known to be cross-reactive with chicken egg.

How to Read a Label for a Shellfish-Free Diet

All FDA-regulated manufactured food products that contain a crustacean shellfish as an ingredient are required by U.S. law to list the specific crustacean shellfish on the product label.

Avoid foods that contain shellfish or any of these ingredients:

crab
crawfish *(crayfish, ecrevisse)*
lobster *(langouste, langoustine, scampo, coral, tomalley)*
prawn
shrimp *(crevette)*

Mollusks are not considered major allergens under food labeling laws and may not be fully disclosed on a product label.

Your doctor may advise you to avoid mollusks or these ingredients:

abalone
clams *(cherrystone, littleneck, pismo, quahog)*
cockle *(periwinkle, sea urchin)*
mussels
octopus
oysters
snails *(escargot)*
squid *(calamari)*
Shellfish are sometimes found in the following:
bouillabaisse
cuttlefish ink
fish stock
seafood flavoring *(e.g., crab or clam extract)*
surimi

Keep the following in mind:

- Any food served in a seafood restaurant may contain shellfish protein due to cross-contact.
- For some individuals, a reaction may occur from inhaling cooking vapors or from handling fish or shellfish.

How to Read a Label for a Tree Nut-Free Diet

All FDA-regulated manufactured food products that contain a tree nut as an ingredient are required by U.S. law to list the specific tree nut on the product label.

Avoid foods that contain nuts or any of these ingredients:

almonds
artificial nuts
beechnut
Brazil nuts
butternut
cashews
chestnuts
chinquapin
coconut
filberts/hazelnuts
gianduja *(a chocolate-nut mixture)*
ginkgo nut
hickory nuts
litchi/lichee/lychee nut
macadamia nuts
marzipan/almond paste
Nangai nuts
natural nut extract *(e.g., almond, walnut)*
nut butters *(e.g., cashew butter)*
nut meal
nut paste *(e.g., almond paste)*
nut pieces
nutmeat
pecans
pesto
pili nut
pine nuts *(also referred to as Indian, pignoli, pigñolia, pignon, piñon, and pinyon nuts)*
pistachios
praline
shea nut
walnuts

Tree nuts are sometimes found in the following:

black walnut hull extract *(flavoring)*
natural nut extract
nut distillates/alcoholic extracts
nut oils *(e.g., walnut oil, almond oil)*
walnut hull extract *(flavoring)*

Keep the following in mind:

- Mortadella may contain pistachios.
- There is no evidence that coconut oil and shea nut oil/butter are allergenic.
- Many experts advise patients allergic to tree nuts to avoid peanuts as well.
- Talk to your doctor if you find other nuts not listed here.

Source: © 2009 The Food Allergy & Analphylaxis Network, used with permission.

SUMMARY

Interviewing the patient and/or caregiver provides information that you sometimes cannot find in the chart. You can develop trust with the patient during the interview, and the interview provides a foundation on which to build or develop a treatment plan. Phrase questions properly to avoid confusion and ambiguity. Interviews conducted in the patient's primary language produce better results. In some Spanish-speaking groups, similar words have different meanings. Pay special attention to the patient's body language, culture, and religion and be respectful at all times.

REVIEW QUESTIONS

1. Patient SH is a 55-year-old man who came to the emergency department with visible bruising on his left arm. He denies falling or hitting his arm anywhere. Medical history reveals heart attack 8 months ago, at which time the patient was placed on Coumadin. Upon interviewing the patient, he reveals he has been taking omega-3 fatty acids and niacin as recommended by his friends to help with his heart condition. What could be the possible cause for the bruising on his arm?
2. JT is a 13-year-old boy who was rushed to the hospital for anaphylactic shock after eating homemade cookies at his friend's home. He knows he has an allergy to nuts, but his friend's mom said there were no nuts in the cookies. Outline a list of questions that you would use to track the source of the allergen.

REFERENCES

American Dietetic Association. (2005). Practice paper of the American Dietetic Association: Dietary supplements. *Journal of the American Dietetic Association, 105*(3), 460–470.

American Liver Foundation. (2006). *Hepatitis B: What you need to know.* Retrieved October 1, 2009, from www.liverfoundation.org/downloads/alf_download_22.pdf

Campo, L. C., Calabuig, A. J. R., Aquilar J. J., & Alonso, E. (2004). Skeletal, anifestation of Gaucher's disease. *Anales de Medecina Interna, 21*(4), 179–182.

Charney, P., & Malone, A. M. (2009). *ADA pocket guide to nutrition assessment* (2nd ed.). Chicago: American Dietetic Association.

Christie, L., Hine, J. R., Parker, J., & Burks, W. (2002). Food allergies in children affect nutrient intake and growth. *Journal of the American Dietetic Association, 102,* 1648–1651.

Cuellar, N. G., Cahill, B., Ford, J., & Aycock, T. (2003). The development of an educational workshop on complementary and alternative medicine: What every nurse should know. *Journal of Continuing Education in Nursing, 34*(3), 128–134.

Drago, L. (2008). *Best culturally competent communication tool.* Retrieved January 15, 2009, from http://hispanicfoodways.com/professionals_education/

Drago, L. (2004, October). *Effective teaching strategies for dietetic professionals counseling Hispanics with diabetes.* Paper presented at the American Dietetic Association's Food and Nutrition Conference and Expo, Anaheim, CA.

Fertility Treatment Center. (2009). *Preimplantation genetic diagnosis: Breaking the "family curse" of genetic disease.* Retrieved September 16, 2009, from http://www.fertilitytreatmentcenter.com/pgd.htm

Food and Drug Administration. (2002, March 25). Consumer advisory: Kava-containing dietary supplements may be associated with severe liver injury. Retrieved September 15, 2009, from http://www.fda.gov/Food/ResourcesForYou/Consumers/ucm085482.htm

Food and Drug Administration. (2005, July). Liqiang 4 dietary supplement capsules. Retrieved September 15, 2009, from www.fda.gov/Safety/MedWatch/SafetyInformation/SafetyAlertsforHumanMedicalProducts/ucm150476.htm

Food and Drug Administration. (2007, August). FDA warns consumers to avoid red yeast rice products promoted on Internet as treatments for high cholesterol found to contain unauthorized drug. Retrieved September 15, 2009, from http://www.fda.gov/NewsEvents/Newsroom/PressAnnouncements/2007/ucm108962.htm

Gibson, R. (2005). *Principles of nutritional assessment* (2nd ed.). New York: Oxford University Press.

National Institute of Allergy and Infectious Diseases. Retrieved October 1, 2009, from http://www3.niaid.nih.gov/topics/foodAllergy/understanding/whatIsIt.htm

Piscitelli, S. C., Burstein, A. H., Welden, N., Gallicano, K. D., & Falloon, J. (2002). The effect of garlic supplements on the pharmokinetics of Saquinavir. *Clinical Infectious Diseases, 34,* 234–238.

Shane-McWhorter, L. (2002, November 4). Interactions between complementary therapies or nutrition supplements and conventional medications. *Diabetes Spectrum, 15,* 262–266.

Waibel, R. A. (2004). Religion and Dietary Practices. In *Gale Nutrition and Well-Being A to Z.* Retrieved June 1, 2009, from http://www.healthline.com/galecontent/religion-and-dietary-practices

ADDITIONAL RESOURCES

Food Allergy and Anaphylaxis Network: http://www.foodallergy.org

Food and Drug Administration: http://www.fda.gov

National Center for Complementary and Alternative Medicine: http://www.nccam.nih.gov

Tate, D. M. (2003, September–October). Cultural awareness: Bridging the gap between caregivers and Hispanic patients. *The Journal of Continuing Education in Nursing, 34*(5).

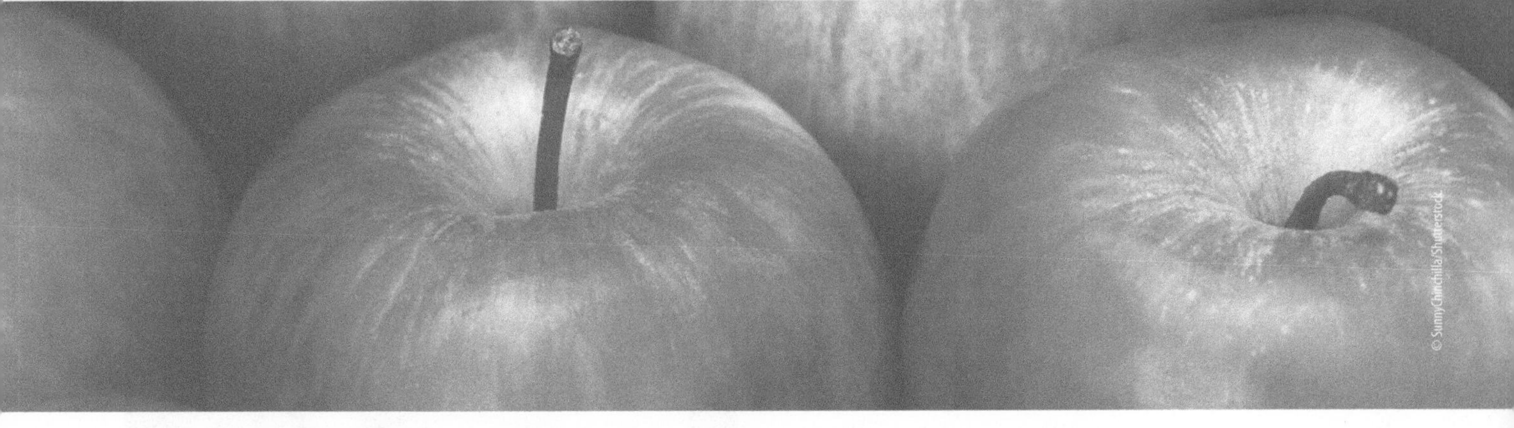

Computerized Food and Nutrition Analysis Systems

Lona Sandon, PhD, MEd, RDN

CHAPTER OUTLINE

- Introduction
- Dietary-Intake Assessment Methods
- Innovative Technologies in Nutrition Assessment
- Selecting a Computerized Diet-Analysis System for the Research Nutritionist
- Computer-Based Diet-Assessment Applications
- Internet-Based Diet-Analysis Applications
- Chapter Summary

LEARNING OBJECTIVES

After reading this chapter, the learner will be able to:

1. Discuss the advantages and disadvantages of dietary assessment methods commonly used in nutrition research and clinical practice, including food records, 24-hour dietary recall, food-frequency questionnaires, and screeners.
2. Describe three types of innovative technologies that can be used to enhance the collection of dietary data for more-accurate and objective nutrient analysis.
3. Evaluate the appropriateness of a computerized diet analysis, based on factors to consider in selecting a computerized diet-analysis application for nutrition research.
4. Choose a computer-based diet-analysis application to meet clinical or research needs.
5. Select an Internet-based diet-analysis application to meet clinical or research needs.

▶ Introduction

Researchers and clinicians in the United States and Great Britain have been interested in determining dietary intake since the 1930s, when the first reports of dietary records appeared in the literature.[1] These early records revealed discrepancies in results coming from the method used to capture the dietary intake and determine the amount of food eaten. In addition to the challenge of accurately recording the actual foods and amount of foods consumed, accurately determining the actual food composition is another concern in dietary-intake assessment.[1] Until the advent of the computer, clinicians and researchers analyzed and calculated dietary intake by hand. As computers became more widely available in the 1980s and 1990s, the need for calculating nutrient intake manually was nearly eliminated, although many clinicians still use quick methods such as the exchange system to quickly assess an individual's dietary intake. Nonetheless, the difficulty of determining the nutrient composition of the total diet and foods available for consumption persists.

As technology continues to advance, so has the number of foods and beverages available for consumption. Early database systems for dietary-intake analysis may have only included a few hundred food items and limited nutrient data to select nutrients. Today's databases are capable of searching hundreds of thousands of food items and are much more robust, with a wider array of nutrient-composition data for individual food items. Nutrient-composition databases can contain information from multiple sources, including the US Department of Agriculture (USDA), research databases, food manufacturers, and restaurant menus and webpages.

Although early computerized nutrient-analysis systems sped up calculating nutrient intake, they did not address the inherent problems and bias in methods used to collect dietary-intake data that truly represents the usual diet. Clinicians and researchers are well aware that one day's record of food intake is not sufficient to determine an individual's usual nutrient intake; multiple days or weeks are required. In addition, bias influences the validity of records of dietary intake.

Current technology can introduce new methods and enhance traditional methods of collecting dietary-intake data to improve accuracy and reduce bias in the data-collection process. Technology may also reduce researcher, clinician, and participant burden associated with dietary-intake data collection, data entry, analysis, and reporting. This chapter discusses traditional dietary-intake assessment methods, evolving technologies for capturing dietary-intake data, existing **computer-based diet-assessment applications**, **Internet-based diet-assessment applications**, and factors to consider in choosing an assessment tool to meet the needs of the researcher or clinician.

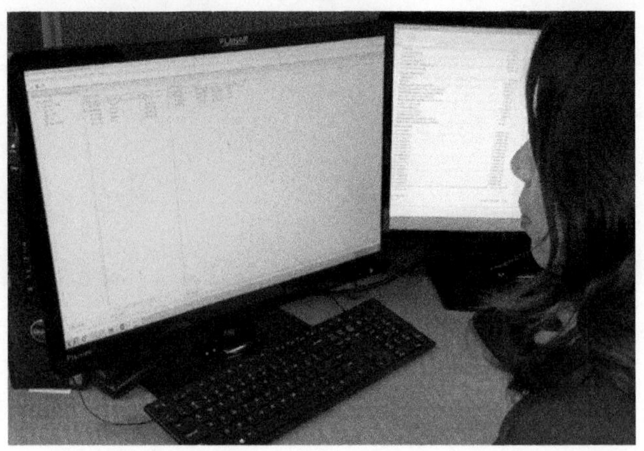

Dietary-Intake Assessment Methods

Preview Dietary-intake assessment relies on self-reported data in both clinical and research settings. Traditional tools used to capture dietary-intake data include dietary-history questionnaires, food records, 24-hour dietary recalls (24-hour recall), **food-frequency questionnaires (FFQs)**, and **screeners**. Each method mentioned comes with its own set of potential errors, benefits, and drawbacks to gathering valid and reliable dietary data. The ease and ability of managing and analyzing data differs with each method.

Food Records

A **food record**, also sometimes referred to as a *food diary* (**FIGURE 1**), may be useful for evaluating associations between health outcomes and dietary intake. Food records intend to provide a complete record of all foods and beverages consumed over a designated period, typically including several days of dietary intake. Clients or research participants are instructed to document all food or beverage items consumed during the designated time period; weigh, measure, or estimate portion sizes of items eaten using standard household measurements; provide descriptions of food items and methods of food preparation; state specific brands if applicable; and record the time and place where food items are consumed. The clinician or researcher may review the food record with the client or participant to clarify recorded items and portion sizes, thereby improving the quality of dietary data collected. In the food-record

Food Diary

Date/ Time	Meal	Food item	Serving size	Calories	Notes
	Breakfast				
	Lunch				
	Dinner				
	Snack				

FIGURE 1 Food diary sample

method, participants are supposed to record all foods and beverages at the time they are consumed. Recording at the time of intake reduces reliance on memory, which leads to better-quality intake data. This is one strength of the food-record method over other intake-assessment methods.[2,3] Weighed or measured food records that account for plate waste or unconsumed portions of food also improve the accuracy of the dietary data. Food records may benefit dietary-intervention studies in which the intent of the intervention is to improve eating behavior. Recording dietary intake can motivate some participants to make better food and beverage choices.[4] However, this is not an advantage if the researcher or clinician is trying to measure participants' usual intake. The food record is the most thorough method of collecting dietary intake.[2,3]

The process of obtaining dietary data through food records has several limitations. First, participants must be literate enough and have the language skills to record their own dietary intake. Second, participants must be willing and motivated to complete food records, and they may not represent the general population.[4] Third, because of the burdensome nature of food records, participants may not record data in real time and instead rely on memory to record data at a more convenient time. This introduces **recall bias** into the method.[2] Participants also may alter their eating habits to make recording intake easier or to be more acceptable to the researcher or clinician; this introduces **reactivity bias** and **social-approval bias** and affects the ability to assess usual intake.[2,3] Also, food records may also not represent usual intake because they are typically limited to a narrow period that represents current intake but does not provide information about past intake.[4] Multiple days are needed to capture variability in daily dietary intake. The more days required, the more respondent burden, which may affect data quality. Traditional food records have been recorded using pen and paper, an arduous process for clients and participants.[3] Food records sometimes underestimate nutrient intake, including energy and protein intake, when compared to biochemical measures of nutrient intake.[2] Furthermore, food records are also labor intensive for researchers. This limits the use of food records in large population studies.[4] Data entry and management for analyzing food records is time-consuming for researchers or clinicians and prevents them from providing immediate feedback to participants. Current technologies including the Internet and smartphones may offer quicker ways to document dietary intake in real time and directly into databases that may lead to both better-quality data and faster analysis.

24-Hour Dietary Recall

A **24-hour recall** uses a structured interview process typically conducted by a trained clinician or interviewer who asks participants to list the foods consumed in the previous 24 hours or a recent 24-hour period. See **FIGURE 2**. The interviewer asks questions to prompt the participant to recall intake details, including portion sizes, brand names, how foods were prepared, condiments added, timing of meals or snacks, and missed items. Use of pictures, food models, and measuring cups or spoons aid memory and improve the estimates of portions consumed. The process is relatively quick, does not require literacy on behalf of the participant, and has no influence on intake as it collects information; there is also little burden put on participants.[3,4] A structured and standardized interview process will likely lead to better data collection and coding of items consumed.[2,3] As Thompson et al.[2] state,

24-Hour Recall	**Instructions:** Record the time, the amount and food item consumed. Describe the food preparation method and document where were you when the food item was consumed. The location can be places such as: home in the kitchen, in front of the TV, at work, in my desk, etc.			
Time	**Amount consumed**	**Food and/or beverage consumed**	**Method of preparation**	**Where consumed (location)**

FIGURE 2 24-hour dietary recall form

"Twenty-four-hour recalls can be used to describe dietary intake, examine associations between diet and other variables such as health, and evaluate the effectiveness of an intervention study to change diet."[2] Data from 24-hour recalls better represent the usual mean intake of a group as opposed to an individual, given the high variability in day-to-day intake and the need for multiple 24-hour recalls from individuals to determine usual intake. This makes the 24-hour recall a good tool for comparing dietary intake between different groups.[3,4]

One drawback of the 24-hour recall is that it relies on the participant's memory. This introduces recall bias and random error and thereby influences data reliability and validity. Underestimation or underreporting of intake is a common problem of 24-hour recalls. In addition, variation in intake from day to day introduces random error. Collecting multiple 24-hour recalls can reduce the potential for error.[2,3] Between eight and 32 days of 24-hour recalls may be needed to reach 80% reliability for energy intake and fruit intake, respectively.[5] Similar to food records, data entry of 24-hour recalls is time-consuming. Existing computer-based technologies help standardize the interview process and allow direct data entry at the time of interview, thereby reducing time and effort for data collection and entry. Current technology also allows for self-administered 24-hour recalls using standardized questions and algorithms to guide the self-administered interview process. However, these self-administered applications may limit the ability to capture complete descriptions of food items sought by a trained interviewer.[4]

Food-Frequency Questionnaires

Food-frequency questionnaires (FFQ) are commonly used in large epidemiological studies because they are less costly than other assessment methods and easier for researchers to administer. See **FIGURE 3**. It is the most objective method for assessing intake because it uses a specific list of foods.[2,4] An FFQ asks questions about the usual frequency of a finite list of foods and beverages consumed over a defined time such as a year, month, or week. An FFQ commonly includes portion-size choices on the questionnaire. The number of items may vary, depending on food and beverage items of interest among the study population, nutrients of interest, and customization for items commonly eaten among specific populations. Generally, an FFQ is self-administered and does not require an interviewer. An FFQ is beneficial for assessing food

Date:

Name:

Instructions: In the past three (3) months did you consume the foods listed below?						
Food Group	**Frequency**					
	Never	Less than one time per week	1-6 times per week	1-3 times per day	4 or more times per day	Serving size
Dairy: milk, cheese, yogurt						
Chicken: grilled chicken, baked chicken, fired chicken, etc.						
Turkey: turkey sandwich, soup, breast, roasted, etc.						
Beef: meatballs, steak, etc.						
Pork: cured ham, fresh ham, ribs, pork chops, pulled pork, etc.						
Fish and seafood: shrimp, scallops, fish, shellfish						
Other Meat: lamb, duck, etc.						
Nuts: walnuts, cashews, peanuts, etc.						
Beans: red beans, chick peas, chili, etc.						
Egg: omelet, hard-boiled egg, etc.						
Vegetables: broccoli, cauliflower, green beans, etc.						
Fruit: banana, strawberry, apple, pear, melon, etc.						
Grains: rice, bread, cereal, etc.						
Sweets: cakes, cookies, pies, etc.						
Beverages: coffee, tea, sodas, juices, etc.						

FIGURE 3 Food frequency questionnaire

groups and dietary patterns of certain foods and beverages and their relationships to disease outcomes. Variability in daily intake does not influence an FFQ, which also takes into account seasonal variation in intake.[2,3] Moreover, an FFQ is the preferred instrument for use in retrospective case-controlled studies. It is the only instrument that asks about long-term past dietary intake.[2]

As with other methods, the reliability and validity of data from an FFQ may be affected by recall bias and the inability to capture total dietary intake because of missing intake items that might be common to the population of interest. The inability to assess the total diet makes the FFQ a poor instrument for clinical settings or settings in which adequacy of nutrient intake is important for assessing individual intake. It is less precise than other methods.[4] In a study comparing an FFQ to a seven-day diet record, the FFQ underestimated sodium and overestimated macronutrient and energy intake. Only weak correlations were found between the FFQ and 24-hour recalls before adjusting for within-person variation, which improved correlations slightly.[6] This calls into question the validity and reliability of FFQ dietary data. Similar to 24-hour recalls, FFQs are subject to social-approval bias—that is, expected norms for behavior influence participants' reported intakes. Miller et al. demonstrated in a randomized blinded study that intervention participants who received prompts related to recommended intake and the benefits of consuming fruits and vegetables were more likely to report higher intakes of fruit and vegetables on an FFQ and 24-hour recall.[7] Underreporting of intake can also be a limitation when using FFQs, which underestimate energy and protein intake when compared to biochemical markers to determine the validity of self-reporting of intake.[2] Underreporting or overreporting of intake can occur if portions listed on the questionnaire are different from what the participant usually consumes.[4] Lastly, traditional paper-based FFQs increase researcher time and effort for data entry and analysis. Technology-based FFQs may decrease the time and effort needed to administer, enter data by the researcher or clinician, and analyze data. Technology also enhances the ability to incorporate food images into the questionnaire, which may help respondents better estimate portion sizes and improve validity.

Screeners

Dietary screeners are more cost-effective and present less burden for participants than previously described intake-assessment methods. Screeners are similar to FFQs but differ by including a shorter list of questions typically related to specific dietary behaviors (**FIGURE 4**). This tool is used to convey gross estimates of the intake of specific dietary components such as fruits and vegetables or usual beverage intakes in both adults and children.[8,9,10] When accurate levels of intake are required, avoid using screeners because they do not assess total diet.[8] Self-administered screeners are easy to use and implement in large cross-sectional studies to determine mean intake of certain dietary components, and they are comparable to 24-hour recalls or FFQs in terms of determining frequency of intake.[2,8] England et al. conducted a review of 47 studies describing 35 different brief questionnaires (having fewer than 35 items) that were designed to assess fat intake, Mediterranean-diet compliance, patterns of healthy eating, and intake of fruits and vegetables.[11] They concluded that validated and reliable brief instruments could guide clinical decision-making when carefully selected to match the client population with the sample population.[11] Short questionnaires allow clinicians and researchers to assess dietary intake quickly. Screeners or brief questionnaires have the advantage of quick and easy scoring. Innovative technologies may further improve the ease of scoring screeners and provide immediate feedback to participants, clinicians, and researchers.

Technology in Nutrition Assessment

Researchers have called for improvements to current methods or the development of new methods of obtaining and analyzing dietary information. Innovative technologies developed in the past decade offer the opportunity to improve on dietary data-collection methods and add objective data. Potential benefits of incorporating the use of technology into dietary-intake data collection include greater ability to standardize the data-collection process: question sequencing, automated and rapid dietary analysis allowing immediate access to results, and improved data management with direct entry and

Fruits, Vegetables, and Grains	Less than 1/WEEK	Once a WEEK	2-3 times a WEEK	4-6 times a WEEK	Once a DAY	2+ a DAY
Fruit juice, like orange, apple, grape, fresh, frozen or canned. (Not sodas or other drinks)	○	○	○	○	○	○
How often do you eat any fruit, fresh or canned (not counting juice?)	○	○	○	○	○	○
Vegetable juice, like tomato juice, V-8, carrot	○	○	○	○	○	○
Green salad	○	○	○	○	○	○
Potatoes, any kind, including baked, mashed or french fried	○	○	○	○	○	○
Vegetable soup, or stew with vegetables	○	○	○	○	○	○
Any other vegetables, including string beans, peas, corn, broccoli or any other kind	○	○	○	○	○	○
Fiber cereals like Raisin Bran, Shredded Wheat or Fruit-n-Fiber	○	○	○	○	○	○
Beans such as baked beans, pinto, kidney, or lentils (not green beans)	○	○	○	○	○	○
Dark bread such as whole wheat or rye	○	○	○	○	○	○

FIGURE 4 Fiber screener

ease of data processing and transfer. The use of technology also affects the time costs of interviewer-led 24-hour recalls and increases acceptability among younger populations.[2,12,13,14] Technology also can add more layers of contextual information such as meal timing and location and eating patterns, as well as more food images to improve reporting of portion sizes. This allows multiple databases to increase the specificity of foods consumed and integration this information with biochemical data.[2] Disadvantages of incorporating innovative technologies include participants' technological literacy; older adults may not be familiar with newer technologies or have difficulty using them because of factors associated with aging (difficulty seeing or hearing). Disabilities can also be a limitation if keyboard or mouse skills are required. Access to technology may limit participation for some socioeconomic groups. Lastly, technology can be more expensive to use than survey instruments that use pen and paper.[12,14]

Incorporating technology into nutrient intake assessment has its advantages and disadvantages. See **TABLE 1**.

Recap Frequent criticism of traditional methods of dietary-intake assessment result from the known systematic errors in data collection, including recall, reactivity, and social-approval bias as well as poor sensitivity to changes in dietary intake.[2,12] Some researchers believe that no dietary data collected from memory recall can be trusted and that only objective data should be used to assess intake. Thompson et al. recommend the use of objective biochemical measures in addition to self-reported data for validation of dietary-intake assessment.[2] In addition, traditional methods that rely on survey tools requiring pen and paper or interviewer-administered instruments limit researchers in their ability to assess larger populations and hard-to-reach populations. They also require more time, money, and effort of researchers and clinicians to obtain, enter, manage, and analyze dietary-intake data. The introduction of technology into nutrition assessment offers the benefits of reaching larger populations; improving data collection, management, and analysis; and potential increased objectivity in data collection.

TABLE 1 Advantages and disadvantages of using technology in nutrition assessment

Advantages		Disadvantages
▪ Reduced cost of labor for data collection ▪ Increased time effectiveness: data can be automatically stored; no data entry is needed ▪ Higher acceptance among some populations (e.g., adolescents, young adults) ▪ Able to assess larger populations with minimal extra cost ▪ Ability to standardize the data-collection process, including question sequencing ▪ Automated and rapid dietary analysis	▪ Prevent incomplete or implausible data entry ▪ Immediate access to results ▪ Improved data management with direct entry and electronic transfer to central database ▪ Capture of contextual information (meal timing, location, eating patterns) ▪ Greater number of real food images to improve reporting of portion sizes ▪ Help features assist users ▪ Incorporate multiple databases to increase specificity of foods consumed ▪ Integrate biochemical data	▪ Self-report bias still exists with new technology ▪ Requires technological literacy of the participants ▪ May require keyboard or mouse skills ▪ Older adults may not be familiar with newer technologies or have difficulty using them because of aging factors (e.g., difficulty seeing or hearing, arthritis) ▪ May not be easily accessible to individuals with physical impairments ▪ Accessibility of technologies may limit participation of some socioeconomic groups ▪ Technology can be more expensive to use than survey instruments requiring pen and paper

Data from Thompson FE, Kirkpatrick SI, Subar AF, et al. The National Cancer Institute's Dietary Assessment Primer: A resource for diet research. *J Acad Nutr Diet.* 2015; 115:1986–1995. Long JD, Littlefield LA, Estep G, et al. Evidence review of technology and dietary assessment. *Worldviews Evid Based Nurs.* 2010;7(4):191–204. Boushey C, Kerr D, Wright J, Lutes K, Ebert D, Delp E. Use of technology in children's dietary assessment. *Eur J Clin Nutr.* 2009;63(Suppl 1): S50–S57. Probst YC, Tapsell LC. Overview of computerized dietary assessment programs for research and practice in nutrition education. *J Nutr Educ Behav.* 2005;37(1):20–26.

▸ Innovative Technologies in Nutrition Assessment

Preview Broad categories of current technologies in use or development for clinical or research-based dietary-intake assessment includes computer or Internet-based applications. The technology can be utilized in handheld devices, mobile phones with cameras, audio or video recording devices, and other scanner- or sensor-based devices.[2,12]

Image-Assisted Dietary Assessment

Image-assisted dietary assessment (IADA) is a new approach to dietary-intake capture. See **FIGURE 5**. It has been described as any "method that uses images/video of eating episodes to enhance self-report of traditional methods or uses images/video as the primary record of dietary intake."[16] New technology in the form of handheld devices with built-in cameras such as smartphones and wearable cameras or sensors have made it easier to objectively capture dietary intake as opposed to relying solely on self-report. Captured images support traditional methods by aiding recall, identifying misreporting, and uncovering unreported food items, and it may increase the validity of energy-intake estimates.[16] Other purported benefits are the reduced burden of recording for the participant, increased engagement in record keeping, and better estimation of food portions.[2] A drawback of this method is that users must remember to capture images of meals before and after eating. The images also must be of adequate quality for assessment. Not meeting these criteria leads to underestimation of dietary intake and reduces the method's reliability and validity.[16]

Gemming categorized IADA as either an active or a passive approach, depending on the type of technology used. The active approach requires the participant to use a handheld device to capture food and beverage items before and after each eating episode. In most instances, participants must include a reference marker in the image view to assist with either manual or automated analysis. Depending on the software used, the participant may add supplementary text or an audio recording to confirm information about the food items such as type, preparation, and portions. For reliability and validity of the dietary data, it is critical that participants capture the image before food intake at each eating episode.

The passive approach uses wearable cameras that automatically record images of dietary intake and require little or no input from participants. No manual recording is necessary, and recorded images can aid recall. This approach also captures activities unrelated to eating, and no reference marker is included to aid in analysis.[16] The lack of a reference marker may affect the validity and reliability of determining the correct portion sizes of foods.

Dietitian-Assessed Food Photographs

Handheld devices and mobile phones with integrated cameras offer a means of gathering dietary-intake data with less recording burden on the user. See **FIGURE 6**. Methods include recording images of food and beverages before and after eating, along with audio- or text-recorded data about the meal. Images are sent to the researcher or clinician for analysis.

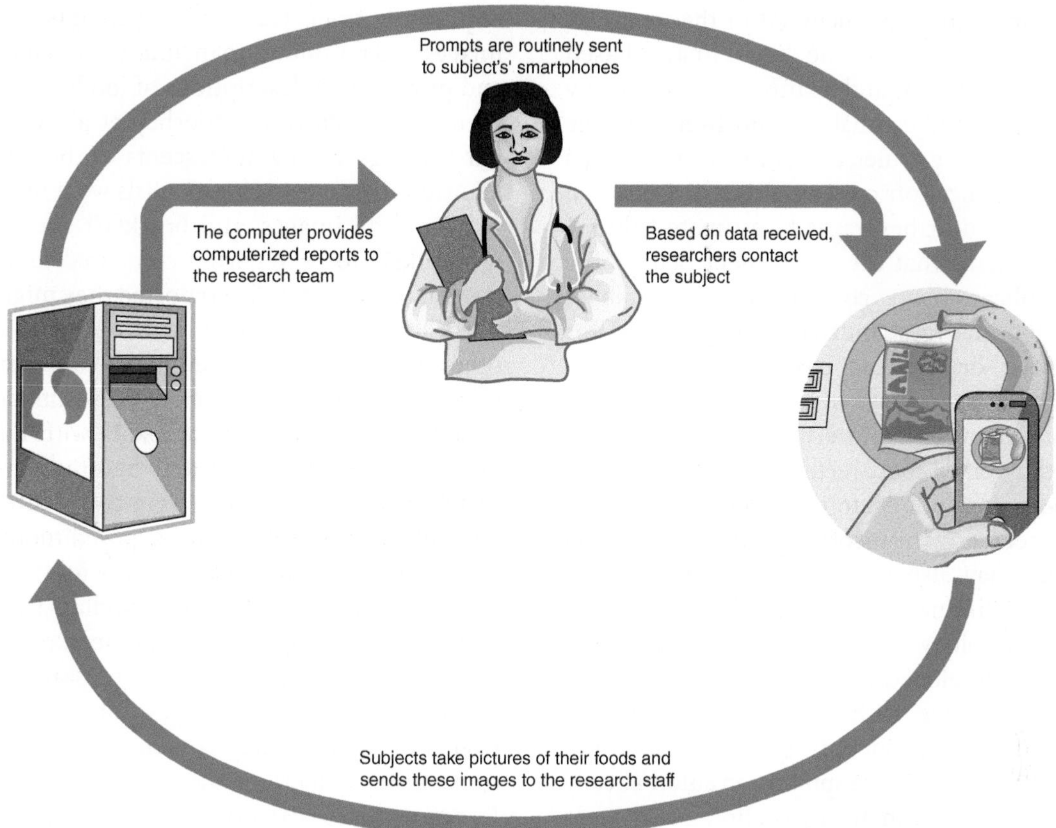
Prompts are routinely sent
to subject's' smartphones
The computer provides
computerized reports to
the research team
Based on data received,
researchers contact
the subject
Subjects take pictures of their foods and
sends these images to the research staff

FIGURE 6 Food photographs used in intake assessment

Modified from Research Gate. https://www.researchgate.net/figure/51846531_fig3_Figure-2-The-Remote-Food-Photography-Method-RFPM-uses-ecological-momentary-assessment Retrieved 7/4/17.

Multiple studies have attempted to validate the IADA method. At least three studies have compared the Wellnavi method to a weighed-food record. The Wellnavi method requires participants to capture food images with a visual reference marker from a 45-degree angle and provide written text describing foods and ingredients. Registered dietitian nutritionists (RDN) then manually analyze images with incorporated text. Two studies found no significant differences between energy or macronutrient intake when comparing the Wellnavi method to a weighed food-record, and the third study (Kikunaga) significantly underestimated macronutrient intake and underestimated energy intake using the Wellnavi method, thereby affecting validity.[17,18,19] Reasons for the results of the later study may have been the lack of text descriptions with the food images. Other studies have documented similar results and noted difficulties with capturing clear images, remembering to capture images before and after eating occasions, and including corresponding text or voice recordings.[16]

Rollo et al. conducted a study comparing energy intake obtained from a 3-day food record using the Nutricam Dietary Assessment Method (NuDAM) to energy expenditure measured by the doubly labeled water (DLW) technique.[20] A weighed food record was used to determine relative validity. Both the NuDAM and weighed food-record methods significantly underestimated energy intake compared to total energy expenditure determined by DLW, indicating the validity of the method is a concern. Moderate correlations were found between the weighed food record and NuDAM for energy, carbohydrate, protein, and alcohol. Interrater reliability was also assessed among three dietitians. Agreement on estimates of nutrients between dietitians was lower than agreement between NuDAM and the weighed food-record.[20] Assessing nutrient intake based on images does not appear to be superior to traditional methods of gathering and assessing dietary data.

Automated Food-Photograph Analysis

More-advanced technology exists to recognize food and beverages from digital images based on their shapes, colors, or textures. The mobile phone food record (mpFR) captures multiple digital images of foods and beverages before and after a meal or snack. Estimating volume typically requires more than one image and an item of known size, or a reference marker must be included in the image. A server receives and analyzes the digital images based on features such as color and texture to automatically identify the food and estimate the portion size. The reference marker (e.g., ruler, card, or USB stick) helps the software application create a three-dimensional image of the food or beverages to estimate volume. The user confirms that the items identified by the imaging application are correct. Next, a database automatically analyzes nutrient composition for the researcher or clinician based on the analysis of the image and estimate of portion size.[21] When participants forget to capture images during eating episodes, they enter food-record data into an electronic food record built into the mobile phone.[16] In addition to reducing the recording burden, capturing food images may also increase reporting accuracy and reduce or eliminate recall bias in food reporting.

The Technology Assisted Diet Assessment (TADA) tool, developed at Purdue University, uses a single food image with a reference marker—a checkerboard card—to identify and quantify foods. The image-analysis software application automatically separates foods in the image by outlining each item and labeling it by food type. Items must not overlap. The geometric shape of the food is used to determine the volume. The user can confirm the type of food and volume. The food is analyzed for nutrient content by connecting with a database.[1] Researchers validated the TADA tool by comparing it against known portion sizes and nutrient contents of food items. The mean percentage error ranged from 1% to 10%, indicating good validity and accuracy.[22]

Children and adolescents are challenging populations when considering accurate assessment of nutrient intake. The accuracy of dietary-intake reporting and recording among children and adolescents is generally poor. Better methods are needed to assess nutrient intake in these populations. Some researchers hypothesize that mobile technologies are more acceptable and easily adopted by adolescents, although challenges still exist. Six et al. found that adolescents were open to using the mpFR technology but require additional training to improve the accuracy of food-image capturing.[21] A small study of children aged 11 to 14 years asked them to keep an mpFR for three to seven days; fewer than half of those studied were able to correctly follow instructions for capturing food images before and after eating. Participants recorded an average of 3.2 days and an average of 2.2 meals per day. Of the meals captured, many did not include all foods or the required reference marker. The results indicate that children of this age are capable of using an image-based food record. This might require additional training and prompts for capturing images and reminders to include the reference marker and provide text descriptions of foods to increase the accuracy of analysis.[23] Boushey et al. reported similar findings among adolescents of the same age, in addition to other findings.[13] Girls were more likely to capture food images, and breakfast and lunch were more likely to be reported compared to snacks and dinner. Adolescents also reported they might be more likely to use the mpFR if it incorporated a game or other form of entertainment.[13] An earlier study evaluated usability among both adolescents and adults. Researchers provided participants with instructions on how to capture food and beverage images correctly. Adults were more likely to capture all foods and beverages in the image, required more attempts, and found remembering to capture food images easy. Both groups had difficulty including the reference marker in the images. As with others, results suggest that training and practice are necessary to increase accuracy of capturing images correctly to improve results of dietary analysis using an mpFR.[24] Validation studies using the mpFR are yet to be published.[16] Its correct use is essential for future validity and reliability testing.

Food Intake and Voice Recorder

The Food Intake and Voice Recorder (FIVR) is another mpFR tool. The FIVR captures food images along with a reference marker to estimate food volume using the three best images. The camera uses a three-dimensional point cloud method to detect the shape and area of the food for volume estimation. Food-recognition software receives the data and calculates the volume. Users also provide a voice recording that includes the name and a description of each food consumed. The food names are compared with color and texture of foods detected in the image and the database of foods available in the software system. The foods are then matched with a nutrient-composition database for analysis.[1,25]

Dietary Data Recorder System is another tool. This tool eliminates the need for a reference marker by using a laser beam to detect the size of the food portion. The laser beam displays a grid over the food item in the image, which the researcher uses to identify the food item, the portion size, and the composition.[1]

Wearable Image-Capturing Systems

SenseCam

SenseCam is a wearable camera attached to a lanyard worn around the neck. The camera captures and stores images automatically on a continuous cycle for

HIGHLIGHT

Bite-Counting Technology

Bite counters are a new technology for monitoring portion intake and estimating the energy intake of foods consumed. Bite counters are worn on the wrist like a watch or embedded in a fork or spoon. Each time the hand with the bite counter is lifted toward the mouth, the device counts a bite based on the movement of an internal gyroscope or accelerometer. Therefore, bite counters may offer an objective and possibly more accurate measure of food intake. Salley et al. conducted a study to evaluate the accuracy of a bite-based estimate of energy intake compared to estimates of energy intake by participants when energy information is available or not available. Researchers measured bite count and energy intake among study participants who consumed a meal in a cafeteria. After the meal, study participants estimated their energy intake with or without a menu containing caloric information. Both age and gender predicted energy per bite, and the number of bites better estimated energy intake compared to participants' estimation of intake with or without the help of caloric information. Bite count may be a suitable objective measure of energy intake in a free-living population.[1]

References

1. Salley JN, Hoover AW, Wilson ML, Muth ER. Comparison between human and bite-based methods of estimating caloric intake. *J Acad Nutr Diet.* 2016; 116:1568–1577.

12 to 16 hours. The researcher downloads the images from the camera to analyze the recorded dietary intake.[16] One study found that reviewing SenseCam data increased estimates of energy intake by 12% to 23% when compared to food record alone, by revealing unreported and misreported food items. Difficulties with the SenseCam included poor quality images in poor lighting and users not wearing the device correctly.[26] When used correctly, this technology offers the opportunity to improve validity of dietary-intake assessment.

eButton

The **eButton** is a device worn on the chest like a pin. The eButton contains a miniature camera, an accelerometer, a GPS unit, and other sensors that passively capture images of food intake and other health behaviors. The eButton does not require additional self-reporting. Its camera automatically captures images of each eating event every two seconds. Using captured images, the software detects the shapes of plates, bowls, and utensils. It segments food items based on their texture, color, and complexities. The software estimates the volume of food based on the shape of a food-specific model. The food-specific model, which is a virtual wire-mesh frame of known volume sized to the food on the plates. A nutrient database analyzes dietary intake using the software-captured data.[27] Researchers compared the eButton data to manual visual rating of food images and physical measurement of 100 foods to determine the accuracy of its estimated food portions. The error was no more than 30% on 85 food items for the computer analysis. The computer estimates showed less bias and variability than the manual raters did. Irregularly shaped foods or poor-quality images were more likely to cause errors. Overall, the eButton estimates were more accurate for food volume than were visual-rater estimates.[28]

Crowdsourcing Image-Based Assessment Applications

At least two mobile phone applications, Meal Snap and Platemate, are available and promise to deliver estimated energy intake of a food item based on a single image using crowd sourcing. Crowd sourcing relies on a group of individuals, trained or untrained, who are willing to provide information about the food image. The user simply captures an image of the food item and sends it to a server location for analysis. Analysis is relatively rapid and occurs within a matter of minutes. However, validity and reliability are questionable because it is not known who is providing the information and where the information came from. Informal testing has shown inconsistency in the ability to provide accurate data through crowdsourcing using a single image.[1] At this time, it cannot be recommended for use in research or clinical applications.

Recap Adding images to food records and food recalls appears to increase estimates of energy intake and identify unreported or misreported foods. Images may also improve portion-size estimates and better identify types of foods consumed. However, images do not capture ingredients such as added fats and sugar that may increase energy content, so relying only on images as the only source of dietary-intake information will likely lead to inaccuracies in assessing true intake.[16]

Selecting a Computerized Diet-Analysis System for the Research Nutritionist

Preview Several factors should be considered when choosing a computerized diet-analysis application for nutrition research. First, the researcher must keep in mind the purpose and objectives of the nutrition research and the level of detail of dietary information needed to answer the study questions.[2] Other factors to consider include the cost of the analysis application, ease of use by the researchers or study participants, ability to import or export data for statistical analysis, the source of the nutrient data, reports that can be generated, and the number of food items and nutrients available in the database for analysis.[29]

Types of Research and Study Questions

Before selecting a diet-analysis application, consider the type of research that will be conducted and the study questions that will need answering. The application you choose must be able to capture the type of data needed to answer your research questions. Therefore, your first step is to define your research objectives and dietary variables of interest. A 24-hour recall will provide details about the total diet and nutrient intake, whereas an FFQ or screener may be limited to only a few components of the diet.

The Dietary Assessment Primer, developed by the National Cancer Institute (NCI), provides guidance on the type of dietary assessment methods deemed most appropriate for differing study designs and research objectives. Common research objectives for dietary assessment include determining usual dietary intake of a group, identifying associations between dietary intake and health outcomes, identifying associations between group characteristics (age, race, socioeconomics) and dietary intake, and determining the effect(s) of dietary interventions.[2,30] If your research objective were to describe the usual dietary intake of a group, compare usual dietary intake between groups, or determine the prevalence of individuals meeting a specified level of dietary intake, then an application capable of collecting multiple 24-hour recalls from each study participant would be optimal. A computerized FFQ might be useful but would provide less dietary detail and is not useful for determining the proportion of individuals meeting dietary intake criteria. The recommendation is to use multiple 24-hour recalls when evaluating health outcomes related to dietary intake in cross-sectional and prospective studies. Retrospective studies must rely on FFQs to look for relationships between diet and health outcomes. The NCI recommends using multiple 24-hour recalls for prospective and cross-sectional studies evaluating relationships between study-participant characteristics and their influences on dietary-intake variables.

A single 24-hour recall at each observation time point is useful for intervention studies that aim to examine change in intake over a period of time, look for a difference in the change of usual intake between groups, and compare post-intervention intake between groups. To determine change in the prevalence of individuals or differences in prevalence between groups meeting specific dietary criteria, multiple 24-hour recalls at each measurement time point are recommended.[30]

Required Levels of Dietary Detail

The degree of detail needed for diet analysis is a factor in determining the most appropriate dietary-analysis system. Whether you plan to use the analysis software for clinical nutrient assessment or metabolic diet research will help you determine the level of detail needed. Questions the clinician or researcher must answer before selecting a system include the following:

- Can the application assess dietary patterns?
- Does the application assess total diet nutrient intakes?
- Does the application assess intake by meal, day, and/or multiple days?
- Does the application assess standard nutrients or food components not typically assessed (i.e., oxalates, bioactive food components?

Applications that only include FFQ or screeners capture less detail. The USDA Automated Multiple-Pass Method

(AMPM) and the Automated Self-Administered 24-Hour Dietary Assessment Tool (ASA24) assess both total nutrient intake and dietary patterns. Less commonly assessed nutrients and food components such as oxalates will likely require an application designed specifically for food and nutrition research centers, such as the Nutrient Data System for Research (NDSR) application.

Accuracy and Quality of the Nutrient Database

Researchers and clinicians must consider how accurately the system captures dietary-intake information. Validity and reliability testing prior to use in a research study is ideal. The ability of users to search for food items consumed, correctly identify them, and correctly estimate portion sizes will influence reliability and validity of data. Nutrient-analysis systems are capable of automatically checking for implausible data entry and providing memory prompts to increase the likelihood of including all foods and beverages consumed. The quality of the database, and quantity of the food items and nutrients found in the database of the computerized system, is a key factor for accuracy in dietary analysis as well. Missing data and missing food items will detrimentally affect validity. For research purposes, food and nutrient databases need to be accurate, complete, up to date, include a large number of food and beverage items, incorporate brand names or restaurant items to help select correct food items, and have the ability to analyze a wide variety of nutrients of interest to the researcher. A system should be in place by the application developer to make regular updates to the food and nutrient database. In addition, the ability of the researcher, clinician, or user to add new foods and recipes to the database improves the ability to assess a participant's dietary intake accurately. The nutrition researcher should be able to determine the source of the food and nutrient database, the frequency of updates to the database, and the nutrients assessable before selecting an application.[29]

Research-quality databases commonly used by computerized dietary assessment applications include the USDA's Food and Nutrient Database for Dietary Studies (FNDDS), the Food Pattern Equivalent Database (FPED), and the NDSR from the Nutrition Coordinating Center of the University of Minnesota. The USDA FNDDS is the nutrient database used for determining nutrient intake of the nutrition-assessment portion of the National Health and Nutrition Examination Survey (NHANES). It is also the main database used for the SuperTracker, the NCI's Dietary History Questionnaire II (DHQ II), and the Automated Self-Administered 24-hour recall (ASA24). The FNDDS includes 8,536 main food descriptions and codes and an additional 12,128 food descriptions related to the main foods, along with 64 nutrients or food components (USDA Agricultural Research Service: https://www.ars.usda.gov).[31] The FPED uses the FNDDS as the source of nutrient values to convert foods and beverages into 37 different USDA food pattern components using portion equivalents to compare to the *Dietary Guidelines for Americans* 2015–2020. For example, the FPED database converts the reported dietary intake of fruits and vegetables into cup equivalents.[31] Lastly, the NDSR boasts more than 18,000 food items, 8,000 brand name items, 23 common restaurant menu items, and 165 nutrients and food components. It also has the capacity to assess food-group equivalents. The main source of nutrient values for the NDSR is the National Nutrient Database for Standard Reference, maintained by the USDA to provide nutrient-composition data. Additional nutrient data are obtained from other databases and published research.[32]

Technology Requirements

When selecting an application for dietary analysis, determine and consider required network capabilities, Internet connection speed, type of browser, and hardware and software requirements. Some applications may run on a network system instead of individual computer hard drives or vice versa. When installed on individual computers, hardware memory capabilities must be sufficient for storing data and running the application. Operating systems (Microsoft Windows, MAC-OSX, Linux), personal computer (PC) or Macintosh, for example, also must be capable of running the application. Internet connection speed is important for Internet-based applications and the ability to quickly enter, analyze, download, and generate reports based on dietary intake. Note the type of web browser best suited for using Internet-based applications. Ideally, these applications are usable with multiple current versions of web browsers. Whether the Internet-based application can be accessed using mobile phone or tablet devices may also be of interest, because this offers greater flexibility for users. Applications such as the ASA24 is an example of a web-based system that eliminates the need for the researcher to meet specific hardware and software requirements, but requires the researcher and the research participant to access the application from an Internet connection using a web browser anytime, anywhere.

Cost

Cost is another consideration in choosing a dietary assessment application. Consideration should be given to the cost of equipment needed (i.e., computers, handheld devices, and sensors) and staff and administration costs for data collection and analysis.[15] Handheld devices such as the SenseCam and mobile camera phones cost hundreds of dollars and therefore may be prohibitive for large studies. Image-based food records that do not include automated methods for identifying and analyzing food items will require significant labor costs for expert analysis. Furthermore, most computerized or Internet-based applications require an initial licensing fee that may vary, depending on the number of application users, and they may require an annual renewal fee. The licensing fee may or may not include regular updates to the database or software, and this should be clear before purchasing. In addition, there may be a fee associated with technical support of the system and data storage on a network server or cloud-based system. The amount of data needing storage often determines the fees. Regular updates, technical support, and sufficient data storage are benefits often worth purchasing. Some systems may require payment for analysis of the results, which can be costly. Diet-analysis applications developed with federal grant funds may be free to use but likely come with less support. These include the NCI's DHQ II and the ASA24.

Data-Management Efficiency

A primary reason for the development of computerized diet-analysis systems is to make collecting and analyzing dietary-intake data more efficient and therefore reduce the burden on researchers, clinicians, and respondents. Applications that allow for self-administration of 24-hour recalls or FFQs and direct entry of food records improve time efficiency by eliminating the need for data entry by the researcher or clinician from traditional paper-based records. This greatly reduces administration time and effort by the researcher and clinician. In addition, systems that use built-in algorithms that allow for skipping unnecessary questions based on previous answers reduces the burden on respondents.[15] This shortens the number of questions that the participant is required to answer and therefore may lead to better-quality data by reducing the fatigue associated with long questionnaires. Internet-based applications that allow data entry anytime, anywhere without requiring the participant to travel to a research center reduces respondent burden as well.

Another important factor regarding data-management efficiency includes coding, transferability, and storage. The efficiency of coding data by automated systems reduces time and effort by the researcher or clinician. The exportability or importability of data to statistical-analysis applications without additional data handling also improves efficiency. Finally, how and where the data will be stored are important considerations. Data should be easily stored on a secure system to prevent loss of confidentiality and easily backed up to prevent loss of data. Internet-based applications typically use a server or cloud-based system to store and retrieve data. This system will generally have in place a method for regularly backing up data.

Applicability

The researcher or clinician must consider the population for which they intend to collect dietary-intake, and whether or not it is necessary to collect multiple measures of dietary intake. The target population must have the ability to access the technology-based system. Although mobile phones and Internet access are widely available, some target populations such as low-income groups or older adults may not have access to or be comfortable using the technology. The population size also matters. Some systems may limit the number of users or number of data-set entries. In the case of 24-hour recalls in which multiple recalls are beneficial to better estimate usual intake, the computerized system must be capable of handling multiple entries by the same users.

Usability

In choosing a technology-based dietary assessment method, usability is a factor for researchers, clinicians, and participants. Cognitive effort, time for completion, necessity of training, level of literacy required, and computer skills are all usability items identified by Illner et al. as important to assess.[15] Usability among differing age groups is another consideration because not all age groups will be appropriate for some forms of technology or dietary assessment methods. Different age groups may be more accepting of certain technologies and more comfortable using technology and therefore require less training. One could expect that the lesser the learning curve on using technology in dietary assessment, the better the outcomes. As previously discussed, the user's ability to correctly follow instructions and capture images using a mobile-phone food-recording system influenced the quality and quantity of dietary data collected. How easily the system can be incorporated into a user's lifestyle may also make a difference. Self-administered systems must be easy for the participant to access, navigate, search for food items, and correctly enter information. The researcher should look for applications that are intuitive to users and include help features such as multiple food images in varying portion sizes, avatars, or help wizards. Applications should also allow the user to choose from multiple measurement options (cups, ounces, tablespoons, grams) for ease of portion-size determination and multiple food-preparation methods for food selection, thereby improving quality of data entered. The majority of dietary-analysis applications available on the market allow researchers and clinicians to access a demonstration version of the application to evaluate ease of use prior to purchasing and implementation.

Reports and Data Analysis

Another factor to consider in selecting a dietary-analysis system is data reporting and analysis. Consider the types of reports you want to generate, such as daily menus for production of metabolic meals, summary of nutrients over multiple days, single-meal or single-day nutrient intake reports, or summary reports of group mean intakes of dietary data. The quality of the report format and layout on the screen or in print is important for easier interpretation of results. The ability to save the reports as a common file type, such as a portable document format (PDF), assists in the ability to share data with other researchers, clinicians, and participants. Other questions to consider include are: What types of analysis will the application provide? Can the raw data be easily exported and imported for statistical analysis by statistical software applications?

Data Security and HIPAA Compliance

Dietary-analysis systems may allow for the entry and collection of data that includes personal health information and therefore is protected information through the Health Information Portability and Accountability Act (HIPAA). The researcher must consider if the dietary assessment system meets HIPAA compliance standards. Institutional research boards and clinical facilities will most likely require that any computerized systems used to collect participant information and dietary data comply with HIPAA. Any dietary data-collection system should have a means of ensuring data are stored in a secure location to prevent data breaches and maintain confidentiality. Individual researcher, clinician, and user passwords are means to protecting access to the data.

TABLE 2 provides a summary of factors to consider in choosing a technology for dietary-intake assessment.

Recap In summary, many factors must be considered when selecting a computerized dietary assessment application. Start with identifying your research objectives and variables; this will help determine the most appropriate dietary assessment method to choose, thereby narrowing the choice of assessment applications. Quality of the food and nutrient database and the number of foods and nutrients included for analysis are also important factors for accuracy of assessment. Cost, ease of use, technology requirements, and ability to analyze data are other considerations for the nutrition researcher. Finally, data security is of utmost importance to protect confidentiality.

▸ Computer-Based Diet-Assessment Applications

Preview A computer-based diet-assessment application requires specific hardware and software components for use. They were initially introduced in the last few decades of the 20th century with the advent of the personal computer. Illner et al. contends that their use does not necessarily change the methodology of data collection but enhances it by increasing the potential of increased cost-effectiveness of dietary assessment. It also reduces the time and effort needed for data collection and analysis. For these reasons, it may be a more acceptable means of collecting dietary data. Dietary intake can be collected by a trained interviewer who enters the participant's response directly into the computer application. Otherwise, the dietary interview can be self-administered using standardized, structured prompts and a question sequence in which the participant directly inputs responses.

Automated Multiple-Pass Method

The USDA developed the Automated Multiple-Pass Method (AMPM) based on the science-based methodology of the 24-hour recall commonly used in surveys to evaluate dietary intake in the American population. The AMPM is used for collecting data during the NHANES dietary interview portion.[33] It is

TABLE 2 Summary of factors to consider when choosing a technology-based dietary assessment instrument

Selecting a Technology-Based Dietary Assessment Instrument	
Type of Research and Research Question	Define the type of research and research variables Research objective(s) and question(s) Determine the level of dietary detail required
Level of Detail Required	Analyze for dietary patterns or individual foods Analysis by meal, day, or multiple days Type and number of nutrients or food components available for analysis
Technology Requirements	Network-based or computer-workstation–based Internet-based, web-browser requirements Internet connection speed Hardware and software requirements Handheld or tablet capabilities
Accuracy and Quality of the Database	Individual or group validity and reproducibility Food identification Automatic check for implausible data Incorporation of memory prompts Number of foods and beverages included Portion-size estimation Completeness of the database
Costs	Equipment and licensing Database or software updates Staff and administration cost Data analysis or storage fees Technical support
Data-Management Efficiency	Data-collection duration and entry Transfer of data Data coding Data storage, retrieval, and backup
Applicability	Population size Target specific groups Repeated measures
Usability	Required training Cognitive effort Time to complete Literacy Computer skills
Reports and Analysis	Ease of generating reports Types of reports and analysis Variety of file formats for reporting Format of report
Data Security and HIPAA Compliance	Secure data storage and access Meets HIPAA requirements for electronic data

Data from Thompson FE, Kirkpatrick SI, Subar AF, et al. The National Cancer Institute's Dietary Assessment Primer: A resource for diet research. *J Acad Nutr Diet.* 2015;115:1986–1995. Illner AK, Freisling H, Boeing H, Huybrechts I, Crispim SP, Slimani N. Review and evaluation of innovative technologies for measuring diet in nutritional epidemiology. *Int J Epidemiol.* 2012;41:1187–1203. Vozenilek, G. Choosing the best nutrient analysis software for your needs. *J Amer Diet Assoc.* 1999;99(11):1356–1358.

designed to be interviewer administered in person or by telephone and is respondent driven. Participants are asked to list foods they consumed in a recent past 24-hour period. The interviewer probes for eating events and commonly forgotten foods or additions to foods and then reviews the list of foods. The companion Food Model Booklet is used to help estimate portion sizes during the recall. The AMPM is programmed to adjust questioning based on participant responses. Foods can be added, edited, or deleted at any time during the interview, and automated data checks look for potential errors in data entry. The AMPM links with two other systems that allow for coding and editing of food items, reformatting, review, and nutrient analysis. The Food and Nutrient Database for Dietary Studies serves as the source of nutrient values of foods and beverages.[33,34]

To assess validity, Blanton et al. compared the AMPM to the Block FFQ and the NCI's DHQ using the DLW technique for measuring total energy expenditure and a 14-day food record for nutrient intake.[35] Energy intake assessed by the AMPM and food record was not significantly different from DLW results. The FFQ and DHQ were found to underestimate energy intake. The AMPM most closely estimated absolute nutrient intakes by the food record, whereas the questionnaires significantly underestimated nutrient intake.[35] These results support the validity of the use of the AMPM in dietary assessment.

In another study, the AMPM was evaluated for its accuracy in assessing reported energy intake by comparison to energy expenditure determined by the DLW technique. Study participants were given the DLW technique at the start of the two-week study. Participants completed three 24-hour recalls, one in person and two by telephone. Compared to total energy expenditure as determined by the DLW, energy intake was underreported by 11%. Normal-weight participants were less likely to underreport energy intake compared to those who were overweight. Obese participants were more likely to report low energy intakes. Acceptable energy intake was reported by 78% of men and 74% of women.[36] These results conclude that the AMPM is an acceptable method of evaluating energy intake and that the validity of reporting of energy intake is influenced by body weight and gender. Future studies using biometric measures alongside the AMPM dietary assessment are necessary to validate its use in nutrition research.

Nutrition Data System for Research

The NDSR, from the Nutrition Coordinating Center (NCC) at the University of Minnesota, is a software application designed for collecting and analyzing dietary-intake information for research purposes. This Microsoft Windows-based software application allows the entry of food records, 24-hour recalls using a guided multipass method, recipes, and development of menus for immediate analysis. Reports of nutrients can be generated for individual ingredients, foods, meals, and days. More than 18,000 foods and brand name items are included in the NCC Food and Nutrient Database, which is updated annually. The USDA's National Nutrient Database serves as a primary source of data for the database. As the researcher enters food items into the software, the database searches for and automatically codes foods for analysis and converts the quantities into grams. The conversion is typically needed for metabolic diet development and production. Data are available for 165 nutrients, food components, and nutrient ratios. An additional module is available for purchase to assess dietary supplement intake.[32] A free demo of the software is available on request from the NCC website (http://www.ncc.umn.edu/). **FIGURE 7** shows an example of the report that can be generated through this system.

ProNutra

ProNutra is another research-quality software application aimed at meal planning for metabolic feeding studies and analyzing dietary intake in research centers. As food items are entered to create a metabolic diet, nutrient data are immediately calculated and can be seen alongside preset nutrient parameters required for the study's diet protocol. This allows for quick comparisons of nutrients and adjustments in food items and portion sizes. Reports can be generated for meal production, menus, labels, and analysis of dietary intake. Furthermore, data can be exported to statistical software for further analysis. The source of nutrient data is the USDA's Nutrient Database for Standard Reference and the Food and Nutrient Database for Dietary Studies[37]. **FIGURE 8** shows a sample report for the ProNutra database.

The Food Processor

The Food Processor nutrition analysis software, from Esha Research, has a large database of 72,000 foods that includes the USDA's Nutrient Database for Standard Reference. It can analyze for 163 nutritional components and includes an exercise database with more than 900 individual activities, according to information provided on the company's website. It is designed primarily for use in a healthcare setting. Clinicians can manage

NDSR 2015 Nutrient Totals Report

Project Abbreviation: 961DS027
Participant ID: 961DS027 | Date of Intake: 03/13/2016

Primary Energy Sources	
Energy (kilocalories)	1129 kcal
Total Fat	31.953 g
Total Carbohydrate	193.581 g
Total Protein	24.709 g
Animal Protein	12.695 g
% Calories from Fat	25.056 %
% Calories from Carbohydrate	66.706 %
% Calories from Protein	8.470 %
Fat and Cholesterol	
Cholesterol	80 mg
Solid Fats	26.356 g
Total Saturated Fatty Acids (SFA)	16.104 g
Total Monounsaturated Fatty Acids (MUFA)	10.288 g
Total Polyunsaturated Fatty Acids (PUFA)	3.027 g
Total Trans-Fatty Acids (TRANS)	1.572 g
Total Conjugated Linoleic Acid (CLA 18:2)	0.113 g
Omega-3 Fatty Acids	0.501 g
% Calories from SFA	12.676 %
% Calories from MUFA	8.047 %
% Calories from PUFA	2.359 %
Polyunsaturated to Saturated Fat Ratio	0.188
Cholesterol to Saturated Fatty Acid Index	20.261

FIGURE 7 Nutrient data system for research nutrient totals report

unlimited individual client data; analyze intake; analyze and print labels for recipes; and generate reports for clients, diets, and menus. The clinician is able to compare recommended nutrient intake to client intake, customize and track nutrient intake and weight goals, and monitor physical activity. It also has the ability to add the capacity for clients to enter food and activity data via the Internet.[38]

Nutritionist Pro

The Nutritionist Pro software is also designed for healthcare settings and can be used in research settings. It is a PC-compatible application that can be used on a standalone computer or network system. The database includes more than 80,000 foods from the United States and other countries, fast-food items, ethnic foods, and medical foods. Foods and recipes can be added to the database. Similar to other applications, an unlimited number of clients can be managed and monitored for nutrient intake, weight goals, and physical activity. Reports can be generated for nutrient-intake summaries, deficiencies, MyPlate analyses, weight-tracking graphs, nutrient-intake graphs, diet plans, menus, food and shopping lists,

Low Phosphorus 1800

Modified: November 10, 2015; Last Used: May 05, 2014
Description: 700 mg Pho, 1000 mg Ca, 2 gm Na, 3000 mg K

Food Item	Food Code	Database	Amount	Measure	Weight (g)	Energy (kcal)	Protein (g)	Total lipid (fat) (g)
- Breakfast								
Bread, white, commercial	18069	Custom Da	50.00	gram	50.00	133.50	4.10	1.80
Margarine-like spread, tub	81103080	FNDDS Ve	5.00	gram	5.00	26.55	0.03	3.00
Egg, whole, raw, fresh	01123	Custom Da	40.00	gram	40.00	59.60	5.00	4.01
Salt, table	02047	USDA Cust	0.30	gram	0.30	0.00	0.00	0.00
Orange juice, with calcium	61210250	FNDDS Ve	240.00	gram	240.00	108.00	1.63	0.14
Applesauce, canned	09019	Custom Da	100.00	gram	100.00	43.00	0.17	0.05
- Lunch								
Spaghetti, dry, enriched	20120	Custom Da	50.00	gram	50.00	185.50	6.39	0.79
Spaghetti sauce, meatless	74404050	FNDDS Ve	100.00	gram	100.00	109.00	1.80	4.80
Beef, ground, 80% lean meat	23572	USDA Stan	60.00	gram	60.00	152.40	10.30	12.0
Beans, snap, green, frozen	11060	Custom Da	75.00	gram	75.00	24.75	1.35	0.16
Bread, white, commercial	18069	Custom Da	25.00	gram	25.00	66.75	2.05	0.90
Pineapple, raw	09266	Custom Da	50.00	gram	50.00	24.50	0.20	0.22
Margarine-like spread, tub	81103080	FNDDS Ve	10.00	gram	10.00	53.10	0.06	6.00
Salt, table	02047	USDA Cust	0.40	gram	0.40	0.00	0.00	0.00
- PM Snack								
Cookies, chocolate chip	18164	Custom Da	1.00	1 medium	12.00	59.04	0.59	2.71
- Dinner								
Pork, fresh, loin, top loin	10063	Custom Da	85.00	gram	85.00	198.05	23.65	10.78
Spices, MRS. DASH Original		USDA Cust	1.00	gram	1.00	0.00	0.00	0.00
Rice, white, long-grain, regular	20044	Custom Da	50.00	gram	50.00	182.50	3.56	0.33
Carrots, frozen, unprepared	11130	Custom Da	50.00	gram	50.00	19.50	0.55	0.11
Bread, white, commercial	18069	Custom Da	25.00	gram	25.00	66.75	2.05	0.90
Margarine, regular, liquid, soy	04105	Custom Da	10.00	gram	10.00	72.10	0.19	8.06
Pears, canned, juice pack	09254	Custom Da	90.00	gram	90.00	45.00	0.31	0.06
Salt, table	02047	USDA Cust	0.45	gram	0.45	0.00	0.00	0.00
- HS Snack								
Crackers, saltine	54325000	FNDDS Ve	8.00	1 cracker	24.00	104.16	2.21	2.83
Cheese, cheddar	01009	Custom Da	14.00	gram	14.00	56.36	3.49	4.64

	Energy (kcal)	Protein (g)	Total lipid (fat) (g)	Carbohydrate, by difference (g)	Water (g)	Cacium, Ca (mg)
Diet Target	1800.00	67.50	60.00	247.50	3000.00	700.00
Diet Actual	1790.11	69.66	64.28	233.88	786.17	702.69

FIGURE 8 ProNutra metabolic diet development and analysis tool

Reproduced from ProNutra. Viocare. www.viocare.com/pronutra.html. [Accessed September 18, 2016].

and recipe analyses; these can be exported in a variety of formats similar to those offered by other applications. Clinicians can view nutrients of food items as they are added to dietary-intake analysis, recipes, and menus. The client group feature allows tracking of nutrient data among participants in a research study group, and the data-extraction tool quickly pulls data for statistical analysis.[39]

HIGHLIGHT

Steps of the Automated Multiple-Pass Method

1. Quick list: List all foods and beverages consumed the previous day.
2. Forgotten foods: Probe for forgotten foods.
3. Time and occasion: Obtain time and eating occasion for each food.
4. Detail cycle: Obtain detailed description and amount for each food and any additions. Review reported items.
5. Final probe: Inquire about any missed items.

Information Collected by the AMPM

- For each food record:
  - Description of food item
  - Additions to food items (e.g., milk or cream added to coffee)
  - Combination code for foods commonly eaten together (e.g., bread with butter)
  - Quantity of food consumed (e.g., 1 cup, 2 tablespoons, 1 ounce)
  - Time of day eaten
  - Name of eating occasion (breakfast, lunch, dinner, snack)
  - Where food was obtained (grocery store, sit-down restaurant, fast-food restaurant)
  - Was the food eaten at home or away from home?
- Amount of water (bottled or tap) consumed
- Use of salt in food preparation or at the table
- The amount of food consumed on the recall day was usual, more than usual, or less than usual
- Following a diet for weight loss or special diet for health reasons

Modified from U.S. Department of Agriculture.https://www.ars.usda.gov/northeast-area/beltsville-md/beltsville-human-nutrition-research-center/food-surveys-research-group/docs/ampm-usda-automated-multiple-pass-method/.

Recap Computer-based diet-assessment applications described in this chapter are some of the most frequently used in research and clinical settings. These applications are designed for use by nutrition researchers and nutrition professionals. They are not intended for general-public use. The applications mentioned offer similar features but may vary in the number of foods included in the database, number of nutrients available for analysis, ease of use, and cost. The validity and reliability of the dietary-intake data is only as good the data entered and the underlying food composition database.

Internet-Based Diet-Analysis Applications

Preview An Internet-based diet-analysis application does many of the same functions as computer-based applications. The main differences are in how the application is accessed and how data are stored and retrieved. For the nutrition researcher, the Internet offers the opportunity to reach a greater number of individuals and to reach groups of individuals previously considered unreachable because of geographical constraints. For the clinician, the Internet makes it possible to collect dietary data for analysis and rapid feedback to improve clinical outcomes.

Automated Self-Administered 24-Hour Dietary Recall (ASA24)

The Automated Self-Administered 24-hour dietary recall system (ASA24), developed by the National Cancer Institute of the National Institutes of Health, is designed for research studies assessing dietary intake among adults and large-population studies. It is available for free to researchers, teachers, and clinicians without cost.[40] The latest version, ASA24-2016, allows researchers or clinicians to collect both single-day and multiple-day food records. It is currently available in both English and Spanish and in a Canadian version, and it is under development for use in other countries. Researchers or clinicians access the researcher website to set the options available for data collection, manage user accounts, obtain reports to monitor progress of participants, and access analysis files. Analysis for American versions is based on the FNDDS. Users are provided with a website link and login information to access the respondent site for data entry. Guidance through the application is provided through written or audio prompts using the multipass methodology for 24-hour recall. Users enter the eating occasion and the time this meal or snack was eaten; then they search for food and beverage items consumed, including supplements, type of food, and preparation method.[40] Real food images in multiple portion sizes are used to help users accurately estimate the portions consumed. Real food images also act as prompts triggering any missing items or modifying food and drink items. Data on where meals were consumed, sources of foods, whether eaten alone or with company, and if computer or television use occurred during meals can be collected if desired. Multiple recalls or food records can be collected from individual users. The maximum number of recalls is set by the researcher. Lastly, the ASA24 system can be used with computer-screen readers for individuals with disabilities and is accessible with most common web browsers. The ASA24-2016 version is also accessible on mobile devices.[40]

The ASA24 has good potential for use in research or clinical settings for collecting dietary data. When compared to observed intake and plate-waste measurements, the ASA24 performed almost equivalently to dietary recall by AMPM.[41] In addition, Thompson et al. compared the performance of the ASA24 to that of the AMPM with adults across three health systems.[42] There were four groups with each participant completing two recalls: (1) ASA24 and AMPM, (2) AMPM and ASA24, (3) ASA24 and ASA24, and (4) AMPM and AMPM. Study participants preferred the ASA24, and lower attrition was observed among participants who experienced the ASA24 before the AMPM or experienced the ASA24 on both recalls. In addition, energy and nutrient intakes were similar.[42] The greater acceptability, greater retention, and reduced time and cost benefits of using a self-administered system may outweigh the minor differences found between self-administered and interviewer-administered recalls. Note that in a study (in press at the time of writing this chapter) involving this author, adult participants with limited literacy and computer skills had some difficulties using the ASA24 without assistance. Further research is needed to assess the feasibility of use and validity among adult users with limited literacy and computer skills. **FIGURE 9** shows an example of the "Add Details" tab indicating portion size for a food item in a 24-hour recall using the ASA24 free demonstration site.

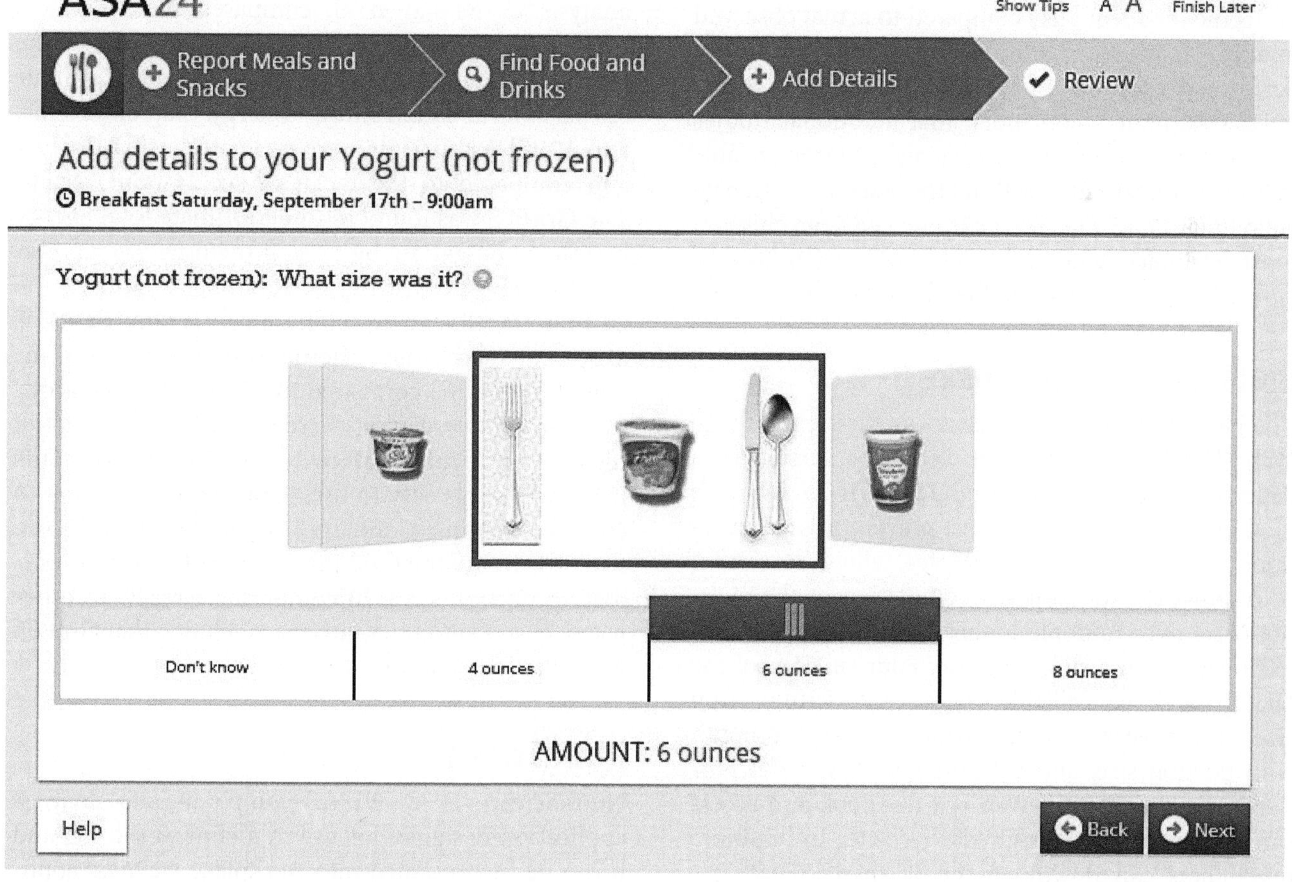

FIGURE 9 ASA24 "Add Details" tab for portion size

Reproduced from Automated Self-Administered 24-Hour Dietary Assessment Tool. National Institutes of Health, National Cancer Institute. epi.grants.cancer.gov/asa24/. [Accessed September 18, 2016]

Automated Self-Administered 24-Hour Dietary Recall: ASA24Kids

The ASA24Kids was developed based on the same methodology and features of the ASA24 for use with children 10 years of age and older and is free for use by researchers. Modification for use with children included simplifying wording, removing food and drink items not reported by children in national food and nutrition surveys, removing alcoholic drinks, and removing probing questions that children might not understand or know how to answer. "School" was added as an option for eating location. Obtaining valid and accurate dietary data from children is difficult. In a crossover study, overall matches for reported food intake between the ASA24Kids and an interviewer-led 24-hour recall among children 8 to 13 years old were less than 50%. Younger children had significantly lower matches and were more likely to omit foods and need help with the ASA24Kids.[43] Diep et al. conducted a validation study of the ASA24Kids 2012 version with children ages 9 to 11 years, comparing the web-based self-administered recall to 24-hour recalls conducted by trained interviewers and direct observation of meals consumed.[44] Both modes of obtaining dietary recalls performed inadequately compared to actual observed intakes. Interviewer-administered 24-hour recalls performed only slightly better than the ASA24Kids 2012. Researchers concluded that additional studies are needed to determine at what age children are able to provide dietary data without the assistance of a parent or guardian.[44] Dietary data collected from children must be interpreted cautiously, and automated systems may need to be simplified for children.

Diet History Questionnaire II–Web

The NCI's web-based Diet History Questionnaire II–Web (DHQII) is simply an electronic version of a paper-based FFQ. However, the DHQII–Web is able to skip unnecessary questions, prevent missed questions and inconsistent responses, allow correction of responses, and allow for completion of the questionnaire over multiple logins as opposed to having to finish within a single session. Four versions of the DHQII–Web are available: (1) past year with portion size, (2) past year without portion size, (3) past month with portion size, and (4) past month without portion size. The DHQII–Web is a free tool, and access can be requested through the website. In addition, researchers can download the PC-based Diet*Calc companion software designed specifically to analyze the DHQII–Web data. The software will provide estimates of nutrient intake and food groups. To date, the DHQII–Web has not been validated separately from the paper-based version. However, usability studies have been conducted and have demonstrated the ease of use. Results indicate that the web version is less time-consuming than the paper version.[45] **FIGURE 10** shows an example of questions relating to the frequency of consumption and portion size consumed of a food item from the DHQII free demonstration site.

VioScreen

VioScreen is a HIPAA-compliant, web-based, self-administered, graphical FFQ designed for research purposes. VioScreen uses branching logic to avoid unnecessary questions based on user responses, thereby reducing respondent burden, and checks for errors or implausible responses in real time to prevent inaccurate data entry. Users receive memory prompts and are able to choose from food images of differing portion sizes to help them report more accurately. In addition, the FFQ can be completed in English or Spanish. Reports of dietary behavior, estimated nutrient intakes, and food patterns are available instantly. Data can be exported for use in other statistical software applications for further analysis.[46,47] Kristal et al. compared the Graphical Food-Frequency System (GraFFS) to dietary-intake data collected by telephone-administered 24-hour recalls in a validation study.[47] Energy, macronutrients, and 17 micronutrients were estimated using GraFFS and compared to the mean of six 24-hour recalls. The GraFFS was found to underestimate total energy by 9%, carbohydrate by 12%, protein by 5%, and fat by 15%. However, it provided similar results to the 24-hour recalls when comparing macronutrients as a percent of calories. Micronutrients were overestimated in GraFFS compared to 24-hour recalls. Moderate to high correlations were found for the test-retest reliability of GraFFS. Moreover, 100% of participants felt GraFFS was easy to use, 98% would be willing to complete the questionnaire if requested by a doctor, and 80% found the food images to be helpful for estimating portion sizes. In comparing GraFFS to other paper-based FFQs, the authors concluded that GraFFS was equally as good.[47]

NutraScreen

NutraScreen is a HIPAA-compliant diet-analysis application designed for use in a clinical setting, and it can be incorporated into workplace wellness applications and platforms. It is a web-based application that allows users to enter dietary information using any computer or tablet with an Internet connection.

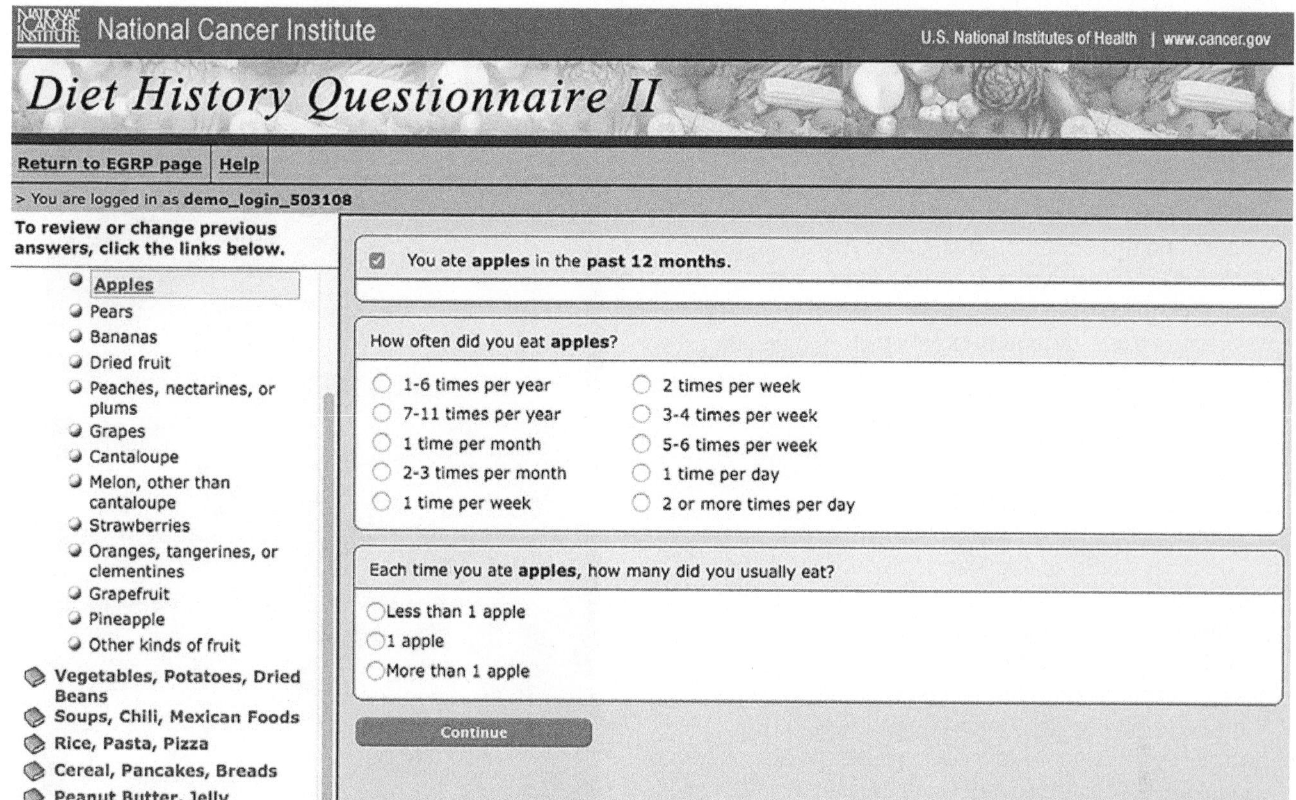

FIGURE 10 DHQII–web questionnaire sample frequency and portion-size questions

Reproduced from Diet History Questionnaire II and Canadian Diet History Questionnaire II: Web-based. National Institutes of Health, National Cancer Institute. epi.grants.cancer.gov/dhq2/. [Accessed October 29. 2016]

Data entry is enhanced by real food photos to assist with portion-size estimates and to allow for quick entry. Results are available immediately for viewing by healthcare providers and users. User data are compared to dietary recommendations, and reports indicate areas needing improvement. A Healthy Eating Index score is also calculated.[48]

NutritionQuest's Data-on-Demand

Data-on-Demand is a web-based nutrition and physical activity assessment and analysis system developed by NutritionQuest, the source of the well-known and validated Block FFQs. Nutrition researchers may choose any of the Block FFQs or food- or nutrient-specific (e.g., fat, sugar, fruit, vegetable, calcium, sodium) screening questionnaires to deliver on the Data-on-Demand system. Data-on-Demand allows for direct online entry of dietary-intake information for interviewer- or self-administered questionnaires. For the latter, the participant is provided a website address and a login to complete the questionnaire. Researchers may also choose to upload offline data and scanned paper questionnaire data into the system. Data are automatically analyzed when questionnaires are completed, allowing the researcher to see trends in the data before the study is complete. The data are stored online and backed up daily. The researcher accesses results and manages data through a private, password-protected account. Reports can be printed and data downloaded at any time in batches; for individual subjects, the researcher can track which subjects have completed questionnaires. Automatic transfer of data to a study server is also possible. Like others, the FFQ application uses algorithms to adjust questions based on user responses and skips unnecessary questions, thus reducing time for completion. The Block FFQs, screeners, and physical activity assessment tools have been validated in a variety of studies and groups, as well as used in many research studies assessing dietary intake. A list of validation studies of FFQs and screeners for use with both adults and children is available on the NutritionQuest website.[49]

Nutribase Cloud Edition

The Nutribase Cloud Edition, by CyberSoft, Inc., is a robust nutrient-analysis application designed for the individual nutrition professional and could be incorporated into methods for collecting dietary intake for research studies. It includes nutrient data on more than 500,000 food items and research-quality databases from

VIEWPOINT

Apps

Randi S. Drasin, MS, RDN

What's trending in nutrition and fitness? Why, it's "apps," of course! Having an app to track your fitness and nutrition is the newest hot topic and one of the simplest ways to store, analyze, and track your daily routine. So, what is an app?

An app is defined as a self-contained program or piece of software designed to fulfill a particular purpose—an application, especially as downloaded by a user to a mobile device. **FIGURE A** shows the Calorie Counter and Diet Tracker app.

In other words, an app is an application! It can be used on any electronic device, but in today's world we see them being used mostly on smartphones or as wearable units. And these days it seems as if everyone has a smartphone or smart device. Whether it's in your hand, on your wrist (as a watch or a bracelet), in your pocket, in your purse, in your car, in your backpack, on your nightstand, or on your desk, it's usually never far from reach.

And these devices all have the ability to download one or more apps to track your every move, whether it's your steps, your calories burned, the number of floors climbed, your nutrient intake, your health record, your weight, your favorite healthy restaurant down the road, recipes to make the foods you like to eat, or tracking your heart rate, sleep patterns, or blood sugar. There is an app for almost anything you need or want to track.

So where do you start? That is a great question. As nutrition professionals, we want to make sure we are providing our clients with applications that are not only useful to that particular client, but also one that meets them at their literacy level as well as his or her stage of change. We wouldn't want to recommend an app to a client who is not comfortable with advanced technology, nor would we want to provide a client with an app that demands more than they are willing to engage in. **FIGURE B** shows the EaTracker app.

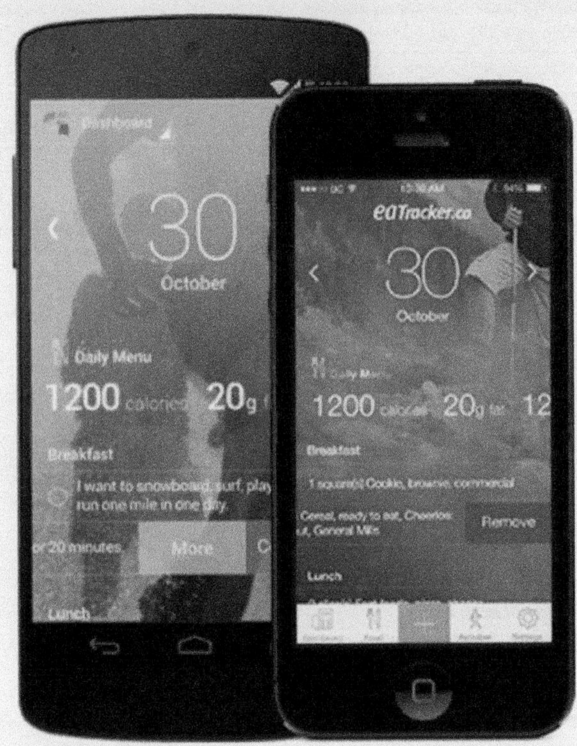

FIGURE B EaTracker App

Reproduced with permission from eaTracker.

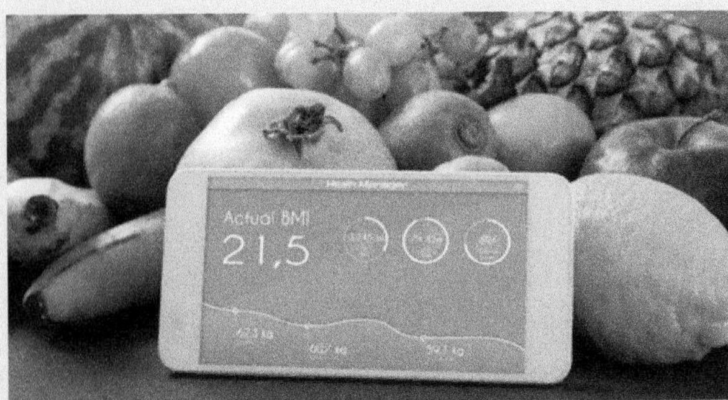

FIGURE A Calorie Counter and Diet Tracker app

So, what are our best resources? Well, best practice would be to try out several apps yourself to see what you like, what works, and what doesn't. Ask yourself questions: Would my client be able to use this? Is it easy to handle? Confusing? Too detailed? Not detailed enough? Does it have the tracking program that would benefit the client? What is my client trying to accomplish?

Bottom line, is it user-friendly? And what benefit would it be to you as the clinician? Are you actually analyzing the data your clients are tracking? Or is it mainly to encourage self-awareness? Either way, research, research, research and make sure you know the outcome you want to achieve.

Check out the app reviews by three RDNs at the Academy of Nutrition and Dietetics. **TABLE A** shows a few of the top-rated apps with four- and five-star ratings!

Resource List

The Academy of Nutrition and Dietetics: www.eatrightpro.org

The Academy of Nutrition and Dietetics Food and Nutrition Magazine: www.FoodandNutrition.org

TABLE A Free Apps available for mobile technology as reviewed by the Academy's spokespeople

App Name	Rating	Description
EaTipster	5 stars	Tips to increase healthy eating, fight chronic diseases, and support a healthy weight. Addresses common food and nutrition questions.
GluCoMo	4 stars	An electronic diary to track blood sugar levels, insulin intake, and carbohydrate intake.
Calorie Counter & Diet Tracker by MyFitness Pal	4.5 stars	Tracks weight loss and fitness goals with calorie intake and exercise output. Database of more than 350 exercises with calories burned.
Gluten Free Daily	4.5 stars	Provides resources for following a gluten-free diet.
Calorie Counter: Diets & Activities	4 stars	Tracks calories, water, and fitness along with carbohydrates, protein, fat, cholesterol, saturated fat, and fiber. Offers the ability to create user's own diet and physical-activity plan.
Calorie Tracker by Livestrong.com	4 stars	Food and fitness diary. Tracks calories, fat, cholesterol, sodium, carbohydrates, sugars, fiber, and protein. Is a companion tool for members of The Daily Plate.

Created by Randi Drasin, from info obtained by the Academy's spokespeople: Marisa Moore, MBA, RD, LD; Jessica Crandall, RD, CDE; Sarah Krieger, MPH, RD, LDN.

both the United States and Canada. It works with multiple smartphone apps for connecting with clients and allows direct entry of dietary intake and physical activity by the client. The cloud-based system makes it easy to synchronize data from any computer. Features of the application include publication-quality food labels, the ability to search food names or brand names, add food items, drag and drop columns of nutrient data and order them according to preference, sort foods from high to low and vice versa based on specific nutrients, send messages to clients, monitor clients' activity at any time, and much more. Data can be backed up and restored on different computers, and backed up to external media such as a flash drive. An extensive list of features and a comparison to other commonly used nutrient-analysis applications is available on the company website at www.nutribase.com.[50] Nutribase may be the most comprehensive application available to date. Previous versions of Nutribase have been used in research studies to analyze self-reported dietary intake. No studies are available assessing its validity and accuracy compared to other methods.

SuperTracker

Developed by the USDA, the SuperTracker was designed as a consumer-based application for diet tracking and analysis; it also includes a meal-planning tool. The SuperTracker allows for allows for personal goal setting and physical activity and weight tracking encouraging health behavior change through self-monitoring and self-regulation. One of the features of the SuperTracker is the ability for health professionals or nutrition researchers to create private groups with as many as 150 members. Each group member must create a login and is invited to the group by the leader through email or provided an access code for joining the group. The group leader can generate reports of average group intake or individual group members that include age, gender, height, weight and weight history, food intake, physical activity, personal goals, and account activity such as login frequency. Reports can be exported as Excel, Word, or PDF files. Leaders can also send messages and develop healthy eating challenges.[51] This feature allows a new opportunity for nutrition researchers or clinicians to collect and analyze dietary and physical-activity data over time. Incorporating healthy eating challenges or sending messages to the group may serve as an intervention for food and activity behavior changes. The tool could be used with individual or group-based lifestyle interventions and incorporated into analysis to determine the effectiveness of applications for lifestyle changes. Research on feasibility and validity of

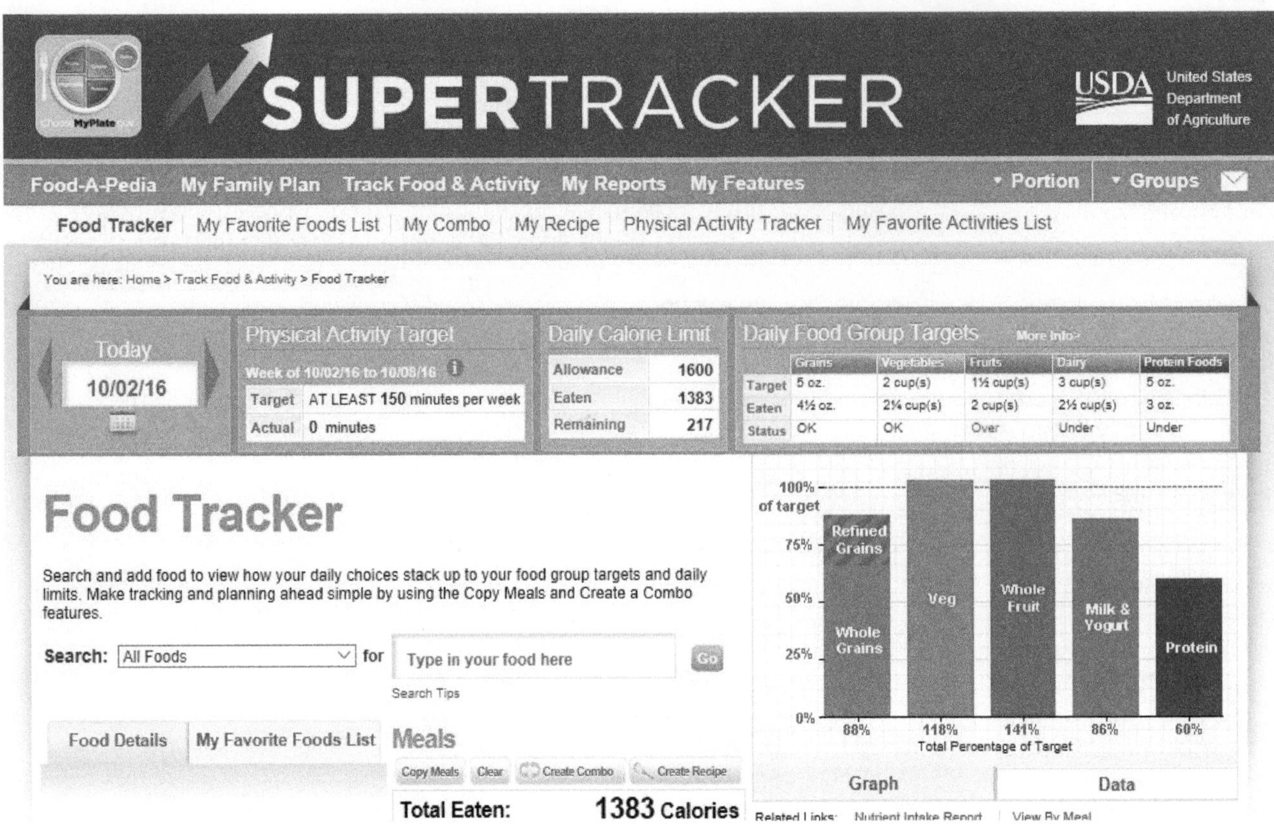

FIGURE 11 SuperTracker food-intake entry page

Reproduced from SuperTracker. United States Department of Agriculture. www.supertracker.usda.gov. [Accessed September 18, 2016].

using SuperTracker in this way is needed. **FIGURE 11** shows the food-intake entry page of the SuperTracker along with the bar graph report indicating percent of target for recorded intake of key food groups.

> **Recap** Internet-based dietary assessment applications offer more flexibility for nutrition researchers and professionals. The Internet removes some of the barriers that nutrition researchers face, including reaching certain populations and having greater numbers of participants in nutrition studies. Research participants can provide dietary-intake data without having to travel to the research center, which saves time for both the participants and researchers. The Internet can help remove barriers for clinicians as well, allowing them to connect with patients outside the clinical setting. Clinicians can track food and beverage intake along with weight and exercise goals of clients as they submit information online and provide more immediate feedback to help them meet their nutrition goals. This could lead to improved patient outcomes. Researchers and clinicians may also use these applications to gather data to determine the effectiveness of nutrition interventions.

Chapter Summary

Researchers and clinicians have been interested in determining true dietary intake and evaluating its relationship to health outcomes for decades. The ability of traditional methods to collect valid and accurate dietary intake has been criticized because of the known potential for error, primarily recall bias. Traditional methods are also labor intensive and burdensome. There are several advantages with current technologies when it comes to collecting dietary-intake data for analysis. This includes reducing the cost and the time and effort required, providing automatic data storage and rapid analysis, preventing incomplete and implausible data, and incorporating memory prompts and help features. Both computer-based and Internet-based applications improve the dietary interview process by using standardized questions and question sequencing based on the user's response. These applications may also help reduce bias in memory recall and reporting by incorporating multiple real food images and portion sizes, larger databases of food items to correctly identify foods consumed, and reduce the burden of recording dietary intake. Use of computerized technology in nutrition research may increase the objectivity of data collection and allow for larger sample sizes, therefore improving the ability to make stronger conclusions about the relationship of dietary intake to health and disease. Computerized nutrition analysis may also improve assessment in clinical settings and enhance clinical decision making and the provision of care that leads to improved outcomes.

Disadvantages of using technology in dietary assessment include the need for technological literacy on behalf of the participant as well as the research or clinician, keyboard and mouse skills for data entry, a lack of familiarity with or inability to use technology (older adults and the physically impaired may have difficulty using technology), and higher cost than pen-and-paper instruments. In addition, some socioeconomic groups may have limited access to technology. Newer technologies with the capacity to record images of foods consumed can improve the objectivity of reporting intake, aid in memory recall, and reduce recording burden, and they may be more acceptable to users and thus help correct misreporting. However, there is room for improvement in image-based food records and automated analysis of food items. Image-based food recording also may require more training for the user. Overall, incorporation of technology into dietary assessment has not changed the underlying methodology. Still, in many cases, technology has enhanced the dietary assessment methodology.

Computerized technology is constantly changing and advancing. What is available today will likely change in the near future. Nutrition professionals must be prepared to adopt computerized food and nutrient-analysis systems in any setting and adapt to new technology as it becomes available. This will require acquiring skills in using technology for nutrient intake analysis. In addition, technology-savvy nutrition professionals can lead initiatives to improve systems and work with technology developers to advance systems.

CASE STUDY

You are a postdoctoral fellow working with a prominent senior investigator on a project examining risk factors for dementia.

Nearly one in three Americans are living with hypertension; certain ethnic groups are more affected than others. Lifestyle behaviors, including diet and physical activity, can affect individual risks for developing hypertension, which is itself a risk factor for some leading causes of morbidity and mortality such as cardiovascular disease and stroke. A goal of *Healthy People 2020* is to improve cardiovascular health by controlling risk factors, including hypertension and improving dietary patterns,

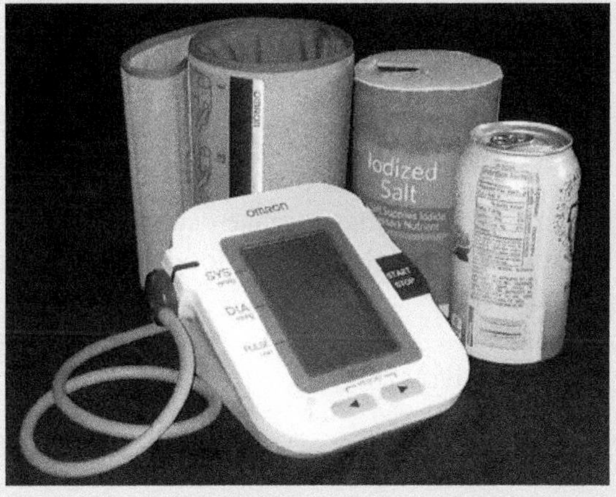

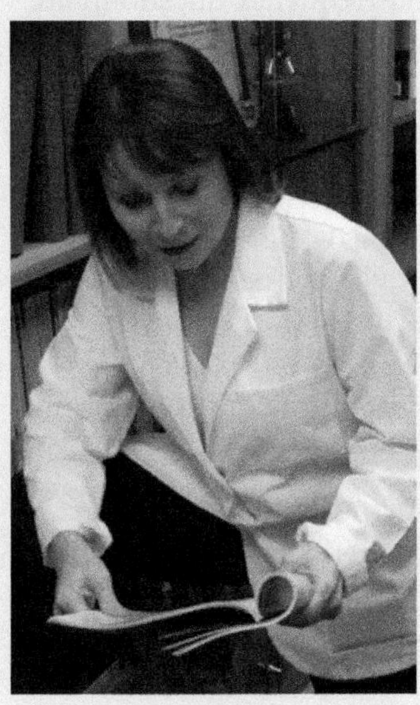

among Americans. Dr. Casas, PhD, RDN, is interested in studying the effects of such dietary components as sodium, phosphorous, and added sugars on hypertension. She wants to know the average intake of these nutrients among a large population of African Americans and Hispanics living in Dallas, Texas. She also plans to conduct a metabolic diet study using diets varying in nutrient composition among a subset of this population.

Question:

1. Looking back through the information in this chapter, which nutrition assessment method would you recommend for the study procedures, and which tool(s) would be most appropriate, and why?

Learning Portfolio

Key Terms

24-hour recall
Computer-based diet-assessment application
eButton
Food-frequency questionnaire (FFQ)
Food record
Image-assisted dietary assessment (IADA)
Internet-based diet-assessment application
Reactivity bias
Recall bias
Screeners
SenseCam
Social-approval bias

Study Questions

1. Which of the following is an advantage of using a food record to collect dietary-intake information?
   a. Low respondent burden
   b. Quick and easy to analyze
   c. Does not rely on memory
   d. Requires literacy skills
2. Which method of collecting dietary-intake data is considered the most thorough?
   a. Food record
   b. 24-hour recall
   c. Food-frequency questionnaire
   d. Dietary screener questionnaire
3. What is the type of bias in which the respondent changes dietary-intake patterns because of having to record or report food and beverages consumed?
   a. Recall
   b. Reactivity
   c. Social
   d. Recording
4. In what type of bias does the respondent report dietary intake consistent with expected norms or expectations but does not represent true intake?
   a. Recall
   b. Reactivity
   c. Social-approval
   d. Recording
5. Which method of gathering dietary-intake data relies on a structured interview process to obtain information about recently consumed foods?
   a. Food-frequency questionnaire
   b. Food record
   c. Dietary screener questionnaire
   d. 24-hour recall
6. What method of gathering dietary-intake data would be best when working with a population with low literacy levels?
   a. Food-frequency questionnaire
   b. Food record
   c. Dietary screener questionnaire
   d. 24-hour recall
7. Which of the following is a drawback of using the 24-hour recall method for collecting dietary-intake data?
   a. High respondent burden
   b. Introduces recall bias into the data
   c. Requires little time and effort from the researcher
   d. Includes a finite list of foods consumed
8. Which method of obtaining dietary-intake data asks participants to identify how often and sometimes the amount of a specific list of foods they consumed over a period of time, such as a year or month?
   a. Food-frequency questionnaire
   b. Food record
   c. 24-hour recall
   d. Dietary screener questionnaire
9. Which of the following is a benefit of using a food-frequency questionnaire?
   a. It is not affected by variability in daily intake.
   b. It is limited to a specific list of foods.
   c. It can be used to assess the total diet.
   d. It is good for quickly assessing intake of a few food groups.
10. What method of obtaining dietary-intake data is best for retrospective studies?
    a. Food record
    b. Dietary screener questionnaire
    c. Food-frequency questionnaire
    d. 24-hour recall

11. Which method of obtaining dietary-intake data is least burdensome for the participant and provides the least detail?
    a. Food record
    b. Dietary screener questionnaire
    c. Food-frequency questionnaire
    d. 24-hour recall

12. What method would be best to choose for quickly assessing calcium intake among a group of high-school female athletes to determine if an intervention is needed to encourage higher intakes of high-calcium foods?
    a. Food record
    b. 24-hour recall
    c. Food-frequency questionnaire
    d. Dietary screener questionnaire

13. What is a criticism of pen-and-paper methods of gathering dietary-intake data?
    a. It limits the researcher's ability to reach larger populations.
    b. It requires little time and effort for data entry and management.
    c. It is a more objective measure of intake.
    d. Literacy level is not a consideration among study participants.

14. What is a benefit of incorporating technology into dietary assessment methods?
    a. It is easily accessible by all populations.
    b. It is less costly than pen-and-paper methods.
    c. It allows for direct data entry.
    d. It can be easily adapted for people with disabilities.

15. Which of the following is a disadvantage of using technology for gathering dietary assessment data?
    a. Data are automatically analyzed in real time.
    b. A lack of technological literacy among some groups may require more training.
    c. It is more acceptable to use by adolescents.
    d. It limits the amount of data that can be collected because of storage capacity.

16. Image-assisted dietary assessment:
    a. Uses photographs or food models to aid in recall of foods eaten and portions consumed.
    b. Uses images of eating occasions to objectively capture dietary-intake data.
    c. Uses food packaging to estimate portion size of foods consumed.
    d. Requires expensive technology not available to most people.

17. Which of the following is a benefit of using image-assisted dietary assessment for research purposes?
    a. It allows for a more passive approach to collecting dietary data.
    b. It reduces the burden of analysis for the researcher.
    c. It aids in identifying unreported foods.
    d. It it is easier for participants to remember to capture images of foods than to write them down.

18. An example of a passive technology that can be used to capture dietary intake without the participant having to manually record dietary information is:
    a. SenseCam.
    b. A mobile-phone food record.
    c. A mobile voice recorder.
    d. An automated food-photograph analysis.

19. The ____________ method requires that participants include (a) a reference marker along with the food in the photograph taken at a 45-degree angle and (b) written text describing the food and ingredients for analysis by an RDN.
    a. SenseCam
    b. NuDAM
    c. Wellnavi
    d. TADA

20. This image-assisted dietary assessment method was found to underestimate energy intakes when compared to the doubly labeled water technique.
    a. SenseCam
    b. NuDAM
    c. Wellnavi
    d. TADA

21. This uses multiple images of foods before and after eating to create a three-dimensional model for estimating nutrient intake.
    a. Dietitian-assessed food photographs
    b. Automated food-photograph analysis
    c. Wearable image-capturing systems
    d. Automated 24-hour recall

22. Which age group likely requires additional training to correctly capture foods and beverages when using the mobile-phone food record for obtaining dietary-intake data?
    a. Adolescents
    b. Adults
    c. Adolescents and adults
    d. No additional training is needed

23. What is a common problem among users of automated food-photograph analysis systems that affects the ability to accurately analyze nutrient-intake data?
    a. Using the wrong reference marker
    b. Forgetting to take images before and after eating
    c. Inability to accurately identify food items
    d. Including too many high-quality food images

24. This tool creates a three-dimensional point cloud and uses recognition software to estimate the volume of food based on three images captured by video recorder.
    a. eButton
    b. Technology Assisted Dietary Assessment
    c. Food Intake and Voice Recorder
    d. Dietary Data Recorder System

25. The _______________ eliminates the need to include a reference marker along with food images by displaying a laser-beam grid over the food items in the image.
    a. eButton
    b. Technology Assisted Dietary Assessment
    c. Food Intake and Voice Recorder
    d. Dietary Data Recorder System

26. Users can wear this on the chest to automatically capture food images without additional self-reporting.
    a. eButton
    b. Technology Assisted Dietary Assessment
    c. Food Intake and Voice Recorder
    d. Dietary Data Recorder System

27. Why is it important to consider the type of research and research questions before you choose a dietary assessment method?
    a. The method will determine the cost of data collection.
    b. The method must be able to capture the data needed to answer research questions.
    c. The method will determine the level of detail needed.
    d. The method will determine the accuracy of the data.

28. If your research objective were to evaluate health outcomes related to dietary intake in cross-sectional and prospective studies, what type of dietary assessment method would be most appropriate?
    a. Food-frequency questionnaire
    b. Food record
    c. Multiple 24-hour recalls
    d. Single 24-hour recall

29. Which of the following can affect the ability to accurately obtain dietary-intake data when using a nutrient-analysis system?
    a. Ability to search for and identify correctly the foods consumed
    b. Cost: Lower-cost systems include fewer food and beverage items.
    c. Efficiency with which data are managed.
    d. The variety and quality of reports available

30. Which of the following is *not* a factor in choosing a computerized nutrient-analysis system?
    a. Cost
    b. Quality of database
    c. Data security
    d. Participant preference

31. Which factor in selecting a computerized diet-analysis system would be most important to evaluate if you have limited time and personnel for data collection, entry, and analysis?
    a. Accuracy and quality of the database
    b. Technical requirements
    c. Data-management efficiency
    d. Usability

32. What is a key difference of computer-based diet-assessment applications versus Internet-based diet-analysis applications?
    a. Computer-based applications are more secure.
    b. Internet-based applications allow access anytime, anywhere.
    c. Computer-based applications require a trained interviewer.
    d. Internet-based applications analyze data in real time.

33. What is the method and system used for gathering dietary-intake data for the National Health and Nutrition Examination Survey?
    a. Diet History Questionnaire II
    b. Nutrient Data System for Research
    c. Automated self-administered 24-hour recall
    d. Automated Multiple-Pass Method

34. Which of the following Internet-based diet-analysis applications are available free of cost for nutrition researchers?
    a. ASA24
    b. ASA24Kids
    c. DHQ II–Web
    d. All of the above

Discussion Questions

1. Compare and contrast methods of dietary-intake assessment, and give an example of a scenario in which it would be most appropriate to use each method.
2. Describe how you can use technology to improve the collection of dietary-intake data.
3. Choose three computer- or Internet-based diet-analysis applications and create a table comparing the factors to consider in selecting a system.
4. You want to assess dietary intakes of specific nutrients and patterns of food groups among individuals coming to the outpatient cancer center. Which computer-based diet-assessment application(s) would best help gather the data from this population, and why?
5. You are working on a research team across multiple study sites nationwide and are responsible for obtaining data for determining commonly consumed foods and food patterns. Which Internet-based diet-analysis application would best meet your needs, and why?

Activities

1. Access the ASA24 demonstration site (https://asa24.nci.nih.gov/demo/) and complete at least one 24-hour dietary recall. Note how much time it takes you to complete one 24-hour recall. Reflect on how easy the tool was to use, and provide an example of a research setting in which the tool's use would be appropriate and advantageous.
2. With a group of your peers, brainstorm new ways of using existing technology or ideas for new technology for collecting dietary-intake information. How would your new methods or technology improve the validity and reliability of dietary-intake assessment?

Online Resources

The ASA24 demonstration site allows clinicians and researchers to experience how user data are entered using the online 24-hour recall system: https://asa24.nci.nih.gov/demo/

The Axxya Systems video "How to use Nutritionist-Pro in a Research Study" can help researchers evaluate whether the application will meet their study needs: https://www.youtube.com/watch?v=GKGoBECue7A

The Dietary History Questionnaire II web demo allows clinicians and researchers to experience entering food-intake data and determine whether the tool is appropriate for their needs: http://epi.grants.cancer.gov/dhq2/webquest/demos.html

This article describes advances made to the eButton health monitor for automatically identifying and quantify food intake: https://www.sciencedaily.com/releases/2013/09/130909131224.htm

This video describes the development and uses for the Microsoft Research Sensecam: https://www.youtube.com/watch?v=g2-FfYCVr_s

This video demonstrates how the SenseCam can be used as a memory aid: https://www.youtube.com/watch?v=gYMQsi7cLqA

References

1. Stumbo PJ. New technology in dietary assessment: A review of digital methods in improving food record accuracy. *Proc Nutr Soc.* 2013; 72:70–76.
2. Thompson FE, Kirkpatrick SI, Subar AF, et al. The National Cancer Institute's Dietary Assessment Primer: A resource for diet research. *J Acad Nutr Diet.* 2015; 115:1986–1995.
3. Boyle MA. *Community Nutrition in Action: An Entrepreneurial Approach.* 7th ed. Boston, MA: Cengage Learning; 2017.
4. Monsen ER, Van Horn L. *Research: Successful Approaches.* 3rd ed. Chicago, IL: Academy of Nutrition and Dietetics; 2008.
5. St. George SM, Van Horn ML, Lawman HG, Wilson DK. Reliability of 24-hour dietary recalls as a measure of diet in African-American youth. *J Acad Nutr Diet.* 2016; 116:1551–1559.
6. Yuan C, Spiegelman D, Rimm EB, et al. Validity of dietary questionnaire assessed by comparison with multiple weighted dietary records or 24-hour recalls. *Am J Epidemiol.* 2017; 185:570–584.

7. Miller TM, Abdel-Maksoud MF, Crane LA, Marcus AC, Byers TE. Effects of social approval bias on self-reported fruit and vegetable consumption: A randomized controlled trial. *Nutr J.* 2008; 7:18.
8. Yaroch AL, Tooze J, Thompson FE, et al. Evaluation of three short dietary instruments to assess fruit and vegetable intake: The National Cancer Institute's Food Attitudes and Behaviors (FAB) Survey. *J Acad Nutr Diet.* 2012; 112(10):1570–1577.
9. Hedrick VE, Savla J, Comber DL, et al. Development of a brief questionnaire to assess habitual beverage intake (BEVQ-15): Sugar-sweetened beverages and total beverage energy intake. *J Acad Nutr Diet.* 2012; 112(6):840–849.
10. Lora KR, Davy B, Hedrick V, Ferris AM, Anderson MP, Wakefield D. Assessing initial validity and reliability of beverage intake questionnaire in Hispanic preschool-aged children. *J Acad Nutr Diet.* 2016; 116(12):1951–1960. doi: 10.1016/j.jand.2016.06.376.
11. England CY, Andrews RC, Jago R, Thompson JL. A systematic review of brief dietary questionnaires suitable for clinical use in the prevention and management of obesity, cardiovascular disease and type 2 diabetes. *Eur J Clin Nutr.* 2015; 69:977–1003.
12. Long JD, Littlefield LA, Estep G, et al. Evidence review of technology and dietary assessment. *Worldviews Evid Based Nurs.* 2010; 7(4):191–204.
13. Boushey C, Kerr D, Wright J, Lutes K, Ebert D, Delp E. Use of technology in children's dietary assessment. *Eur J Clin Nutr.* 2009; 63(Suppl 1):S50–S57.
14. Probst YC, Tapsell LC. Overview of computerized dietary assessment programs for research and practice in nutrition education. *J Nutr Educ Behav.* 2005; 37(1):20–26.
15. Illner AK, Freisling H, Boeing H, Huybrechts I, Crispim SP, Slimani N. Review and evaluation of innovative technologies for measuring diet in nutritional epidemiology. *Int J Epidemiol.* 2012; 41:1187–1203.
16. Gemming L, Utter J, Mhurchu CN. Image-assisted dietary assessment: A systematic review of the evidence. *J Acad Nutr Diet.* 2015; 115:64–77.
17. Wang DH, Kogashiwa M, Kira S. Development of a new instrument for evaluating individuals' dietary intakes. *J Am Diet Assoc.* 2006; 106(10):1588–1593.
18. Wang DH, Kogashiwa M, Ohta S, Kira S. Validity and reliability of a dietary assessment method: The application of a digital camera with a mobile phone card attachment. *J Nutr Sci Vitaminol.* 2002; 48:498–504.
19. Kikunaga S, Tin T, Ishibashi G, Wang DH, Kira S. The application of a handheld personal digital assistant with camera and mobile phone card (Wellnavi) to the general population in a dietary survey. *J Nutr Sci Vitaminol (Tokyo).* 2007; 53(2):109–116.
20. Rollo ME, Ash S, Lyons-Wall P, Russell AW. Evaluation of a Mobile Phone Image-Based Dietary Assessment Method in Adults with Type 2 Diabetes. *Nutrients.* 2015; 7(6):4897–4910. doi:10.3390/nu7064897.
21. Six BL, Schap TE, Zhu FM, et al. Evidence-based development of a mobile telephone food record. *J Am Diet Assoc.* 2010; 110(1):74–79. doi:10.1016/j.jada.2009.10.010.
22. Zhu F, Bosch M, Boushey CJ, Cel EJ. An image analysis system for dietary assessment and evaluation. *Proceedings/ICIP. International Conference on Image Processing.* 2010; 1853–1856.
23. Casperson SL, Sieling J, Moon J, Johnson L, Roemmich JN, Whigham L. A mobile phone food record app to digitally capture dietary intake for adolescents in a free-living environment: Usability study. Eysenbach G, ed. *JMIR mHealth and uHealth.* 2015; 3(1):e30. doi:10.2196/mhealth.3324.
24. Daugherty BL, Schap TE, Ettienne-Gittens R, et al. Novel technologies for assessing dietary intake: Evaluating the usability of a mobile telephone food record among adults and adolescents. Eysenbach G, ed. *J Med Internet Res.* 2012; 14(2):e58. doi:10.2196/jmir.1967.
25. Weiss R, Stumbo PJ, Divakaran A. Automatic food documentation and volume computation using digital imaging and electronic transmission. *J Amer Diet Assoc.* 2010; 110(1):42–44.
26. O'Loughlin G, Cullen SJ, McGoldrick A, et al. Using a wearable camera to increase the accuracy of dietary analysis. *Am J Prev Med.* 2013; 44(3):297–301.
27. Sun M, Burke LE, Mao Z-H, et al. eButton: A wearable computer for health monitoring and personal assistance. *Proceedings/Design Automation Conference.* 2014; 2014:1–6.
28. Jia W, Chen HC, Yue Y, et al. Accuracy of food portion size estimation from digital pictures acquitted by a chest-worn camera. *Public Health Nutr.* 2014; 17(8):1671–1681.
29. Vozenilek, G. Choosing the best nutrient analysis software for your needs. *J Amer Diet Assoc.* 1999; 99(11):1356–1358.
30. National Institutes of Health, National Cancer Institute. Dietary Assessment Primer. https://dietassessmentprimer.cancer.gov. Accessed September 18, 2016.
31. US Department of Agriculture. Automated Multiple-Pass Method. https://www.ars.usda.gov/northeast-area/beltsville-md/beltsville-human-nutrition-research-center/food-surveys-research-group/docs/ampm-usda-automated-multiple-pass-method/. Accessed September 18, 2016.
32. University of Minnesota, Nutrition Coordinating Center. NDSR. http://www.ncc.umn.edu/products. Accessed September 18, 2016.
33. Falomir Z, Arregui M, Madueno F, Corella D, Coltell O. Automation of food questionnaires in medical studies: A state-of-the-art review and future prospects. *Comput Biol Med.* 2012; 42:964–974.
34. US Department of Agriculture. Food and Nutrient Database for Dietary Studies. https://www.ars.usda.gov/northeast-area/beltsville-md/beltsville-human-nutrition-research-center/food-surveys-research-group/docs/fndds/. Accessed September 18, 2016.
35. Blanton CA, Moshfegh AJ, Baer DJ, Kretsch MJ. The USDA Automated Multi-Pass Method accurately estimates group total energy and nutrient intake. *J Nutr.* 2006; 136:2594–2599.
36. Moshfegh AJ, Rhodes DG, Baer DJ, et al. The US Department of Agriculture Automated Multi-Pass Method reduces bias in the collection of energy intakes. *Am J Clin Nutr.* 2008; 88:324–332.
37. Viocare. ProNutra. http://www.viocare.com/pronutra.html. Accessed September 18, 2016.
38. Esha Research. The Food Processor. www.esha.com. Accessed September 25, 2016.
39. Nutritionist Pro. Nexgen. https://nexgen1.nutritionistpro.com/shop/product-detail/nutritionist-pro-diet-analysis-software-13. Accessed September 25, 2016.
40. National Institutes of Health, National Cancer Institute. Automated Self-Administered 24-Hour Dietary Assessment Tool. http://epi.grants.cancer.gov/asa24/. Accessed September 18, 2016.
41. Kirkpatrick SI, Subar AF, Douglass D, et al. Performance of the Automated Self-Administered 24-hour recall relative to a measure of true intakes and to an interviewer-administered 24-h recall. *Am J Clin Nutr.* 2014; 100:233–240.

42. Thompson FE, Dixit-Joshi S, Potischman N, et al. Comparison of interviewer-administered and Automated Self-Administered 24-hour dietary recalls in 3 diverse integrated health systems. *Am J Epidemiol.* 2015; 181(12):970–978.
43. Baranowski T, Islam N, Baranowski J, et al. Comparison of a web-based versus traditional diet recall among children. *J Acad Nutr Diet.* 2012; 112(4):527–532.
44. Diep CS, Hingle M, Chen T, et al. The automated self-administered 24-hour dietary recall for children, 2012 version, for youth aged 9 to 11 years: A validation study. *J Acad Nutr Diet.* 2015; 115:1591-1598.
45. National Institutes of Health, National Cancer Institute. Diet History Questionnaire II and Canadian Diet History Questionnaire II: Web-based. http://epi.grants.cancer.gov/dhq2/webquest/. Accessed October 29, 2016.
46. Viocare. VioScreen. http://www.viocare.com/vioscreen.html. Accessed September 18, 2016.
47. Kristal AR, Kolar AS, Fisher JL, et al. Evaluation of web-based, self-administered, graphical food frequency questionnaire. *J Acad Nutr Diet.* 2014; 114:613–621.
48. Viocare. NutraScreen. http://www.viocare.com/nutrascreen.html. Accessed September 18, 2016.
49. NutritionQuest. Data-on-Demand. http://nutritionquest.com/assessment/data-on-demand/. Accessed September 18, 2016.
50. Cybersoft. Nutribase Cloud Edition. www.nutribase.com. Accessed September 25, 2016.
51. United States Department of Agriculture. SuperTracker. https://www.supertracker.usda.gov. Accessed September 18, 2016.

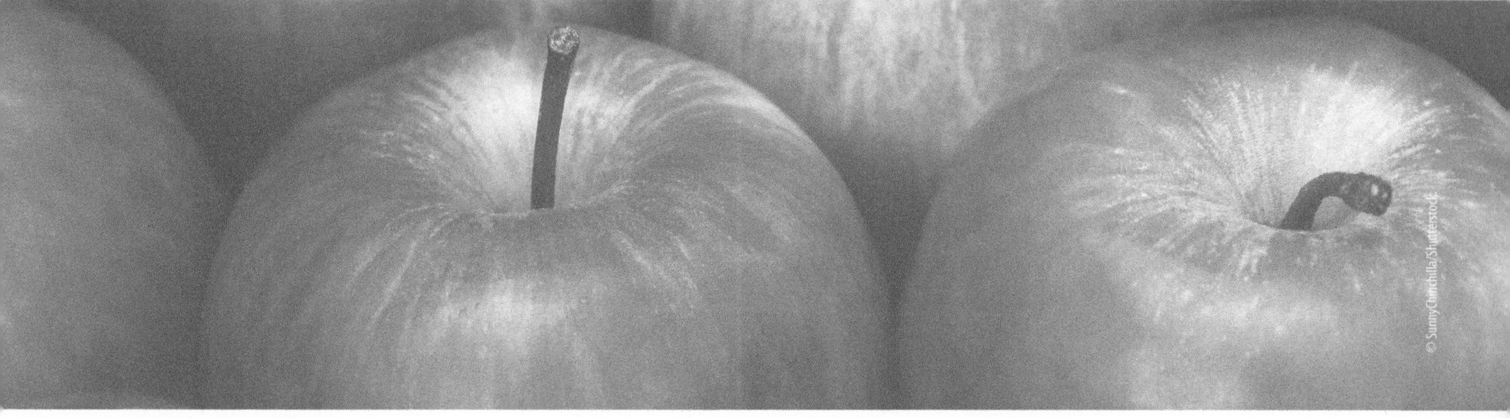

Anthropometry

Patricia G. Davidson, DCN, RDN, CDE, LDN, FAND
Dwight L. Davidson, PhD, LMHC

CHAPTER OUTLINE

- Introduction
- Anthropometric Indicators and Cutoffs
- Plotting and Interpreting Measurements in Children
- Additional Anthropometrics
- Body Composition
- Chapter Summary

LEARNING OBJECTIVES

After reading this chapter, the learner will be able to:

1. Define anthropometric measures and their use in assessing metabolic disease risk.
2. State and describe age-appropriate anthropometric measurements throughout the life cycle.
3. Demonstrate how to calculate and accurately evaluate body mass index.
4. Evaluate a person's metabolic fitness and nutritional status based on body composition.
5. Compare and contrast methods for assessing body composition.
6. Accurately measure height, weight, and waist circumference.

Introduction

Anthropometric measurements are useful in establishing normative data and standards, assessing efficacy of treatments, and determining the impact of disease states. As a tool, it is useful in establishing normative data and standards, assessing efficacy of treatments, and determining the impact of disease states.

History

The human body has been measured since antiquity because it was essential to the figurative arts of painting and sculpture. Eventually, these systematic measurements were adopted by anthropologists to identify basic "aspects" of human morphology. The term anthropometria dates back to naturalists of the 17th century.[1] The manual *Anthropometria* by Johann Sigismund Elsholtz appears as the earliest recorded effort to investigate and measure the human body for scientific and medical purposes. It brought a quantitative approach to acquiring data concerning variations and changes in the human form, and it described the relationship between the human body and disease.[2]

As a measurement of physiological and developmental human growth, anthropometrics appeared in clinical practices, which used instruments to assess and record individual data and begin establishing norms. The importance of these measurements grew from several intricately linked concepts, including nutrition and infection, psychological and social stress, and food contaminants. Variables linked to socioeconomic conditions indicated that body size was a sign of quality of life. Thus, **anthropometry** became a tool for social welfare. The role of anthropometrics in the pediatric population became the foundation of both research and clinical interventions, with techniques and technologies initially focused on this group. Certain measures were developed, but in practice were limited to the assessment, diagnosis, and intervention of childhood development and disease states.[1]

Accurately assessing a person's nutritional status involves more than just evaluating what a person eats. It also involves determining his or her **body composition** and comparing the person's growth and development to accepted standards. Measuring, monitoring, and accurately evaluating body composition are important skills to define and trend the health status of a person, as well as the population, throughout the life cycle. Overweight and obesity and associated comorbid conditions have been clinical concerns since the 1980s. The health implications associated with these conditions have further stimulated the need for accurate assessment of weight and body composition to determine the risk for such metabolic diseases as diabetes mellitus and cardiovascular disease (CVD), as well as a person's metabolic fitness.

Definition of Anthropometry

As the science of nutrition has expanded, the need for accurate measures of nutritional status has become essential when performing a nutrition-focused physical assessment. Assessing a person's body composition, protein status, muscle strength, and body fat is crucial for identifying malnutrition and a response to medical nutrition therapy intervention. Anthropometric assessment is an essential nutrition-evaluation tool. It reveals malnutrition, overweight, and obesity; it also quantifies the loss of muscle mass, increases in fat mass, and redistribution of adipose tissue.

These techniques and methodologies make up the area of **anthropometrics**, which is defined as "the study of human body measurements, especially on a comparative basis."[3] Anthropometrics includes measurements of body weight, stature, composition, and a focus on specific area measurements such as circumference (waist and hip), skinfold (SF), and bone dimensions. Some provide direct measurements (e.g., height and weight), and others are derived (e.g., body composition).[4] The anthropometric measures in common use for adults and children include weight, height, waist circumference (WC), **skinfold thickness** (as measured at different body sites), and a set of weight-for-height indices, such as **body mass index (BMI)**. Often such measures, or a combination of them, are used to determine **body composition (BC)**—for example, percentage of body fat (%BF).

Studies have been conducted to assess the validity of anthropometric measures such as BMI, WC, and skinfold thickness to estimate body fat and using **dual-energy x-ray absorptiometry (DXA)** as the reference. Results indicate modest to excellent agreement. Other studies found that measures of skinfold thickness are better predictors of %BF than other, simpler anthropometric methods such as BMI.[5]

Anthropometric Indicators and Cutoffs

Preview Anthropometric measurements have two requirements: an anthropometric indicator (measurement) and a cutoff point. By applying statistical analyses to the compiled body measurements of study groups of children, the cutoff points were established.

Anthropometric measurements require: (1) an **anthropometric indicator** and (2) a **cutoff point**. The anthropometric indicator, also known as an *anthropometric index*, is a measurement or measurements (such as height and weight) or a combination of additional data with measurements (e.g., age).

A cutoff point is established below which either individuals or populations will require an intervention or therapy. The application of universal cutoff points has the dual advantage of allowing comparisons between populations and preventing bias on the part of staff when performing an initial assessment or follow-up of patients.[6,7] In addition, cutoff points can be used to characterize changes and trends within a population and identify persons at a higher risk for adverse outcomes.[6,8] The cutoff point of 0.5 has been recommended for waist-to-height ratio (WHtR) to classify central obesity in adults and children and as well as different ethnic groups.[9]

Cutoff thresholds are used to explicate variations in age, gender, ethnicity, and other technical factors that affect anthropometrics alone or in conjunction with social or health causes or outcomes, as well as in policy formulation and advocacy. In growth references, certain *Z*-scores and percentiles have been chosen for cutoff points to classify problematic growth and nutritional status.[10]

Body Measurements: Foundations in Pediatrics

The clinical outcomes of alterations in body composition should be a necessary component of any physical assessment, even more so in the care of children. Body measurements are essential in the analysis of the development or progression of disease and for monitoring the efficacy of treatment. Accurate measurement of changes in BC because of interventions is vital in planning nutritional care and the management of developmental and aging processes, disease progression, and rehabilitation efforts. The need for better quantification of what constitutes an excessive deviation from normative standards has sparked a growth in the technologies for measurement of human body composition.[11]

In pediatrics, the essential, static measurements for infants up to age 2 years are length, weight, head circumference (HC), and weight for length. For ages 3 years and older, they are height, weight, and BMI.[7,12]

Height and Length in Children

To accurately measure a child's height, we must first think in terms of length for those too young to stand. The child should be placed supine on a measuring device or board, and the measurement should be recorded to the nearest 0.1 cm (**FIGURE 1**).

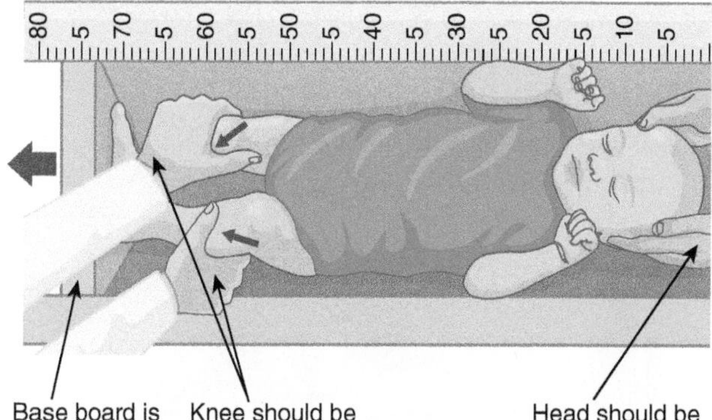

FIGURE 1 Infant length measured using a standard measuring board

For children unable to stand for reasons other than age, alternative methods are used, including knee height or upper-arm length.[13] The knee height is measured with the specific caliper from the top of the patella to the bottom of the foot, with both knee and foot at a 90-degree angle. The following gender and racial specific formulas are used for calculating the child's height for ages between 6 and 18 years.

White children:

Boys: height = 40.54 + (2.22 × knee height)
Girls: height = 43.21 + (2.15 × knee height)

Black children:

Boys: height = 39.60 + (2.18 × knee height)
Girls: height = 46.59 + (2.02 × knee height)

These values must be compared to specific standard curves designated for knee-height calculations.

To evaluate suspected short or tall stature, accurate measurements of height and weight are plotted on the appropriate age growth chart.[14] Infants and toddlers should have their length, weight, and head circumference plotted on a growth curve at every well or sick visit to the physician. The Centers for Disease Control and Prevention (CDC) and the American Academy of Pediatrics recommend using the World Health Organization (WHO) growth charts for children younger than two years and the CDC growth charts for children older than two years.[15,16]

For patients 2 to 20 years of age, weight, height, and body mass index should also be plotted. Short stature is determined when plotted height is more than two standard deviations below the mean for age, or less than the third percentile. Height in children older than two years should be measured using a wall-mounted stadiometer[14,17,18,19] (**FIGURE 2**).

In the United States, use the WHO growth charts to monitor growth for newborn infants and children up to two years of age. Use the CDC growth charts

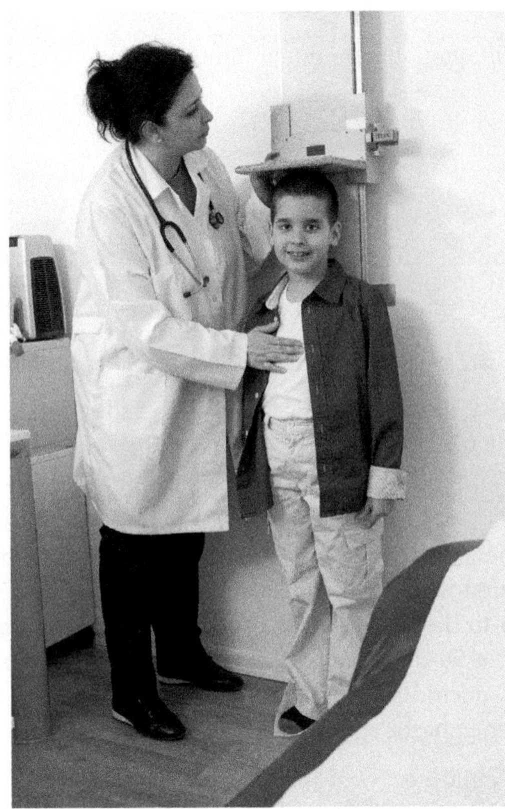

FIGURE 2 Standing-height measurement technique

to monitor growth for children ages 2 years and older.[18,19]

Percentiles and *Z*-Scores

Widely used in the assessment of children's nutritional status and growth performance are two indicators: percentiles and ***Z*-scores**. Both are interchangeable, but their respective cutoff points may not be identical.[14,20]

Percentiles

A **percentile** is defined as the position of an individual on a given reference distribution of 100 points, and it is easier to understand and use in practice by professionals and the public. In addition, a percentile designates the expected percentage of a population that should fall above or below it. Age-specific and sex-specific percentiles are often used to assess growth and nutritional status in children as based on anthropometric measures. There is a growing consensus on using BMI percentiles as cutoffs instead of WHt *Z*-scores in assessing overweight and obesity in children more than two years old. The most widely used percentiles are the 3rd, 5th, 50th (median), 85th, 95th, 97th, and 99th. The term *percentile* and the related term *percentile rank* are often used in descriptive statistics and are frequently represented graphically with a normal curve.[21–23]

Z-Scores

Several considerations support the use of *Z*-scores. First, they are calculated from the distribution [both mean (μ) and the standard deviation (σ)] of the reference population. Second, *Z*-scores are standardized measures and comparable across ages, genders, and measures. Third, a group of *Z*-scores is subject to the measures of statistics such as μ and σ and thus can be studied as a continuous variable. Finally, *Z*-scores can be used to quantify the growth status of those children falling outside the percentile ranges. In clinical settings, growth references and standards are useful for monitoring populations and research projects.[10]

Recap To address non-normative data obtained from children, whether from malnutrition, disease, or genetic conditions, it is plotted on the growth charts developed by the WHO and the CDC. The resultant percentiles and *Z*-scores permit the quantification of the measurements in relation to the anticipated parameters.

Plotting and Interpreting Measurements In Children

Preview The use of established growth charts facilitates the interpretation of growth data in children. Height and stature can be projected from the height velocity as determined over time.

To plot the growth of a child, first the appropriate growth chart (**FIGURE 3**) is selected from either the WHO or CDC. The measurements should be taken at each visit to the physician and recorded by first locating the child's age on the horizontal axis and using a ruler/straight edge to draw a line from the age. Then on the vertical axis locate the particular measurement (weight, height, BMI, and HC) and draw a line across placing a circle where the age and measurement intersect to determine the percentile. The percentile rank is used for assessing nutritional risk base on age/gender/population cutoff value. It is also used as a comparative standard for the child in that it identifies shifts or changes between visits and the need for further evaluation. For example, if the intersect is plotted the 5th percentile, it means that 95 of

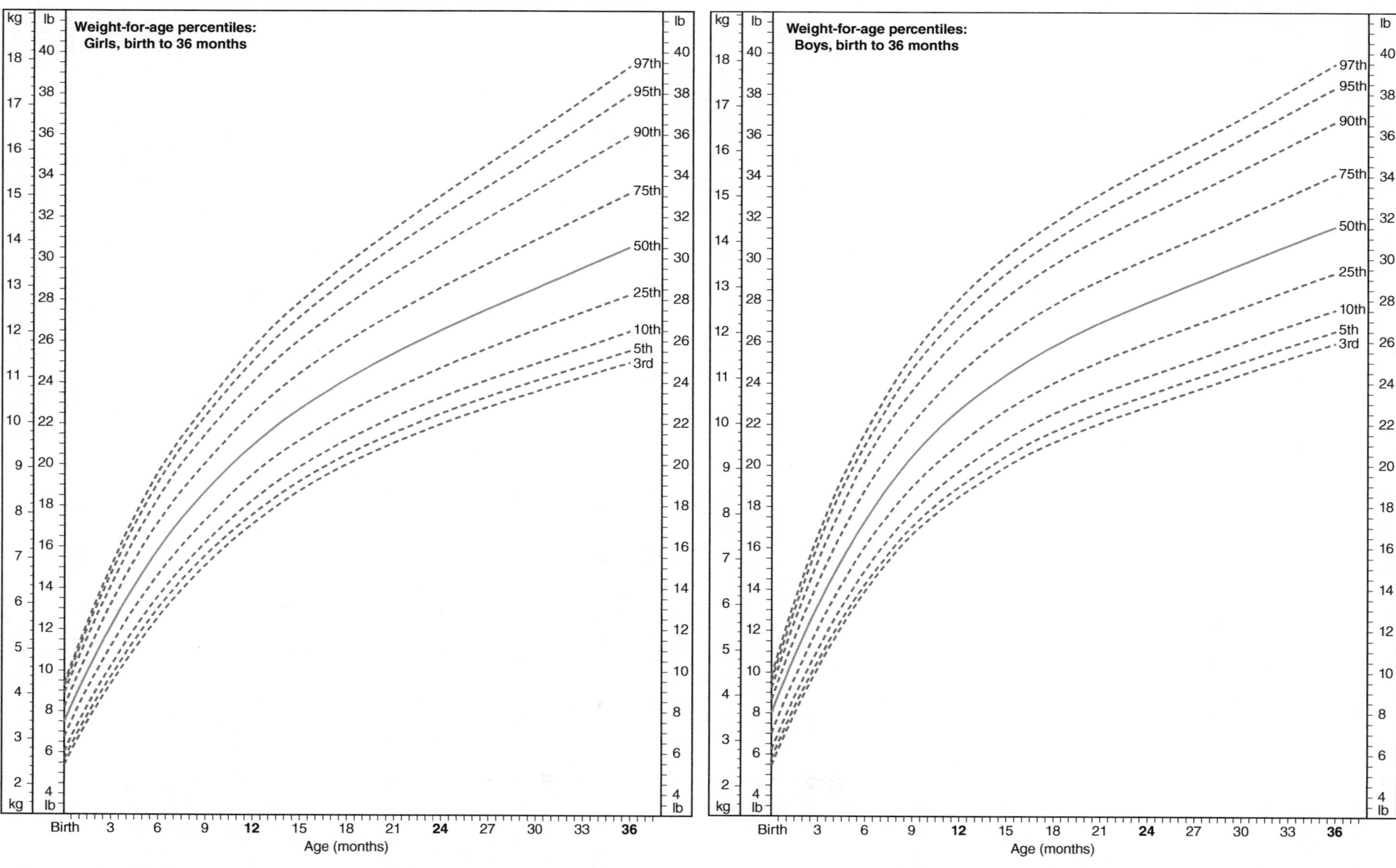

FIGURE 3 Growth charts girls (birth to 36 months) and boys (birth to 36 months)

Data from the National Center for Health Statistics in collaboration with the National Center for Chronic Disease Prevention and Health Promotion (2000).

100 children (95%) of the same age and gender have a lower for-age measurement (Figure 3).

Height Velocity

The most sensitive measurement in detecting growth abnormalities early in the course of all types of chronic illness is **height velocity**.[24] If a child more than two years of age has a height velocity of less than 4 cm/year, he or she should be carefully monitored for nutritional deficits or other causes of short stature, as 95 percent of children have a height velocity more than 4 cm/year.[25] Peak height velocity occurs in puberty, with boys growing 6 to 12 cm/year and girls growing 5 to 10 cm/year; there is a substantial variability in the age of peak height velocity.

Adult Stature

Height and weight are often used in combination to assess nutritional status, thinness, and fatness. Therefore, height-measurement accuracy is important and should be measured with an accurate stadiometer with a fixed vertical ruler and an adjustable sliding horizontal headpiece. The person being measured, while standing on a hard floor, is requested to stand up straight, look forward with relaxed arms at the sides, straight legs close together, and feet flat with the heels together. The head is positioned by the technician, taking the measurement in the Frankfort horizontal plane in which the lower eye lid or socket is horizontally level with the top of the ear. If a person is unable to stand or is bedridden, then using demispan, knee height (KH), or ulna length (UL) (**FIGURES 4, 5,** and **6**) for estimating a person's height are options.[26,27] The demispan measures from the sternal notch to the web between the middle and ring fingers, and the knee height is measured using a sliding broad-blade caliper while both the knee and ankle are at a 90-degree angle. Using a standard formula for gender, age, and either knee height or demispan, a person's height is calculated.

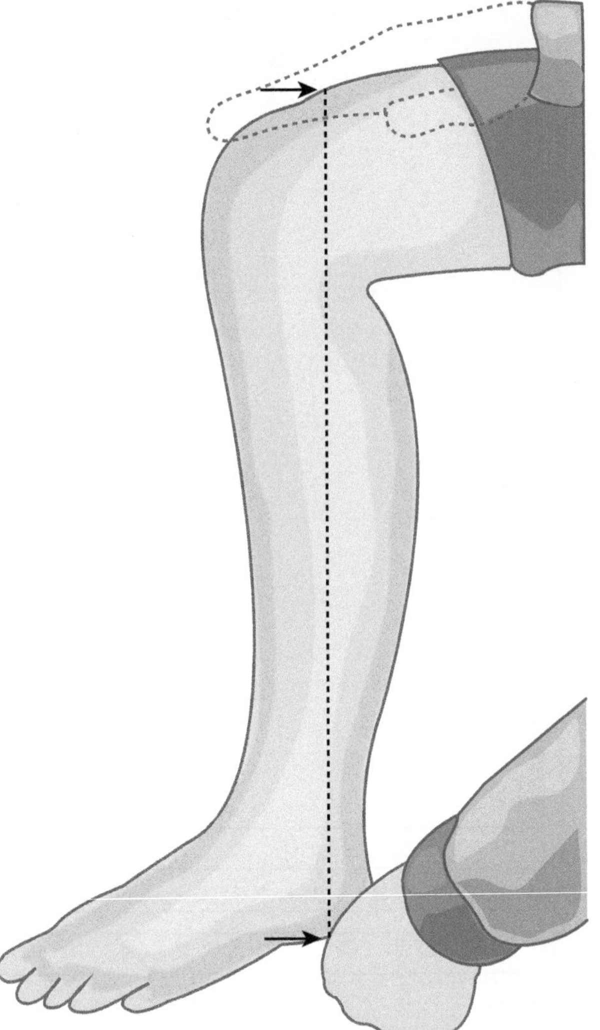

Females
Height in cm = 84.88 – (0.24 × age) + (1.83 × knee height)
Males
Height in cm = 64.19 – (0.04 × age) + (2.02 × knee height)

FIGURE 5 Knee-height calculation

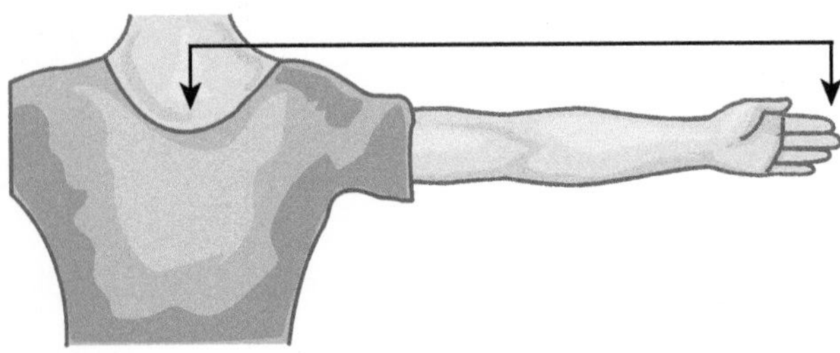

Females
Height in cm = (1.35 × demispan in cm) + 60.1
Males
Height in cm = (1.40 × demispan in cm) + 57.8

FIGURE 4 Demispan height calculation

For ulna-height measurement, the forearm is measured using an anthropometric tape while the person's left arm is bent across the chest with the hand flat on the chest and fingers pointing toward the right shoulder (Figure 6).[28] The measurement is taken on a bare arm from the tip of the elbow (olecranon process) to the styloid process (prominent bone of the wrist). It is a useful tool because it is low cost and does not require special equipment, but it has been noted to overestimate height for certain ethnic groups such as healthy Asians and blacks.

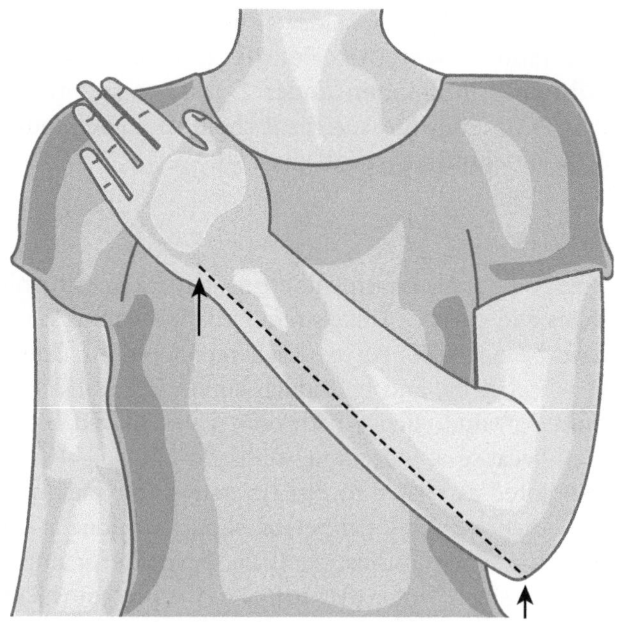

Females

Height in cm = 95.6 + (2.77 × ulna length in cm)

Males

Height in cm = 79.2 + (3.60 × ulna length in cm)

FIGURE 6 Ulna predicted height calculation

Advantages and Limitations

Like other anthropometric measures, height is influenced by a variety of factors, including racial and ethnic differences, because both of these can affect the actual height measure and interpretation as well as the relationship between them. As people age, height decreases, beginning sometime between ages 30 and 50, and varies by gender, with women's height decreasing more rapidly with age. Factors affecting height measurements include postural changes, decrease in vertebrae height, and conditions limiting the ability to stand straight (such as **kyphoscoliosis** or disease-related curvature of the spine and arthritis). All of these can limit accurate height assessment and result in poor interpretation of BMI and its associated health risks. Alternative height measures have limited agreement with the exact height because they estimate maximal height, not current height, and are based on a healthy, younger population and do not correlate with hospitalized adults 65 years of age and older.[26] Demispan is considered to be the best alternative height measure because it does not decline like standing height (SH) and is a better measurement to use for calculating BMI for health risk, particularly in the older adults at least 65 years of age.[29] Knee height has limitations, especially for people who are bedridden, preventing appropriate positioning of the leg and requiring specific anthropometric calipers, but KH estimates are closer to SH than to UL. Similar trends are noted when calculating BMI using KH. It is recommended to add 1.8kg/m^2 if calculating the BMI with UL, especially if using the BMI to assess for malnutrition.[30]

Head Circumference

Measurement of head circumference, also known as **frontal-occipital circumference**, is vital in children 3 years old and younger because this corresponds to the period of greatest brain growth. Correct measurement requires a flexible tape measure (usually paper or vinyl) applied at the maximum head diameter, along the supraorbital ridge to the occiput (**FIGURE 7**). The value should be recorded to the nearest 0.01 cm and also be plotted on a standardized growth chart. Because children grow in spurts, two measurements at least three to six months apart and preferably 6 to 12 months apart are needed to

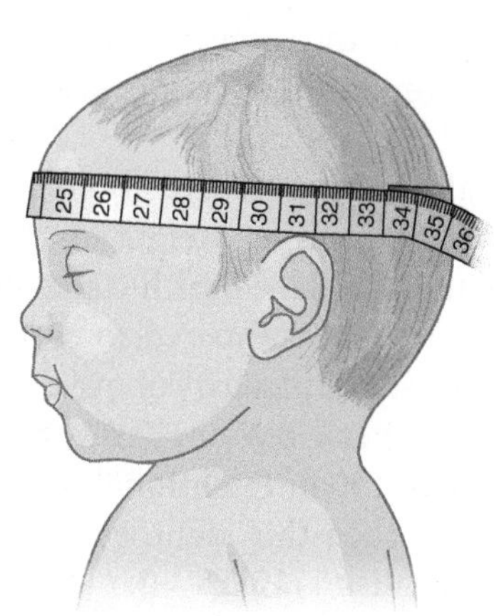

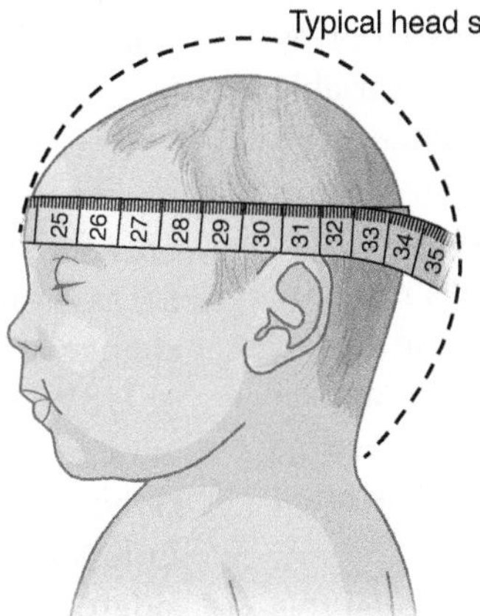

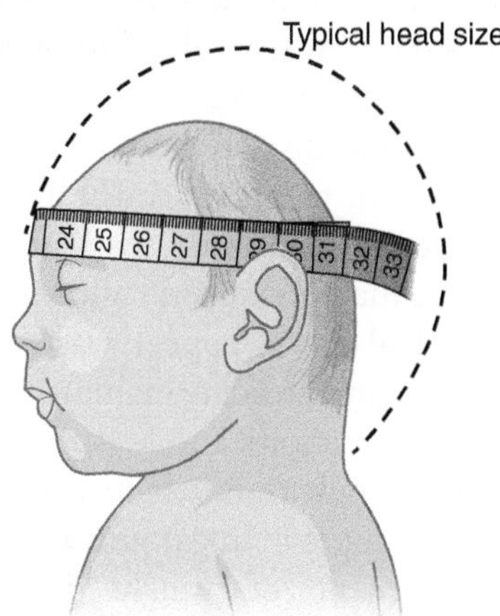

FIGURE 7 Head-circumference measurement comparison

Reproduced from Centers for Disease Control and Prevention. Congenital Zika syndrome and other birth defects. https://www.cdc.gov/zika/hc-providers/infants-children/zika-microcephaly.html.

accurately determine growth velocity. Measurement of head circumference rarely occurs after 16 years of age in a clinical setting.[7,12] Clinically, accurate and ongoing measurement of the HC is important, particularly in tall and short-statured children, because HC has been shown to correlate with both height and weight through adolescence but is particularly strong in the first couple of months of infancy.[31,32]

HC measurement and its strong association with brain development make it an essential component for assessing growth and development in infants and toddlers.[33] Cranial development is influenced not only by age and gender but also by ethnicities; therefore, the measurement needs to be compared to the appropriate HC growth chart.[34] For comparative age, gender, and population, it is considered an abnormal measurement if it is two standard deviations above the mean (macrocephaly) or two standard deviations below the mean (microcephaly). See Figure 7. A positive percentile deviation from the comparative age standard is suggestive of hydrocephalus, which is a condition caused by increased pressure on the brain related to excess cerebrospinal fluid in the brain. Craniostenosis is indicated by negative standard deviation, indicating a premature closure of the skull suture(s), thus limiting the growth of the brain and changing the shape of the skull. Rapid changes in cranial growth have also been linked to brain developmental changes and related to the overall growth pattern.[33]

Weight and Stature: Children and Adults

Children

Weight and stature are key for assessing growth patterns and determining deviations from the norms for a specified population.[7,22,23] Abnormal growth patterns can signify changes in nutritional status, either because of nutrient malabsorption caused by a disease such as cystic fibrosis and inflammatory bowel or by poor nutritional intake. Malnutrition has variable effects, but clinically these can be noted in changes in anthropometric measures, including height, weight, and changes in lean body mass and adipose tissue. With severe malnutrition, a child's growth is not only stunted but also will appear wasted because of BC changes. In contrast, acute malnutrition will be apparent by BC alterations and wasting, as compared to chronic undernutrition, which will be demonstrated by pattern changes in linear growth.

Measurement of weight in all populations should be taken on a calibrated scale. The infant or toddler should be weighed sans clothing or diaper. The measurement is recorded to the nearest 0.1 kg. The ratio of **weight-to-length** is used to predict **adiposity** in children under 2 years of age, rather than BMI. This measurement should also be plotted on a standardized growth chart.[7,12]

Adults

Adult weight measurements are usually taken with only shoes and coats or jackets removed. Specialized scales have been developed to weigh mobile adults, adults in wheelchairs, and bedridden adults. Scales that are moved around, such as bathroom scales, should not be used because of inaccurate calibration. If weight is be monitored as related to disease state or for malnutrition, then weighing the person should be done at the same time of day. Adjustments are also made for amputations using a factor that estimates the percent weight for the amputated limb, using the following formula:

$$(\text{Weight}/100 - \%\ \text{amputation}) \times 100$$

Being that weight includes an overall measurement of the body compartments, it is important to include it as a general measure as part of the nutrition assessment. Establishing a reference weight, either by calculating the ideal body weight (IBW) or usual body weight (UBW), is important in assessing a person's nutritional status. In some cases, the 1983 Metropolitan Life Insurance charts have been used as a guide for IBW comparison. These charts are based on weight ranging, incorporating three skeletal frame sizes, and morbidity and mortality. In theory, some use the midrange for determining IBW, but this could potential underestimate IBW and overestimate the excess body weight in a person being evaluated for bariatric surgery.[35] A common formula used for calculating the IBW or reference weight is the Hamwi formula (**FIGURE 8**), developed in the 1960s. The main criticism for using IBW is that it does not consider ethnicity, age, or body frame size or the changes in anthropometric trends—that is, increases in both height and weight.[11]

Accurate weight references are important not only for setting weight goals for weight loss but also for assessing nutritional risk or health status. Weight change and current weight compared to either IBW or UBW are indices used clinically. For example, if an adult is <70% of his or her UBW or IBW or has experienced a greater than 5% unintentional weight loss in less than a month, then this adult would be considered at nutritional risk (**TABLES 1**, **2**, and **3**). The same would be considered for unintentional weight gain as well.

Males:

106 for 5 feet + 6 lbs per inch over 5 feet

Example: 72" (6 feet) = 12 × 6
= 72 + 106 = 178 lbs

Females:

100 pounds for 5 feet + 5 lbs per inch over 5 feet

Example: 64" (5 feet 4 in) = 4 × 5
= 20 + 100 = 120 lbs

Determine range: Add/subtract (±) 10% to account for body frame size

Adjust for persons less than 5' and >18 yrs

Subtract 1.55 lbs/inch for women

Subtract 1.76 lbs/inch for men

FIGURE 8 Hamwi formula

TABLE 1 Percent of IBW or UBW

% IBW = Current weight ÷ IBW × 100%	%UBW = Current weight ÷ UBW × 100%
Example: IBW 166#; current wt 142#	Example: UBW 129#; current weight 101#
142# ÷ 166# × 100 = 85.5%	101# ÷ 129# × 100 = 78.5%

TABLE 2 Nutritional status and weight change (unintentional)

Time	Significant (%)	Severe Weight Loss (%)
1 week	1.0–2.0	> 2.0
1 month	5.0	> 5.0
3 months	7.5	> 7.5
6 months	10.0	> 10.0
1 year	20.0	> 20.0

Modified from White JV, Guenter P, Jensen G, et al. Consensus statement of the academy of nutrition and dietetics/American Society for Parenteral and Enteral Nutrition: Characteristics recommended for the identification and documentation of adult malnutrition (undernutrition). *J Acad Nutr Diet*. 2012;112(5):730-738.

TABLE 3 UBW and IBW nutritional status

Index	Mild Deficit (%)	Moderate Deficit (%)	Severe Deficit (%)
IBW	80–90	70–79	< 70
UBW	85–95	75–84	< 75

Modified from White JV, Guenter P, Jensen G, et al. Consensus statement of the academy of nutrition and dietetics/American Society for Parenteral and Enteral Nutrition: Characteristics recommended for the identification and documentation of adult malnutrition (undernutrition). *J Acad Nutr Diet*. 2012;112(5):730-738.

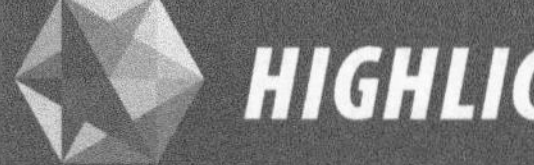

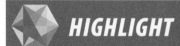

HIGHLIGHT

Estimating Energy Requirements

Indirect calorimetry is considered the gold standard by the Academy of Nutrition and Dietetics for calculating the energy needs of patients in the clinical setting, particularly the critically ill. This method is more accurate than using a predictive equation because it closely estimates actual energy expenditure and accounts for the effects of stress, trauma, and the disease state, thus eliminating the need for adding in a stress factor. If resting energy expenditure cannot be measured by indirect calorimetry, then it may be estimated by a predictive equation, including the Harris-Benedict, Mifflin-St. Jeor, and Ireton-Jones equations. To calculate needs using these equations, an accurate weight in kilograms, height in centimeters, and age in years are needed. Then to determine total energy expenditure or needs, multiply by a stress factor, ranging from 1.3 to 1.5, to indicate additional energy needs associated with activity, fever, trauma, and malnutrition. Both equations consider a decrease in energy needs associated with aging, and separate equations are derived for males and females. A potential source for error in these equations is the lack of distinction between fat and lean mass; in addition, the Harris-Benedict equation is known to overestimate needs by 5% to 15%. The Academy has concluded that the Harris-Benedict equation is not accurate enough to estimate energy expenditure in critically ill patients and does not recommend its use for that purpose.

Mifflin-St. Jeor, the predictive equation, is recommended by the Academy because it demonstrates increased accuracy over Harris-Benedict. This equation calculates total energy expenditure by calculating requirements based on age, weight, height, and stress factor.

Mifflin-St. Jeor:

Men: EEE = 9.99 × (weight in kg) + 6.25 × (height in cm) − 4.92 × (age in years) + 5

Women: EEE = 9.99 × (weight in kg) + 6.25 × (height in cm) − 4.92 × (age in years) − 161

Example: For a 30-year-old man standing 170 cm tall and weighing 70 kg:

Mifflin-St. Jeor EEE = 9.99 × (70) + 6.25 × (170) − 4.92 × (30) + 5 = 1,619 kcal

Harris-Benedict:

Men: EEE = 66.5 + 13.8 × (weight in kg) + 5.0 × (height in cm) − 6.8 × (age in years)

Women: EEE = 655.1 + 9.6 × (weight in kg) + 1.9 × (height in cm) − 4.7 × (age in years)

Example: For a 30-year-old man standing 170 cm tall and weighing 70 kg:

Harris-Benedict EEE = 66.5 + 13.8 × (70) + 5.0 × (170) − 6.8 × (30) = 1,679 kcal

Activity Factors

Based on general activity level

Range: 1.0–1.2 sedentary, 1.3 ambulatory, 1.4 lightly active, 1.5 moderately active, 1.7 very active, 1.9 extra active

Stress Factors

1.0 fever, 1.2 pneumonia, 1.3 major injury, 1.5 severe sepsis, burns (15% to 30% TBSA), 1.5–2.0 burns (31% to 49% TBSA), 1.8–2.1 burns (> 50% TBSA)

TBSA = total body surface area; EEE= estimated energy expenditure

Modified from Determination of Resting Metabolic Rate: Individual Equations. ADA Evidence Analysis Web site. http://www.adaevidencelibrary.com/topic.cfm?cat=4311. Accessed November 1, 2016.

Recap Anthropometric data is only as reliable as the measurements are consistent, both in technique and instrumentation. Whether measuring height, head circumference, weight, or stature, the standardization of the techniques and the plotting of the data necessitate attention to detail.

Additional Anthropometrics

Preview The anthropometric study of the body now moves from the quantitative (physical measurement) to the qualitative projective (interpolation from specific component measurements).

Waist-to-Height Ratio

The waist-to-height ratio was developed as an indicator of central obesity and for risk of CVD. However, scant data are available on the utility of WHtR in assessing abdominal obesity and related cardiometabolic risks among children of normal weight or those overweight or obese, as categorized according to BMI values.[36] In theory, this measurement takes into consideration a person's size by dividing the WC by height. There are concerns that this index does not adjust for age, particularly during periods of growth, or for gender. For some ethnicities in which BMI may not identify a person as overweight or obese, WHtR has the potential to identify metabolic abnormalities and risk. WHtR has been studied as a simple anthropometric index in the detection of central obesity and in the assessment of associations between cardiometabolic risk factors and central intra-abdominal obesity.[9] Adult studies have shown that this measure has the ability to identify adverse cardiometabolic risk profiles not only in those with normal weight but also in those with normal metabolic risk profiles in the overweight or obese classifications.[37] The WHtR and obesity risks are listed in **TABLE 4**.

Measures of Adiposity

Body Mass Index

Central adiposity functions as a complex and active endocrine organ, producing a variety of hormones and cytokines. They play an important role in the dysregulation of inflammatory, metabolic, and hemodynamic processes through various mechanisms, including hepatic lipogenesis and hepatic insulin resistance and release of free fatty acids from adipocytes.[38]

TABLE 4 Waist-to-height ratio and obesity risk

WHtR Category	Male (%)	Female (%)
Underweight	<43	<42
Healthy weight	43–52	42–48
Overweight	53–62	49–57
Obese	>63	>58

Modified from Wildman RP, Muntner P, Reynolds K, McGinn AP, Rajpathak S, WylieRosett J, Sowers MR: The obese without cardiometabolic risk factor clustering and the normal weight with cardiometabolic risk factor clustering: prevalence and correlates of 2 phenotypes among the 8 US population (NHANES 1999-2004). *Arch Intern Med 2008*; 168:1617–1624.

BMI is determined from the measurements of height and weight, calculating the relative proportion between the two. It is a valid predictor of adiposity.[39] BMI will vary based on gender, age, and pubertal stage. The calculation is as follows:

$$\text{BMI} = (\text{Weight in kg}) / (\text{Height in m})^2$$

BMI is recommended in the clinical setting as the most appropriate single indicator of overweight and obesity in the pediatric population. In comparison to other anthropometric measurements, such as waist circumference and **triceps skinfold thickness (TSF)**, BMI is a stronger data point for estimating %BF in children and adolescents.[40,41] The required measurements to calculate BMI are routine, noninvasive, and inexpensive. BMI values are plotted on a BMI reference chart; a child with a BMI above the 85th percentile is overweight, and a child with a BMI above the 95th percentile is obese. A child with a BMI below the 5th percentile is underweight.[7,12] BMI is identified as the best choice among available measures that can be easily assessed at low cost, and it is strongly associated with body fat and health risks. However, as an indirect measure of adiposity, BMI has several limitations, especially when used for children. In children, BMI measures should be expressed as *Z*-scores or percentiles relative to age and gender because BMI is strongly related to growth and maturation.[36] Children's maturation statuses and growth patterns affect their BC and BMI. BMI is positively associated with height in children. Although there is a correlation between BMI for overweight children and percent fat mass (FM), there is only a weak relationship in thin children, although the data were not analyzed for ethic differences.[41] In contrast, a study evaluating the correlation of BMI strongly correlated with the %BF determined by DXA for a variety of ethnic groups.[42]

In a systematic review of 25 population-based studies, Simmonds et al. found that BMI correctly detected obesity in children (81.9%) compared to reference standards (95% confidence interval [CI], 73-93.8), with a false-positive rate of only 4%, but detected fewer children as overweight (76.3% sensitivity; 95% CI, 70.2–82.4) with a higher false-positive rate of 7.9%. The referenced studies used various methods: five used densitometry, one used deuterium dilution, and the rest used DXA.[5] In comparisons with classification of obesity by comparing %BF to BMI, BMI demonstrated a low sensitivity, although it does have a high specificity. Results also showed that BMI does not always correlate to central obesity.

In adults, BMI has historically been used to assess both risks for obesity-related diseases as well as nutritional risk. As noted, it does not depict BC, but is a good indicator of both ends of the spectrum and the need for further assessment. There are several features for a good measure of body fatness, and BMI possesses a majority of them, including low cost and its value as an easy assessment tool for health risk and body adiposity. However, it does not distinguish the type of fat or account for growth, gender, ethnicity, or athletes, all of which confound the association of BMI to adiposity. It is among several methods used to estimate BC but is not reasonable for daily clinical use.[4]

With a strong association shown between body stores or adiposity and a need for a quick, noninvasive assessment measure, the WHO established classifications to be used for underweight, overweight, and obesity. Adults with a BMI ≤18.5 are classified as underweight and BMI ≥25 as overweight. In general, a BMI between 18 and 25 kg/m^2 for adults is considered healthy.

Using BMI in a hospital setting can allow for early recognition of malnutrition and thus influence the disease course, decrease the length of stay, and decrease mortality. Established norms for BMI can allow the clinician to estimate morbidity and mortality.

BMI and its association to muscle mass can vary considerably between people of the same height. Bodybuilders and participants in other strength-related sports, are among those who can be incorrectly assessed by BMI typically possessing lower %BF but presenting with a BMI in the overweight or even obese index.[43,44] In contrast, a lower BMI in an adult could be attributed to a loss of **fat-free mass**

(FFM) (lean tissue) caused by **sarcopenia**, increased adipose tissue, or shifts in both. The BMI measure does not distinguish the BC changes and could lead to an incorrect BMI classification or delay in nutrition intervention. If an adult's BMI is determined as nonobese but with unintentional lean body mass weight loss, unintentional loss in lean body mass, the risk for malnutrition could be missed. In contrast, if the weight loss was because of FM, the nutrition risk is less.

BMI is often cited as a correlate of key health indicators of cardiovascular and metabolic disease. However, as BMI cannot differentiate between FFM and adiposity and cannot indicate the distribution of these components in the body, it leads to misclassification on the individual level and has low sensitivity in determining excess adiposity.[45]

The effectiveness of BMI as an assessment tool for adiposity and as a predictor of health complications must be evaluated for cultural and ethnic differences. An analysis of data from some 900,000 participants in 57 prospective studies on four continents confirms that obesity, as measured by BMI, is associated with increased total mortality in both men and women in age classifications ranging from 35 to 89 years.[46] However, even though BMI has been the most widely applied phenotypic technique in measurement of human adiposity, close scrutiny has led to the observation that correlations with adult adiposity are generally modest and that other factors such as age, race, and physical activity levels perplex efforts to correlate BMI and adiposity.[47]

Because BMI does not distinguish between FM and lean (nonfat) mass or FFM, it can vary considerably between individuals of the same height. Data suggest different health effects of FM and FFM. When only BMI is used, these disparate associations cannot be distinguished.[48]

Clearly, the relationship between BMI and FM% differs among ethnic groups and populations. Among Asians of many ethnicities (Chinese, Indians, Indonesians, Malaysians, Japanese), differences in the BMI-FM% relationship have repeatedly been documented when compared with Caucasians.[49] With as much as 5% higher body fat at any BMI value, as well as higher risks of type 2 diabetes and cardiovascular diseases at lower BMIs, Asian Indians consistently demonstrated greatest deviations from Caucasians. These ethnic groups also have their BMIs affected by differences in frame size and relative leg length (relative sitting height).[48,50] To date, the WHO has not redefined the cutoff points in any specific Asian populations.[51]

Research has suggested some ethnic differences in the associations among BMI, %BF, fat distribution, and health risks. Different BMI cutoff points have been recommended for some Asian and Pacific populations. There are biological differences between ethnic groups and populations in BC, the relationships between BMI and %BF, and those between BC and morbidity.[52,53]

There are two sets of international BMI cutoff points in addition to other classifications: one recommended by the WHO and another by the International Obesity Task Force (IOTF). The IOTF values have been used widely worldwide.[54]

The FFM and FM indices (FFMI and FMI) are comparable notions to the BMI (the denominator is the same) and result from the partitioning of BMI into two subcomponents using BC, namely:

$$\text{BMI (kg/m}^2\text{)} = \text{FFMI (kg/m}^2\text{)} + \text{FMI (kg/m}^2\text{)}$$

Thus,

$$\text{FFMI} = (\text{BMI} - \text{FMI}); \text{FMI} = (\text{BMI} - \text{FFMI})$$

Therefore, FFMI, FMI, and BMI use similar ratios for their calculation, the difference being that the numerator is composed of FFM or FM (in kg) rather than body weight. Interpretation of BMI and FM% may fail to allow a clinician to detect the presence of protein-energy malnutrition (PEM). Calculation of FFMI, however, does allow for the identification of an individual as malnourished.[48]

Hull et al. investigated the presence of FFMI differences in 1,339 healthy adults (ages 18–110 years) of different races and ethnicities (Caucasian vs. African American, Hispanic, and Asian). They found that among the four ethnic groups for both genders (males > females), FFMI did differ, with FFMI lowest in Asians and greatest in African Americans. This demonstrated racial disparities in BC and infers that identification by race will show greater susceptibility for disease relative to loss of FFM.[55]

Waist Circumference

Internationally (WHO and the International Diabetes Federation) and in the United States, WC has been accepted as a valid anthropometric measure for identifying central and visual adiposity as well as an established component of metabolic syndrome, a predictor of risk for cardiovascular disease, and type 2 diabetes.[56] Because of gender, age, and ethnic variations in body fat distribution, consideration for different cutoffs or indices are recommended in assessing health risk. In theory, circumference differences represents FM-to-FFM proportions for any area of

VIEWPOINT

BMI: The Weight Categories for Older Adults Are Different

Robin B. Dahm, RDN, LDN

Eating healthfully and getting adequate physical activity contribute significantly to how well we maintain a healthful weight—one that is neither too high nor too low. A healthful weight is an optimal goal at any age and protects against numerous health problems. Being underweight increases the risk for immediate and acute health challenges such as skin breakdown and chronic diseases. Carrying excess weight also can cause clear and present dangers such as joint and respiratory problems. In addition, overweight adults are statistically likely to develop several diseases associated with aging.[1] Body mass index is a key screening tool for determining weight status and is based on a person's weight-to-height ratio. **Figure A** lists some of the conditions associated with being overweight.

- High blood pressure (hypertension)
- High levels of LDL cholesterol, low levels of HDL cholesterol, or high levels of triglycerides (dyslipidemia)
- Type 2 diabetes
- Coronary heart disease
- Stroke
- Gallbladder disease
- Osteoarthritis (a breakdown of cartilage and bone within a joint)
- Chronic inflammation and increased oxidative stress
- Some cancers (endometrial, breast, colon, kidney, gallbladder, and liver)

FIGURE A Some chronic diseases associated with overweight

Modified from Centers for Disease Control and Prevention. About Adult BMI. https://www.cdc.gov/healthyweight/assessing/bmi/adult_bmi/index.html. Accessed February 2, 2017.

Older Adults Are Not the Same as Younger Adults

The BMI weight classifications for adults are based specifically on associations between BMI and chronic disease and mortality risk in healthy, ***young*** adults (20 years and older) populations.[2] What kind of a skew does this create? Consider an older adult whose atherosclerosis (a precursor to cardiovascular disease) began at age 55 years versus a younger adult whose atherosclerosis began at age 20 years. The younger adult is statistically more likely to manifest full-blown cardiovascular disease by age 55 years, whereas the older adult at this age has only the precursor to cardiovascular disease. The 55-year-old is also statistically less likely to develop cardiovascular disease even within her next few years of life because its onset was later in life (which is statistically protective). Yet the BMI population chart treats all adults as a single population, with no distinction between younger adults and older adults and their differing statistics for developing diseases later in life.

A main use of BMI for adults is to determine chronic disease risks associated with higher BMI values. The standard BMI categories are less applicable as age increases; the concept that mortality risk increases as weight increases does not seem to hold as true for older adults.[2]

Older Adults and Underweight

The BMI weight categories require some adjustment to address health statistics associated with older adults. At a higher BMI, for example, a person at least 65 years of age has a lower mortality risk, whereas the *opposite* is true for younger adults![1,2]

BMI cannot distinguish between lean tissue, fat, and bone mass. Yet as we age, our bodies tend to develop more fat, which increases BMI values. In addition, mortality statistics for older adults show that somewhat higher BMIs are protective.[2] **Figure B** shows how how BMI status for older adults is "more lenient" than for younger adults.

Why is underweight more of a concern for older adults than for their younger counterparts? Underweight older adults might be more susceptible to certain undernutrition-related health problems that often go unrecognized. These include physiologic changes, chronic disease, polypharmacy, and psychosocial changes. Such combinations of underweight and unrecognized conditions may have a stronger effect on older adults than on younger adults.[2,3]

For older adults, carrying "a few extra pounds" can temporarily compensate for unplanned weight loss and hold off the development of secondary conditions that weight loss can trigger such as loss of bone-mineral density.[4]

Practical Application

Currently, BMI weight classifications do not differentiate between older adults and younger adults. Healthcare practitioners who use the right-shifted BMI weight categories can more appropriately address the health needs of their older adult clients and patients.

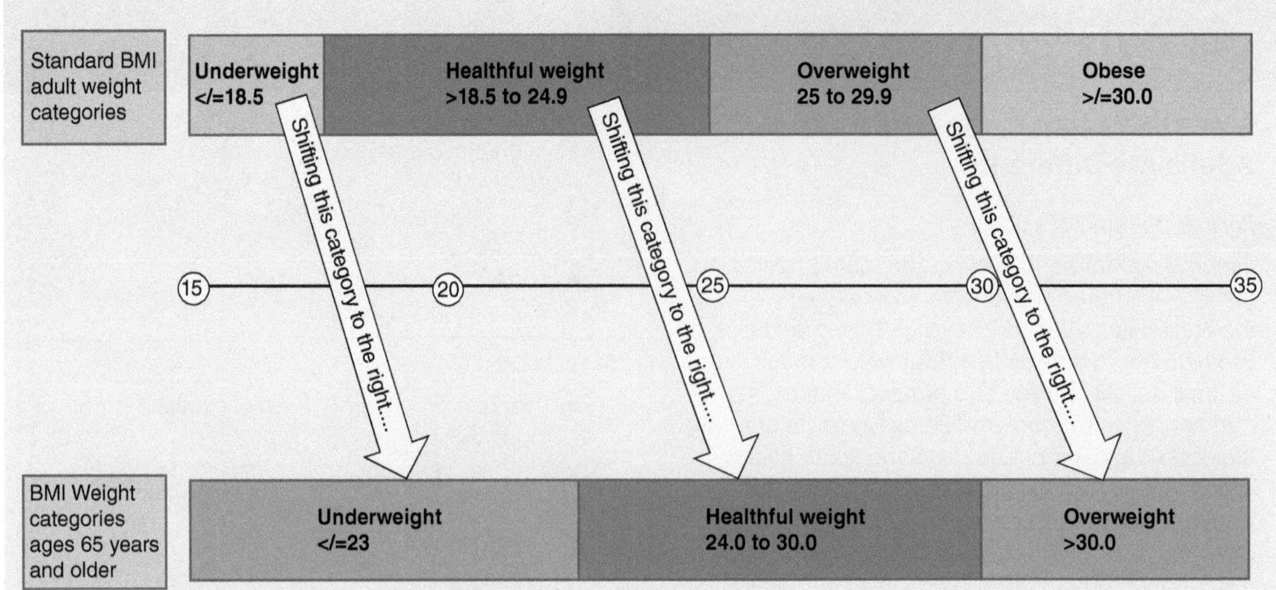

FIGURE B Shifting BMI weight categories to the right for adults ages 65 years and older more accurately represents the health statistics associated with this subpopulation.

Modified from Using Body Mass Index. Queensland Government. https://www.health.qld.gov.au/__data/assets/pdf_file/0031/147937/hphe_usingbmi.pdf. Accessed February 2, 2017.

References

1. Department of Health and Human Services, Centers for Disease Control and Prevention. Body mass index: Considerations for practitioners. https://www.cdc.gov/obesity/downloads/BMIforPactitioners.pdf. Accessed February 2, 2017.
2. Raeburn ED. Higher BMI may be better for older adults. *MedPage Today*. 2014; March 19. http://www.medpagetoday.com/Endocrinology/General Endocrinology/44843. Accessed February 2, 2017.
3. Winter JE, MacInnis RJ, Wattanapenpaiboon N, Nowson CA. BMI and all-cause mortality in older adults: A meta-analysis. *Am J Clin Nutr.* 2014; April; 99(4): 875-890. http://ajcn.nutrition.org/content/99/4/875.long. Accessed February 2, 2017.
4. MedlinePlus. Body mass index. https://medlineplus.gov/ency/article/007196.htm. Accessed February 2, 2017.

the body, with larger measures reflecting a higher percentage of body fat. Circumference measures are taken with a flexible measuring tape and can be performed at the waist, hip, and thigh to assess body fat distribution. Adiposity of the abdomen, as measured by WC, is useful in diagnosing cardiovascular risk factors and metabolic syndrome. Exact location of the WC measurement is necessary. Common WC sites are (1) just beneath the lowest or floating rib, (2) at the midpoint between the iliac crest and the lowest or floating rib, (3) the narrowest point of the abdomen as visualized, and (4) just above the iliac crest. Sites using bony landmarks are preferable (see **FIGURE 9**).

In both adults and children, BMI has been the accepted method to identify the overweight and obese; however, visceral fat strongly mediates the association between obesity and weight-related diseases. WC measurement has emerged as a useful clinical measure in the assessment of those so identified. Specific waist circumference cutoff points have been established to identify overweight and obese adults, but values are not so clearly defined for children, where waist circumference differs between genders and varies with age as well.[57]

WC correctly detected obesity in children (83.8%) compared to reference standards, with a false-positive rate of 3.5%. WC correctly detected overweight in children (73.4%), with a false-positive rate of 5.3%.[3]

WC is particularly useful in adult patients who are categorized as normal or overweight on the BMI scale. Waist circumference has little added predictive power of disease risk at BMIs of at least 35. Therefore, there is no benefit to measuring waist circumference in adults with BMIs of at least 35.[22]

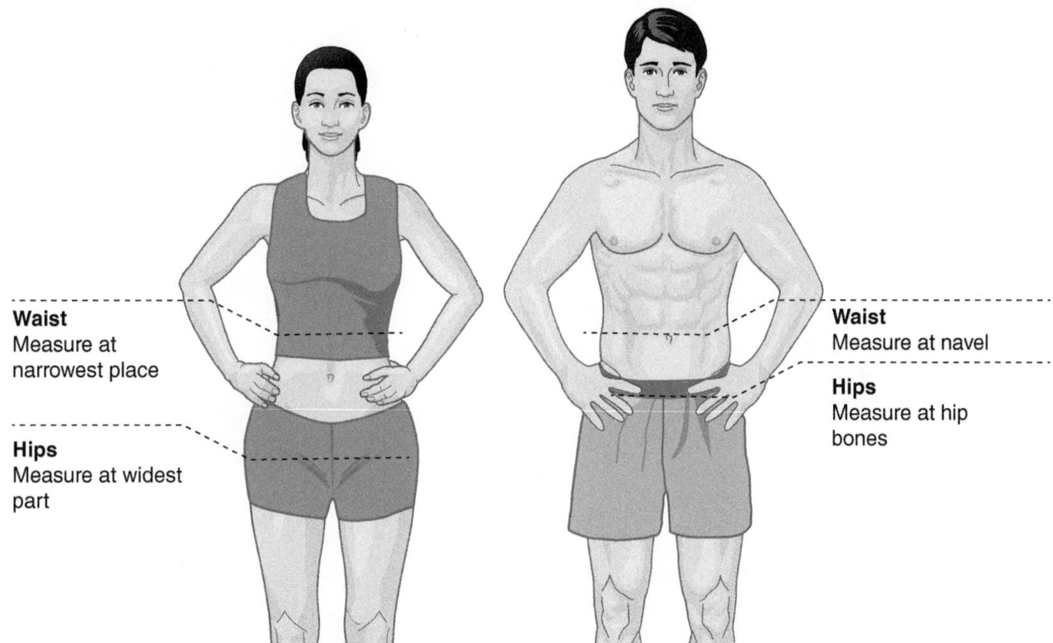

FIGURE 9 Waist circumference measurement female and male

The WHO has identified ethnic groups for which waist circumference may reflect more body fat at a given BMI level. Studies investigating BC and association with health outcomes in Asia have focused on Chinese, Japanese, Korean, or South Asian (or Indian). Some have viewed these ethnic groups as a homogeneous population labeled "Asians" and found a higher %BF in Asians at lower BMIs and an increased prevalence of truncal fat compared to Caucasians.[58]

European men and women display less visceral adipose tissue for a given waist circumference than do Chinese and South Asians (Indians).[59] Correspondingly, an increase %BF across a range of WC values has been recorded in East Asia.[60] Comparisons of indigenous or aboriginal peoples and Caucasians in North America have reported no difference between visceral adipose tissue and BMI, total body fat, or WC.[61] Black women in South Africa, compared to European women, have a slightly lower BMI at a given %BF, but they also have less abdominal adipose tissue as determined by DXA at the same WC.[62] In a few small studies, African women reportedly had less visceral adipose tissue than do white women.[63–65]

One study reported that visceral adipose tissue at a specific WC was not appreciably different in Hispanics than in whites.[66] There have been reports that Pacific Islanders have more muscle mass and less %BF than Europeans have at similar BMIs.[62,67]

Although there is substantial evidence of age and gender variations in WC, there is less evidence for demonstrable ethnic differences. Asian populations have more visceral adipose tissue, and African populations—with possibly Pacific Islanders—have less visceral adipose tissue or %BF at any given waist circumference compared to Europeans. If higher levels of abdominal fat for a WC are reflected in associations with health outcomes, then lower thresholds for these indicators might be needed for the affected ethnicities than for Europeans. Data from Africans and Pacific Islanders are possible indications for more cutoffs than those used for Europeans. Because the objective is to predict disease risk, drawing conclusions about cutoffs based solely on observed risks is not pertinent.[61]

Skinfold Thickness

One of the earliest techniques used for estimating %BF is skinfold (SF) measurements using specially designed calipers to measure the subcutaneous fat (see **FIGURE 10**).[4] Skinfold thickness measurements are based on an assumption that subcutaneous fat is approximately 50% of total body fat. SF measurements are obtained in a minimum of three and as many as nine areas of the body, including subscapular, triceps, biceps, suprailiac, and abdominal; these measurements indirectly predict %BF through population-specific (gender-specific and

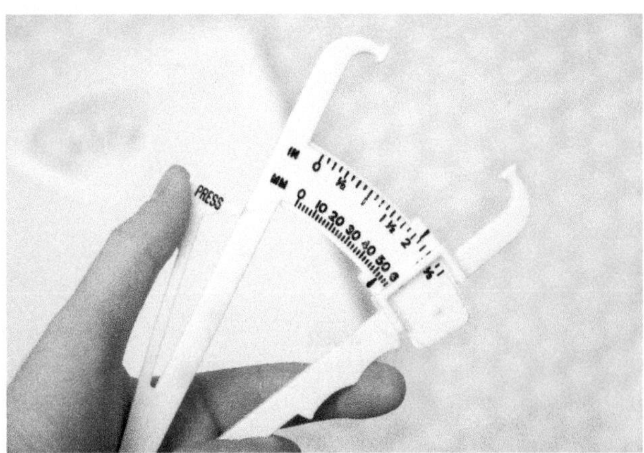

FIGURE 10 Skinfold calipers

age-specific) equations.[68] All measurements for skinfolds are taken using skinfold calipers. To begin, the examiner needs to carefully mark the point for performing the skinfold measurement—either the specified midpoints for the arms and legs or the designated boney points for the trunk of the body. To improve comfort when taking measurements, the procedure should be explained to the child or adult and demonstrated on the patient's hand. Before applying the caliper, a fold of skin along with the **subcutaneous adipose tissue (SAT)** is grasped between the thumb and index finger. Caution should be taken to ensure there is distinction between the fold and the underlying muscle, with the two sides close to parallel. While holding the skinfold, the jaws of the caliper are placed perpendicular to the fold length and measured to the nearest 0.1 mm. the reading is taken within three seconds after the caliper is released. Most calipers can measure up to 44 mm.

The skinfold caliper measurement is prone to interrater error because of difficulty separating the fold of skin from the muscle. The procedure requires that the skinfold include the adipose tissue below and two thicknesses of skin.[7] However, with practice, the interrater error can be as low as 5% if standard protocol is followed and measurements are taken in the same areas.[69,70,71]

Adults

Measurement recommendations can be gender specific, with only three measurements. For men, measurements include chest, abdomen, and thigh; for women, the measurements include, triceps, suprailiac, and thigh (**FIGURE 11**). In addition, site-specific correlations have been established with triceps SF estimating %BF as compared to subscapular skinfolds, with total body fat (TBF) and health risk.[72]

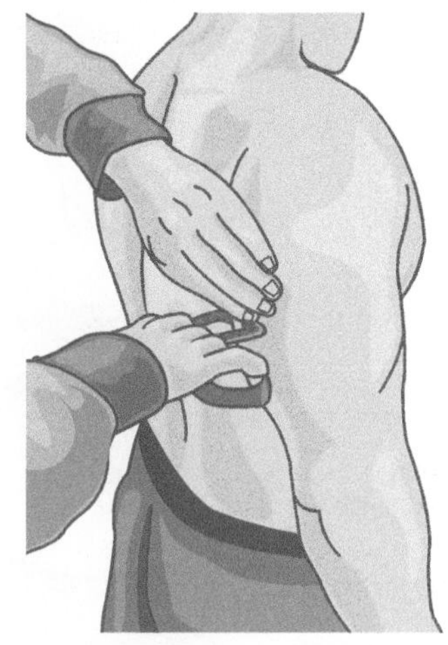

(a)

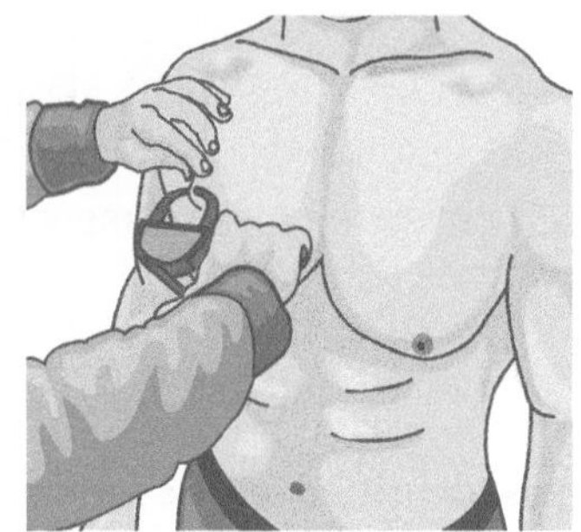

(b)

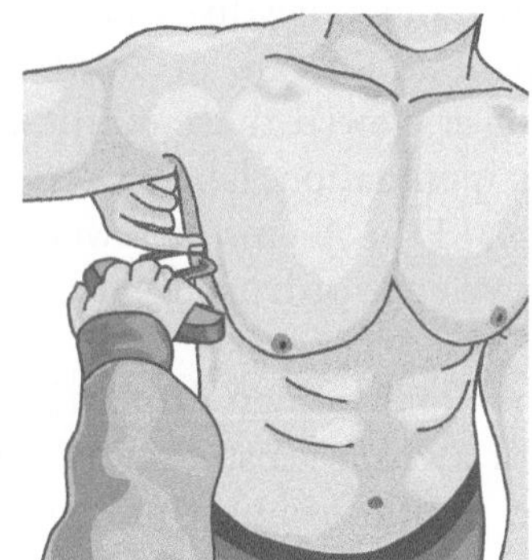

(c)

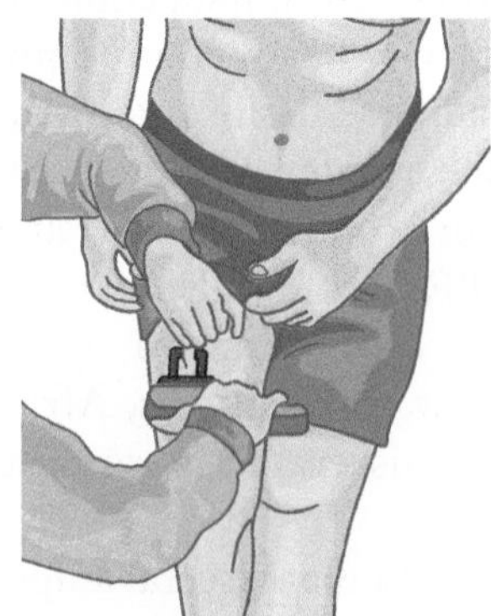

(d)

FIGURE 11 Skinfold sites: (a) triceps (b) chest (c) supraillic (d) thigh

Although SF thickness is inexpensive and easy to measure, it is limited by the training of the of the person performing the assessment, the type of calipers used, and the appropriate selection of the equations to match the population.[68,72] From estimating the TBF percentage, it is possible to calculate lean tissue weight by using the following formula:

Lean tissue weight = Total body weight –
(Total body weight × %BF)

Following protocol is essential, particularly the timing for conducting the test. It should be avoided after the person has been swimming, showering, or exercising, all which increase blood flow and skinfold thickness.[8] Other limitations include compression of subcutaneous adipose tissue; variability of the elasticity of the tissues, specifically in elderly and obese individuals; and inaccuracy of site placement, which can alter measurement results by 1 centimeter.[73,74] All of these can decrease the accuracy of measured SAT, with site placement at 39% and site compressibility ranging from 25% to 37%.[74] This emphasizes the importance of training and having the same clinician perform the measurements by following the measurement protocol.

Children

Skinfold thickness tests correctly detected obesity in children (72.5%) compared to reference tests, with a false-positive rate of 6.3%, and correctly detected overweight in children (78%), with a false-positive rate of 9.7%.[5]

Mid-Upper-Arm Circumference

Another method to quickly assess for malnutrition, particularly protein and energy reserves, is the mid-upper-arm circumference (MUAC). This is an inexpensive, simple measurement that can be implemented for a variety of populations across the life cycle as well as across ethnicities. MUAC requires minimal equipment and calculations compared to weight and height measurements for calculation of BMI, or other anthropometrics such as skinfold thickness. This measurement can be used from the age of 2 months onward. In children, MUAC is useful for assessing nutritional status, predicting mortality, and in some studies, predicting death in children better than any other anthropometric indicator.[75]

A nonelastic measuring tape is used to measure the posterior surface of the upper left arm, with the person standing, weight even on both feet, and facing away from the examiner. The elbow of the left arm is bent at a 90-degree angle, left palm facing up. The upper-arm length is then measured. The tape is placed at the acromion process (shoulder blade) and extended to the olecranon process (elbow). With the tape in place, the examiner places a mark on the posterior surface as the midpoint of the arm (see **FIGURE 12**). The measuring tape is positioned at the midpoint and wrapped flush around the arm, snugly but without causing a compression of the skin, and is measured to the nearest 0.1 cm. An alternative method has the person in a sitting position with the left arm hanging relaxed during the measurements.[76] When the measurement is taken on an infant, a similar procedure is completed with the infant upright, not supine. Numerous studies have shown that MUAC correlates well with BMI in adult populations.[77–79]

In situations when an accurate weight or height is unobtainable, indirect measures are used, leading to poor estimates of the BMI and poor assessment of nutritional status. The MUAC is an anthropometric measurement that correlates with BMI and can be an alternative measure for nutritional status in clinics, the field, and hospitals.[80]

Both the WHO and the United Nations Children's Fund (UNICEF) propose to define nonedematous severe acute malnutrition (SAM) by either an MUAC of <115 mm or by a weight-for-height *Z*-score (WHtZ) of less than −3.[10] The Academy of Nutrition and Dietetics (the Academy), in conjunction with the American Society for Parenteral and Enteral Nutrition (ASPEN), recommend the MUAC as a measure for detecting and documenting pediatric malnutrition.[81]

Studies with children and adults have documented that MUAC is as good a predictor for mortality as BMI is. Since 2007, because of its specificity for identifying high mortality risks in children, MUAC has been the measurement of choice as the single diagnostic anthropometric measure in the community setting for identifying SAM.[10,61] Briend et al. compared the sensitivity and specificity of using MUAC or WHtZ measurements alone or in combination in 5,751 children; it confirmed that MUAC is a more specific and more sensitive measurement for identifying high-risk children, and that including WhtZ brought no added value.[10] Even though combining the two measures increased specificity, the sensitivity for appropriately identifying children at high risk for SAM decreased. Assessment of nutritional status for children typically uses *Z*-scores for height and weight for age as well as weight for height. A WHO Mulicentre Growth Reference study not only

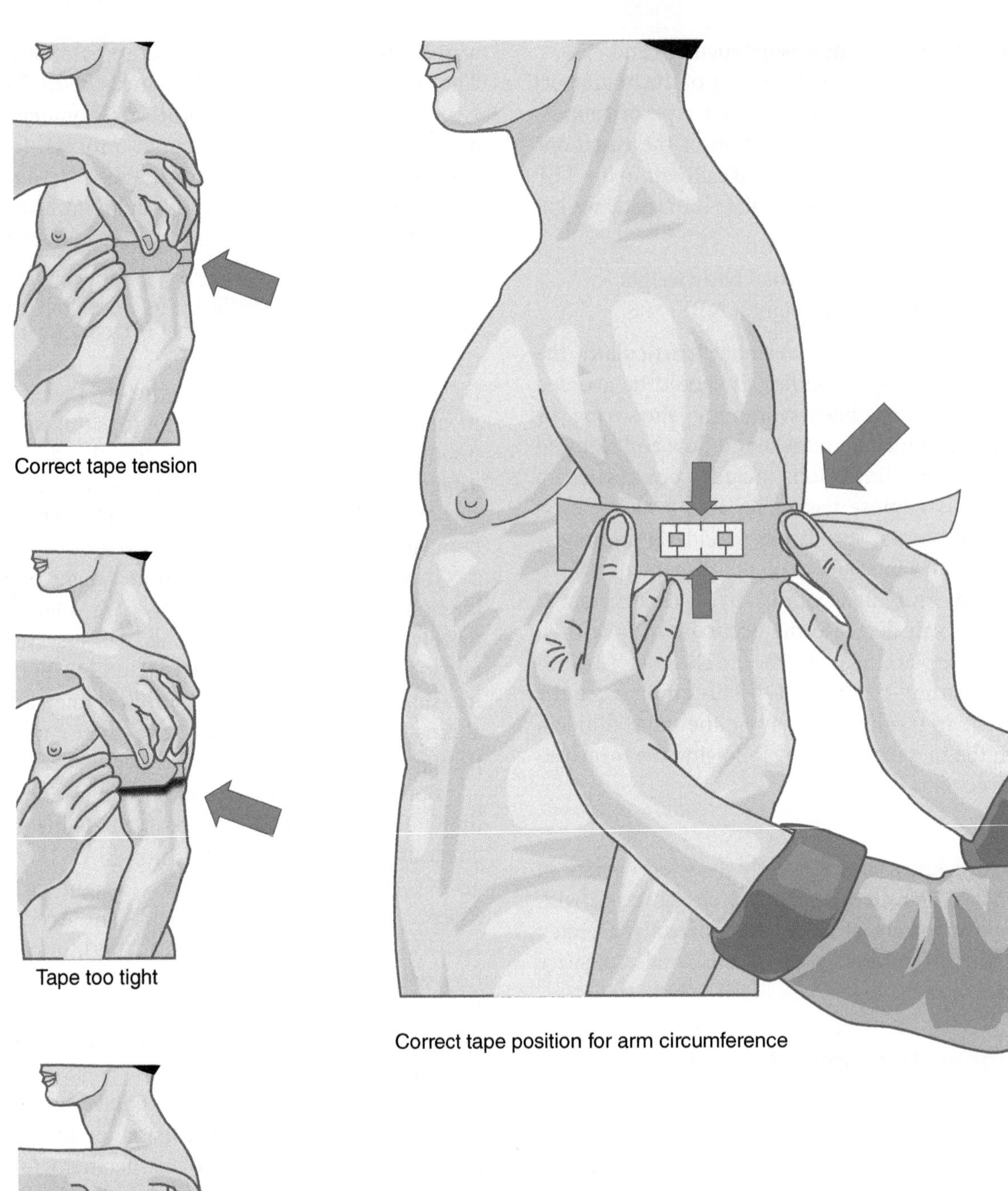

FIGURE 12 Appropriate measurement of mid-upper-arm circumference

evaluated height and weight measures, but included multi-age Z-score for MUAC for children, starting at three months of age.[22,23] A comparison between the use of the MUAC and MUAC Z-score in infants (six to 35 months of age) predicted equally short-term morality risk, with no significant difference in the prevalence of malnutrition or severe malnutrition between the two measures.[82] In lower-income and underdeveloped countries, almost 20 percent of the population are adolescents, underscoring the importance of establishing a cost-effective and rapid anthropometrical measurement for identifying the nutritional status of this population. As an anthropometric measure, MUAC has been shown to have a strong positive correlation with nutritional or protein status with biochemical markers such as serum albumin and serum retinol, confirming its value as a measure of muscle and fat status.[83] Similarly, MUAC, based on its reflecting both muscle and fat stores, is beneficial in obesity screening and determining body fat distribution.[84]

MUAC is beneficial in assessments for weight restoration in children and adolescents being treated for eating disorders. Weight can be of limited value in assessing progress because of time-of-day variability and manipulation by weight loading. Even though peripheral edema caused by fluid restoration following dehydration can affect MUAC, neither rapid water loading nor intense biceps exercising affect the accuracy of this measurement.[85] Research suggests that for children and adolescents being clinically treated for anorexia, MUAC benefits are twofold: First, they confirm the accuracy of weight changes; second, they are better tolerated and produce less anxiety as compared to SF or weight.[86] In adults, MUAC is strongly associated with BMI, but there are no established cutoffs used for identifying malnutrition in the adult population like there is for children. A MUAC at or below 23.5 cm, which indicates an increased risk of low birthweight and poor pregnancy outcomes, has been consistently documented in cross-sectional and longitudinal studies.[84] In healthy, nonpregnant adults and the elderly, a correlation was found between a low BMI (< 18.5) and MUAC (< 24 cm, with women < 22 cm and men < 23 cm) and nutritional risk, with an overall specificity and sensitivity of 70%.

In summary, MUAC has proven to be an accurate, quick method to assess nutritional status and identify acute malnutrition among children and adults, particularly in lower-income environments. It has become one of the main screening indices recommended by the WHO and UNICEF for identifying and starting early treatment for SAM from infancy (three months) to childhood (five years of age).[61] More research is needed for establishing specific MUAC cutoffs to identify not only the risk for malnutrition in adults but also a possible spectrum from moderate to severe, as well as to identify those who will not respond to treatment or are at an increased risk for mortality related to acute malnutrition.

Mid-Upper-Arm Muscle Area

An indirect measure for estimating midarm muscle (MAMA) and fat (MAMF) combines the TSF and MUAC. These measures, compared to NHANES reference tables, can estimate muscle adequacy and wasting (see **TABLE 5**). Estimating MAMA is an evaluation of overall muscle mass and is based on the following assumptions: (1) Arm muscle and bone are circular, and (2) the TSF measurement is twice the thickness of fat and bone. MAMA as a calculated value has historically been overestimated by 15% to 25% but can estimate somatic protein and fat stores.

Midarm muscle or arm muscle area is determined from the MUAC and TSF:

$$\text{MAMA} = \text{MUAC} - (3.14 \times \text{TSF})$$

The MUAC and MAMA can be easily applied to a subject anywhere and at any time by a trained examiner

TABLE 5 Midarm muscle circumference and muscle status

Percentage of Standard Measurement	Muscle Status Category
50	Wasted
60	Below average—depleted
75	Average—marginal
100 ± 20	Adequate
> 120	High muscle

Reproduced from National Health and Nutrition Examination Surveys I and II;: Anthropometric reference data for children and adults: United States, 2003–2006. Natl Health Stat Report Oct 22 (10): 1–48, 2008.(pgs 24-26.) https://www.cdc.gov/nchs/data/nhsr/nhsr010.pdf

with a flexible tape measure and a caliper. Reference tables for MUAC and MAMA have been published in the United States, the United Kingdom, and Japan (see the resources provided in "Online Resources" section). Two-dimensional MAMA is a better indicator of three-dimensional muscle mass when compared with one-dimensional MUAC.[76]

Calf and Thigh Circumference

Similar to the MUAC, calf and thigh circumferences can be measured to assess muscle mass. The loss of skeletal muscle and its associated effects on physiological and functional decline occurring with aging has led to the need for quick and accurate noninvasive methods predicting functional capacity, balance issues or risks for falls, and bone-mineral density (BMD).

Calf Circumference

Because of the complexity and impracticality of using dual-energy x-ray absorptiometry, the National Institute of Aging recommends the use of anthropometric measures such as calf circumference (CC) to assess muscle mass and bone density. Currently, as part of the Mini Nutritional Assessment for Malnutrition and the need for care using either BMI or CC in assessing functional status, the World Health Organization states that CC is a better anthropometric measure and has higher sensitivity than both BMI and MUAC in the older adult.[22] In addition, the CC measurement better depicts body-composition changes, reflecting lower-extremity muscle loss and atrophy contributing to decreased mobility and risk of falling.[87,88] Various cutoffs have been reported in the literature ranging from 29 cm to 33 cm for men and 27 cm to 31 cm for women, with a general cutoff for both of 31 cm as predictive of disability, sarcopenia, and BMD.[89] Higher CC has shown an inverse relationship between CC and frailty and functionality in community-dwelling older adults.[88] Along with the CC as a strong predictor of BMD, particularly for the hip and spine, a higher CC also correlates with structural changes and strength of the hip.

While sitting with feet gently resting on the floor and knee and ankle flexed in a 90-degree angle, the calf circumference is measured using a flexible, nonelastic measuring tape at the bulk area, or the greatest circumference area, of the nondominant leg (i.e., the right leg for a left-handed person); this is most often the midpoint between the patella and the ankle. To be sure the maximum circumference area is being measured, the examiner should take measurements up and down the calf. For the most accurate measurement and to prevent compressing the subcutaneous fat, the tape measure is pulled snuggly but should not constrict the skin; the value is recorded to the nearest 0.1 cm.[7]

Thigh Circumference

Like CC, thigh circumference (TC) is an alternative marker of muscle mass and a predictor of risk for bone fracture because of its linear correlation with BMD and hip strength.[89] TC alone inconsistently predicts bone strength, and it is speculated that the higher fat content of the thigh may influence the measurement.[90] This higher fat composition limits the TC's strength as a predictor of total lean body mass as compared to CC and MUAC. There is an inverse relationship for TC and risk of cardiovascular disease, with two times the risk in those with a TC <55 cm.[91] The TC is measured to the nearest 0.1 cm using a flexible nonelastic measuring tape at the midpoint of the dominant leg (i.e., the right leg for a right-handed person) while the person stands with the weight shifted onto the nondominant leg.[7]

In summary, there is a strong positive correlation of both CC and TC to muscle mass and its value as a predictor of BMD and disability. However, more studies are needed to validate its use for predicting sarcopenia and BMD that take into consideration the influence of changes in the distribution of fat and skin elasticity occurring with aging, with the potential to affect the accuracy of CC and other anthropometric measures.[92] Assessing for muscle mass by using a simple, quick anthropometric measure such as CC is beneficial in a variety of healthcare settings and community living situations for predicting need for care, early interventions, and improving functionality in the aging adult.[93] Also, consideration for population and gender-specific cutoffs, including ethnicity, race, and age, is recommended.

TABLE 6 provides benefits and limitations associated with the use of anthropometric measurements.

Recap Anthropometrics shift to a predictive milieu. Through standardized techniques, repeated measures provide reliable estimates of the percent of fat in the body. These same methodologies allow for the development of population and cultural norms.

TABLE 6 Summary of the benefits and limitations of anthropometric measurements

Benefits	Limitations
Low cost: most require only minimal financial investment	Time of day variances: successive measurements in some methods will vary if not conducted at similar time of day
Ease of training: no special skill sets are needed nor extensive training required	Variations in location or site of measurement: sites on the body must be marked and recorded to ensure accurate replications
Noninvasive: none of the common techniques are invasive	Observational subjectivity: Measurements—especially of length, height, Circumference—can be altered by strength of pull or elasticity of the measuring tape

Data from McDowell MA, Fryar CD, Ogden CL, Flegal KM. Anthropometric reference data for children and adults: United States, 2003–2006. *Natl Health Stat Rep*. 2008; Oct 22 (10);1–48: 24-26. https://www.cdc.gov/nchs/data/nhsr/nhsr010.pdf.

Body Composition

Preview Anthropometrics now shift to qualitative measurements, techniques, and technologies that can provide data on actual body composition.

Assessing changes in BC can augment strategies for the prevention and treatment of disease. BC can be influenced by physical activity, lifestyle choices or interventions, and dietary patterns, as well as by nutritional intake. Accurately assessing and monitoring BC can provide important clinical information for making intervention decisions in disease prevention and in managing and accessing treatment outcomes. As discussed, BMI only assesses a person's weight status or risk for disease and does not portray what proportion or distribution is fat-free mass such as bone and lean mass or adiposity and water.

This section will discuss BC in relation to health and different methods used for assessing BC, including hydrodensity, air-displacement phlethysmography (ADP), **bioelectrical impedance analysis (BIA)**, skinfolds, and densitometry. Depending on the setting, some methods are more applicable for the research, hospital, or community setting. Selecting a technique to use not only depends on the setting but also on its validity, reliability, cost, complexity of what it measures, and practicality.

Body-Composition Models: Reasons to Measure

To fully realize the nutritional status of a person, a measurement or evaluation of the discrete components of BC, including adiposity (body fat), FFM (bone and lean mass), and water are required. All of these can be influenced by disease status and affects a person's health risks. Both the quantity and distribution of adiposity and FFM vary by age, gender, ethnicity, weight changes (loss and gain), growth, activity level, and disease state(s). They also reflect the impact of nutritional intake and tissue losses and gains over time. Determining a person's BC can lead to the development of comparative standards that are gender-, age-, and disease-specific. An individual's BC can support improved understanding of body changes that are occurring, such as decreasing bone density and increasing adiposity in elderlies, or FFM and adiposity changes from malnutrition, a disease state, exercise, or medications.

Understanding and using BC techniques is important in both research and clinical practice. In research, they are used to assess changes in these components as they relate to age, growth, disease risk, and assessment standards.[94,95] For the clinician, BC comparative standards that are disease, gender, and age specific are used in determining treatment strategies, monitoring the effects of an intervention, and achieving improved outcomes. They are important to consider when selecting the method to use, its reproducibility, its accuracy for the population, and how simple it is to perform. Being able to quantify changes in body weight, particularly FFM and assessing for malnutrition, is critical to improving disease management and decreasing healthcare costs. In contrast to BMI and weight-loss percentage, assessing BC (particularly FFM and FM) is a stronger indicator of clinical outcomes and relationships with mortality.[96,97]

Body fat composition varies throughout the life cycle but begins at 10% to 15% in early infancy and increases to 30% at six months.[98] During adolescence, adiposity increases in females compared to males in which there is a rapid increase in FFM. The difference between genders when comparing body fat to FFM continues into adulthood, with females having a higher percentage of **essential fat** and storage fat (**FIGURE 13**).

The rate of increase in body fat slows during early and middle adulthood and is followed by a decline in FFM. It is not clear if there is a true increase in %BF in the elderly or if it just reflects a decrease in FFM caused by sarcopenia or **cachexia**. By definition, sarcopenia is a condition characterized by both a decrease in muscle mass (myopenia) and strength (dynapenia).[92] Depending on the cause, it is classified as either primary (age related) or secondary (related to changes in activity, disease, or nutritional intake).[92] Cachexia differs from sarcopenia because it is a wasting condition occurring concomitantly with a disease state such as cancer, heart

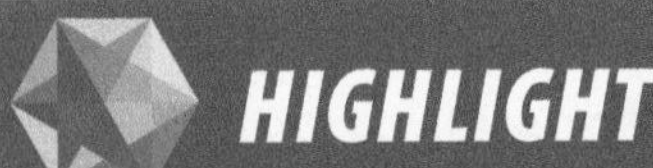

Anthropometrics and Malnutrition: Why Assess?

Malnutrition, or undernutrition, is a problem that occurs not only in the hospital but also in the community. Identifying malnutrition is difficult because it can be the result of inadequate intake or poor nutrient utilization; thus, *malnutrition* and *undernutrition* are synonymous. The prevalence of undernutrition in the hospital setting ranges from 20% to 50% internationally and is a strong factor for extended hospital stays, acute illness, morbidity, mortality, and decreased functionality and quality of life. Since the late 1990s, the Joint Commission—which is an independent, not-for-profit organization, that accredits and certifies nearly 21,000 health care organizations and programs in the United States—has required that institutions assess patients for malnutrition within 24 hours of their admission to a hospital. According to the 10th revision of the *International Classification of Disease*, malnutrition can be identified as a BMI < 18.5 kg/m^2 or by unintentional weight loss because of an intake of less than estimated needs. Anthropometric data are simple to acquire and are part of the six characteristics—energy intake, weight loss, body fat, muscle mass, fluid accumulation, grip strength—for identifying malnutrition by the Academy of Nutrition and Dietetics and the American Society for Parenteral and Enteral Nutrition, including weight, grip strength, body-composition fat, and muscle (see **TABLE A**). Accurate measurements of height and weight are essential for estimating energy needs (EENs) and comparing EENs to a person's recent food intake. Consuming less than 75% of EEN is classified as moderate malnutrition if a person is acutely ill for more than seven days or chronically ill for a month or more. Severe malnutrition is consuming less than 50% of energy needs for five or more days in acute illness and one month or more in chronic illness. Whether in a hospital or community setting, weight loss as a percentage of baseline usual body weight over a period of time should be assessed and monitored regularly. Body composition by both physical signs (around the eyes, face, and rib area) and skinfold measurement (triceps, biceps, subscapular, and suprailiac) can identify subcutaneous fat loss, a sign of malnutrition with mild loss being moderate malnutrition in both acute and chronic illness, and moderate loss equaling severe malnutrition in acute illness, and severe loss for severe malnutrition in chronic illness. Why assess? Early identification and intervention leads to better health outcomes and decreased length of stay and overall health costs. Table A shows how to identify malnutrition.

TABLE A Identifying malnutrition

Criteria	Severe	Moderate/Nonsevere
Estimated energy needs	≤50% for ≥5 days	<75% for >7 days
Loss of body fat	Moderate	Mild
Loss of muscle mass	Moderate	Mild
Reduced grip strength	Reduced based on nomogram	Normal

Modified from White, J. V., Guenter, P., Jensen, G., Malone, A., and Schofield, M. (2012). Consensus statement of the academy of nutrition and dietetics/American Society for Parenteral and Enteral Nutrition: Characteristics recommended for the identification and documentation of adult malnutrition (undernutrition). Journal of the Academy of Nutrition and Dietetics. 112(5). pp. 730–738.

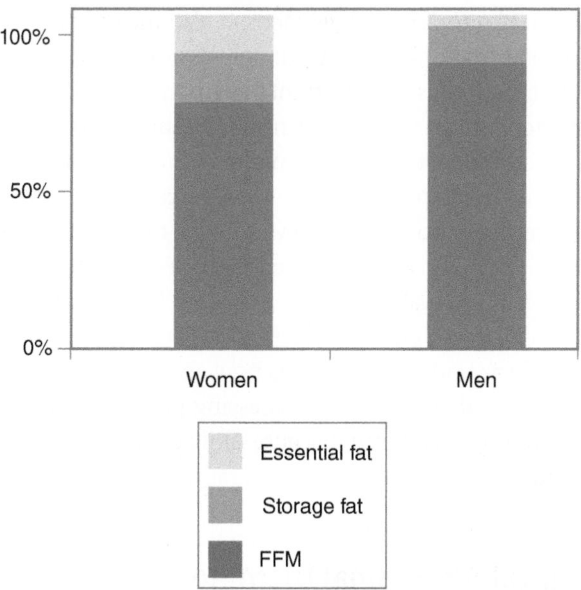

FIGURE 13 Body-composition differences, women and men

Data from Heo M, Faith M, Pietrobelli A, Heymsfield S. Percentage of body fat cutoffs by sex, age, and race-ethnicity in the US adult population from NHANES 1999–2004. *Am J Clin Nutr*. 2012; 95(3):594–602.

failure, or end-stage renal or liver disease. In general, those with cachexia are sarcopenic but not vice versa.[99]

Over the past decade, body fat composition has been considered an important health risk indicator. Body fat composition and distribution appear to be associated with metabolic changes and as a strong predictor for disease risk and not obesity alone.[100] Research demonstrates that the distribution of adipose tissue sets the systemic pathway for increasing the risk for disease development.[100] Body fat is stored in two predominant compartments, **visceral adipose tissue (VAT)** and subcutaneous adipose tissue. VAT makes up 85% of total body adiposity and is located intra-abdominally, surrounding organs. SAT constitutes 10% of total body fat and is found between the muscle and subcutaneous tissue (hypodermis). There are predominantly two body types: **android**, or apple shaped, and **gynoid**, or pear shaped. In the typical android shape, larger fat cells are primarily in the upper part of the body such as the abdomen, which is more common in males and associated with an increased risk for such metabolic diseases as diabetes and cardiovascular disease.[101,102] In the gynoid shape, there are smaller fat cells in the hip and thigh area, which is more common in females. It is not only associated with lower risk for metabolic disease but also may be cardioprotective, especially if located in the thighs, buttocks, and lower abdomen—and is difficult to lose.[103,104] It is possible that the comorbid conditions associated with obesity are related to the visceral fat opposing the expansion of the protective subcutaneous fat, leading to deposition of fat within the organs such as the liver. Recently, the concept of a VAT:SAT ratio has been studied and found to correlate with increased cardiometabolic risk and as a stronger predictor than BMI or VAT. Thus, evaluating where the fat is stored, along with the ratio, may be more useful in determining a person's health risk.[100]

Body-Composition Measurements and Models and Techniques

Body composition can be measured both indirectly and directly. Most of the methods used are indirect measures based on assumptions derived from research and cadaver data on expected components for human BC.[4] FFM contains potassium and is as much as 74% water. Potassium content varies between males and females and is expressed in grams/kilogram of FFM.[4,44] Models for determining BC focus on the components measured. The **two-components model** evaluates only body fat mass and FFM, the **three-components model** adds bone, and the **four-components model** adds bone and total body water (**FIGURE 14**).

Methods also vary in complexity for what is measured from the whole body (BMI, weight, anthropometry), molecular, cellular, and tissue (blood, bone, adipose tissue, skeletal muscle), or **body cell mass (BCM)**. Models measuring the body tissues are used more in the clinical setting because they are less expensive, noninvasive, and fairly simple to use; these include bioelectrical impedance BIA analysis,

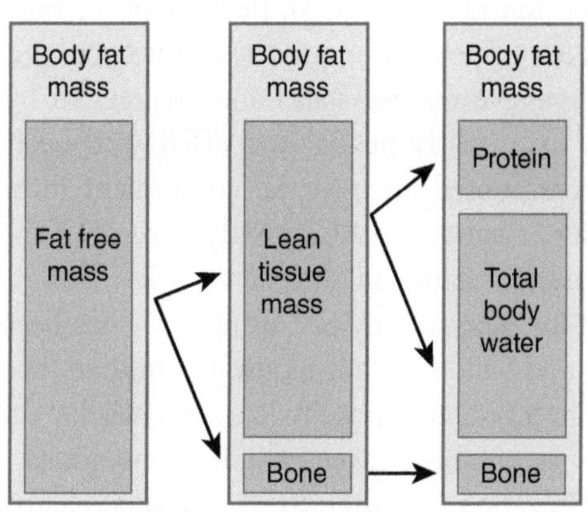

FIGURE 14 Two-, three-, and four-compartment body-composition models

Courtesy Nancy Munoz

Reference: Kuriyan R, Thomas T, Ashok S, J J, Kurpad AV. A 4-compartment model based validation of air displacement plethysmography, dual energy X-ray absorptiometry, skinfold technique & bio-electrical impedance for measuring body fat in Indian adults. *The Indian Journal of Medical Research*. 2014;139(5):700–707.

TABLE 7 Body-composition and anthropometric measures for nutritional assessment	
Protein Status	Mid–arm-muscle circumference Grip strength Plasma proteins
Fat Stores	Triceps skinfold BMI DXA BIA MR or CT Ultrasound Waist circumference Waist to height
Body Water	BIA Weight change Abdominal girth (waist circumference)

dual-energy x-ray absorptiometry, and **computerized tomography (CT)** (**TABLE 7**).[105]

Body Cell Mass

Body cell mass (BCM) is a way to assess body composition. This method evaluates the cellular functions of muscles, viscera, blood, and the brain—in other words, the functioning components of the body. Assessing the BCM is considered important clinically because it can demonstrate the effects of disease, medications, and changes in nutritional status or physical activity at an earlier point.[106] The vast majority of the body's potassium (98%) is found in the BCM. Because of the body's tight regulation of potassium and the fact it remains constant in progressive disease states and changes in hydration status, **total body potassium (TBK)** had been historically considered an essential component in assessing nutritional status and BC.[107] Sixty percent of the body's potassium is found in skeletal muscle (SM). An adult model for determining SM using TBK has been established and validated, but its use in children, because of their lower SM, is uncertain. Research has documented a difference of TBK between children and adults, with an SM:TBK ratio in children (0.0071 6 0.0008 kg/mmol) as compared to SM (kg) 0.0082 TBK (mmol) in adults.[107] Using the WBC method for determining TBK is not only safe and noninvasive but also has a lower standard estimated error at 1.5 kg, as compared to other anthropometric and body-composition measures, which range from 2.2 kg to 2.5 kg. This method also measures BCM and total body protein. Accurately assessing BCM and protein status has an important place in the public-health nutrition arena for evaluating BC changes following nutritional interventions for malnutrition and catch-up growth.[107] BC is often expressed as a percentage of fat and FFM or as a ratio of fat to FFM. Using a two-component model may not be specific enough because the FFM includes bone, water, muscle, and other tissues and thus may not detect significant fluctuations in body protein or loss of lean body mass. TBK is now again being considered as a viable method for assessing protein accretion, particularly in children, because of its potential to more accurately measure protein status rather than FFM or BF percentages.[108]

Sagittal Abdominal Diameter

In clinical practice, adipose tissue—specifically, abdominal adiposity—correlates with a person's risk for metabolic diseases such as diabetes as well as morbidity and mortality.[103] Gold-standard methods, including computerized tomography, **magnetic resonance imaging (MR)**, and DXA, are expensive and not used as an ongoing assessment method because of radiation exposure.[44,109] For clinical practice and ongoing assessment, waist circumference and sagittal abdominal diameter are more applicable for measuring abdominal obesity.[110,111,112] There are four sites identified for measuring WC and SAD: (1) the narrowest point between the thorax and waist, (2) the midway or slimmest point between the last rib and the iliac crest, (3) the highest point or just above the iliac crest, and (4) the umbilical level. In comparison to SAD, WC is a less reliable measure because the measurement can be influenced by anatomical site used, age, and weight. SAD is measured using a standardized sliding beam abdominal caliper with the subject in the supine position, knees bent. Flaccidity of the abdominal muscles can lead to an overestimation of adipose tissue, and site identification can be masked in those who are have prominent abdominal obesity, thus making it hard to identify the thinnest point for measurement, particularly with WC. Accuracy in SAD measurement is increased by placing the person supine, which effectively redistributes subcutaneous fat along the sides of the abdomen, revealing true abdominal height and allowing accurate assessment of visceral fat.[113]

Measuring SAD midpoint or at the highest point of the iliac crest best predicts AT, particularly VAT, no matter the person's age, gender, level of obesity, or cardiometabolic risk.[110,111] In contrast, WC correlates with SAD. Lack of established population-specific reference ranges and cut points is a primary limiting

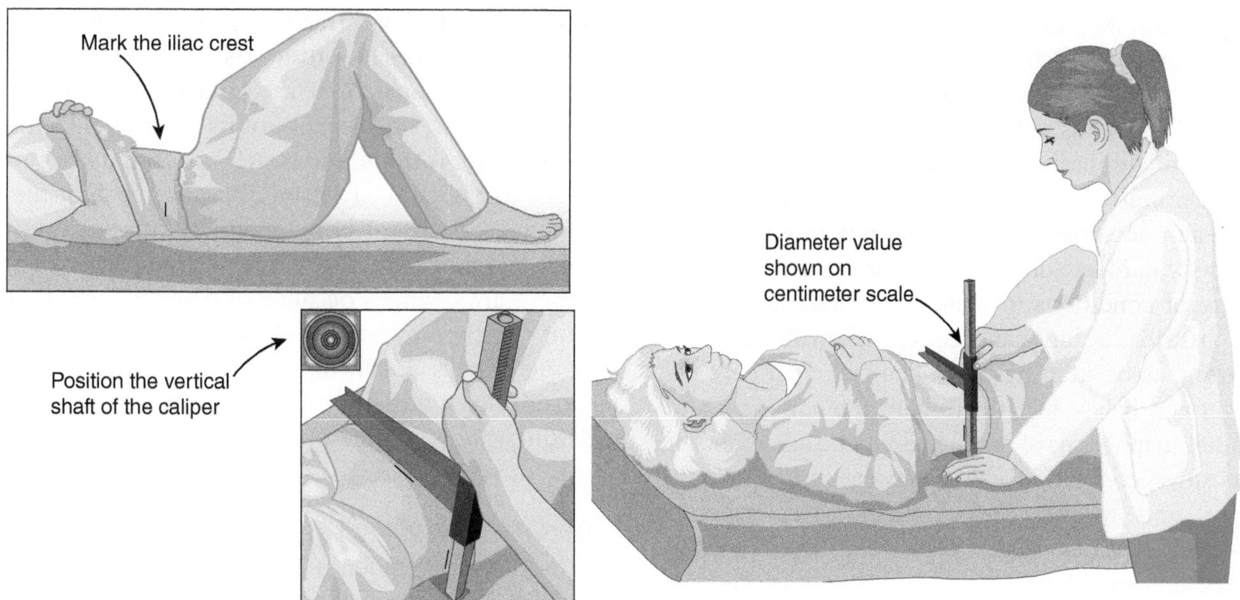

FIGURE 15 Sagittal abdominal diameter measurement

Reproduced from Kahn HS, Gu Q, Bullard KM, Freedman DS, Ahluwalia N, et al. (2014) Population Distribution of the Sagittal Abdominal Diameter (SAD) from a Representative Sample of US Adults: Comparison of SAD, Waist Circumference and Body Mass Index for Identifying Dysglycemia. PLoS ONE 9(10): e108707. doi:10.1371/journal.pone.0108707 Link: https://stacks.cdc.gov/view/cdc/25540/Share

factor to using SAD for nutrition assessment in clinical practice.[4] See **FIGURE 15**.

Handgrip Strength

Handgrip strength (HGS) is a quick, quantitative index for assessing upper-body strength and a good predictor of health changes, morbidity, and mortality for adults as well as children. It has become a valid, acceptable measure for muscle strength and a biomarker for identifying sarcopenia.[92] Clinically, HGS is being used to detect a decrease in muscle strength a because low grip strength (GS) strongly suggests pending cognitive decline, physical disability, and morbidity.[114] A **dynamometer** is used to assess GS and can be isokinetic, electrical, digital, or electronic. See **FIGURE 16**. Grip strength is a measure of the static force exerted in kilograms and pounds when the hand squeezes the dynamometer. Normative data for comparison are used to assess a person's strength and are stratified by age and gender. Male grip strength is greater than for females, and it peaks between the ages of 30 and 40 years and then declines in a linear direction equally in both genders.[115]

The equipment and procedures used for measuring HGS varies, leading to difficulty in interpreting results and establishing standard protocols and comparative standards. In general, the Jamar dynamometer is the most commonly used device, measuring in kg or pounds in 2-kg (5-lb) increments and rounding to the closest kilogram. There are five positions for the handle; hand size determines where the handle is positioned. The second position is the most used and reliable, with handle positions one and five providing the least reliable measurements. HGS is reduced by fingernail length, that extends from 0.5 cm to 1 cm beyond the fingertip for positions one and two, respectively, because it reduces joint movement. In general, the strength of the dominant hand is 10 percent higher than for the nondominant hand for right-handers but not for left-handers, whose hand strength is equal. Factors affecting the accuracy of the HGS measurement include hand size, posture, joint position and nails, time of day for testing, testing frequency, and hand dominance. Providing encouragement during the testing can influence the results, particularly from the tone and volume of the instructions.

A systematic review shows that HGS predicted mortality, extended length of stay in the hospital, and

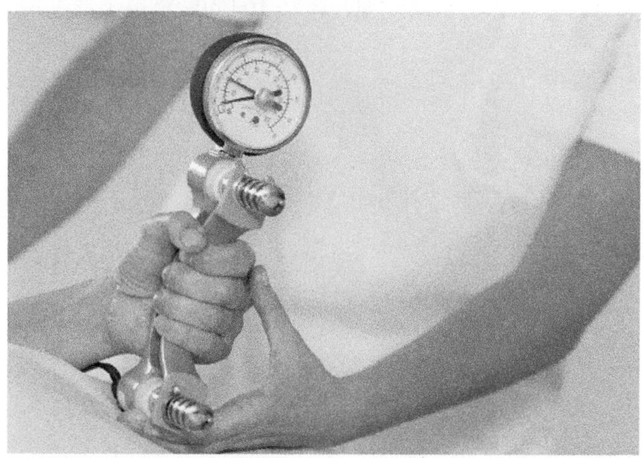

FIGURE 16 Dynamometer

complication risks in older adults better than did other clinical measures such as WHtR, weight loss, and even serum albumin. It is considered to be a strong marker of nutritional status and frailty.[116] Lower HGS is strongly correlated with impaired mobility and is considered a better clinical measure than muscle mass for predicting health outcomes. HGS is used not only in assessing frailty in older adults but also for evaluating a large variety of conditions in children, including rheumatoid arthritis, trauma, and congenital malformations. A strong association has been demonstrated between weight and height in HGS in both the dominant and nondominant hands of both children and adolecents.[117] A positive correlation exists between grip strength, height, and weight. HGS growth curves generate age-specific values, which allows for developmental observation and evaluation of interventions (normative data).[118] Because of its reliability, simplicity, and ease of use in a variety of settings, HGS is considered important as a screening tool for pediatric and adult populations.

Densitometry

Various **densitometry** methods have been used typically to evaluate body volume (BV) and body density, and extrapolated to predict %BF and FFM.[4] The two most commonly used methods, based on the two-compartment model, are underwater weighing or hydrodensity weighing (HW) and air-displacement phlethysmography (**FIGURE 17**).

Both methods assume a consistent body chemical composition, FM density, and FFM density. Variability in bone mineral or water content of the FFM occurring in different conditions or populations inhibits these methods as the reference standard. HW is considered the gold standard for BV measurements, but because of its poor applicability for use in some populations, ADP is used more commonly in the clinical setting. Because both of these assume a consistent body chemical composition of water, minerals, and protein, inaccuracies can occur if there are changes because of disease state, treatment, or therapy and if study population-density characteristics do not apply or are varied (gender, age, ethnicity, athleticism).[109] Each method involves dividing body volume into the body mass and controls for residual lung volume.[7]

Hydrostatic Weighing

Performing HW requires a large tank of water maintained at 37 degrees Celsius. The person being assessed is lowered into the tank while sitting in a basket or on a platform attached to a scale. While completely underwater, the person being measured expels as much air as possible. Using Archimedes' principle, the volume of displaced water determines the volume of the weight loss by calculating the difference in the body weight (dry weight) before submersion from the weight after submersion. The following formula is used to calculate body density:

$$Wa / [(Wa - Ww) / Dw) - (RV + 100cc)]$$

Note that density of the water (Dw) and residual air volume (RV), as well as air volume can be trapped in the intestine. The %BF is then calculate using the Siri equation:

$$(495 / \text{body density}) - 450$$

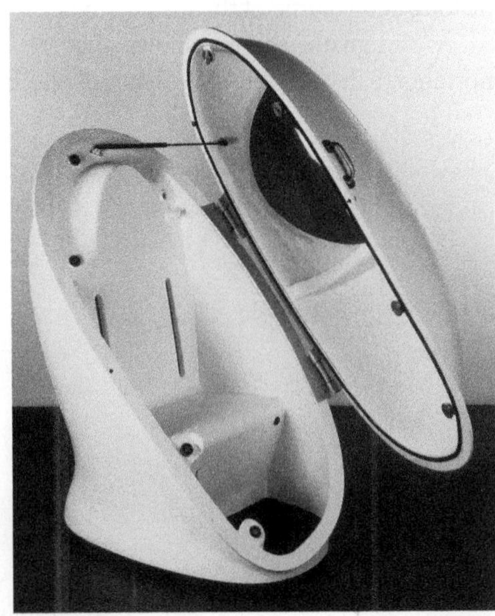

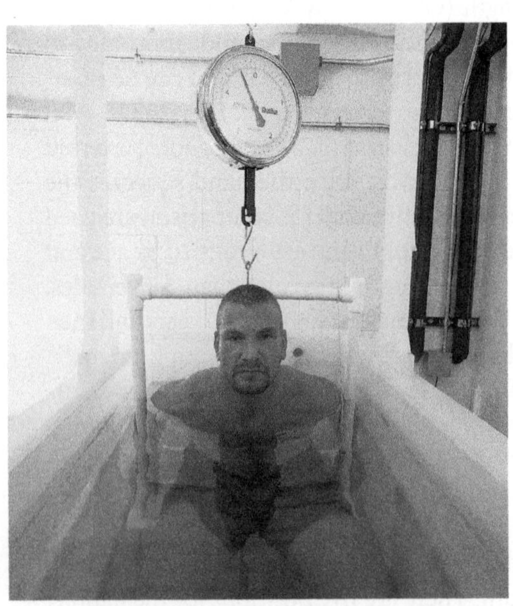

FIGURE 17 BOD POD and underwater weighing

Courtesy of COSMED USA, Inc.

This is the same equation used for skinfold calculations.[7] Even though the body fat estimates are reproducible, this method is not used, because of the test's complexity and problems it presents for some populations, including nonswimmers and those with pulmonary disease, the elderly, and children.[4,109]

Displacement Plethysmography

ADP is conducted using similar principles as the HW for determining body density and is an alternative for a wider population. Commercially, for adults between 35 and 200 kg it is known as the BOD POD. For infants up to 8 kg it is known as the PEA POD.[119] This device measures BV by determining air displacement or changes between when the capsule is empty and when the person is sitting inside it. It applies Poisson's law that, at a constant temperature, pressure is inversely related to volume. ADP is a sealed air capsule in which there are two chambers, a test chamber in the front and a reference chamber at the back, connected by a diaphragm that is not only airtight but also flexible. Small volume changes are caused by the vibrating diaphragm in the test chamber, to which both chambers respond. Before entering the capsule, the person is weighed and then sits for two minutes breathing normally in the capsule before performing a breathing exercise. To calculate residual lung volume, the volume of air the person displaces is estimated by the difference between the air pressure when the capsule is occupied and when it is empty. Because of the effects of clothing and hair altering chamber temperature, the person wears minimal clothing such as a bathing suit and a swim cap. In comparison, HW and ADP calculate body density similarly for normal and obese adults and children (10–15 years old).[120,121] Drawbacks to using ADP include its expense, its need for well-trained technicians, and limited size (greater than 35 kg and less than 200 kg for the BOD POD and up to 8 kg for the PEA POD). In general, ADP use for measuring body composition has good within- and between-day measurements. However, ADP has shown some bias in measuring fat mass and has a total error %BF measurement, which can range from 2% to 6%, particularly if there is uncertainty that temperature conditions are met. Variability determining BC has been demonstrated between HW and ADP for athletes and gender, overestimating body fat percent in males by 2% and underestimating it in females by 8%.[44] It is recommended that both of these densitometry methods be combined with other multicompartment methods to confirm the accuracy of body fat estimations.[109,120] As with other BC methods, strict adherence to protocol is essential, including fasting, no exercise within 12 to 24 hours preceding the test, and maintaining normal hydration.

Dual-Energy X-Ray Absorptiometry

DXA, a three-compartment method, is one of the most versatile methods for assessing body composition in adults and children, providing both regional and whole-body measurements for bone-mineral density, bone-free FFM, and FM. DXA machines transmit low-dose x-rays of different energy peaks. Measuring the amount of x-rays that pass through the bone and bone-free mass, bone density and FFM can be determined by the calculated attenuation ratios (R-values) of the absorption of the two energy frequencies through soft tissue (fat and lean) and bone mineral. The soft-tissue R-value is lower than the bone minerals. A faulty assumption in using DXA is that fat and FFM remain stable, leading to an overestimation of fat in those who are obese and an underestimation in those with lower body fat such as athletes.[122,123] Fluid or hydration status does not seem to affect the DXA BC measurement, but intermachine variability has been documented for both overestimating and underestimating FM.[124] Size and positioning of the person can also lead to errors in body-composition measures.[125,126] Clinical studies have documented limited-effect FM calculations in hemodialysis or in ascites paracentesis but document variations in the measurement in body fat in obese adolescents.[127–129] Also in DXA, comparisons in a four-compartment model indicated good correlations and with no effect of hydration status on body fat measurements.[109,127] Estimating VAT is a recent application of the DXA. This involves measuring SAT width in the abdominal region, along with a geometrically derived formula. The SAT width us subtracted from the total FM to equal the VAT in the abdominal region. There is a concern that DXA overestimates VAT in proportion to increased weight and is not recommended over CT or MRI.

DXA is considered the gold-standard method in determining bone density and for diagnosing osteopenia and osteoporosis.[130] A *T*-score is calculated based on the bone density of a healthy 30-year-old. This reference population is used because this is the age when bones have reached peak development and are at their strongest. The lower the ***T*-score**, the weaker or thinner the bones, detecting osteoporosis, a condition characterized as porous, fragile bone resulting from the loss of the calcium hydroxyapatite and collagen matrix. Osteoporosis is diagnosed when BMD is 2.5 standard deviations below the reference population. Because of documented differences for gender and ethnicity, a *Z*-score is calculated and represents values derived from a reference population that is age, gender, and ethnicity matched.[130] Often a decreased BMD *T*-score will occur with the *Z*-score remaining stable; thus, the *Z*-score more accurately depicts the BMD changes. BMD is considered to be the most prominent assessment for bone health and fracture risk because the risk for fracture increases with every reduction in standard deviation. Typical DXA focus on the spine and hip because peak bone is reached in these areas by 30 years of age and then declines. Peripheral DXA (P-DXA) scans arms and legs and may not detect changes or risk. The International Society for Clinical Densitometry and the US Preventive Screening Task Force for Osteoporosis recommend the spine and hips (femoral neck or total proximal femur) as the recommended scanning sites.[131,132] Kalkwarf et al. conducted a three-year longitudinal study examining bone-mineral content (BMC) and bone-mineral density (BMD) in children and adolescents.[133] Baseline *Z*-scores were predictive of the *Z*-scores at three-year follow-ups, with those at below average scores at baseline continuing with low BMC and BMD at follow-up, indicating screening for BMD earlier using gender- and age-specific *Z*-scores. These scores, along with clinical risk factors such as smoking, family history, and lifestyle factors, led to the computerized screening algorithm used in the **WHO fracture-risk assessment tool (FRAX)** for men and women.[134]

Bioelectrical Impedance Analysis

Bioelectrical impedance analysis (BIA) is another method used to determine BC. This method uses measurements of resistance and reactance or impedance of electrical conductivity of the body. In theory, electrical current passes through the low-resistance electrolyte-containing water portion of the body. BIA systems can be single frequency or multi-frequency. Electrodes are placed on the body to transmit a signal that is measuring the opposition of body tissues to the flow of a small (< 1 mA) varying current.[44] The paired placement of electrodes can be arm-leg, leg-leg, or arm-arm (see **FIGURE 18**).

The arm-leg pairing is the most commonly used, with four total electrodes, two on the arm and two on the leg, usually on the right side of the body. The leg-leg method concurrently measures weight and impedance and does not estimate FFM as accurately, because

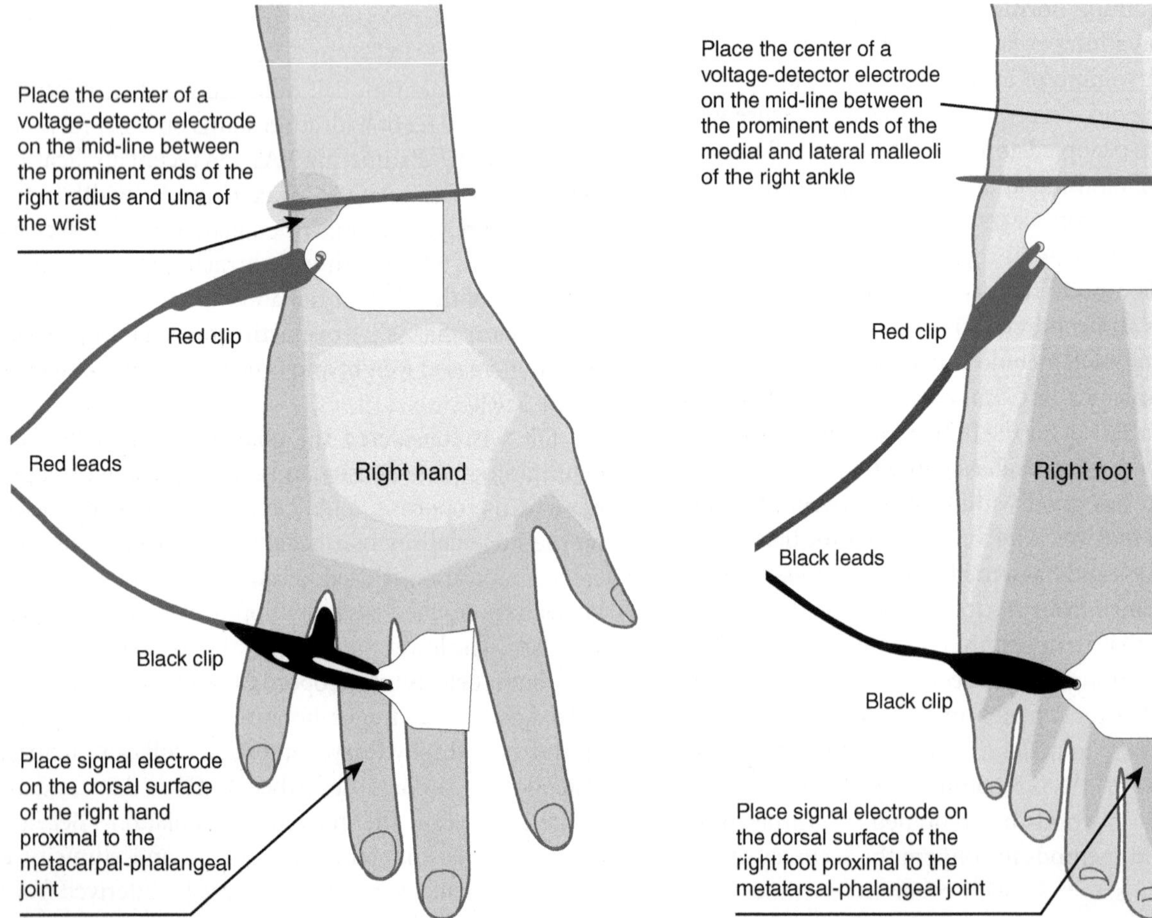

FIGURE 18 Placement of electrodes

Data from Cheryl Winter. DiabeteStepsRX.com. http://diabetestepsrx.com/product/medgem-metabolic-analysis-body-composition-analysis-package/

it only measures the legs and part of the abdomen. Similarly, the arm-arm method measures the arms and part of the abdomen. BIA measurements (resistance versus reactance) are calculated based on how resistance correlates with the amount of body water and lean tissue, thus determining the TBW and FFM. The impedance is caused by two vectors: (1) resistance to the tissues, along with (2) the reactance to the strength of the cell membranes, the nonionic tissues, and tissue membrane. Like the other methods described, FFM is calculated with the assumption that hydration status is stable. Total body fat is then determined as the difference between a person's TBW and FFM. In comparison to other methods, BIA is similar, with a margin of error of 3% to 4% for HW, and 2% to 2.5% for ADP.[44,109,120,121] Advantages of using this method include its ease of use in both clinical and research settings, its low expense, and its portability. It also does not require extensive training to operate. Clinically, BIA, particularly multifrequency, is effective in quantifying fluid shifts (extracellular and intracellular) in disease states in patients with renal disease and heart failure.[135] It should not be used if hydration status is not stable—that is, during growth, pregnancy, following exercise, in the morbidly obese, for athletes, and for the undernourished.[44,136,137]

Total Body Water: Hydration Status

For all BC assessment techniques, understanding hydration status and its effect on accurately determining body fat and FFM is important.[44,138] Errors in the estimation of hydration status from changes in body mass can occur as a result of changes in tissue osmolality due to substrate metabolism and the release of water bound to muscle glycogen.[138] Water is 50% to 70% of total body mass, with lean tissue being predominantly water (70% to 80%) and fat mass (~20%). Alterations in body water can be affected by a disease state, with losses up to 1 liter/hour as in acute diarrhea or in vomiting, and even as much as 3 liters/hour during exercise in hot and humid environments. Disease states that change the metabolism of water, such as malnutrition or edema, can skew hydration calculations. Hydration can be as high as 75% with severe protein malnutrition; similar results are seen with edema. In athletes such as bodybuilders, because of their expanded muscle mass, the hydration constant can increase by 3%.[139] For example, body fat composition estimation can increase by almost 22% with a 10% loss of body water. Both FFM and TBW are both used to determine hydration status, both dehydration and overhydration.[140] Water isotopes such as deuterium oxide used in the deuterium dilution process are the main techniques used to determine total body water. Bromide is used for extracellular water, and radioactive potassium isotope is used for intracellular water. All of these are expensive and cannot be used to clinically assess short-term fluid shifts. Other less-expensive methods have been used, including urinary tests for color, urine specific gravity and osmolality, plasma osmolarity, and sodium concentration, with urine tests being more reliable in detecting mild to moderate changes in hydration status.

Imaging

Magnetic resonance imaging and computed tomography are two imaging techniques that provide the most precise and specific tissue-level analyses, including measures of total adipose tissue, subcutaneous adipose tissue, visceral adipose tissue, and intestinal adipose tissue.[44,109] MRI is a noninvasive method that uses strong magnets and radio waves to construct an image; it can provide high-resolution images of vessels as small as 2 mm in diameter, which enables the detection of an occlusion or tumors in difficult-to-access areas. CT is a radiographic technique, with or without intravascular injection of a contrast material, to display a cross-sectional image of targeted areas.

Magnetic Resonance Imaging

The MRI provides an in-depth view of the chemical composition of body tissue. It is not used to quantify body composition but to form images of organs, structures, and tissues using magnetic fields and radio waves that interact with hydrogen nuclei in the body.[141] To perform this test, a person is placed in a closed system or under a strong magnetic field. The hydrogen nuclei absorb the energy from a radio frequency (RF) pulse and align with the magnetic field. When the energy is released from the nuclei, the nuclei realign and release RF, which are captured to produce an image. In contrast, magnetic resonance spectrometry expands the view to distinguish chemical structures in the area, such as fat from muscle. Both focus on producing images of the body's soft tissues. The MRI is used for a variety of medical purposes, including diagnoses, disease detection, staging, and monitoring treatment. It is used to provide information on something discovered in an ultrasound scan or CT—the causes for bleeding, for example. Segmental MRIs are less expensive and take less time, and research shows they correlate with whole-body tissue measures in cancer and sarcopenic obesity.[109,141]

Computed Tomography

Complementing both ultrasound and x-ray, computed tomography involves an x-ray tube and a receiver that attenuates the x-rays to produce an image made of pixels, each measuring a unit of attenuation in relation to water and air or Hounsfield unit (HU). The HU value represents the density of the tissue, with adipose tissue equaling −190 to −30 and skeletal muscle 30 HU to 100 HU. The person undergoing the CT scan lays on an examination table that slides in and out of the box- or tunnel-like scanner. Each cross-sectional segment of tissue is calculated. Because of the risk of high radiation exposure, whole-body scans are not done. Similar to the MRI, the CT is a diagnostic test used to detect the presence of a tumor, as well as its size and location, and vascular diseases related to a stroke, pulmonary embolism, or aortic aneurysm.[141,142]

Using an MRI offers several advantages. It is noninvasive, does not use dyes or ionizing radiation, provides good-quality images of soft tissue, and distinguishes the amount and location of body fat, making it a better option than the CT. Also, key minerals can be imaged, including phosphorus, sodium, hydrogen, and potassium. Its biggest disadvantages are cost and that it cannot be used with people who are claustrophobic. The CT has limited use in the assessment of body composition and is not recommended for children, women of childbearing age, and for multiple scans of the same person. For regular everyday use, neither MRI nor CT are recommended for body-composition assessment.

Ultrasound

Another technique used for assessing body composition is the **ultrasound** transducer, also known as color Doppler imaging (CDI), either A mode or B mode. The A mode scans for the continuity of the area, and CDI involves the use of a brightness-mode ultrasound device (B mode) with a pulsed Doppler flow detector to provide a two-dimensional color image of the of the area being scanned.[143] Often both are used together. The differences in velocity are represented by variations in the colors and their brightnesses. This scanning method allows for isolating and identifying body fat and lean tissue based on sound reflected from ultrasound waves and differences in the acoustic impendence between the tissues, with stronger sound being produced from muscle than from fat. The scanning process uses a bonding gel on the skin or the transducer to improve the sound reflection or decrease sound artifacts. Depending on the reason for the test, the ultrasound technician slides the transducer over the area to be evaluated, ranging from as little as +/−5 mm. To measure body tissue thickness, a two-dimensional picture is produced that shows stronger images or interfaces in white for subcutaneous fat to skin and muscle to bone but weaker images for the interface between fat and muscle. There are no established protocols for the use of ultrasound for measuring body composition in general. In comparison to other techniques, there is inter-rater variability, similar to but slightly higher than with skinfold measurements, and equal predictive capability of BF% as the DXA, with one-site abdomen measurement for healthy adults and athletes.[73,144] Leahy et al. developed equations, including lower-limb measurements with the abdomen, for men and women, with highly predictive accuracy of body composition.[145]

The advantages of for ultrasound outweigh the limitations, including quick test, non-invasive, portability, low cost, ability to obtain regional and segmental measurements, and to determine muscle and bone tissue thickness. The primary limitation is the interpretation. Results interpretation can be more subjective and difficult because the image that appears contains both continuous, bright, light interfaces (skin-fat, fat-muscle, or muscle-bone) and fascia light streaks which can be confused as body composition interfaces. It is important that the technician be trained to identify the interfaces correctly. There are no standard protocols for ultrasound procedure, but consideration of the site and force of the transducer applied by the technician can vary the subcutaneous adipose tissue by 25% to 37%, and scanning longitudinally is better than scanning vertically.[73]

Summary of Body Composition Methods

Clinically, DXA or ultrasound appear to be the best measures of sarcopenia, while ultrasound has the added advantage of being able to measure changes in tendons. CT or MRI give excellent measurements of muscles and can delineate fat infiltration, but they are very expensive as capital outlays and in operating and staffing costs. Due to the uncertainty regarding levels of hydration in the subjects, Bioelectrical Impedance BIA measures have questionable value. Both MUAC and calf circumference are inexpensive but inaccurate measures of muscle mass.

Recap These evolving technologies facilitate the non-invasive analysis of body composition. Whether modified from earlier predictive techniques, or innovative adaptations of imaging or applied physics, the barriers to qualitative physical assessment are being removed.

Chapter Summary

Since the days of Johann Sigismund Elsholtz and the publication of his *Anthropometria*, there has been a concerted effort to investigate and measure the human body for scientific and medical purposes. Since that time, there has been a quantitative approach to acquiring data concerning variations and changes in the human form, and describing the relationship between the human body and disease. These measurements found a ready application in the assessment of a person's nutritional status, involving more than just evaluating what a person eats, but also in determining his or her body composition and comparing this person's growth and development to accepted standards. Anthropometric assessment rapidly evolved into an essential feature in conducting a nutritional evaluation for determining malnutrition; in defining overweight status and obesity; and in quantifying loss of muscle mass, increase in fat mass, and in the redistribution of adipose tissue.

Anthropometrics includes measurements of body weight, stature or composition; or a focus on specific area measurements, such as circumference (waist and hip), skinfold, and bone dimensions. Some provide direct measurements (i.e., height and weight); others are others derived (i.e., body composition). The application of universal cut-off points has the dual advantage of allowing comparisons between populations and also the prevention of bias on the part of staff when performing initial assessment or follow-up of patients. Additionally, cut-off points can be used to characterize changes and trends within a population and identify persons at a higher risk for adverse outcomes. Body measurements are essential in the analysis of the development and/or progression of disease and also to monitor the efficacy of treatment. Accurate measurement of changes in body composition due to interventions is vital in planning nutritional care and the management of developmental and aging processes, disease progression, and rehabilitation efforts.

In order to evaluate suspected short or tall stature, accurate measurements of height and weight are plotted on a standardized, appropriate-age growth chart. Age-sex-specific percentiles are often utilized to assess growth and nutritional status in children, based on anthropometric measures. Weight and stature are key for assessing growth patterns and determining deviations from the norms for a specified population. Being that weight includes an overall measurement of the body compartments, it is important it be included as a general measure as part of the nutrition assessment.

BMI is determined from the measurements of height and weight; calculating the relative proportion between the two, it is a valid predictor of adiposity. BMI is recommended in the clinical setting as the most appropriate single indicator of overweight and obesity in the pediatric population. Established norms for BMI can allow the clinician to estimate morbidity (chronic-disease risk) and mortality.

Waist circumference has been accepted internationally as a valid anthropometric measurement for identifying central/visual adiposity as well as an established component of metabolic syndrome, a predictor of risk for cardiovascular disease and type 2 diabetes. Skinfold measurement uses specially designed calipers to measure the subcutaneous fat, the original but still useful method for assessing body composition. Additional methods have been developed, including mid-upper-arm circumference, to assess nutritional status, predict mortality, and, in some studies, predict the death of children better than any other anthropometric indicator. MUAC has proven to be an accurate and quick method to assessing nutritional status and identifying acute malnutrition among children and adults, particularly in lower-income environments.

More complex and impractical methods such as DXA have been recommended by various organizations. Ultrasound scanning, another technologically intense method, allows an examiner to isolate and identify body fat and lean tissue based on sound reflected from ultrasound waves and differences in the acoustic impedance between tissues. Even as the technology evolves, the desired outcome remains constant: to best assess the health and growth of the person through accurate, quantifiable, and qualitative measurements.

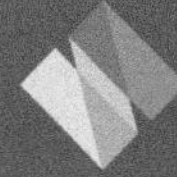

CASE STUDY

Daniel is a 74-year-old male, of height 5'9" (69"), weight 130 lbs (58.9 kg), and usual body weight 175 lbs (79.37 kg). He is a widower who lives in an apartment of a large continuing-care retirement community (CCRC). Daniel has lived there for many years and gets along quite well. He was diagnosed as having thyroid cancer 1 year ago; in the past 6 months, his weight has gradually decreased to his current 130 lbs. He is seen in the CCRC clinic an average of every three months for regular follow-ups. The facility has a congregate meal program, but lately, he refuses to eat there. Staff members bring him food from the grocery store, and he buys foods that he likes. Much of this goes

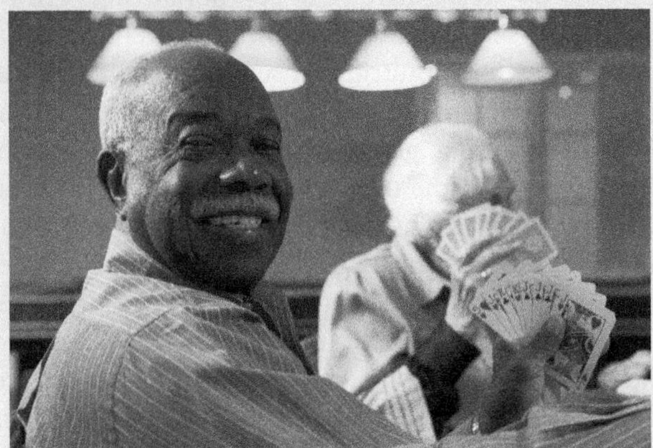

© Monkey Business Images/Shutterstock.

uneaten, however. His labs reveal that his visceral proteins are depleted (low serum albumin). Daniel's triceps skinfold measurement reveals a body fat value that is 50% of the standard. His oral intake ability has decreased gradually; he can only take sips of a high protein supplement (such as Ensure) and occasional bites of food.

Questions:

1. Daniel's current weight is what percentage of his usual body weight?
2. His current weight is what percentage of his ideal body weight?
3. Calculate the percentage loss of body weight from usual weight.
4. Calculate his BMI at his usual weight. What is his BMI at his current weight? Interpret his current BMI and compare it to his usual weight.
5. Explain what his triceps percentile means as compared to his weight-loss pattern and BMI.
6. What degree of undernutrition is he exhibiting? Explain why you would classify him as exhibiting malnutrition.

Additional Anthropometrics

Have students perform the triceps skinfold, mid-upper-arm circumference, sagittal abdominal diameter, calf circumference, and waist-circumference measures.

1. Have the students calculate their BMI and WHtR values.
2. Using these measurements, have the students discuss what the numbers mean regarding body composition and health risk.

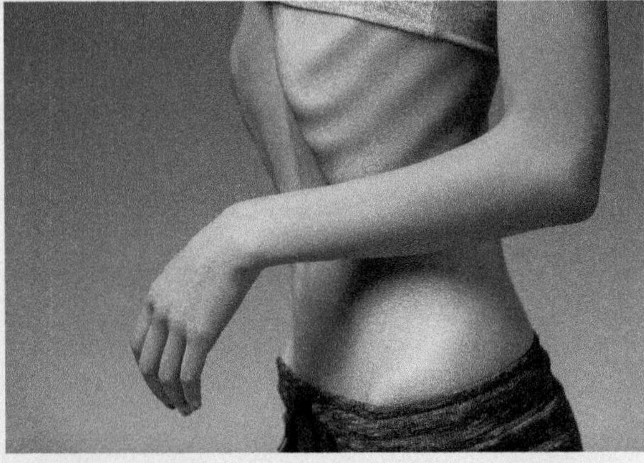

© Vgstockstudio/Shutterstock.

3. Discussion should include outlining the difference between TSF and MUAC. Is one of them better?

Class Case Study

Barbara is a 30-year-old female, 5'1" (61") tall and weighs 85 lbs (38.5 kg). She has a long history of eating disorders and substance abuse. She calls in sick from her job at the hospital, where she works as a cook. When working, she has the benefit of one free meal on the days she works. She eats most of her other meals out and prepares few meals at home. Because she frequently missed work—this was the third time this month—Barbara's employer insists she bring verification from her doctor that she is cleared to return to work. Her doctor is concerned about her dietary pattern and that she appears undernourished. He calculates the following:

- Ideal weight from the Hamwi equation is 105 lbs. Weight ranges from 94 to 105 lbs.
- BMI: 16.1
- Waist: 20 cm
- Waist-to-height ratio: 33

Measure	Value	Percentile
TSF (mm)	6	< 5th
MAFA (mm^2)	746	< 5th
MUAC (mm)	258	10th to 25th
MAMA (mm^2)	4554	> 75th

Explain what the percentiles mean for her mid-arm fat area, mid-arm muscle area, and TSF. What conclusions do you have about her body composition from these measurements? What interpretations would you make regarding her body composition and nutritional risk? Would you recommend any other anthropometric measurements? Will the doctor clear her to go back to work?

Questions:

1. Discuss the innovative adaptations of imaging or applied physics and barriers to qualitative physical assessment.
2. Summarize and discuss the differences between the methods reviewed in the chapter.
3. What is the most accurate method for measuring fat-free mass versus fat mass?
4. Are the techniques appropriate for a hospitalized patient? What about an outpatient in an ambulatory care setting?

Plotting Case Study

Calculate the percentiles (use growth charts to plot) for a baby boy with the following data, born June 1, 2016.

1. What is the growth velocity at 21/2 months of age? Is it average, below, or above average?
2. What is the growth velocity between 9 and 12 months of age? Is it average, below, or above average?

Learning Portfolio

Key Terms

Adiposity
Android
Anthropometric indicator
Anthropometrics
Anthropometry
Bioelectrical impedance analysis (BIA)
Body cell mass (BCM)
Body composition (BC)
Body mass index (BMI)
Cachexia
Computerized tomography (CT)
Cutoff point
Densitometry
Dual-energy x-ray absorptiometry (DXA)
Dynamometer
Essential fat
Fat-free mass (FFM)
Frontal-occipital circumference
Four-components model
Gynoid
Handgrip strength (HGS)
Height velocity
Kyphoscoliosis
Magnetic resonance imaging (MRI)
Percentile
Sarcopenia
Skinfold thickness
Subcutaneous adipose tissue (SAT)
Two-components model
Three-components model
Total body potassium (TBK)
Total body water
Triceps skinfold thickness (TSF)
T-score
Visceral adipose tissue (VAT)
Ultrasound
Weight to length
WHO fracture-risk assessment tool (FRAX)
Z-score

Study Questions

1. ________ is a measurement(s) including height and weight assessed in combination with age and gender.
   a. Anthropometric index
   b. Percentile
   c. Cutoff
   d. BMI
2. The purpose of cutoffs is:
   a. To make a change based on the examiner's judgment.
   b. To make comparisons between populations and decrease assessment bias.
   c. Not used for trending data.
   d. Arbitrarily determined by ethnicity and race.
3. A patient has a BMI of 30. This is considered to be:
   a. Obese.
   b. Normal.
   c. Underweight.
   d. Protein energy malnutrition.
4. The IBW range for a female who is 5'7" tall is:
   a. 155 ± 10%.
   b. 135 ± 10%.
   c. 125 ± 10%.
   d. 165 ± 10%.
5. If a patient has a UBW of 200 lbs and now weighs 150 lbs, what is the percentage weight loss?
   a. 25%
   b. 24%
   c. 20%
   d. 15%
6. The patient has experienced an unintentional weight loss of more than 10% in six months. This weight loss is considered:
   a. Moderate.
   b. Severe.
   c. Normal.
   d. Healthy.
7. The TSF:
   a. Measures muscle protein directly.
   b. Represents visceral fat.
   c. Is an index for body fat stores.
   d. Represents visceral protein.
8. Mid-upper-arm circumference:
   a. Measures muscle protein (lean muscle).
   b. Represents visceral fat.
   c. Is an index for body fat stores.
   d. Represents visceral protein.

9. A person who has >85% arm muscle area is considered:
   a. Above average for muscle and excess fat.
   b. Average for muscle and excess fat.
   c. At a deficit for muscle and excess fat.
   d. Below average for muscle and excess fat.

10. A person's basal metabolic rate is directly related to:
   a. Body fat.
   b. Muscle mass.
   c. Total body cell mass.
   d. Fluid mass.

11. Body mass index:
   a. Is synonymous with obesity.
   b. Measures obesity by considering both weight and height.
   c. Measures lean body mass relative to fat mass.
   d. Of 27 corresponds to morbid obesity.

12. A body weight (as a percentage of usual body weight) of 89% is considered to be:
   a. Healthy
   b. Mildly malnourished.
   c. Moderately malnourished.
   d. Severely malnourished.

13. Percent usual body weight is calculated as:
   a. Percent body weight = (current weight/usual weight) × 100.
   b. Percent body weight = (current weight/usual weight) × 50.
   c. Percent body weight = (usual weight/current weight) × 100.
   d. Percent body weight = (ideal body weight/usual weight) × 25.

14. The weight distribution of women who carry most of their weight in the hips is described as:
   a. Android obesity.
   b. Gynoid obesity.
   c. Anthropometry.
   d. A high metabolic health risk.

15. A skinfold assessment is a method for determining total body fat by measuring ________ body fat.
   a. Visceral
   b. Subcutaneous
   c. Essential fat
   d. The ratio of visceral to subcutaneous fat.

16. The most common site used for obtaining skinfold thickness measurements is the:
   a. Biceps skinfold
   b. Fluteal skinfold
   c. Subscapular skinfold
   d. Triceps skinfold

17. ________ fat is the type that is needed by the body to function optimally and protect its organs.
   a. Essential
   b. Storage
   c. Nonessential
   d. Somatic

18. What body-composition measurement technique involves the use of a device that measures the body's resistance to an electrical current?
   a. DXA
   b. BOD POD
   c. PEA POD
   d. BIA

19. In terms of BC measurement, what body tissue is a good conductor of electricity?
   a. Bone
   b. Muscle
   c. Fat
   d. Connective tissue

20. What anthropometric device assesses body composition by displaced air?
   a. DXA
   b. BOD POD
   c. Hydrostatic weighing
   d. BIA

21. What anthropometric device assesses body composition by displaced water?
   a. DXA
   b. BOD POD
   c. Hydrostatic weighing
   d. BIA

22. What anthropometric device assesses body composition by using x-ray technology?
   a. DXA
   b. BOD POD
   c. PEA POD
   d. BIA

23. Which of the following is the most suitable anthropometric measurement for the clinical setting?
   a. BIA
   b. DXA
   c. Air displacement
   d. Underwater weighing

24. ________ fat is considered stored fat.
   a. Subcutaneous
   b. Adipose
   c. Visceral fat
   d. All

25. The fat stored around the organs is known as:
   a. Adipose tissue.
   b. Visceral fat.
   c. Subcutaneous fat.
   d. Topical fat.
26. If a person's weight distribution is characterized by fat stored in the abdominal region and upper body, it is called:
   a. Android.
   b. Gynnoid.
   c. Nonmetabolic.
   d. Protective.
27. Lean mass includes all:
   a. Muscle, bone, and tissue.
   b. Essential fat, tissue, and bone.
   c. Muscle and stored fat.
   d. Stored fat, essential fat, and bone.
28. What is compared when determining body composition?
   a. Muscle to bone
   b. Adipose tissue to muscle
   c. Fat-free mass to muscle
   d. Fat mass to adipose tissue
29. ________ are calculated from the distribution using the mean and standard deviation of the reference population.
   a. Percentiles
   b. *Z*-scores
   c. *T*-scores
   d. Beta scores
30. ________ is a quantitative index for assessing upper-body strength, a good predictor of measure for muscle strength, and a biomarker for identifying sarcopenia
   a. Waist circumference
   b. Handgrip strength
   c. Demispan
   d. Ulna measurement

Discussion Questions

1. How did the study of anthropometrics transition from the world of art to the world of health?
2. Compare and contrast the differences between anthropometric indicators and cutoff points. Explore NHANE's website (https://www.cdc.gov/nchs/nhanes/) and provide examples of how they are used.
3. Discuss why it is important to use established growth charts. What are the benefits of plotting the data?

Activities

1. Plotting case study
   At what percentiles (use growth charts to plot) is a baby boy (date of birth June 1, 2016) with the following data:
   a. What is the growth velocity at 2½ months old? Is it average, below average, or above average?
   b. What is the growth velocity between 9 and 12 months? Is it average, below average, or above average?
      (1) At birth: Wt 3.9 kg, Lt 51 cm, HC 35 cm
      (2) At August 15, 2016: Wt 6.18 kg, Lt 60.5 cm, HC 40.5 cm, Wt/Ht:
      (3) At March 1, 2017: Wt 7.9 kg, Lt 71 cm, HC 44.4 cm, Wt/Ht:
      (4) At June 1, 2017: Wt 8.6 kg, Lt 73 cm, HC 45 cm, Wt/Ht:
      (5) At December 1, 2017: Wt 9.0 kg, Lt: 78 cm, HC: 46.1 cm, Wt/Ht:
2. Determining BMI and waist circumference
   Accurately measure your height, weight, and waist circumference. Using the information provided in this chapter, calculate your BMI.
   a. What is your BMI classification?
   b. Based on your BMI classification, what is your health status?
   c. What is your waist circumference classification?
   d. What is your disease-risk classification?

Online Resources

CDC Growth Charts:
http://www.cdc.gov/growthcharts/who_charts.htm

WHO Growth Standards:
http://www.who.int/childgrowth/en/

Medscape Nutrition and Growth Measurement Technique:
http://emedicine.medscape.com/article/1948024-technique

FRAX® Fracture Risk Assessment Tool:
https://www.shef.ac.uk/FRAX/

Anthropometric Reference Data for US Children and Adults, 2007–2010:
https://www.cdc.gov/nchs/data/series/sr_11/sr11_252.pdf

Nutri Stat—Nutritional Anthropometry Program:
https://nutristat.codeplex.com/

Human Factors and Anthropometric Data:
http://researchguides.library.tufts.edu/humanfactors/anthropometric

FANTA:
https://www.fantaproject.org/sites/default/files/resources/MUAC%20Systematic%20Review%20_Nov%2019.pdf

Anthropometric Procedures:
https://www.youtube.com/watch?v=1ajuqBQOFXg

Arm Circumference:
https://www.youtube.com/watch?v=myaB4eZDBBc

References

1. Albrizio A. Biometry and anthropometry: From Galton to constitutional medicine. *J Anthro Sci.* 2007; 85:101–123.
2. Ercan I, Ocakoglu G, Sigirli D, Özkaya G. Statistical shape analysis and usage in medical sciences: Review. *Turkiye Klinikleri J Biostat.* 2012; 4(1): 27–35.
3. Merriam-Webster dictionary [online]. http://www.merriam-webster.com/dictionary/anthropometry. Accessed November 8, 2017.
4. Toomey CM, Cremona A, Hughes K, Norton C. A review of body composition measurement in assessment of health. *Top Clin Nutr.* 2015; 30(1):16–32.
5. Simmonds M, Llewellyn A, Owen CG, Woolacott N. Simple test for the diagnosis of childhood obesity: A systematic review and meta-analysis. *Obes Rev.* 2016; 17(12):1301–1315.
6. Woodruff BA, Duffield A. Assessment of nutritional status in emergency-affected populations—Adolescents. UN ACC/Subcommittee on Nutrition. Geneva. UN Statistics Division. 2003. Demographic Yearbook Special Census.
7. ISAK. *International Standards for Anthropometric Assessment* (manual). Marfell-Jones M, Olds T, Stewart A, Lindsay Carter LE, eds. Underdale, South Australia, Australia: International Society for the Advancement of Kinanthropometry; 2012. http://www.ceap.br/material/MAT17032011184632.pdf.
8. FAO. *Uses of Food Consumption and Anthropometric Surveys in the Caribbean.* http://www.fao.org/docrep/008/y5825e/y5825e00.htm. Accessed November 2016.
9. Nambiar S, Hughes I, Davies PS. Developing waist-to-height ratio cut-offs to define overweight and obesity in children and adolescents. *Public Health Nutr.* 2010; 10(10):1566–1574.
10. Briend A, Maier B, Fontaine O, Garenne M. Mid-upper arm circumference and weight-for-height to identify high-risk malnourished under-five children. *Matern Child Nutr.* 2012; 8:130–133.
11. Fryar CD, Gu Q, Ogden CL. Anthropometric reference data for children and adults: United States, 2007–2010. National Center for Health Statistics. *Vital Health Stat.* 2012; 11(252):1-48.
12. Flaherty-Hewitt M, Kline MW, et al. Nutrition and growth measurement technique. *Medscape.* http://emedicine.medscape.com/article/1948024-technique. Accessed November 22, 2016.
13. Bell C, Davies PSW. Prediction of height from knee height in children with cerebral palsy and nondisabled children. *Ann Hum Biol.* 2006; 33(4):493-499. https://www.ncbi.nlm.nih.gov/pubmed/17060071.
14. World Health Organization. *Training Course on Child Growth Assessment.* Geneva: WHO; 2008.
15. Grummer-Strawn LM, Reinold C, Krebs NF. Use of World Health Organization and CDC growth charts for children aged 0–59 months in the United States. Centers for Disease Control and Prevention. [Published correction appears in *MMWR Recomm Rep.* 2010; 59(36):1184.]
16. *MMWR Recomm Rep.* 2010; 59(RR-9):1–15.
17. Barstow C, Rerucha C. Evaluation of short stature and tall stature in children. *Am Fam Physician.* 2015; 91(1):43–50.
18. Centers for Disease Control and Prevention. WHO growth standards are recommended for use in the US for infants and children 0 to 2 years of age. http://www.cdc.gov/growthcharts/who_charts.htm. Accessed November 2016.
19. World Health Organization. The WHO child growth standards. http://www.who.int/childgrowth/en/. Accessed November 2016.
20. World Health Organization. *Physical Status: The Use and Interpretation of Anthropometry.* Report of a WHO Expert Committee. Technical Report. Series No. 454. Geneva: WHO; 1995: 1–452.
21. Wang Y, Moreno LA, Caballero B, Cole TJ. Limitations of the current World Health Organization growth references for children and adolescents. *Food Nutr Bull.* 2006; 27: S175–S188.
22. WHO Multicentre Growth Reference Study Group. WHO child growth standards. Geneva: World Health Organization; 2006.

23. WHO Multicentre Growth Reference Study Group. Assessment of differences in linear growth among populations in he WHO Multicentre Growth Reference Study. *Acta Pediatr.* 2006;450(Suppl.):56–65.
24. Kanof ME, Lake AM, Bayless TM. Decreased height velocity in children and adolescents before the diagnosis of Crohn's disease. *Gastroenterology*; 1988; 95:1523–1527.
25. Tanner JM, Davies PS. Clinical longitudinal standards for height and height velocity for North American children. *J Pediatr.* 1985; 107:317–329.
26. Hirani V, Mindell J. A comparison of measured height and demi-span equivalent height in the assessment of body mass index among people aged 65 years and over in England. *Age Ageing.* 2008; 37: 311–317.
27. Hickson M, Frost G. A comparison of three methods for estimating height in acutely ill elderly population. *J Hum Dietet.* 2003; 16:13–20.
28. Madden AM, Tsikoura T, Stott DJ. The estimation of body height from ulna length in healthy adults from different ethnic groups. *J Hum Nutr Diet.* 2012; 25:121–128.
29. Hirani V, Aresu M. Development of new demi-span equations from a nationally representative sample of older people to estimate adult height. *J Am Geriatri Soc.* 2012; 60:550–554.
30. Lorini C, Collini F, Dastagnoli M, et al. Using alternative or direct anthropometric measurements to assess risk for malnutrition in nursing homes. *Nutrition.* 2014; 30(10): 1171–1176.
31. Geraedts EJ, van Dommelen P, Calibe J, et al. Association between head circumference and body size. *Horm Res Pediatr.* 2011; 75:213–219.
32. Saunders CL, Lejarraga H, del Pino M. Assessment of head size adjusted for height: An anthropometric tool for clinical use based on Argentinian data. *Ann Hum Biol.* 2006; 33: 415–423.
33. Lampl M, Johnson ML. Infant head circumference growth is saltatory and coupled to length growth. *Early Hum Dev.* 2011; 87:361–368.
34. Rollins JD, Collins JS, Holden KR. United States head circumference growth reference charts: Birth to 21 years. *J Pediatr.* 2010; 156:907- 913.
35. Kammerer M, Porter MM, Beekley A, Tichansky DS. Ideal body weight calculation in bariatric surgery population. *J Gastrointest Surg.* 2015; 19: 1758–1762.
36. Mokha JS, Srinivasan SR, Das Mahapatra P, et al. Utility of waist-to-height in assessing central obesity and related cardiometabolic risk profile among normal weight and overweight/obese children: The Bogalusa Heart Study. *BMC Pediatrics.* 2010; 10:73–80.
37. Wildman RP, Muntner P, Reynolds K, et al. The obese without cardiometabolic risk factor clustering and the normal weight with cardiometabolic risk factor clustering: Prevalence and correlates of 2 phenotypes among the 8 US population (NHANES 1999-2004). *Arch Intern Med.* 2008; 168: 1617–1624.
38. Després JP, Lemieux I, Bergeron J, et al. Abdominal obesity and the metabolic syndrome: contribution to global cardiometabolic risk. *Arterioscler Thromb Vasc Biol.* 2008; 28:1039–1049.
39. Malone SK, Zemel BS. Measurement and interpretation of body mass index during childhood and adolescence. *J Sch Nurs.* 2015; 31(4): 261–271.
40. Reilly JJ, Dorosty AR, Ghomizadeh NM, et al. Comparison of waist circumference percentiles versus body mass index percentiles for diagnosis of obesity in a large cohort of children. *Int J Pediatr Obes.* 2010; 5:151–156.
41. Freedman D, Ogden CL, Blanck HM, Borrund LG, Dietz WH. The abilities of body mass index and skinfold thickness to identify children with low or elevated levels of dual energy X-ray absorptiometry-determined body fatness. *J Pediatr.* 2013; 163:160–166.
42. Tuan NT, Wang Y. Adiposity assessments: Agreement between dual-energy x-ray absorptiometry and anthropometric measures in US children. *Obesity*; 2014; 22:1495–1504.
43. Neovius M, Rasmussen F. Evaluation of BMI-based classification of adolescent overweight and obesity: Choice of percentage body fat cutoffs exerts a large influence—The COMPASS study. *Eur J Clin Nutr.* 2008; 62:1201–1207.
44. Ackland TR, Lohaman TG, Sungot-Borgen J, et al. Current status of body composition assessment in sport. Review and position statement on behalf of the ad hoc working group on body composition health and performance, under the auspices of the IOC Medical Commission. *Sports Med.* 2012; 42(3):227–249.
45. Okorodudu DO, Jumean MF, Montori VM, et al. Diagnostic performance of body mass index to identify obesity as defined by body adiposity: A systematic review and meta-analysis. *Int J Obes (Lond).* 2010; 34(5):791–799.
46. Whitlock G, Lewington S, Sherliker P, et al. Body-mass index and cause-specific mortality in 900 000 adults: Collaborative analyses of 57 prospective studies. *Lancet.* 2009; 373:1083–1096.
47. Snijder MB, van Dam RM, Visser M, Seidell JC. What aspects of body fat are particularly hazardous and how do we measure them? *Int J Epidemiol.* 2006; 35:83–92.
48. Dulloo AG, Jacquet J, Solinas G, Montani J-P, Schutz Y. The BMI–FM% relationship may contribute to these racial differences in trunk-to-leg-length ratio, slenderness, and muscularity *Int J Obes.* 2010; 34:S4–S17.
49. Wulan SN, Westerterp KR, Plasqui G. Ethnic differences in body composition and the associated metabolic profile: A comparative study between Asians and Caucasians. *Maturitas.* 2010; 65:315–319.
50. Heymsfield SB, Scherzer R, Pietrobelli A, Lewis CE, Grunfeld C. Body mass index as a phenotypic expression of adiposity: Quantitative contribution of muscularity in a population-based sample. *Int J Obes.* 2009; 33:1363–1373.
51. WHO Expert Consultation. Appropriate body-mass index for Asian populations and its implications for policy and intervention strategies. *Lancet.* 2004; 363:157–163.
52. Yu Z, Han S, Chu J, Xu Z, Zhu C, Guo X. Trends in overweight and obesity among children and adolescents in China from 1981 to 2010: A meta-analysis. *PLoS ONE.* 2012; 7(12):e51949. doi:10.1371/journal.pone.0051949.
53. Davis J, Juarez D, Hodges K. Relationship of ethnicity and body mass index with the development of hypertension and hyperlipidemia. *Ethn Dis.* 2013; 23(1):65–70.
54. Alqahtani N, Scott J. Childhood obesity estimates based on WHO and IOTF reference values. *J Obes Weight Loss Ther.* 2015; 5:249–251.
55. Hull HR, Thornton J, Wang J, et al. Fat-free mass index: Changes and race/ethnic differences in adulthood. *Int J Obes (Lond).* 2011; 35(1):121–127.
56. Bao Y, Lu J, Wang C, et al. Optimal waist circumference cutoffs for abdominal obesity in Chinese. *Atherosclerosis.* 2008; 201(2):378–384.
57. Sabin MA, Wong N, Campbell P, Lee KJ, McCallum Z, Werther GA. Where should we measure waist circumference

in clinically overweight and obese youth? *J Ped Child Health.* 2014; 50:519–524.
58. Wu CH, Heshka S, Wang J, et al. Truncal fat in relation to total body fat: Influences of age, sex, ethnicity and fatness. *Int J Obesity.* 2007; 31(9):1384–1391.
59. Lear SA, Humphries KH, Kohli S, et al. Visceral adipose tissue accumulation differs according to ethnic background: Results of the Multicultural Community Health Assessment Trial (MCHAT). *Am J Clin Nutr.* 2007; 86(2):353–359.
60. Kagawa M, Binns CB, Hills AP. Body composition and anthropometry in Japanese and Australian Caucasian males and Japanese females. *Asia Pac J Clin Nutr.* 2007; 16(Suppl 1): 31–36.
61. Waist Circumference and Waist-Hip Ratio Report of a WHO Expert Consultation GENEVA, 8–11 December 2008.
62. Rush EC, Goedecke JH, Jennings C, et al. BMI, fat, and muscle differences in urban women of five ethnicities from two countries. *Int J Obesity.* 2007; 31(8):1232–1239.
63. Punyadeera C, van der Merwe MT, Crowther NJ, et al. Weight-related differences in glucosemetabolism and free fatty acid production in two South African population groups. *Int J Obes Relat Metabol Disord.* 2001; 25(8):1196–1205.
64. Punyadeera C, van der Merwe MT, Crowther NJ, et al. Ethnic differences in lipid metabolism in two groups of obese South African women. *J Lipid Re.* 2001; 42(5):760–767.
65. van der Merwe MT, Crowther NJ, Schlaphoff GP, et al. Evidence for insulin resistance in black women from South Africa. *Int J Obes Relat Metabol Disord.* 2000; 24(10):1340–1346.
66. Carroll JF, Chiapa AL, Rodriquez M, et al. Visceral fat, waist circumference, and BMI: Impact of race/ethnicity. *Obes (Silver Spring).* 2008; 16(3):600–607.
67. Rush EC, Freitas I, Plank LD. Body size, body composition, and fat distribution: Comparative analysis of European, Maori, Pacific Island and Asian Indian adults. *Brit J Nutr.* 2009; 102(4):632–641.
68. Leahy S, O'Neill C, Sohun R, Toomey C, Jakeman P. Generalized equations for the prediction of percentage of body fat anthropometry in adult men and women aged 18–81 years. *Br J Nutr.* 2013; 109(4):678–658.
69. Fryar CD, Gu Q, Ogden CL. Anthropometric reference data for children and adults: United States, 2007-2010. National Center for Health Statistics. *Vital Health Stat.* 2012; 11(252).
70. Ramírez-Vélez R, López-Cifuentes MF, Correa-Bautista JE, et al. Triceps and subscapular skinfold thickness percentiles and cut-offs for overweight and in a population-based sample of schoolchildren adolescents in Bogota, Colombia. *Nutrients.* 2016; 8:595–610. doi:10.3390/nu8100595.
71. Freeman, DS, Katzmarzyk PT, Dietz WH, Srinivasan SR, Berenson GS. Relation of body mass index and skinfold thicknesses to cardiovascular disease risk factors in children: The Bogalusa Heart Study. *Am J Clin Nutr.* 2009; 90:210–216.
72. NHANES, 2011. Freeman D, Ogden C, Kit BK. Interrelationships between BMI, skinfold thicknesses, percent body fat, and cardiovascular disease risk factors. *BMC Ped.* 2015; 15(1):188–197.
73. Toomey C, McCreesh K, Leahy S, Jakeman P. Technical considerations for accurate measurement of subcutaneous adipose tissue thickness using B-mode ultrasound. *Ultrasound.* 2011; 19(2):91–96. https://doi.org/10.1258/ult.2011.010057.
74. Hume P, and Marfelli-Jones M. The importance of accurate site location for skinfold measurements. *J Sports Sci.* 2008; 26:1333–1340. doi: 1080/02640410802165707.
75. Sachdeva S, Dewan P, Shah D, Malhotra RK, Gupta P. Mid-upper arm circumference v. weight-for-height *Z*-score for predicting mortality in hospitalized children under 5 years of age. *Public Health Nutr.* 2016; 19(14):2513–2520.
76. Saito R, Ohkawa S, Ichinose S, Nishikino M, Ikegaya N, Kumagai H. Validity of mid-arm muscular area measured by anthropometry in nonobese patients with increased muscle atrophy and variation of subcutaneous fat thickness. *Eur J Clin Nutr.* 2010; 64:899–904.
77. Mazicioglu MM, Yalcin BM, Ozturk A, Ustunbas HB, Kurtoglu S. Anthropometric risk factors for elevated blood pressure in adolescents in Turkey aged 11–17. *Pediatr Nephrol.* 2010; 25:2327–2334.
78. Gueresi P, Miglio R, Cevenini E, Gualdi Russo E. Arm measurements as determinants of further survival in centenarians. *Exp Gerontol.* 2014; 58:230–234.
79. Aparecida Leandro-Merhi V, Luiz Braga de Aquino J, Gonzaga Teixeira de Camargo J. Agreement between body mass index, calf circumference, arm circumference, habitual energy intake and the MNA in hospitalized elderly. *J Nutr Health Aging.* 2012; 16(2):128–132.
80. Kondrup J, Rasmussen HH, Hamberg O, Stanga Z. Nutritional risk screening (NRS 2002): A new method based on an analysis of controlled clinical trials. *Clin Nutr.* 2003; 22(3): 321–336.
81. Becker PJ, Carney LN, Corkins MR, et al. Consensus statement of the Academy of Nutrition and Dietetics/American Society for Parenteral and Enteral Nutrition: Indicators recommended for the identification and documentation of pediatric malnutrition (undernutrition). *J Acad Nutr Diet.* 2014; 114:1988–2000.
82. Rasmussen J, Anderson A, Fisker AB, et al. Mid-upper arm circumference and mid-upper arm circumference *z*-score: The best predictor of mortality? *Eur J of Clin Nutr.* 2012; 66:998–100.
83. Kulathinal S, Freese R, Korkalo L, Ismael C, Mutanen M. Mid-arm circumference is associated with biochemically determined nutritional status indicators among adolescent girls in Central Mozambique. *Nutr Res.* 2016; 36: 835–844.
84. Tang AM, Dong K, Deitchler M, et al. *Use of Cutoffs for Mid-Upper Arm Circumference (MUAC) as an Indicator or Predictor of Nutritional and Health-Related Outcomes in Adolescents and Adults: A systematic Review.* Washington, DC: FHI 360/ FANTA; 2013.
85. Fernernandez-del-Valle M, Larumbe-Zabala E, Graell-Berna M, Perez-R. Anthropometric changes in adolescents with anorexia nervosa in response to resistance training. *Eating Weight Disord—Stud Anorexia, Bulimia Obes.* 2015; 20(3):311–317.
86. Lam PY, Marshall SK, Harjit GD, Coelho JS, Cairns J. Pinch, or step: Evaluating the effectiveness and acceptability of mid-upper arm circumference measurements in adolescents with eating disorders. *Eat Behav.* 2016; 22:72–75.
87. Portero-McLellan KC, Staudt C, Silva FR, Delbue Bernardi JL, Baston Frenhani P, Leandro Mehri VA. The use of calf circumference measurement as an anthropometric tool to monitor nutritional status in elderly inpatients. *J Nutr Health Aging.* 2010; 14:266–270.
88. Landi F, Onder G, Russo A, et al. Calf circumference, frailty and physical performance among older adults living in the community. *Clin Nutr.* 2014; 33:539–544.
89. Singh R, Gupta S. Relationship of calf circumference with bone mineral density and hip geometry: A hospital-based cross-sectional study. *Arch Osteoporos.* 2015; 10:17–26.
90. Kwon HR, Han KA, Ahn HJ, Lee JH, Park GS, Min KW. The correlations between extremity circumferences with total

and regional amounts of skeletal muscle and muscle strength in obese women with type 2 diabetes. *Diabetes Metab J.* 2011; 35(4):374–383.

91. Min JY, Cho JS, Lee KJ, Park JB, Mi KB. Thigh circumference and low ankle brachial index in US adults: Results from them National Health and Nutrition Examination Survey 1999–2004. *Int J Cardiol.* 2013; 163:40–45.
92. Cruz-Jentoft AJ, Baeyens JP, Bauer JM, et al. Sarcopenia: European consensus on definition and diagnosis; Report of the European Group on Sarcopenia in older people. *Age Ageing.* 2010; 39:412–423.
93. Hsu WC, Tsai AC, Wang JY. Calf circumference is more effective than body mass index in predicting emerging care needs of older adults: Results of a nation cohort study. *Clin Nutr.* 2016; 35:735–740.
94. Chung JY, Kang HT, Lee HR, Lee Y. Body composition and its association with cardiometabolic risk factors in the elderly: A focus on sarcopenic obesity. *Arch Gerontol Geriatr.* 2013; 56:270–278.
95. Christensen HM, Kistorp C, Schou M, et al. Prevalence of cachexia in chronic heart failure and characteristics of body composition and metabolic status. *Endocrine.* 2012; 43:626–634.
96. Thibault R, Le Gallic E, Picard-Kossovsky M, Darmaun D, Chambellan A. Assessment of nutritional status and body composition in patients with COPD: Comparison of several methods. *Rev Mal Respir.* 2010; 27:693–702.
97. Nordén J, Grönberg AM, Bosaeus I, et al. Nutrition impact symptoms and body composition in patients with COPD. *Eur J of Clin Nutr.* 2015; 69:256–269.
98. Carberry AE, Colditz PB, Lingwood BE. Body Composition From Birth to 4.5 Months in Infants Born to Non-Obese Women. *Pediatr Res.* 2010; 68(1):84–88. doi: 10.1203/00006450-201011001-00161.
99. Muscaritoli M, Anker SD, Argiles J, et al. Consensus definition of sarcopenia, cachexia, and pre-cachexia: Joint document elaborated by Special Interest Group (SIG) "cachexia-anorexia in chronic wasting disease" and "nutrition in geriatrics." *Clin Nutr.* 2010; 29:154–159.
100. Booth A, Magnuson A, Foster M. Detrimental and protective fat: Body fat distribution and its relation to metabolic disease. *Horm Mol Biol Clin Invest.* 2014; 17(1):13–17.
101. Koutsari D, Ali AH, Mundi MS, Jensen MD. Storage of circulating free fatty acid in adipose tissue of postabsorptive humans quantitative measures and implications for body fat distribution. *Diabetes.* 2011; 60:2032–2040.
102. Messier V, Karelis AD, Prud'homme D, Primeau V, Brochu M, Rabasa-Lhoret R. Identifying metabolically healthy but obese individuals in sedentary postmenopausal women. *Obesity.* 2010; 18:911–917.
103. Fox CS, Massaro JM, Hoffman U, et al. Abdominal visceral and subcutaneous adipose tissue compartments: Association with metabolic factors in the Framingham Heart Study. *Circulation.* 2007;116:39–48.
104. Porter SA, Massaro JM, Hoffmann U, Vasan RS, O'Donnel CJ, Fox CS. Abdominal subcutaneous adipose tissue: A protective fat depot? *Diabetes Care.* 2009; 32:1068–1075.
105. Thibault R, Genton L, Pichard C. Body composition: Why, when and for who? *Eur Soc Clin Nutr Metabol.* 2012; 31:435–447.
106. Murphy AJ, Ellis KJ, Kurpad AV, Preston T, Slater C. Total body potassium revisited. *Eur J Clin Nutr.* 2014; 68:153–154.
107. Wang A, Heshka S, Pietrobelli A, et al. A new total body potassium method to estimate total body skeletal muscle mass in children. *J Nutr.* 2007; 137: 1988–1991.
108. Murphy AG, Davies PSW. Body cell mass index in children: Interpretation of total body potassium results. *Br J Nutr* 2008; 100:666–668.
109. Fosbol MO, Zerahn B. Contemporary methods of body composition measurement. *Clin Physiol Funct Imaging.* 2015; 35:81–97.
110. Pou KM, Massaro JM, Hoffmann U, Lieb K. Patterns of abdominal fat distribution: The Framingham Heart Study. *Diabetes Care.* 2009; 32:481–485.
111. Yim JY, Kim D, Lim SH, et al. Sagittal abdominal diameter is a strong anthropometric measure of visceral adipose tissue in the Asian general population. *Diabetes Care.* 2010; 33(12): 2665–2670. http://dx.doi.org/10.2337/dc10-0606.
112. de Souza NC, de Oliveira EP. Sagittal abdominal diameter shows better correlation with cardiovascular risk factors than waist circumference and BMI. *J Diabetes Metabol Disord.* 2013; 12:41–46.
113. Dahlén EM, Bjarnegård N, Länne T, Nystrom FH, Östgren CJ. Sagittal abdominal diameter is a more independent measure compared with waist circumference to predict arterial stiffness in subjects with type 2 diabetes: A prospective observational cohort study. *Cardiovasc Diabetol.* 2013; 2:55–63.
114. Leong DP, Teo KK, Rangarajan S, et al. Prognostic value of grip strength: Findings from the Prospective Urban Rural Epidemiology (PURE) study. *Lancet.* 2015; 386: 266–273.
115. Roberts HC, Denison HJ, Martin HJ, et al. A review of the measurement of grip strength in clinical and epidemiological studies: Towards a standardised approach. *Age Ageing.* 2011; 40: 423–429.
116. Bohannon RW. Hand-grip dynamometry predicts future outcomes in aging adults. *J Geriatric Phys Ther.* 2008; 31(1):3–10.
117. Ploegmakers JJ, Hepping AM, Geertzen JH, Bulstra SK, Stevens M. Grip strength is strongly associated with height, weight and gender in childhood: A cross sectional study of 2241 children and adolescents providing reference values. *J Physiother.* 2013; 59:255–261.
118. de Souza MA, de Jesus Alves de Baptista CR, Baranauskas Benedicto MM, Pizzato TM, Mattiello-Sverzut AC. Normative data for hand grip strength in healthy children measured with a bulb dynamometer: A cross-sectional study. *Physiother.* 2014; 100:313–318.
119. Life Measurement Inc., Concord, CA, USA. www.bodpod.com. Accessed December 1, 2016.
120. Fosbol MO, Zerahn B, Noreen EE, Lemon PW. Reliability of air displacement plethysmography in a large, heterogeneous sample. *Med Sci Sports Exerc.* 2006; 38:1505–1509.
121. Hillier SE, Beck L, Petropoulou A, Clegg ME. A comparison of body composition measurement techniques *J Hum Nutr Diet.* 2014; 27: 626–631.
122. Bredella MA, Gill CM, Keating LK, et al. Assessment of abdominal fat compartments using DXA in premenopausal women from anorexia nervosa to morbid obesity. *Obes (Silver Spring).* 2013; 12:2458–2464.
123. Breithaupt P, Colley RC, Adamo KB. Body composition measured by dual-energy X-ray absorptiometry half-body scans in obese children. *Acta Pediatr.* 2011; 100: e260–e266.
124. Malouf J, Digregorio S, Del RL, et al. Fat tissue measurements by dual-energy x-ray absorptiometry: cross-calibration of 3 different fan-beam instruments. *J Clin Densitom.* 2013; 16:212–222.

125. Hangartner TN, Warner S, Braillon P, Jankowski L, Shepherd J. The official positions of the International Society for Clinical Densitometry: Acquisition of dual-energy x-ray absorptiometry body composition and considerations regarding analysis and repeatability of measures. *J Clin Densitom*. 2013; 16: 520–530.
126. Libber J, Binkley N, Krueger D. Clinical observations in total body DXA: Technical aspects of positioning and analysis. *J Clin Densitom*. 2012; 15:282–289.
127. LaForggia J, Dollman J , Dale MJ, Withers RT, Hill AM. Validation of DXA body composition estimates in obese men and women. *Obes (Silver Spring)*. 2009; 17:821–826.
128. Fosbol MO, DuPont A, Alslev L, Zerahn B. The effect of (99m) Tc on dual energy x-ray absorptiometry measurement of body composition and bone mineral density. *J Clin Densitom*. 2012; 16:297–301.
129. Lee S, Kuk JL. Changes in fat and skeletal muscle with exercise training in obese adolescents: Comparison of whole-body MRI and dual energy X-ray absorptiometry. *Obes (Silver Spring)*. 2013; 21:2063–2071.
130. Carey JJ, Delaney MF. T-scores and Z-scores. *Clinic Rev in Bone Min Metab*. 2010; 8(3):113–121.
131. Schoushoe JT, Shepherd JA, Bilezikian JP, Baim S. Executive summary of the 2013 International Society for Clinical Densitometry position development conference on bone densitometry. *J Clin Densitom*. 2013; 16(4):455–466.
132. Nelson HD, Haney EM, Dana T, Bougatsos C, Chou R. Screening for osteoporosis: An update for the US Preventive Services Task Force. *Ann Intern Med*. 2010; 153(2):99–111.
133. Kalkwarf HJ, Gilsanz V, Lappe JM, et al. Tracking of Bone Mass and Density during Childhood and Adolescence. *J Clin Endocrinol Metab*. 2010; 95(4):1690–1698.
134. FRAX® fracture risk assessment tool. https://www.shef.ac.uk/FRAX/. Accessed December 1, 2016.
135. Wabel P, Chamney P, Mossi U, et al. Importance of whole body bioimpedence spectroscopy for the management of fluid balance *Blood Purif.* 2009; 27(1):75–80.
136. Vilaça KH, Paula FJ, Ferriolli E, Lima NK, Marchini JS, Moriguti JC. Body composition assessment of undernourished older subjects by dual energy x-ray absorptiometry and bioelectric impedance analysis. *J Nutr Health Aging*. 2011; 15(6):439–443.
137. Haverkort EB, Reijven PL, Binnekade JM, et al. Bioelectrical impedance analysis to estimate body composition in surgical and oncological patients: A systematic review. *Eur J Clin Nutr*. 2015; 69:3–13.
138. Maughan RJ, Shirreffs SM, Leiper JB. Errors in the estimation of hydration status from changes in body mass. *J Sports Sci*. 2007; 25(7):797–804.
139. Sivapathy S, Chang CY, Chai WJ, Ang YK, Yim HS. Assessment of hydration status and body composition of athlete and non-athlete subjects using bioelectrical impedance analysis. *J Phys Ed Sport*. 2013; 13(2):157–162.
140. Jaffrin MY, Morel H. Body fluid volumes measurement by impedance: A review of bioimpedence spectroscopy (BIS) and bioimpedence analysis (BIA) methods. *Med Eng Phys*. 2008;30(10): 1257–1269.
141. Gray C, MacGillivray TJ, Eeley C, et al. Magnetic resonance imaging with k-means clustering objectively measures whole muscle volume compartments in sarcopenia/cancer cachexia. *Clin Nutr*. 2011; 30:106–111.
142. MacDonald AJ, Greig CA, Baracos V. The advantages and limitations of cross-sectional body composition analysis. *Curr Opin Support Palliat Care*. 2011; 5:342–349.
143. Wagner DR. Ultrasound as a tool to assess body fat. *J Obesity*. 2013; 1–9. http://dx.doi.org/10.1155/2013/280713 Accessed November 21, 2016.
144. O'Neil D, Cronin O, O'Neil S, et al. Application of a sub-set of skinfold sites for ultrasound measurement of subcutaneous adiposity and percentage body fat estimation in athletes. *Int J Sports Med*. 2016; 37(05):359–363.
145. Leahy S, Toomey C, McCreesh K, O'Neill C, Jakeman P. Ultrasound measurement of subcutaneous adipose tissue thickness accurately predicts total and segmental body fat of young adults. *Ultrasound Med Biol*. 2012; 38:28–34.

Biochemical Assessment

Katelyn Castro
Kelly Kane

Chapter Outline

CORE CONCEPTS

1. Biochemical assessment is an important component of the nutrition care process, which must be interpreted with other methods (i.e., physical findings, patient history, anthropometrics) for accuracy.
2. Nutrient concentrations in plasma do not reflect the amount of the substance stored in body pools and may be influenced by disease, inflammation, and recent dietary intake.
3. Refeeding syndrome can result in malnourished patients when carbohydrate feedings stimulate insulin, resulting in the intracellular shift of potassium, phosphorus, and magnesium, and fluid retention.
4. Fluid, electrolyte, and acid–base imbalances can lead to serious complications, ranging from metabolic and gastrointestinal problems to cardiovascular, respiratory, and neurological concerns, each requiring careful evaluation, monitoring, and treatment.
5. Visceral proteins can be altered by acute and chronic metabolic stress, making them more accurate indicators of inflammation than indicators of nutritional status.
6. Lipid profile results can be used to assess risk of cardiovascular (elevated low-density lipoprotein, decreased high-density/low-density lipoprotein ratio) and metabolic (elevated triglycerides) disorders, as well as risk of malnutrition (decreased cholesterol) in patients.
7. Deficiencies in iron, vitamin B_{12}, and folate, and toxicities of copper and zinc can all compromise red blood cell functioning and contribute to anemia.

Learning Objectives

1. Describe the role of biochemical assessment in the implementation of the nutrition care process.
2. Identify the causes and treatments of serum electrolyte and fluid imbalances.
3. State the metabolic changes that occur during refeeding syndrome.
4. Compare the causes and treatments of different metabolic and respiratory acid–base imbalances.
5. Specify two biomarkers used to assess each of the following: endocrine, renal, liver, and cardiovascular functioning.
6. Name two protein biomarkers used to assess nutritional status and the advantages and disadvantages of them.
7. Justify the need for careful interpretation of protein markers for malnutrition during inflammation.
8. Identify components of a hematological test and the role of each in diagnosis of anemias.

Introduction

Biochemical assessment is an essential component of nutrition assessment, the first step in implementing the Nutrition Care Process (NCP) in clinical practice. Laboratory tests of patients' blood, urine, feces, and tissue samples are important indicators of nutritional status and organ function. Because disease states, subsequent treatments, and hydration status can have a significant impact on biochemical indices, evaluation of laboratory values is critical in patients with both acute and chronic diseases. While patients with acute illness or injury may experience dramatic changes in laboratory results, patients with chronic illness may develop abnormal lab results more slowly. Comparing patients' laboratory results to reference values and interpreting discrepancies in the context of patients' clinical symptoms and medical history allows clinicians to prevent or diagnose diseases and develop appropriate nutrition interventions. Laboratory values are necessary to monitor effectiveness of medical treatment, evaluate NCP interventions, and adjust the plan of care appropriately. Unlike the other components of nutrition assessment, biochemical assessment is a carefully controlled process and considers only objective data used in the NCP. However, no single laboratory test or panel can be used to make diagnosis of nutritional status and needs.

CORE CONCEPT 1

Biochemical assessment is an important component of the nutrition care process, which must be interpreted with other methods (i.e., physical findings, patient history, anthropometrics) for accuracy.

Specimen Types

There are several types of specimens used for nutrient and nutrient-related analyses. Although the ideal specimens reflect the total body content of the nutrient being assessed, the optimal specimen is not always readily available. The most common specimens utilized for analysis in medical nutrition therapy include the following blood components:

- **Whole blood**: Contains red blood cells (RBCs), white blood cells (WBCs), and platelets suspended in plasma; collected with an anticoagulant when the entire content of the blood is evaluated and none of the elements are removed (Figure 1)
- **Serum**: Fluid remaining in blood after blood has been clotted and centrifuged to remove the clot and blood cells
- **Plasma**: Component of blood composed of water, blood proteins, organic electrolytes, and clotting factors
- **Blood cells**: Measurement of cellular components, separated from anticoagulated whole blood

In addition to blood, other specimens can also be used for analysis:

- **Urine**: Contains a concentrate of excreted metabolites from random samples or timed collection
- **Feces**: Determines composition of gut flora and presence or absence of adequate nutrient absorption, from random samples or timed collection
- **Hair and nails**: Stable, easy to collect, and noninvasive media which determines exposure to toxic metals and is a helpful indicator of levels of trace elements (zinc, copper, chromium, and manganese)
- **Saliva**: Noninvasive medium with high turnover used to evaluate functional adrenal stress and hormone levels
- **Breath tests**: Performed on the air generated from exhalation; less common and less invasive tool to assess nutrient metabolism, use, and malabsorption, particularly of sugars

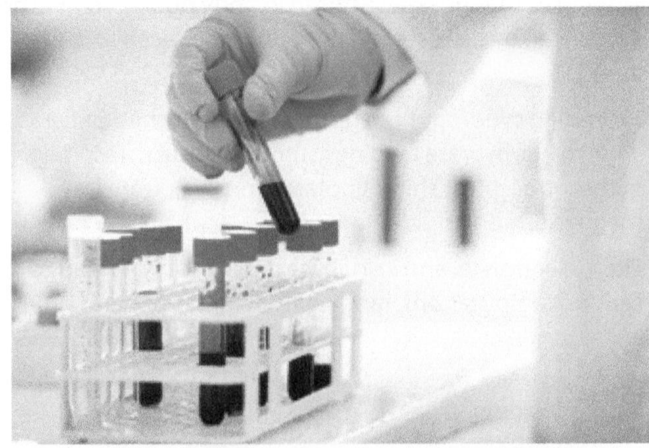

FIGURE 1 **Example of Specimens Collected in Laboratory for Biochemical Assessment**

CASE STUDY INTRODUCTION

Adam is a 68-year-old male admitted to the hospital with a 1-month history of nausea, vomiting, and diarrhea resulting in weight loss and fatigue. He presents tachycardic with abdominal pain, fever, and chills. Adam is a retired engineer and lives at home with his wife.

Anthropometric Data:

Height: 165 cm (65")
Weight: 75 kg (165 lbs)
BMI: 27.5 kg/m²
Weight History
Usual body weight: 82 kg (180 lbs) 1 year ago

Biochemical Data:

Sodium 129 (135-145 mEq/L)
Potassium 3.2 (3.6-5.0 mEq/L)
Chloride 90 (98-110 mEq/L)
Carbon dioxide 43 (20-30 mEq/L)
Blood urea nitrogen 30 (6-24 mg/dL)
Creatinine 0.5 (0.4-1.3 mg/dL)
Glucose 166 (70-139 mg/dL)
Magnesium 1.3 (1.3-2.1 mg/dL)
Calcium 8.0 (8.5-10.5 mEq/L)
Phosphorus 2.7 (2.7-4.5 mg/dL)
Serum osmolality 250 (275-295 mOsm/kg)
Albumin 2.6 (3.5-5.0 g/dL)
Total cholesterol 233 (Desirable <200 mg/dL)
Low-density lipoprotein 41 (Desirable <100 mg/dL)
High-density lipoprotein 52 (Desirable ≥40 mg/dL)
Triglycerides 40 (Desirable <150 mg/dL)
Hemoglobin 11.1 (13.5-17.5 mg/dL)
Hematocrit 36.4 (42%-52%)
White blood cells 6×10^9 ($5\text{-}10 \times 10^9$/L)
Mean corpuscular volume 89 (80-99 fL)
Mean corpuscular hemoglobin concentration 32 (32-36 g/dL)
Red cell distribution width 50 (39-36 fL)

Clinical Data:

Past Medical History: Hypertension, hypercholesterolemia, hypertriglyceridemia, gastroesophageal reflux disease
Medications: Lipitor, Captopril, aspirin, imodium, omeprazole
Vital Signs: Blood pressure 110/50 mm Hg, Temperature 99.6° F, Heart rate 115 beats/min, tachycardic
Nutrition-focused Physical Exam: Patient noted to be pale with dry skin and poor skin turgor. Temporal muscles mildly wasted. Upper arm and lower extremity fat loss evident. Abdomen appears slightly distended. Oral exam notable for a dry tongue and good dentition. No wounds observed and no edema noted. No shortness of breath evident.

Dietary Data:

Dietary History: Normal appetite. Adam reveals he has avoided high-fat foods for the past year, and limits his sodium intake. He reports that he has had minimal intake for 3 to 4 days prior to admission.
Usual Diet Recall:
Breakfast: 8 oz orange juice, hard-boiled egg, ½ bagel with 2 oz cream cheese
Lunch: Sandwich with 3-4 oz turkey or ham and mustard on white bread, canned soup, 1 oz potato chips, 1% milk, apple
Dinner: 4 oz baked chicken, 2/3 cup rice, ½ cup cooked green beans
Diet Prescription: NPO (nil per os or nothing by mouth)

Questions

1. **Describe the possible pathophysiologic etiology associated with Adam's electrolyte abnormalities.**
2. **What are Adam's nutritional risk factors?**
3. **What additional information and labs would you like to obtain?**
4. **What are your priorities for this patient?**

Assay Types

Two types of laboratory assays are available to measure nutrient levels in specimens. A **static assay** is used to measure the actual level of a nutrient in the specimen. This type of assay is specific to the nutrient of interest. Unfortunately the concentration of the nutrient within the specimen does not always reflect its amount stored in body pools and tissues. Serum levels may be influenced by the status of their protein carriers, which may be altered by inflammation. The amount of nutrient found in serum, plasma, or another fluid or tissue is influenced by recent dietary intake in static assays. To address this limitation, overnight (8-12 hour) fasting is recommended when collecting some specimens.[1] Examples of static assays include serum iron and white blood cell ascorbic acid.

In contrast, a **functional assay** measures the specific biochemical or physiological functioning of a nutrient, rather than just the quantity of the nutrient. Usually a functional assay is sensitive for a nutrient at its functional site. Functional assays are not always specific for one nutrient of interest because many physiological and biochemical functions rely on several biological factors beyond the specific nutrient. One example of a functional assay is serum ferritin, which represents the functioning of iron present in the cellular storage pool.[2]

CORE CONCEPT 2

Nutrient concentrations in plasma do not reflect the amount of the substance stored in body pools and may be influenced by disease, inflammation, and recent dietary intake.

PRACTICE POINT

Biochemical assessment values in patients with hemodilution and hemoconcentration must be cautiously interpreted and treated.

Decreased red blood cell concentrations and increased plasma levels (**hemodilution**) and increased red blood cell concentrations and decreased plasma levels (**hemoconcentration**) can result from a gain or loss of plasma volume, respectively. As with abnormalities in fluid volume, an imbalance of plasma volume can contribute to an imbalance in **electrolytes**, or substances that dissolve into ions in solution, and lead to poor interpretation of biochemical assessment tests. For instance, during pregnancy, an increase in total cell and plasma volume can cause hemodilution and create artificial anemia also known as "physiologic anemia of pregnancy." Another example may occur when a patient has extreme edema. Hemodilution may decrease serum sodium levels, providing a false hyponatremia, requiring different treatment than a patient with true hyponatremia.

Routine Medical Laboratory Tests

Most laboratory tests can be ordered as a panel, a grouping of tests, or as individual tests. The most commonly ordered groups of tests include the **basic metabolic panel** (glucose, sodium, potassium, carbon dioxide, chloride, blood urea nitrogen [BUN], and creatinine) and **comprehensive metabolic panel** (all of the above measures plus albumin, total protein, alkaline phosphatase, alanine transaminase, aspartate transaminase, and bilirubin). A **complete blood count** (CBC) provides a count of the cells in the blood and description of red blood cells, while a **differential count** is a CBC for white blood cells. Stool tests can also be performed to assess the presence of blood, pathogens, and gut flora, especially among adults older than 50 years and individuals with unexplained anemia. Stool culture testing may also be ordered for patients with prolonged diarrhea, suspected food-borne illness, chronic gastrointestinal (GI) symptoms, or unexplained weight loss. Several chemical tests in a urinalysis are also commonly performed, including specific gravity, pH, protein, glucose, ketones, blood, and bilirubin. A urine specific gravity test compares the density of urine to the density of water, which can help to determine how efficiently kidneys can dilute urine.

Laboratory values must be used with other assessment data, such as clinical history and physical examination, to confirm diagnosis or monitor effectiveness of treatment. Specific biomarkers used to estimate nutrition availability in biological fluids and tissues often detect deficiencies before clinical or anthropometric changes are recognized. Understanding how to interpret biomarkers and laboratory values for nutrition diagnoses is a critical part of the NCP to provide the most effective and appropriate care for patients. This chapter will focus on interpreting biochemical laboratory values of electrolytes, glucose measures, proteins, enzymes, lipids, hematological tests, and iron studies, and their significance in identifying fluid and electrolyte imbalances, organ dysfunction, and nutritional abnormalities in clinical practice.

PRACTICE POINT

Interpreting changes in laboratory value trends has more clinical significance than simply comparing laboratory values within the established absolute reference ranges.

Fluid and Electrolytes

Bodily fluids can vary greatly in the amount of dissolved substances and their distribution in the body. To maintain an environment necessary for normal cell functioning, different regulatory mechanisms work simultaneously to achieve appropriate electrolyte and fluid balance, regardless of changes in intake. Cells also need acid–base homeostasis because hydrogen ion concentration plays an important role in nearly all biochemical reactions. The presence of both acute injury and chronic illness can alter fluid and electrolyte levels and requirements. Evaluation and treatment of fluids, electrolytes, and acid–base imbalance is critical in practice because disruption in normal levels of these substances can have a significant physiological impact on many organ systems.

Fluid Distribution

Water constitutes approximately 50% to 60% of body weight, with a higher percentage among infants and children and a lower percentage among women, the elderly, and obese individuals. Those with more body fat have proportionally less water because adipose tissue contains less water than lean body mass. As a consequence, total body water is a function of weight, age, sex, and lean body mass. Total body water is divided into three main compartments: intracellular fluid (ICF), extracellular fluid (ECF), and transcellular fluid compartments. Approximately two-thirds of the total body water is found within cells (ICF) and most of the remaining one-third is found outside cells. Only about 1% of total body water accounts for transcellular fluid, which includes specialized fluids such as cerebrospinal fluid, the aqueous of the eye, and secretions of the GI tract. **Table 1** provides the ionic composition of intracellular and extracellular fluid.

ECF is the most clinically important fluid compartment because it contains interstitial fluids (surrounding cells) and intravascular fluid (within blood). The distribution of water between each fluid compartment (**Figure 2**) is primarily determined by **osmotic pressure**, defined as the pressure needed to maintain equilibrium with no net movement of solvent. Each compartment has one major active solute that determines its osmotic pressure and holds water within the compartment. Sodium is the dominant extracellular osmole, potassium is the main intracellular osmole, and plasma proteins are the primary substances in intravascular space. Under normal conditions, the sodium-potassium-adenosine triphosphate (Na^+-K^+-ATPase) pumps maintain the solute compositions of ECF and ICF and play an important role in fluid balance. Serum osmolality is used to express osmotic pressure by calculating the number of osmoles acting to hold fluid within the ECF. Serum osmolality (in mOsm/kg) can be calculated using the following equation:

$$S_{osm} = (2 \times \text{Sodium mEq/L}) + (\text{Glucose mg/dL})/18 + (\text{BUN mg/dL})/2.8$$

Sample Calculation: Sodium 135 mEq/L, Glucose 105 mg/dL, BUN 33 mg/dL

$$S_{osm} = (2 \times 135) + 105/18 + 33/2.8$$

$$S_{osm} = 270 + 5.8 + 11.8$$

$$S_{osm} = 288 \text{ mOsm/kg}$$

Normal serum osmolality ranges from 275 to 295 mOsm/kg.[3] Osmolalities of ECF and ICF are assumed to be equal (**isotonic**) under normal conditions. When cells are exposed to solutions that have an osmolality greater than that of blood (**hypertonic**), fluids move out of cells in an attempt to establish equilibrium and results in cellular dehydration. In contrast, when cells are exposed to solutions with osmolality less than that of blood (**hypotonic**) fluid moves into cells and causes cell swelling. **Figure 3** illustrates the red blood cell responses to solutions of varying tonicities.

To better understand the mechanisms of water distribution to ECF and ICF, consider the composition of commonly used intravenous (IV) fluids administered in practice. For example, when 1,000 mL of 5% dextrose (hypotonic, solute-free water) is infused, the dextrose is metabolized and the free water distributes evenly

TABLE 1 IONIC COMPOSITION OF INTRACELLULAR AND EXTRACELLULAR FLUID

Electrolytes	Extracellular* fluid concentration meq/L	Intracellular† fluid concentration meq/L
Cations		
Sodium (Na^+)	140	13
Potassium (K^+)	5	140
Calcium (Ca^{2+})	5	Minimal
Magnesium (Mg^{2+})	2	7
Total	**151**	**160**
Anions		
Chloride (Cl^-)	104	3
Bicarbonate (HCO_3^-)	24	10
Sulfate (SO_4^{2-})	1	—
Phosphate (HPO_4^{2-})	2	107
Proteins	15	40
Organic anions	5	—
Total	**151**	**160**

* Values are for plasma. Interstitial fluid concentration varies slightly (about 4%).
† Values are for cell water in muscle.
Modified from Shils ME, Shike M, Ross AC, et al., eds. *Modern Nutrition in Health and Disease.* 10th ed. Philadelphia: Lippincott Williams & Wilkins; 2005:149–193.

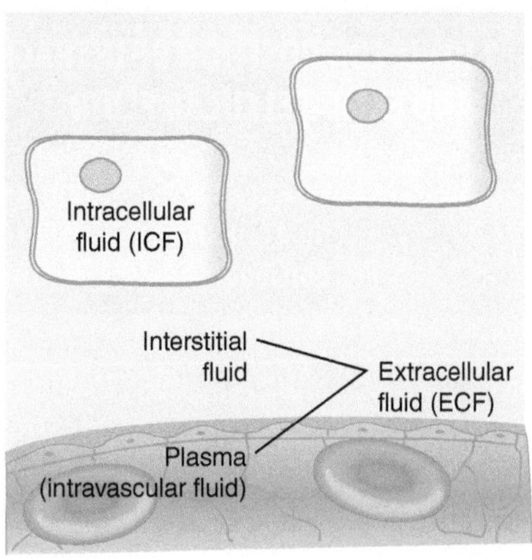

FIGURE 2 **Intracellular Fluid is Found Within Cells** Extracellular fluid includes interstitial fluid and intravasular fluid and is found outside of cells.

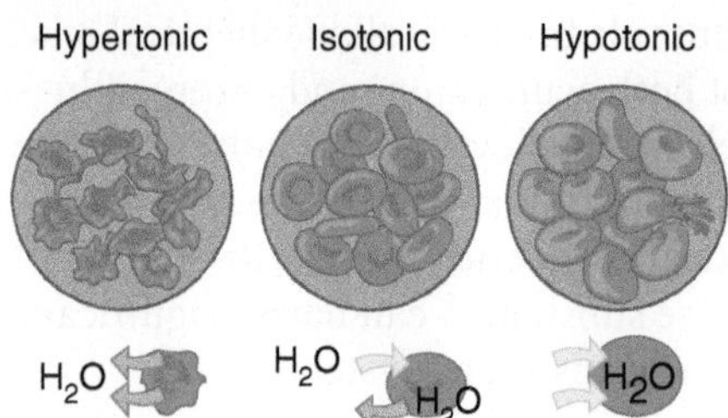

FIGURE 3 **Fluid Distribution Based on Tonicity: Red blood Cells in Hypertonic, Isotonic, and Hypotonic Solution**

across all compartments. That is, two-thirds (667 mL) of the solution goes to the ICF, where water enters the cell, and approximately one-third (333 mL) goes to the ECF. Alternatively, if 1,000 mL of 0.9% sodium chloride (normal saline) is administered, the water is distributed completely to the ECF because sodium is found mainly in the ECF. Approximately 25% (250 mL) will go to intravascular space and 75% (750 mL) will go to interstitial space. In contrast, administration of 3% sodium chloride (hypertonic saline) causes water to move out of cells and into ECF until osmotic equilibrium is reached. The addition of sodium chloride to ECF and the loss of water to ICF eventually would lead to increased osmolalities of both compartments, with the change in volume proportional to the degree of increase in ECF osmolality. Table 2 outlines the composition of commonly used intravenous fluids.

While osmotic pressure determines the distribution of fluid between ECF and ICF, plasma oncotic and hydrostatic pressures influence the movement of fluid between the plasma and interstitial fluid. Under normal conditions these compartments are maintained in a steady state and the pressures are generally balanced, despite large fluid exchanges between compartments.

When disruption in oncotic and/or hydrostatic pressure favors fluid movement from intravascular to interstitial fluid, **third spacing** occurs. Third spacing is the accumulation of fluid in the interstices (edema) or in the potential fluid spaces (effusion) between body cavities. An example of edema can be seen in Figure 4. Third spacing is common during critical illness when capillary permeability increases, causing albumin to leak into interstitial space leading to a decrease in plasma oncotic pressure. Although over a period of days fluid will be absorbed back into extracellular compartments, the acute drop in blood volume can cause severe volume depletion so fluid intake and output should be monitored carefully.

Fluid and Electrolyte Disorders

Disorders in fluid and electrolyte balance can be classified by disturbances of volume, concentration, or

TABLE 2 COMPOSITION OF COMMONLY USED INTRAVENOUS FLUIDS

Commonly Used Intravenous Solutions	Dextrose (g/L)	Sodium (mEq/L)	Tonicity	Free Water
D5W (5% Dextrose)	50	0	Hypotonic	1,000 mL
0.45% NaCl (1/2 Normal Saline)	0	77	Hypotonic	500 mL
0.9% NaCl (Normal Saline)	0	154	Isotonic	0 mL
3% NaCl (hypertonic saline)	0	513	Hypertonic	Negative (Loss of free water)

Modified from Langley, G., & Tajchman, S. (2012). *A. S. P. E. N. Adult Nutrition Support Core Curriculum Chapter 7: Fluids, Electrolytes, and Acid-Base Disorders* (2nd ed., p.100). Washington DC: American Society for Parenteral & Enteral Nutrition.

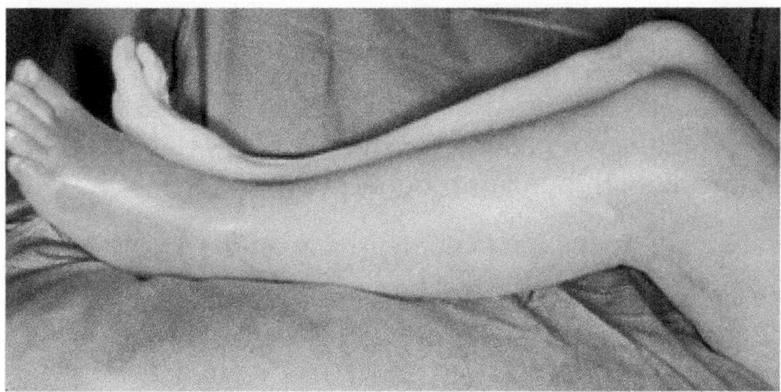

FIGURE 4 **Localized Edema**

composition, which often occur concurrently in clinical practice. Volume overload (**hypervolemia**) and volume depletion (**hypovolemia**) occur when there is a gain or loss in fluid (both water and solute) that alters extracellular fluid volume. The loss of extracellular fluid volume described in circumstances of volume depletion can result from vomiting, diarrhea, diuresis, or GI hemorrhage. Disorders of fluid balance can occur simultaneously with imbalance of electrolytes including sodium, potassium, magnesium, calcium, phosphate, chloride, bicarbonate, or hydrogen ions. For example, a change in sodium concentration leading to a change in plasma osmolality contributes to gain or loss of water (overhydration or dehydration, respectively). Excessive losses from the GI tract and abnormalities in kidney function are often found to be the primary contributors to electrolyte imbalances. Understanding the composition of specific body fluids can be helpful in the management of fluid and electrolyte disorders because many causes of water loss also lead to significant losses of electrolytes.

Management of Electrolyte Disorders

Safe and effective treatment of electrolyte imbalance requires careful assessment of the etiology of the electrolyte imbalance. If laboratory results are inconsistent with the patient's clinical condition, no treatment should be considered before validating the accuracy of the specimen sample. This is a critical step to prevent improper treatment of electrolyte values that may be based on errors in sample collection or handling. Only after laboratory results are validated should clinicians develop a treatment plan.

Generally, when electrolyte levels are above the normal range, removal of exogenous sources or facilitation of elimination of electrolyte is recommended. The severity of the electrolyte disorder and presence or absence of symptoms will determine the most appropriate treatment approach. Treatment may include removal of electrolyte supplementation from IV fluids or parenteral/enteral nutrition, discontinuing medications that may contribute to electrolyte disorder, and/or inducing renal or GI elimination of the electrolyte(s).

When electrolyte levels are below the normal range, electrolyte replacement through oral or IV replacement is appropriate based on patient-specific factors. Intravenous electrolyte replacement is considered optimal for patients with critically low electrolyte levels who are NPO ("nil per os," meaning nothing by mouth) or who have impaired GI functioning or difficulty swallowing. Patients with impaired renal function should receive conservative electrolyte replacement, unless actively receiving renal replacement therapy. Patients with volume overload should receive volume-restricted electrolyte replacement or oral therapy when possible. Identifying peripheral or central venous access is also important because peripheral administration may limit the volume and rate of administration. Tissue damage and potential harm can result from exceeding these limits in patients with peripheral access.

Because patients often have more than one electrolyte abnormality, all electrolyte values should be reviewed. The presence of concurrent electrolyte abnormalities requires clinicians to consider optimizing and minimizing replacement. For example, optimizing treatment should be considered if a patient has both hypomagnesemia and hypokalemia. Because potassium repletion can rarely occur if magnesium is deficient, magnesium should be corrected before potassium to optimize replacement.[3] Minimizing replacement can occur when patients have conditions, such as hypokalemia and hypophosphatemia, where potassium phosphate can be used to correct both of these imbalances simultaneously. Clinicians should also be aware of product availability and shortages to determine whether conservation or alternate therapy may be required.

Sodium

Sodium (Na^+) is the principal cation in the ECF, with a normal serum concentration of sodium range of 135 to 145 mEq/L. Sodium is the major osmotic determinant regulating volume and water distribution in the body, under the direct influence of the kidneys and central nervous system. Maintaining sodium levels requires a careful balance between sodium and water through the renin-angiotensin-aldosterone system, ECF volume, and renal function. Sodium also assists in acid–base balance; activation of enzyme reactions; nerve impulse conduction; and contraction of myocardial, skeletal, and smooth muscles.

Hyponatremia **Hyponatremia**, or low serum sodium, is the most common electrolyte disorder seen in medical care facilities, occurring in about 25% of hospitalized patients.[4]

Signs and Symptoms Evaluation of symptoms, rate of onset, and etiology can help clinicians determine the most effective treatment. Most patients with chronic hyponatremia have values in the range of

CASE STUDY REVISITED

Adam requires treatment for his hyponatremia (Na^+ 129 mEq/L; normal: 135-145 mEq/L). The medical team asks for possible means of correcting his sodium through nutritional modifications of his diet.

Questions

1. **What are the possible causes of Adam's hyponatremia?**
2. **What labs might help you determine its cause?**
3. **How would you recommend his hyponatremia be treated?**
4. **Explain your rationale.**

125 to 135 mEq/L and are asymptomatic or have mild symptoms (nausea, malaise, vomiting, and disorientation). Headaches, lethargy, agitation, confusion, and altered mental status are common symptoms for patients with lower sodium levels in the range of 115 to 125 mEq/L. More severe symptoms, including seizures, coma, respiratory distress, and death, are typically present when serum sodium values are less than 115 mEq/L due to the sodium's inability to maintain blood pressure and support nerves and muscles, which are critical for respiratory and cardiac functioning.

By determining the rate of onset of hyponatremia and assessing medical history and patient symptom information, clinicians can more effectively correct the disorder at a rate similar to that at which it was developed. Acute hyponatremia (developing in <48 hours) is more likely to result in cerebral edema, herniation of the brain, and cardiopulmonary arrest. These rapid adaptations to decreased intracellular osmolality can increase risk of developing **osmotic demyelination syndrome (ODS)** or widespread brain demyelination, which can also develop in patients with chronic hyponatremia when sodium correction is too rapid. Regardless of the severity of symptoms associated with hyponatremia, sodium correction rate should not exceed the target range of 5 to 10 mEq/L per day in order to prevent ODS.[5]

Etiology and Treatment After initial identification of hyponatremia, clinicians should assess serum osmolality to determine etiology and appropriate treatment of hyponatremia. Calculated serum osmolality should be compared to measured serum osmolality. Hyponatremia can occur with high plasma osmolality (hypertonicity), normal osmolality (isotonicity), and low plasma osmolality (hypotonicity). *Hypertonic hyponatremia* (>295 mOsm/kg H_2O) is caused by the presence of other osmotically active substances in the ECF, in addition to sodium. This is most commonly caused by severe hyperglycemia with dehydration or retention of hypertonic infusions of mannitol. To estimate the correction of serum sodium due to hyperglycemia, the following equation can be used:

$$\text{Corrected Sodium} = \text{Serum Sodium (mEq/L)} + 0.016\ [\text{Serum Glucose (mg/dL)} - 100]$$

Sample Calculation: Sodium 125 mEq/L, Glucose 350 mg/dL

$$\text{Corrected Sodium} = 125 + 0.016\ [350 - 100]$$

$$\text{Corrected Sodium} = 125 + 4$$

$$\text{Corrected Sodium} = 129 \text{ mEq/L}$$

The constants in this equation (0.016 and 100) reflect that serum sodium concentration falls approximately 1.6 mEq/L for every 100 mg/dL increment in elevated glucose. For a patient with a serum glucose of 350 mg/dL, the corrected sodium would be 129 mEq/L.

Isotonic hyponatremia (within normal serum osmolality values) occurs when there is a smaller fraction of serum that is composed of water, often resulting from excess plasma proteins or lipids. Normally, serum is 93% water, and the remaining 7% is made up of lipid and proteins. Because there is a larger non-aqueous phase occupied by lipids and proteins, and a smaller aqueous component (and sodium is restricted to the aqueous or water component), the resulting value from laboratory analysis of serum for sodium is low. This condition also called pseudohyponatremia may be caused by hyperlipidemia, hyperproteinemia, infusion of hypertonic solutions, or mannitol, resulting in a larger non-aqueous component to the plasma. Pseudohyponatremia does not reflect true hyponatremia because the concentration of sodium in plasma is normal. Once other laboratory values are corrected, sodium levels return to normal. With laboratory analysis advancing, pseudohyponatremia is less frequently observed in practice.[6] For practical purposes, hyponatremia in the presence of normal serum osmolality is usually attributed to pseudohyponatremia.

Hypotonic hyponatremia (<275 mOsm/kg H_2O) is the most common form of hyponatremia. Once this determination is made, a more detailed assessment of volume status must be done. Hypovolemic (lower than normal ECF volume), hypervolemic (higher than normal ECF volume) and euvolemic (normal ECF volume) hyponatremia each require different treatments.

Hypovolemic hypotonic hyponatremia (low volume, low osmolality) occurs when patients lose more sodium in relation to water. Urine osmolality in these patients is usually greater than 450 mOsm/L because excess sodium in relation to water is excreted in the body's attempt to retain fluid. Common signs of hypovolemia include decreased blood pressure, tachycardia, dry tongue, flattened neck veins, sunken eyeballs, increased body temperature, and acute weight loss. Determining the source of fluid loss is critical. Renal losses are identified by a urine sodium >20 mmol/L and are usually caused by diuretic excess, osmosis diuresis, mineralocorticoid deficiency, salt-wasting nephritis, pseudohypoalderonism, bicarbonaturia, renal tubular acidosis, or ketonuria. Extrarenal losses are commonly associated with a urine sodium <20 mmol/L and can be due to vomiting, diarrhea, fistula output, excess sweating, burns, open wounds, or fluid drains.

Isotonic saline is most often the recommended treatment for most patients with this condition to replenish sodium and water and to increase ECF volume. To calculate sodium deficits in patients, the following equation can be used:

Sodium Deficit (mEq) = [Desired Sodium (mEq/L) – Actual Sodium (mEq/L)] × Weight (kg) × 0.6

Sample Calculation: Desired Sodium: 135 mEq/L, Actual Sodium 129 mEq/L, Weight 70 kg

Sodium Deficit (mEq) = (135 – 129) × 70 × 0.6

Sodium Deficit = 252 mEq

A 70-kg patient with hyponatremia (sodium 129 mEq/L), would require a gradual administration of 252 mEq of sodium (sodium deficit) to obtain the desired serum sodium of 135 mEq/L.

The constant in this equation is 0.6 to reflect the fact that approximately 60% of body weight is water. Note that due to variations of body water with age and sex, some formulas will adjust this constant for females, children, and the elderly. This formula can be used to determine the amount of sodium needed to reach appropriate serum sodium levels. With 154 mEq/L of sodium, isotonic or normal saline increases sodium gradually at approximately 1 mEq/L for each liter administered. Clinicians should be cautious not to replenish sodium too quickly because this can lead to fluid shifts in the brain and cause adverse effects of the central nervous system (CNS). If patients are receiving nutrition support, clinicians should consider changes to fluids or sodium content of formulas.

Sodium can be increased by using a formula with higher sodium content, administering sodium chloride tablets, or replacing water flushes with saline solution. For patients receiving parenteral nutrition (PN), changing the formula can increase both fluid and sodium levels. If diuretics are the cause of hypovolemia, clinicians should consider possible medication changes as part of treatment. Potassium supplementation should be considered in estimating sodium deficit because potassium can increase plasma sodium and osmolality in hyponatremic patients. The following equation can be used to calculate this effect:

Δ Plasma [Sodium] = [Infusate Sodium + Infusate Potassium – Plasma Sodium]/(Body Weight × 0.6 + 1)

Sample Calculation: Infusate Sodium 154 mEq, Infusate Potassium 30 mEq,

Plasma Sodium 129 mEq/L, Body Weight 70 kg

Δ Plasma [Sodium] = [154 + 30 – 129] / (70 × 0.6 + 1)

Δ Plasma [Sodium] = 55 /43

Δ Plasma [Sodium] = 1.3

For a 70-kg patient with hyponatremia (sodium 129 mEq/L), infusing 1 L of normal saline (containing 154 mEq sodium) and 30 mEq potassium will raise the plasma sodium by 1.3 units (to approximately 130 mEq/L).

Euvolemic hypotonic hyponatremia (normal volume and low osmolality) often occurs in patients with syndrome of inappropriate antidiuretic hormone (SIADH), which causes excessive release of antidiuretic hormone (ADH). These patients have stable sodium intake and output but retain large amounts of water due to excess ADH. SIADH can be caused by brain or CNS malignancies, head trauma, lung malignancies, or pneumonia. Urine osmolality >100 mOsm/L and urine sodium >20 mEq/L indicate that kidneys are concentrating urine efficiently. Fluid restriction of 500 to 1,000 mL/day and administration of exogenous salt is the primary treatment for SIADH.[7] Pharmacological therapy with vasopressin-2 receptor antagonists may be required for SIADH refractory to conventional therapy. Other causes of euvolemic hypotonic hyponatremia include psychogenic polydipsia (ingestion of large amounts of water), hypothyroidism, hypopituitarism, medications, and reset osmostat, a condition that occurs when the kidneys adequately concentrate and dilute urine but the threshold for ADH secretion is reset downward. For these conditions, treatment should involve correcting the underlying disorder and fluid restriction.

Hypervolemic hypotonic hyponatremia (high volume and low osmolality) is often present in patients with renal failure, cardiac failure, hepatic cirrhosis, or nephritic syndrome because these conditions result in fluid retention or third spacing. To address water retention and edema, which is a common symptom, the recommendation for medical nutrition therapy is to restrict sodium and water from oral intake, enteral nutrition (EN), or PN. Administration of diuretics may be recommended and vasopressin receptor antagonists may also help to increase serum sodium in cirrhosis and cardiac failure. Figure 5 provides an algorithm to define hyponatremia.

Hypernatremia Hypernatremia, or increased serum sodium, occurs in approximately 2% of hospitalized patients, with values >160 mEq/L associated with increased mortality.[8]

Signs and Symptoms Clinical manifestations of hypernatremia are similar to hyponatremia, including

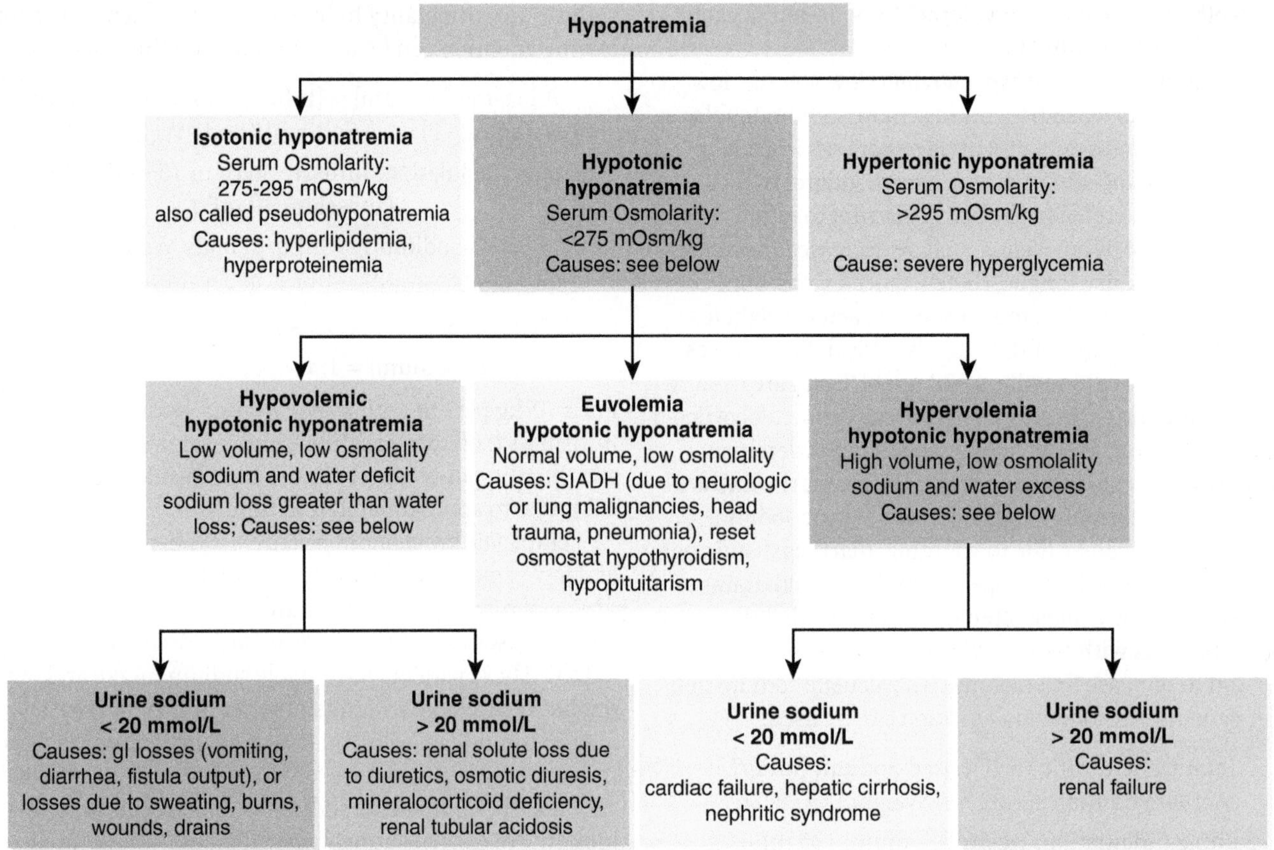

FIGURE 5 Algorithm to Define Hyponatremia

Data from Douglas I. Hyponatremia: Why it matters, how it presents, how we can manage it. *Cleve Clin J Med*. 2006;73(3):S5.

neurologic problems ranging from headaches and dizziness to more severe symptoms of seizures, coma, or death. Similar to hyponatremia, assessment of volume status is the first step in diagnosing hypernatremia.

Etiology and Treatment

Hypovolemic hypernatremia occurs when patients have higher sodium levels relative to fluid volumes. Renal losses due to diuretic use, solute diuresis, or acute tubular necrosis are common causes. Extrarenal losses, such as diarrhea and excessive sweating, are also causes of hypovolemia hypernatremia. Initially, patients need salt and water replacement to perfuse vital organs, which is typically administered via enteral or parenteral routes. Hypertonic solutions are only considered appropriate once volume status is corrected.

Euvolemic hypernatremia occurs when patients have water losses that exceed sodium losses. This is commonly caused by thermal injury, fever, or diabetes insipidus (DI). Central DI, which occurs when there is impairment of ADH secretion, and nephritic DI, which occurs when there is inability of the kidneys to respond to ADH circulating in the serum, lead to excessive water loss via urine. While treatment differs depending on the etiology, all require replacement of water via diet, enteral, or parenteral routes.

Hypervolemic hypernatremia occurs when there is an excess of sodium that is greater than the excess of water. This can be iatrogenic (excess administration of isotonic or hypertonic sodium) or caused by mineralocorticoid excess (exogenous administration, Cushing's syndrome, or adrenal malignancy). Treatment involves correcting the underlying disorder, minimizing fluids, eliminating sodium, and in some cases administering diuretics. To evaluate and treat hypernatremia, free water deficit should be calculated with the following equation where 140 refers to a desired sodium of 140 mEq/L:

$$\text{Free Water Deficit (L)} = \text{Total Body Weight (kg)} \times 0.6 \times ([\text{Serum Sodium mEq/L}/140] - 1)$$

Sample Calculation: Weight 70 kg, Sodium 153 mEq/L

$$\text{Free Water Deficit (L)} = 70 \times 0.6 \times ([153/140] - 1)$$

$$\text{Free Water Deficit (L)} = 42 \times (1.09 - 1)$$

$$\text{Free Water Deficit (L)} = 42 \times 0.09$$

$$\text{Free Water Deficit (L)} = 3.8 \text{ L}$$

A 70-kg patient with hypernatremia (sodium 153 mEq/L) has a fluid deficit of 3.8 L. A gradual infusion of this 3.8-L deficit would be required in order to decrease the serum sodium to normal range of 140 mEq/L sodium.

As with hyponatremia, sodium correction should not exceed 10 mEq/L per day, due to risk of cerebral edema and neurological impairment. Specifically, to prevent cerebral edema and convulsions, the maximal rate to reduce serum sodium levels is 0.5 mEq/L/hour for hypernatremia treatment. Hypotonic saline (1/4 normal saline or 38 mEq Na^+/L), free water, and water replacements with diuretics may be recommended depending on the etiology and patients' condition.

PRACTICE POINT

Sodium is considered as a critical electrolyte because high and low serum sodium can lead to serious, irreversible complications. Careful assessment and monitoring of sodium is critical, especially in the acute care setting.

Potassium

Potassium (K^+) is the major intracellular cation, with 98% of total body potassium located within cells. Normal serum concentration of potassium is 3.5 to 5.0 mEq/L and daily requirements range from 0.5 to 1.5 mEq/kg per day.[9] The most important factors regulating potassium balance include the Na^+-K^+-ATPase pump and the plasma potassium concentration. Extracellular pH, cellular breakdown, exercise, or hormonal secretions (insulin and catecholamines) can also affect potassium distribution indirectly by regulating the activity of the Na^+-K^+-ATPase pump. Potassium plays an important role in cell metabolism, transportation of glucose into the cell, and protein and glycogen synthesis. Although only a small amount of potassium is found in ECF, the ratio of serum potassium levels in ICF and ECF is crucial for neurotransmission and muscle contraction function due to potassium's role in maintaining resting membrane potential. The body strives to maintain potassium levels within a very narrow range because movement of only 1.5% to 2% of cellular potassium to ECF can be fatal.[10]

Hypokalemia

Signs and Symptoms Hypokalemia, or low serum potassium, is found in approximately 20% of hospitalized patients.[11] When this disorder is mild (3.0-3.5 mEq/L), patients are typically asymptomatic but may present with nonspecific symptoms including generalized weakness, lethargy, muscle cramping, anorexia, and constipation. Symptoms in more severe cases are muscle necrosis, ascending paralysis, arrhythmias, and possible death.

Etiology Abnormal potassium loss via urine is one of the most common causes of hypokalemia. Loop diuretics, such as furosemide, increase urine excretion and can contribute to potassium loss. Natural licorice and chewing tobacco, if swallowed, stimulate urinary potassium excretion because they contain an aldosterone compound. Hypokalemia may also result from GI losses, due to vomiting, nasogastric suction, or diarrhea. The compensatory actions in acid–base balance contribute to hypokalemia secondary to GI losses. For example, the loss of gastric acid from vomiting can lead to metabolic alkalosis, which results in sodium retention and potassium excretion. An increase in insulin or catecholamines (epinephrine) can also cause a transcellular shift of potassium from ECF to ICF, decreasing serum potassium levels. Inadequate dietary intake of potassium, common in eating disorders, and certain medications including loop and thiazide diuretics, insulin, corticosteroids, lithium, foscarnet, aminoglycosides, amphotericin B, cisplatin, and laxatives can also contribute to hypokalemia. Cellular shifts due to insulin, metabolic alkalosis, and refeeding syndrome are additional causes of hypokalemia.

Treatment The goals of treatment for hypokalemia include resolving the underlying cause, managing symptoms, restoring serum potassium concentrations, and preventing hyperkalemia. Oral correction of hypokalemia is often preferred due to its safety and the reduced risk of overcorrection and rebound hyperkalemia. Oral supplements of potassium chloride are available as a capsule, tablet, or liquid, although liquid forms may be poorly tolerated, sometimes contributing to nausea, vomiting, and diarrhea, and can also have an unpleasant taste. Clinicians are recommended to administer oral dosages of 40 to 100 mEq/day, divided into two to four doses, to correct deficiency.[12] Diet or oral supplements of potassium are recommended for mild or moderate depletion.

Only patients with severe hypokalemia or GI disturbances require IV potassium supplementation, with doses varying by severity and renal function. Intravenous potassium supplements include chloride, acetate, and phosphate salts. In the presence of metabolic acidosis, potassium acetate is recommended in place of potassium chloride. In general, with every 10 mEq of IV potassium administered, there is an increase in 0.1 mEq/L of serum potassium levels in patients with normal renal function. In most cases, infusion rates should not exceed 10 to 20 mEq/hour, although infusion rates of 40 mEq/hour have been reported and used in emergent cases or severely symptomatic patients.[12] Continuous cardiac monitoring is recommended if infusion rates exceed 10 mEq/hour to detect potential signs of hyperkalemia. A central venous catheter is the preferred administration route to minimize phlebitis and burning. It is recommended that clinicians not administer more than 40 to 100 mEq/day of total daily potassium supplementation. Some patients with severe potassium wasting, however, may require 200 mEq/day or higher, with careful cardiac monitoring.[13] Table 3 provides guidelines for hypokalemia treatment through IV replacement.

To avoid worsening hypokalemia, clinicians should use saline as the diluent instead of dextrose, because dextrose can promote an intracellular shift of potassium due to increased insulin release. In addition, magnesium

TABLE 3 EMPIRICAL TREATMENT OF HYPOKALEMIA	
Serum Potassium Concentration (mEq/L)	Intravenous Potassium Dose (mEq)
3–3.4	20–40
2.5–2.9	40–80
<2.5	80–120

Data from Kraft MD, Btaiche IF, Sacks GS, Kudsk KA. Treatment of electrolyte disorders in adult patients in the intensive care unit. *Am J Health Syst Pharm*. 2005;62(16):1663.

deficiency should be corrected if present. Treatment of hypomagnesemia is critical because magnesium deficiency can result in refractory hypokalemia due to increased potassium loss or impairment of Na^+-K^+-ATPase pump activity.

Hyperkalemia

Hyperkalemia, or increased serum potassium, rarely occurs in healthy individuals due to the body's efficient regulatory mechanisms. Individuals are often asymptomatic until serum potassium concentration exceeds 5.5 mEq/L.[14]

Signs and Symptoms Signs and symptoms of hyperkalemia are related to changes in neuromuscular and cardiac functions, including muscle twitching, cramping, weakness, ascending paralysis, electrocardiogram changes, and arrhythmias. These clinical manifestations are due to inactivation of electrical transmissions across the membrane. Other electrolyte imbalances, such as hypocalcemia or hyponatremia, or acid–base imbalance, can enhance the adverse effects of hyperkalemia.

Etiology The most common cause of hyperkalemia is inadequate potassium excretion due to renal insufficiency or severe burns. Excessive use of potassium-sparing diuretics, often used to treat hypertension, can also result in inadequate potassium excretion.

A shift in potassium from ICF to ECF can also result in hyperkalemia. This can be due to metabolic acidosis, tissue catabolism, and pseudohyperkalemia. Metabolic acidosis occurs when extracellular potassium shifts to maintain electroneutrality when some of the excess hydrogen atoms are buffered intracellularly. In general, potassium increases by 0.6 mEq/L for every 0.1 change in pH. Cellular shifts can also result from insulin deficiency and hyperosmolality. Tissue catabolism and strenuous exercise can also cause hyperkalemia due to the release of intracellular potassium into the ECF. Pseudohyperkalemia can occur when there is an artificial increase in serum potassium resulting from a release of intracellular potassium during or after blood sampling. Trauma during venipuncture is most commonly associated with pseudohyperkalemia, but a blood sample contaminated with infused potassium or that have been hydrolyzed can also cause pseudohyperkalemia. Hemolysis can also lead to falsely elevated serum potassium. If an elevated hyperkalemia is not commonly seen in a patient, a repeat potassium level should be obtained to confirm hyperkalemia diagnosis. Leukocytosis (increased white blood cells) or thrombosis may also increase potassium in ECF when there is increased hemolysis of red blood cells. Drugs including captopril, cyclosporin, digitalis, lithium, propanolol, and spironolactone also increase serum potassium levels.

Although rare, excessive ingestion from consumption of potassium-containing salt substitutes (KCl) can also result in hyperkalemia, especially if patients have renal insufficiency. While a large decrease in total body potassium is required to cause a slight decrease in serum potassium, only a small excess of total body potassium is needed for a significant increase in serum potassium. It should be noted that serum potassium does not always reflect total body potassium. Typically changes in serum potassium are the result of cellular shifting as opposed to changes in total body potassium. Consumption of potassium-containing salt substitutes should be evaluated, especially in renal patients, to prevent or treat hyperkalemia. Blood transfusions and excessive administration of potassium in IV solutions can also cause hyperkalemia.

Treatment Treatment goals differ based on the degree of hyperkalemia and the severity of symptoms. As with other electrolyte disorders, treating the underlying cause is crucial. If patients experience severe cardiac symptoms of hyperkalemia in short-term emergency situations, IV calcium gluconate is recommended to decrease abnormalities in cardiac cells that could lead to cardiac arrest and to restore membrane excitability. If excess exogenous potassium or other medications may have contributed to hyperkalemia, these should be discontinued or decreased if feasible. If a shift in ICF to ECF was the primary etiology, then insulin, dextrose, sodium bicarbonate and $alpha_2$-adreneric agonists can cause potassium to move intracellularly. Diuretics and cation-exchange resins (sodium polystyrene sulfonate) can also be administered to increase potassium excretion. For patients with renal insufficiency, dialysis and a potassium-restricted diet are recommended for long-term treatment. If patients have mild hyperkalemia, 2 g potassium/day dietary restriction is recommended.

Serum potassium levels should be monitored frequently in symptomatic patients during treatment because acute hyperkalemia can cause potassium to be redistributed within the body, without it being removed. After symptom removal, serum potassium should continue to be monitored until potassium levels have returned to normal.

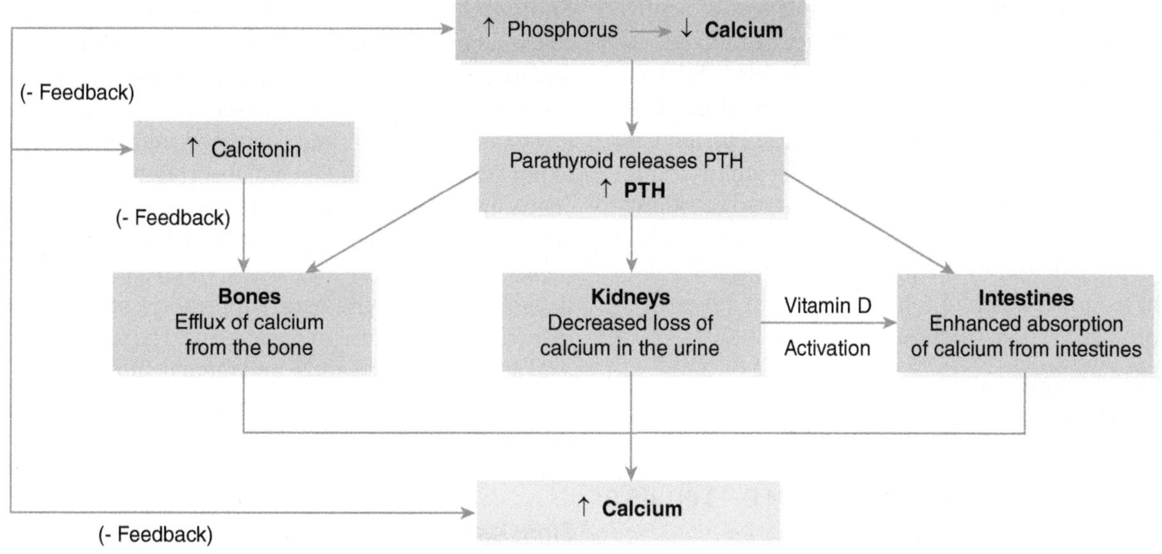

FIGURE 6 Mechanisms Involved in Phosphorus and Calcium Homeostasis

Data from Kraft MD. Phosphorus and calcium: A review for the adult nutrition support clinician. *Nutr Clin Pract.* 2015;30(1):21-33.

Phosphorus and Calcium

Phosphorus (P^{3-}) and calcium (Ca^{2+}) are closely interrelated in the body. Phosphorus and calcium homeostasis can be affected by many factors including disease states, clinical conditions, severity of illness, and medications. Homeostasis of phosphorus and calcium is primarily maintained by the regulation of serum phosphorus levels and ionized calcium levels, and the actions of parathyroid hormone (PTH), vitamin D, and calcitonin. An increase in serum phosphorus levels can lead to a decrease in serum ionized calcium levels, which stimulates release of PTH. The function of PTH is to increase calcium resorption and phosphorus excretion via kidneys, stimulate vitamin D activation in the kidneys, and increase absorption of phosphorus and calcium in the intestine. Vitamin D then upregulates intestinal absorption of phosphorus and calcium, stimulates calcium and phosphorus release from bone, and increases renal calcium resorption and urinary phosphorus excretion. The increase in serum ionized calcium levels and vitamin D will suppress PTH release, decreasing vitamin D activation. The increase in ionized calcium levels will also stimulate release of calcitonin, which inhibits bone resorption and decreases ionized calcium levels as a result. Figure 6 demonstrates the processes involved in phosphorus and calcium homeostasis. Magnesium can also affect calcium homeostasis because it has been found to impair the synthesis and/or release of PTH. Clinicians must understand the relationship between serum phosphorous and serum ionized calcium in order to take measures needed to appropriately prevent and/or correct disorders when they occur, especially in patients who are acutely ill and patients receiving PN and/or EN.

Calcium

Calcium (Ca^{2+}) is the most abundant divalent cation in the body and plays a key role in bone structure, blood coagulation, platelet adhesion, endocrine and exocrine secretory functions, neuromuscular activity, and cardiac and smooth muscle functioning. Figure 7 describes the essential functions of calcium. Calcium is closely regulated by the endocrine system, more specifically PTH, calcitonin, and calcitriol. Most of the body's calcium is located in bones and teeth, while the remaining 1% of calcium is found in body fluids. In serum, 40% of calcium is bound

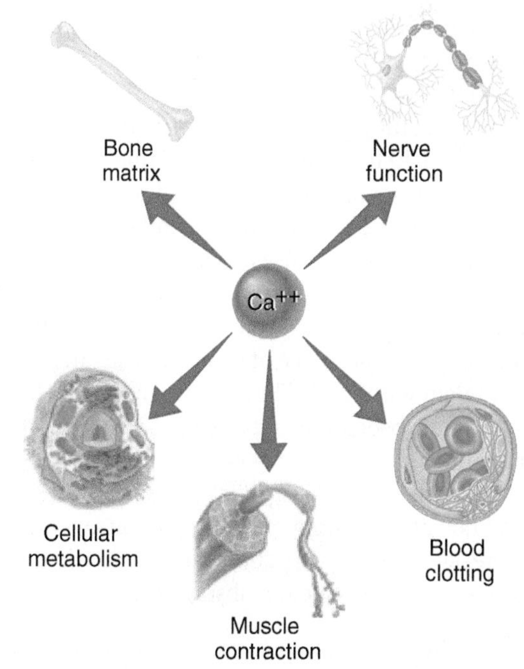

FIGURE 7 Essential Functions of Calcium

to proteins (mostly albumin), 13% is complexed (typically with citrate and phosphate), and 47% is free or ionized. The normal range for total serum calcium levels is 8.5 to 10.5 mg/dL, and ionized calcium has a normal range of 1.12 to 1.30 mmol/L.[15] An equation can be used to correct serum calcium due to hypoalbuminemia. Serum calcium levels must be corrected if a patient has a low serum albumin because a decrease in serum albumin by 1 g/dL will decrease serum calcium by 0.8 mg/dL, on average. To assess total serum calcium in relation to serum albumin levels, a corrected serum calcium formula is used:

$$\text{Corrected Serum Calcium (mg/dL)} = (0.8 \times [4.0 - \text{Albumin Level}]) + \text{Serum Calcium}$$

Sample Calculation: Calcium 8.0 mg/dL, Albumin 3.0 g/dL

$$\text{Corrected Serum Calcium (mg/dL)} = (0.8 \times [4.0 - 3.0]) + 8.0$$

$$\text{Corrected Serum Calcium} = (0.8 \times 1) + 8.0$$

$$\text{Corrected Serum Calcium} = 8.8 \text{ mg/dL}$$

A patient who has an albumin level of 3.0 g/dL, has a corrected serum calcium that is 8.8 instead of 8.0 mg/dL.

The 0.8 in the equation takes into account the 0.8 mg/dL that total calcium concentration decreases with every 1 g/dL reduction in serum albumin concentration while the 4.0 refers to a normal albumin level. Hypoalbuminemia causes a decrease in total serum calcium, but has less of an impact on ionized calcium. Therefore, ionized calcium is considered a better indicator of the functional status of calcium metabolism than serum calcium. In particular, there is a poor correlation between ionized calcium and total calcium in those with hypoalbuminemia, acid–base disorders, and critical illness, resulting in ionized calcium being the preferred indicator of calcium status in these populations.

The recommended adequate intake for calcium is approximately 1,000 to 1,200 mg/day for healthy adults, depending on age and sex. Most EN formulas contain approximately 700 to 1,200 mg/L (~17-30 mmol) of calcium and most adult patients with normal renal function require a dose of 10 to 15 mEq/day for maintenance with PN admixtures. Calcium doses can be adjusted by approximately 20% to 50%, depending on the daily calcium dose, serum calcium levels, responses to dose changes, and underlying clinical conditions. Absorption of calcium from diet and supplements ranges from 25% to 35%, influenced by source, salt form, presence of stomach acid, and whether or not it is taken with food. The recommended individual dose for optimal absorption is ≤500 mg.[16] Calcium citrate is also recommended in place of calcium carbonate because it appears to have better absorption. Calcium citrate is the preferred oral calcium supplement for patients receiving acid-suppression therapy or patients with achlorhydria, who may have reduced calcium absorption.

Hypocalcemia Hypocalcemia, or low serum calcium or low ionized calcium, has been observed in approximately 15% to 88% of hospitalized patients, and has been reported in 21% of critically ill trauma patients.[17]

Etiology Hypocalcemia is rarely a result of low intake of calcium because bone resorption helps maintain normal serum levels for a prolonged period of time despite variation in calcium intake. Hypomagnesemia, hyperphosphatemia, low vitamin D intake, and decreased calcium absorption due to phytate, oxalate, and fat malabsorption can cause hypocalcemia. Increased calcium losses may also contribute to hypocalcemia as a result of a high-protein, high-sodium diet, which increases urinary calcium losses. Altered calcium regulation due to hypoparathyroidism, pancreatitis, or metabolic bone disease can also cause hypocalcemia. Hypoalbuminemia, as well as sepsis, pancreatitis, and renal insufficiency can also lead to hypocalcemia. Medications including loop diuretics, phosphate, dilantin, corticosteroids, citrated blood, fluoride, and contrast dye can also cause hypocalcemia.

Signs and Symptoms Tetany (intermittent muscle spasms) is the most common sign of severe acute hypocalcemia (<7 mg/dL). Mild-moderate hypocalcemia may present other neuromuscular, cardiovascular, and central nervous symptom symptoms, including muscle cramps, paresthesias (tingling, numbness of extremities), seizures, ventricular arrythmias, prolonged QT interval, heart block, and ventricular fibrillation. Patients with chronic hypocalcemia may experience dermatologic manifestations including dermatitis; eczema; brittle, grooved nails; and hair loss.

Treatment

Hypocalcemia treatment involves removing the underlying cause, correcting hypomagnesemia (if present), and taking appropriate calcium supplementation. Because magnesium deficiency may impair release of PTH and/or PTH activity and contribute to hypocalcemia, magnesium supplements can be used to correct deficiency if it is concurrent with calcium deficiency. Phosphate binders may also be recommended if hyperphosphatemia is the underlying cause. Fixed IV doses of calcium gluconate are determined by symptoms and ionized calcium levels, rather than weight-based doses. If ionized calcium is not available, empirical treatment with 1 to 2 g calcium gluconate may be recommended followed by measurement of ionized calcium levels.[11] Calcium gluconate is recommended as the preferred calcium salt for routine calcium maintenance dosing and supplementation, while calcium chloride is recommended for use in urgent and emergency situations only. Severe, symptomatic hypocalcemia (i.e., seizures, tetany, arrhythmias, or refractory hypotension) should be corrected promptly with IV calcium administration over 10 minutes to control symptoms. Calcium gluconate is the preferred salt for peripheral venous administration to avoid extravasation (leakage of liquid into surrounding tissue) and tissue necrosis from calcium chloride. Figure 8 shows an example of extravasation. Clinicians must be careful to prevent dosing errors from confusion about calcium salts and calcium dose, as well as the manner calcium is ordered. Calcium chloride provides three times more elemental calcium than an equivalent of calcium gluconate.[18] To prevent dosing errors, orders should contain dose of calcium, calcium salt, and dose in grams, milligrams, or

Content removed due to copyright restrictions

Content removed due to copyright restrictions

milliequivalents. Clinicians must also be sure not to infuse calcium in the same IV line as solutions containing phosphate due to the risk of calcium-phosphorus precipitation.

In patients with mild-moderate hypocalcemia who are receiving EN or can tolerate oral medication, oral calcium supplements (calcium gluconate, calcium acetate, calcium citrate, or calcium carbonate) may be considered. Vitamin D status and evaluation of PTH may need to be considered prior to oral administration. If patients are receiving PN, adjustments of daily calcium maintenance doses in PN formulations or daily oral supplements may be recommended depending on patient's clinical condition and underlying cause of hypocalcemia.

As discussed earlier, hypoalbuminemia can produce a falsely low serum calcium (pseudohypocalcemia). If a patient has asymptomatic hypocalcemia due to hypoalbuminemia with normal ionized calcium levels, then no treatment is needed to correct hypocalcemia. Although there is debate over the need to correct asymptomatic hypocalcemia, most clinicians treat hypocalcemia to avoid the potential negative consequences of severe hypocalcemia, especially in critically ill patients.

Hypercalcemia Hypercalcemia is increased serum calcium or increased ionized calcium.

Etiology Hypercalcemia most frequently results from increased resorption from bone in malignancies with bone metastases (predominantly breast cancer, lung cancer, and multiple myeloma), and from decreased urinary excretion in patients with primary hyperparathyroidism.[15] Other causes include vitamin A or D toxicity, chronic ingestion of milk and/or calcium carbonate–containing antacids in patients with renal insufficiency (milk-alkali syndrome), or adrenal insufficiency. Immobilization, tuberculosis, Paget's disease, rhabdomyolysis, and medications including thiazide diuretics, estrogens, tamoxifen, and aluminum intoxication are other potential causes of hypercalcemia.

Early signs and symptoms of hypercalcemia are nonspecific and include fatigue, nausea, vomiting, constipation, anorexia, and confusion. Chronic hypercalcemia may lead to calcium-phosphate precipitation, metastatic calcification, and renal failure. Patients with severe cases can experience cardiac manifestations such as bradycardia (slow heart rate) or arrhythmias with electrocardiograph changes. Immediate treatment is required for severe hypercalcemia because acute kidney injury, ventricular arrhythmias, obtundation, coma, and death are potential consequences. Prolonged hypercalcemia can lead to tissue calcification (Figure 9), which can be irreversible.

As with other electrolyte disorders, treatment of hypercalcemia must include treatment or removal of the underlying cause if possible. Mild hypercalcemia (total serum calcium of 10.5-12.9 mg/dL or ionized calcium of 1.31-1.49 mmol/L) does not require immediate therapy; hydration and ambulation are typically effective treatments. Patients receiving PN may benefit from temporary reduction or removal of calcium from the PN prescription, based on the underlying cause and severity of hypercalcemia. Severe hypercalcemia (total serum calcium ≥13 mg/dL or ionized calcium ≥1.5 mmol/L) should be treated immediately with IV hydration to reverse the IV volume depletion caused by hypercalcemia. After hydration is restored, furosemide (40-100 mg) is recommended to enhance renal calcium excretion; however, careful monitoring is necessary to avoid further IV volume depletion.[19] Within the first 48 hours of treatment, saline hydration and furosemide have been found to reduce serum calcium by 2 to 3 mg/dL.[20] Calcitonin inhibits bone resorption and increases renal calcium elimination. This may also be used to treat acute hypercalcemia, although tachyphylaxis (diminishing response of successive doses) limits its effectiveness. In addition, biphosphonates are potential inhibitors of bone resorption and are often recommended for treatment of hypercalcemia in patients with malignancies or critical illness who have accelerated bone breakdown and associated metabolic bone disease. Serum or ionized calcium levels should be monitored every 4 to 8 hours during active treatment of severe hypercalcemia and every 24 to 48 hours after hypercalcemia is treated. Cardiac monitoring is critical for patients receiving treatment of hypercalcemia.

Phosphorus Phosphorus (P^{3-}) is the primary intracellular anion in the body, existing mainly as phosphate (PO_4) in the serum. Phosphate is the key form of phosphorus as it relates to medical nutrition therapy because it is also the primary form ingested in the diet and in exogenous administration of phosphorus. Only a small percentage of total body phosphorus is found in extracellular fluid, with the remaining 99% located in bones and soft tissues.

Phosphorus has many important functions in the body, including bone and cell membrane composition (phospholipids) and maintenance of normal pH. Phosphorus also provides the energy-bonds in the form of adenosine triphosphate (ATP), which supplies energy needed for many cellular processes and functions. Phosphorus is a key component of 2,3-diphosphoglycerate (2,3-DPG), which is essential for oxygen release from hemoglobin and delivery to tissues. Total body phosphorus is necessary for glucose use and glycolysis, protein synthesis, neurological function, and muscular function.

Serum phosphorus concentration is determined by the amount of intestinal absorption, renal excretion, hormonally regulated bone resorption and deposition, and distribution within intracellular and extracellular compartments. Intracellular shifts in phosphorus may be a result of insulin administration, catecholamines, and alkalosis while extracellular shifts may occur from cellular destruction and acidosis. Normal serum phosphorus concentration ranges from 2.7 to 4.5 mg/dL; however, serum phosphorus levels may not correlate well with total body phosphorus as serum phosphorus is only a small percentage of total phosphorus. As a result, clinicians must take a complete assessment of patient and consider factors that may affect serum levels and total body homeostasis of phosphorus including chronic kidney disease, severe malnutrition, and certain medications.

Hypophosphatemia Hypophosphatemia, or low serum phosphorus, has been found to occur in approximately 2% to 3% of hospitalized patients, but is reported in 28% to 80% of critically ill patients.[21]

Etiology Potential causes of hypophosphatemia include decreased intake (diet, PN, IV fluid), malnutrition, vomiting, or diarrhea. Decreased GI absorption due to antacids, vitamin deficiency, malabsorption, and chronic alcoholism or alcohol withdrawal may also cause hypophosphatemia. Many acutely ill and critically ill patients have underlying conditions or receive medications that predispose them to developing hypophosphatemia. Medications that increase urine phosphorus losses include antacids, phosphate binders, sucralfate, insulin, and corticosteroids. Low serum magnesium or phosphorus, osmotic diuresis, hyperparathyroidism, and renal tubular defects can also increase urine losses and cause phosphorus imbalance. Cellular shifts from respiratory and metabolic alkalosis (following treatment of diabetic ketoacidosis) can also result in hypophosphatemia due to decreased hydrogen ion secretion. Many clinicians have reported hypophosphatemia associated with initiation of nutrition support, including oral nutrition, EN, and PN. Hypophosphatemia can be a result of metabolic consequences of refeeding syndrome due to increased phosphorus needs during increased glucose utilization.

Signs and Symptoms Hypophosphatemia can cause a variety of adverse effects on respiratory, neurological, neuromuscular, and cardiopulmonary functions. Severe hypophosphatemia (serum phosphorus concentration <2 mg/dL) has been associated with impaired contractibility of diaphragm, acute respiratory failure, tissue hypoxia, decreased myocardial contractibility, paresthesia, confusion, disorientation, encephalopathy, areflexic paralysis, seizures, coma, and death. Some studies have found that hypophosphatemia is associated with higher mortality, longer hospitalization, and longer mechanical ventilation. Low phosphate levels can also result in mobilization of calcium and phosphorus in bone, contributing to osteomalacia and rickets.

Treatment The magnitude of the abnormality and presence of symptoms must be considered in treatment of hypophosphatemia. Treatment should focus on treating the underlying cause of phosphate abnormality (medically induced, malabsorption, inadequate maintenance dose, etc.). Patients with asymptomatic mild hypophosphatemia can be treated with oral phosphorus supplement if the GI tract is functioning, although absorption may vary among patients and diarrhea may result.

Patients with moderate–severe hypophosphatemia who are symptomatic and cannot tolerate oral supplements can be treated with IV phosphorus supplementation. A fixed IV dose of phosphorus is considered appropriate for patients with normal renal function based on serum phosphorus levels. Estimating doses is largely empirical because serum phosphorus levels may not correlate with total body stores of phosphorus. Patients with persistent hypophosphatemia may require a daily phosphorus supplement, IV supplementation, or increased maintenance phosphorus dose in PN admixtures. The recommended IV phosphorus dose should be provided over 4 to 6 hours to reduce risk of Ca-PO_4 precipitation and minimize infusion-related adverse effects, such as thrombophlebitis.

Hyperphosphatemia

Etiology Hyperphosphatemia, or increased serum phosphorus concentration, is most commonly caused by acute or chronic renal insufficiency, especially in hospitalized and critically ill patients. Decreased urinary phosphorus excretion can also result in patients with hypoparathyroidism and vitamin D toxicity. Excessive IV and/or oral administration of phosphorus could also cause hyperphosphatemia, which would be more likely found in patients with impaired renal function. Cellular shifts resulting from dehydration, hemolysis, rhabdomyolysis, and tumor lysis are also causes of hyperphosphatemia. Metabolic and respiratory acidosis are other potential causes of hyperphosphatemia. Oral and rectal administration of phosphorus-containing laxatives has also been reported to cause hyperphosphatemia. In addition, medications including enemas, salts, diuretics, biphosphonates, and lipid emulsions can lead to hyperphosphatemia.

Signs and Symptoms Many of the signs of hyperphosphatemia are concurrent with signs of hypocalcemia. Flaccid paralysis, mental confusion, hypertension, cardiac arrhythmias, and tissue calcification are common symptoms in patients with prolonged phosphorus toxicity. Due to the risk of calcium-phosphate precipitation, hyperphosphatemia can lead to hypocalcemia, further leading to its clinical manifestations such as altered nerve transmission and tetany. Calcium-phosphorus crystals can also cause further organ damage, particularly in the lungs, myocardium, and blood vessels, and can deposit on soft tissue. Evaluation of individual serum levels of calcium and phosphorus is recommended to guide treatment plans and prevent these complications.

Treatment A complete assessment of the patient is required for appropriate treatment of hyperphosphatemia. Identifying and correcting the underlying cause of this condition should be the first approach, followed by adjustment or restriction of phosphorus intake (reduced daily doses of PN prescription or initiating a renal EN formula). Volume deficit should be corrected if the cause is dehydration. Oral phosphorus binders are also recommended with meals and snacks to control high serum phosphorus levels by binding dietary phosphate. Common phosphate binders include calcium-, aluminum-, and magnesium-containing antacids. Individuals with hyperphosphatemia due to renal failure on renal replacement therapy may require different therapies for hyperphosphatemia treatment because various forms of renal replacement therapy, such as continuous renal replacement therapy, peritoneal dialysis, or intermittent hemodialysis, vary in their ability to remove phosphorus.

Magnesium

Magnesium (Mg^{2+}) is an abundant mineral in the ICF, with approximately 50% to 60% of magnesium located in bones and most of the remaining found within in cardiac muscle, skeletal muscle, and other soft tissues. Magnesium is an important cofactor in more than 300 biochemical processes in the body, including glucose metabolism, fatty acid synthesis, and DNA and protein metabolism. Magnesium also plays an important role in maintenance of the Na^+-K^+-ATPase, which is necessary for nerve impulse conduction, muscle contraction, and normal heart rhythm. Magnesium also is required for the synthesis of glutathione, and is a factor in PTH synthesis, and vasomotor tone.

As an important structural component of bone, magnesium also plays a role in maintaining intracellular potassium and calcium levels. The GI system, kidneys, and bones tightly regulate cellular and extracellular magnesium concentrations. Healthy individuals absorb about 30% to 40% of dietary magnesium; this occurs primarily in the distal jejunum and ileum. Normally about one-third of absorbed magnesium is excreted, but absorption varies with intake to maintain normal serum concentrations. Normal serum magnesium levels ranges from 1.3 to 2.1 mEq/L, but these serum levels do not accurately assess total body magnesium because less than 1% of total magnesium is found in serum. As the majority of magnesium is bound to albumin, hypoalbuminemia can cause a falsely low serum magnesium level.

Hypomagnesemia Hypomagnesemia, or low serum magnesium, has been found in up to 47% of hospitalized patients and in up to 65% of critical care patients.[22]

Etiology Decreased intake or absorption or excessive losses and redistribution into ICF are possible causes of hypomagnesemia. Protein-calorie malnutrition and prolonged administration of magnesium-free IV fluids or PN contribute to decreased intake. Chronic alcoholism or withdrawal of alcohol, malabsorption syndromes, short bowel syndrome, and intestinal bypass surgeries can lead to reduced magnesium absorption and GI losses. Renal losses of magnesium also occur in patients with acute tubular necrosis, renal tubular acidosis, Bartter syndrome, and hyperaldosteronism. Certain medications including cyclosporine, thiazide, loop diuretics, laxatives, cisplatin, amphtericin B, amino-glycosides can also cause hypomagnesemia. In addition, pancreatitis, low serum phosphorus, refeeding syndrome, diabetic ketoacidosis, hyperthyroidism, and myocardial infarction can also cause intracellular shifts of magnesium, decreasing serum magnesium levels.

Signs and Symptoms The primary symptom of magnesium deficiency is neuromuscular hyperexcitability. Latent tetany, muscular weakness, convulsions, and seizures may also occur. Cardiac complications, including electrocardiogram changes, arrhythmias, and increased sensitivity to cardiac glycosides, such as digoxin, are also common with magnesium deficiency. General symptoms may include depression, anorexia, nausea, vomiting, and ileus. Many of the signs and symptoms of hypomagnesemia are difficult to differentiate from those of hypokalemia and hypocalcemia, both of which are refractory to treatment in the presence of hypomagnesemia. Reports indicate that approximately 38% to 61% of patients with hypokalemia and 22% to 28% of patients with hypocalcemia also present with hypomagnesemia.[23]

Treatment Serum levels may not correlate with intracellular concentrations of magnesium or total body magnesium. As a result, hypomagnesemia treatment goals are largely empirical. Treatment should focus on addressing the underlying cause and correcting coexisting electrolyte imbalances following magnesium repletion. Oral salts are recommended for mild to moderate depletion, although they should be used with caution because they may cause diarrhea. For severe depletion or GI impairment, such as short bowel syndrome, IV administration of $MgSO_4$ is often preferred. The slow onset of action and GI intolerance limit the effectiveness oral administration, especially in severe cases of hypomagnesemia. For asymptomatic patients, clinicians should not exceed 1 g/L/hour of magnesium infusion because high levels of magnesium can cause cardiac arrest. In addition, patients with renal impairment should be administered 50% or less of recommended empirical doses to reduce risk of overcompensating and causing hypermagnesemia.

CASE STUDY REVISITED

On hospital day (HD) 3, you visit Adam and learn that he has been NPO since admission due to his medical GI evaluation. Because Adam is feeling better and his GI symptoms have resolved, the medical team has just advanced Adam to a regular diet. Adam reports an excellent appetite and is looking forward to eating.

Anthropometric Data:

Weight: 73 kg (161 lbs)
Last weight: 75 kg (165 lbs) at admission

Biochemical Data: (HD 3)

Sodium 134 (135-145 mEq/L)
Potassium 3.3 (3.6-5.0 mEq/L)
Blood Urea Nitrogen 22 (6-24 mg/dL)
Creatinine 0.2 (0.4-1.3 mg/dL)
Glucose 95 (70-139 mg/dL)
Phosphorus 2.9 (2.7-4.5 mg/dL)
Magnesium 1.4 (1.3-2.1 mEq/L)

Clinical Data:

Medications: protonix, lipitor, captopril

Dietary Data:

Diet Prescription: Regular

Questions

1. **Is Adam at risk for refeeding syndrome? Explain.**
2. **What biochemical indices should be monitored with refeeding syndrome?**
3. **What factors mediate the refeeding process?**
4. **Do you have any recommendations for interventions for Adam?**

Hypermagnesemia Hypermagnesemia, or high serum magnesium, is uncommon, occurring primarily in patients with renal insufficiency.

Etiology

In addition to renal insufficiency, medications interfering with magnesium excretion, such as lithium and spironolactone, and excessive supplementation of magnesium-containing antacids or laxatives (such as Milk of Magnesia) can also contribute to hypermagnesemia.

Signs and Symptoms Dehydration, nausea, vomiting, diaphoresis (excessive sweating), flushing, sensation of heat, drowsiness, depressed mental status, hypotension, and bradycardia are common symptoms of mild–moderate hypermagnesemia. Neuromuscular functions can also be impaired, leading to decreased reflexes, muscle weakness, and paralysis. Severe cases of hypermagnesemia may also cause respiratory paralysis, cardiac arrest, liver dysfunction, coma, and possibly death.

Treatment In mild cases, where medications or supplementation were the cause of hypermagnesemia, discontinuation of medications containing magnesium or supplementation of antacids or laxatives can treat the abnormality. Rehydration is recommended for those with symptoms of dehydration. In patients with asymptomatic hypermagnesemia, the recommended treatment is to remove or restrict other exogenous sources from PN or IV fluids. Patients with more severe symptomatic hypermagnesemia may need to be treated with IV calcium gluconate to alleviate neuromuscular and cardiovascular symptoms. Elimination of magnesium from IV fluids and PN are the preferred treatment; however, clinicians must consider the potential for ECF to ICF shifts when decreasing magnesium in PN. For patients with renal failure, hemodialysis may be recommended. Clinicians may also consider administering diuretics to increase magnesium excretion.

Refeeding Syndrome

Refeeding syndrome is a condition that can occur in malnourished patients during the initiation of concentrated calorie delivery, characterized by several metabolic complications due to derangements in phosphorus, potassium, magnesium, and glucose control. Together, the effects of depletion, repletion, and compartmental shifts in electrolytes, fluids, and other substrates in response to excessive nutritional resuscitation define refeeding syndrome. Patients with malnutrition, history of long-term inadequate intake, and those with minimal intake for several days are considered at risk for refeeding syndrome.

Reintroduction of carbohydrates (oral, enteral, or parenteral) after starvation induces a shift from ketones as the primary energy source to glucose. During this shift to anabolism particularly with the introduction of insulin, phosphorus, potassium, and magnesium shift intracellularly leading to low serum levels. The carbohydrate delivery also suddenly enables massive phosphorylation of ADP to ATP, leading to a rapid depletion of marginal phosphorus stores as well as thiamin. In addition, sodium and water is retained, leading to the potential for fluid overload. Figure 10 outlines the metabolic changes associated with refeeding syndrome. According to case reports, refeeding syndrome can continue up to 5 days after initiation of feedings.[24]

Electrolyte abnormalities in refeeding syndrome can lead to neurologic, respiratory, and cardiac abnormalities, while vitamin deficiencies can cause severe encephalopathy and sodium retention can contribute to pulmonary edema and cardiac decompensation. Many strategies have been suggested to prevent the adverse effects of refeeding syndrome. Any electrolyte abnormalities should be addressed prior to initiating feedings, and sodium and fluids should be closely monitored in severely malnourished patients during the first days of nutrition repletion. By initiating feedings more slowly or at a lower level, clinicians can help prevent or reduce the metabolic effects of refeeding syndrome from occurring in patients. Starting energy intake at 15 to 20 kcal/kg/day, 1,000 kcal/day, or 50% of estimated needs are common recommendations, with a gradual increase to goal over 5 to 7 days.[25] Clinicians must recognize the risks of refeeding syndrome for severely malnourished patients and the dynamic process requiring continual monitoring and modification according to metabolic needs to maintain stability and promote nutritional repletion.

CORE CONCEPT 3

Refeeding syndrome can result in malnourished patients when carbohydrate feedings induce insulin, resulting in the intracellular shift of potassium, phosphorus, and magnesium, and fluid retention.

PRACTICE POINT

Screening patients for malnutrition (i.e., evaluating anthropometrics, functional assessment, diet history) prior to initiating feeds is critical to prevent and reduce the adverse effects of refeeding syndrome. Slow advancement of feeds to 30% to 50% of caloric requirement is recommended.

Chloride

Chloride (Cl^-) is the most abundant anion in the ECF, with approximately 88% found in ECF and only 12% located intracellularly.[26] Normal serum chloride levels range from 98 to 110 mEq/L, with serum chloride levels closely regulated by the kidneys. Chloride is most commonly found in the body as sodium chloride (NaCl) and hydrochloric acid (HCl). With a negative charge, chloride is usually associated with positively charged sodium and is typically regulated in the same proportion of sodium in extracellular fluid. As a result, chloride works closely with sodium to maintain cell membrane integrity via regulation of fluid balance and serum osmolality. The formation of hydrochloric acid also plays a crucial role in digestion and in acid–base balance. High serum chloride results in metabolic acidosis and low serum chloride can lead to metabolic alkalosis. As a large component of gastric

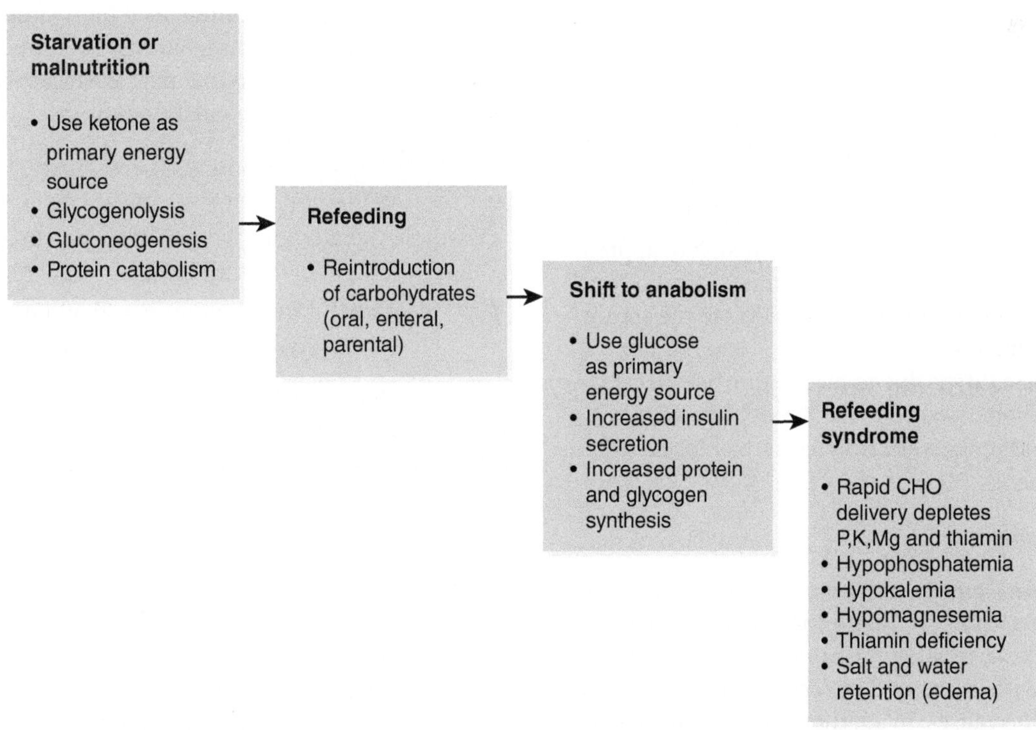

FIGURE 10 **Metabolic Changes Occuring During Refeeding Syndrome**

juice, HCl also alters the pH of the stomach, assists in protein digestion, and activates other digestive enzymes.

Hypochloremia

Etiology Hypochloremia, or low serum chloride, can occur from vomiting, diarrhea, nasogastric suction, GI fistulae, renal failure with salt restriction, and excessive sweating. Chronic respiratory acidosis, metabolic alkalosis, diabetic ketoacidosis, SIADH, adrenal insufficiency, and hyperaldosteronism may cause hypochloremia. Chronic use of laxatives, bicarbonate, corticosteroids, and diuretics may also lead to hypochloremia.

Signs and Symptoms Many people with hypochloremia are asymptomatic, with symptoms only present at extremely low levels. Common symptoms may include dehydration, hyperirritability, tetany, slowed respirations, and hypotension resulting from fluid loss.

Treatment Treatment of hypochloremia must initially address the underlying cause. Assessment of hydration status, severity of hypochloremia, and presence of concurrent electrolyte disorders (hypokalemia, hyponatremia) and metabolic alkalosis is critical. In acute hypochloremia, if the patient is in shock, isotonic fluid, preferably saline, should be administered. Clinicians should treat chronic hypochloremia more slowly because rapid treatment can lead to more serious complications. Intravenous administration of isotonic sodium chloride and potassium chloride is recommended, with doses determined by patients' serum chloride levels. To calculate chloride deficit, the following equation is used:

Chloride Deficit in mEq = (0.27) (Weight in kg) (100 – Chloride level)

Sample Calculation: Weight 70 kg, Chloride 92 mEq/L

Chloride Deficit in mEq = (0.27) (70) (100 – 92)

Chloride Deficit = 151 mEq

The 100 in the equation refers to a desired chloride level and the 0.27 refers to the chloride distribution in the body. A 70-kg patient with hypochloremia (chloride 92 mEq/L) has a chloride deficit of 151 mEq if a chloride level of 100 mEq is desired. Furthermore, an infusion of approximately 1 L normal saline (which contains 154 mEq NaCl) would correct this deficit in order to increase the serum chloride to normal range.

If the abnormality is due to medication use, decrease or remove medication if possible. For hypochloremic acidosis, clinicians should replace electrolytes with chloride salts as primary treatment.

Hyperchloremia

Etiology Hyperchloremia, or increased serum chloride, can also result from a variety of health conditions. Renal failure, nephritic syndrome, renal tubular acidosis, dehydration, overtreatment with saline, and hyperparathyroidism are the most common causes. In addition, diabetes insipidus, metabolic acidosis from diarrhea, respiratory alkalosis, and hyperadrenocorticism can also result in hyperchloremia. Certain drugs including acetozolamide, androgens, hydrochlorothiazide, and salicylates can also cause hyperchloremia.

Signs and Symptoms The most common symptoms of hyperchloremia are weakness and lethargy, with more serious symptoms including unconsciousness and Kussmaul respirations, which are deep and labored breaths often associated with diabetic ketoacidosis or kidney failure.

Treatment Treatment of hyperchloremia varies based on the etiology. If excessive intake or inadequate excretion of chloride causes hyperchloremic acidosis, clinicians should substitute acetate, citrate, or phosphate salts for chloride salts in infusions. To treat GI causes of hyperchloremia, clinicians are recommended to administer saline solutions to treat volume losses and to administer potassium. Acidosis should be treated with bicarbonate-containing solutions with potassium replacement due to the potential consequences of rapid introduction of potassium into cells (cardiac arrhythmias and muscular paralysis). If chronic acidosis is present with hyperchloremia due to diarrhea, long-term therapy with sodium and potassium citrate solutions may be recommended.

Bicarbonate

Bicarbonate is a compound in the blood that works closely with chloride to maintain acid–base balance in the body. Bicarbonate usually refers to HCO_3 or carbon dioxide (CO_2), with normal serum levels ranging from 20 to 30 mEq/L. High serum bicarbonate results in metabolic alkalosis, while low serum bicarbonate causes metabolic acidosis. Treatment for metabolic acidosis is typically sodium bicarbonate ($NaHCO_3$) via IV administration. Due to the instability of bicarbonate in patients receiving PN, acetate, the biological precursor of bicarbonate, is recommended for treatment in these patients, assuming they have normal liver function to convert acetate to bicarbonate. To calculate the bicarbonate deficit in patients, the following calculation is used:

Bicarbonate Deficit in mEq = (0.50)(Weight in kg) (Desired Bicarbonate – Serum Bicarbonate)

Sample Calculation: Weight 70 kg, Serum Bicarbonate 17 mEq/L

Bicarbonate Deficit in mEq = (0.50)(70)(24 – 17)

Bicarbonate Deficit = 245 mEq

The value of 0.50 is used in this equation to calculate the bicarbonate deficit because the bicarbonate volume of distribution is usually 50% of body weight under normal conditions. A 70-kg patient with a serum bicarbonate of 17 has a bicarbonate deficit of 254 mEq if a bicarbonate level of 24 mEq is desired.

Acid–Base Physiology

An acid is any substance that releases hydrogen ions (H^+) in solution, whereas a base is a substance that accepts or combines with H^+. The free hydrogen ion concentration, represented by the pH, determines the acidity of body

CASE STUDY REVISITED

On HD 6, Adam undergoes an urgent laparotomy for a severe gastric ulcer with perforation. On post-operative (postop) day 1/HD 7, you visit Adam for reassessment. He is currently in the ICU on mechanical ventilation with increased drainage from a nasogastric tube.

Anthropometric Data:

Weight: 77 kg (169 lbs) on HD 7
Last weight: 73 kg (161 lbs) on HD 3

Biochemical Data: (postop day 1/HD 7):

Sodium 143 (135-145 mEq/L)
Potassium 3.5 (3.6-5.0 mEq/L)
Chloride 88 (98-110 mEq/L)
Carbon Dioxide 41 (20-30 mEq/L)
Blood Urea Nitrogen 24 (6-24 mg/dL)
Creatinine 0.2 (0.4-1.3 mg/dL)
Glucose 139 (70-139 mg/dL)
Calcium 7.7 (8.5-10.5 mEq/L)
Phosphorus 3.0 (2.7-4.5 mg/dL)
Magnesium 1.4 (1.3-2.1 mEq/L)

Arterial Blood Gas:

pH 7.48 (7.35-7.45)
$PaCO_2$ 48 (35-45 mm Hg)
PaO_2 90 (80-100 mm Hg)
HCO_3 29 (22-26 mEq/L)

Dietary Data:

Diet Prescription: NPO

Questions

1. **Describe Adam's acid–base status.**
2. **What specific acid–base disorder does he have?**
3. **What interventions would you recommend to manage this acid–base imbalance?**

fluids. Because the pH varies inversely with the hydrogen ion concentration, a decrease in hydrogen ion concentration raises the pH and an increase in hydrogen ion concentration lowers the pH. In arterial blood, the pH is normally maintained within the narrow range of 7.35 to 7.45. An increased concentration of hydrogen ion concentration in the blood reflected by a blood pH below 7.35 is called **acidemia**, while a decreased concentration of hydrogen ion concentration in the blood reflected by blood pH above 7.45 is called **alkalemia**. **Acidosis** is the condition of increased hydrogen ion concentration and **alkalosis** is the condition of decreased hydrogen ion concentration. These terms are important to understand when evaluating acid–base disorders in patients because both acidotic and alkalotic processes can coexist. Figure 11 illustrates the pH scale and hydrogen ion concentration range.

As with fluid and electrolyte balance, acid–base balance is critical for many physiologic functions and biochemical reactions. Serum chloride and bicarbonate levels are the most common electrolytes associated with acid–base imbalance. In a healthy individual, the kidneys, lungs, and buffering systems tightly regulate the pH level within the body, despite changes in acidity from diet and tissue metabolism. Metabolic and respiratory disorders can disrupt acid–base balance, resulting in alkalosis and acidosis. Adverse consequences of acid–base imbalance can be life threatening in severe cases. Clinicians must

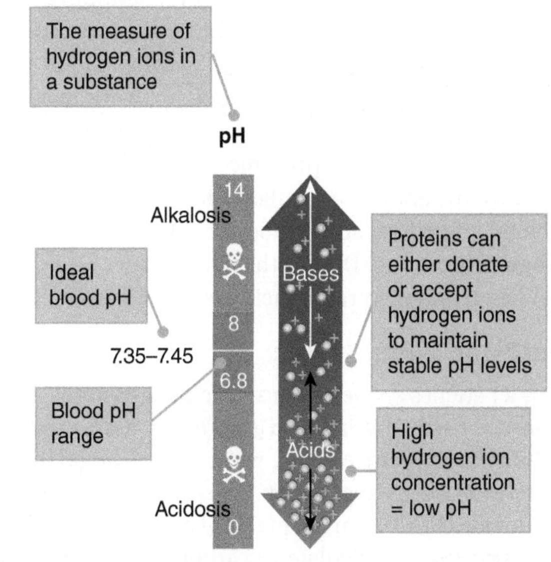

FIGURE 11 **pH Scale in Relation to Hydrogen Ion Concentration**

understand the underlying physiological processes and/or exogenous causes that occur in acid–base disorders to accurately diagnose and determine therapy regarding fluids, PN, and electrolyte managements.

Most hydrogen ions originate as a byproduct or end product of cellular metabolism, although a small amount of acidic substances enter the body via ingested food. Together, carbohydrates and fats produce approximately 15,000 mmol of CO_2, which forms carbonic acid when combined with water. Also, protein metabolism produces 50 to 100 mEq/day of noncarbonic acid.[27] Without tight regulation, progressive accumulation of acids can be detrimental. Hydrogen ion regulation within the body involves three steps: (1) chemical buffering via intracellular and extracellular mechanisms; (2) control of partial pressure of carbon dioxide in blood by changes in rate of alveolar ventilation; and (3) control of plasma bicarbonate concentration by alterations in renal H^+ excretion.

Chemical Buffers (1): Buffering systems prevent large changes in hydrogen ion concentration and are the first line of defense, occurring immediately to resist changes in pH. In general, the buffering systems consist of weak acid and base pairs that can take up or release hydrogen ions to minimize changes in free concentration. The carbonic acid/bicarbonate (H_2CO_3/HCO_3^-) system is the principal buffer system in the body, while the others (proteins, phosphate, and hemoglobin) also contribute to maintain a normal pH.

Lungs (2): The primary role of the lungs in maintaining acid–base balance is to control the pressure exerted by dissolved CO_2 gas in the blood. Among all chemicals impacting respiration, CO_2 is considered the most powerful respiratory stimulant. The rate and depth of ventilation can both be changed to allow diet and cellular metabolism to generate CO_2. Within minutes of acid–base disturbances, the rate and depth of ventilation begins to be compensated. As a result, any condition that impairs respiratory system functioning can lead to acid–base imbalances.

Kidneys (3): Alterations in renal hydrogen ion excretion is the last and slowest mechanism used to maintain acid–base balance within the body. Both the reabsorption of filtered bicarbonate and the excretion of hydrogen ions, which is produced daily from protein metabolism, work to achieve this balance. The acid–base regulatory mechanism of the kidneys is unique from the prior mechanisms because the kidneys have the ability to regulate alkaline substances in the blood and eliminate metabolic acids (organic acids, other than carbonic acid) from the body. Figure 12 outlines the renal and respiratory acid–base regulation.

Arterial Blood Gases

To assess a patient's oxygenation and acid–base status, blood gas values are used. **Arterial blood gases (ABGs)** assess the lung's ability to oxygenate blood, while venous blood gases (VBGs) reflect tissue oxygenation. The partial pressure of carbon dioxide (PCO_2), partial pressure of oxygen (PO_2), oxygen saturation (SaO_2), calculated bicarbonate, pH, and base excess are the most common blood gas measurements used.

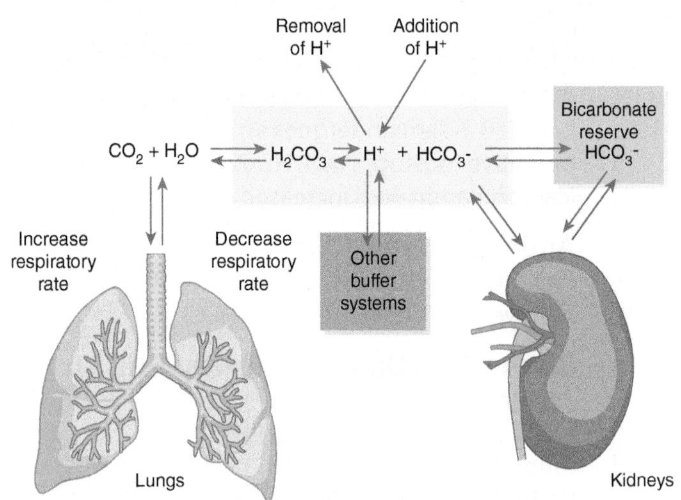

FIGURE 12 **Renal and Respiratory Acid-Base Regulation**

Normal values are listed in the Table 4. The normal ranges of these measurements differ for ABGs and VBGs, and evaluations also differ in aspects of ventilation and perfusion.

The $PaCO_2$ reflects the lung's ability to excrete carbon dioxide. Changes in $PaCO_2$ are associated with respiratory processes that can cause acid–base disorders. Because $PaCO_2$ is the acid component of the carbonic acid/bicarbonate buffer system, an increase in $PaCO_2$ reflects an acidosis and a decrease in $PaCO_2$ reflects an alkalosis. PaO_2 reflects hemoglobin's ability to carry oxygen, and is directly related to hemoglobin saturated with oxygen (SaO_2). When the partial pressure of oxygen is high, oxygen saturation of the blood is also high, and vice versa.

Changes in bicarbonate are associated with metabolic processes that can lead to acid–base disorders. Either calculated bicarbonate reported in blood gas or serum bicarbonate can be used to evaluate acid–base status. Because

TABLE 4 REFERENCE RANGE FOR BLOOD GAS VALUES

Blood Gas Values for Acid–Base Balance		
Laboratory Test	**Normal Arterial**	**Normal Mixed Venous**
pH	7.35-7.45	7.33-7.43
PCO_2	35-45 mm Hg	41-51 mm Hg
PO_2	80-100 mm Hg	35-40 mm Hg
HCO_3^-	22-26 mEq/L	24-28 mEq/L
O_2 saturation	>95%	70-75%
Base excess	−2 to +2	0 to +4

bicarbonate is the base component of the carbonic acid/bicarbonate buffer system, an increase in serum or calculated bicarbonate reflects an alkalosis, and a decrease reflects an acidosis. Base excess is another value that can be calculated and estimates the metabolic component of acid–base disorder. An increase in base excess occurs a metabolic alkalosis, while base deficit occurs in metabolic acidosis.

Acid–base Disorders

Acid–base disorders can be assessed using a systematic approach to avoid misdiagnosis and inappropriate treatment. The following steps can be useful for adequate evaluation for clinicians:

1. Use pH value to determine whether patient is acidemic (pH <7.4) or alkalemic (pH >7.4). A pH of 7.4 should not be excluded from assessment because compensation or a mixed acid–base disorder could contribute to a normal pH range.
2. Assess $PaCO_2$ to determine respiratory status. Elevated $PaCO_2$ indicates respiratory acidosis, while low $PaCO_2$ indicates respiratory alkalosis. (Table 5 highlights the characteristics of primary acid–base imbalances.)
3. Assess HCO_3^- to determine metabolic status. Elevated HCO_3^- indicates metabolic alkalosis, while low HCO_3^- indicates metabolic acidosis.
4. Calculate the anion gap to determine the presence of metabolic acidosis. The anion gap can be calculated using the equation below (normal range is 8-16 mEq/L). Calculating anion gap is critical to assess the etiology of acid–base and determine appropriate treatment:

$$\text{Anion gap} = Na^+ - (Cl^- + HCO_3^-)$$

5. Determine whether the acid–base disorder is an acute or chronic condition and assess whether the acid–base disorder is appropriately compensated. If appropriate compensation is not evident, a mixed acid–base disorder may be present.

TABLE 5 CHARACTERISTICS OF PRIMARY ACID–BASE IMBALANCES

Disorder	pH	Primary Disturbance	Compensatory Response
Metabolic Acidosis	Low	Low HCO_3^-	Low $PaCO_2$
Metabolic Alkalosis	High	High HCO_3^-	High $PaCO_2$
Respiratory Acidosis	Low	High $PaCO_2$	High HCO_3^-
Respiratory Alkalosis	High	Low $PaCO_2$	Low HCO_3^-

Data from Charney P. Ch.7: Clinical: Water, Electrolytes, and Acid-Base Balance. In *Krause's Food & the Nutrition Care Process*. 13th ed. St. Louis, Missouri: Elsevier Saunders; 2012:188.

Respiratory acidosis is characterized by a low pH, high $PaCO_2$, and a variable increase in plasma HCO_3^- concentration. This disorder is most commonly caused by decreased effective alveolar ventilation and not an increase in carbon dioxide production. When there is interference in the ventilation at any step, hypoventilation can occur. In patients with severely impaired CO_2 excretion and/or life-threatening hypoxemia, adequate oxygenation should be provided. The most common causes include central nervous system depression, neuromuscular disorders, chronic obstructive pulmonary disease, and interstitial pulmonary disease. The underlying cause should be treated accordingly (bronchodilators and steroids, adjustment of ventilation, etc.), with sodium bicarbonate reserved for treatment of severely acidotic patients (pH <7.15).

Respiratory alkalosis is characterized by a high pH, low $PaCO_2$, and a variable decrease in plasma HCO_3^- concentration. This often occurs with increased effective alveolar ventilation beyond the level needed to eliminate metabolically produced CO_2, leading to hyperventilation. Common causes of respiratory alkalosis include pulmonary disease, hypoxemia, and increased central stimulation of respiration. See Table 6 for more a complete list of the

TABLE 6 CAUSES OF RESPIRATORY ACID–BASE DISORDERS

Respiratory Acidosis	Respiratory Alkalosis
• Acute respiratory distress syndrome (ARDS) • Aspiration • Asthma • Cardiac arrest • Central depression of respiration • Chronic obstructive pulmonary disease (COPD) • Drugs (opioids, anesthetics, sedatives) • Head injury • Hypoventilation • Hypoxemia • Multiple sclerosis • Perfusion abnormalities • Parenteral nutrition • Pulmonary abnormalities, such as pulmonary edema and severe pulmonary embolism • Sleep apnea • Stroke	• Altitudes (high) • Anemia (severe) • Anxiety • Asthma • Brain tumor • Central stimulation of respiration • Drugs (catecholamines, salicylates) • Fever • Head trauma • Hyperventilation • Hypoxemia • Pain • Peripheral stimulation of respiration • Pregnancy • Pulmonary issues, such as pulmonary edema and pulmonary embolism • Pneumonia • Vascular accident

Modified from Langley G, Tajchman S. *A.S.P.E.N. Adult Nutrition Support Core Curriculum Chapter 7: Fluids, Electrolytes, and Acid-Base Disorders*. 2nd ed. Washington DC: American Society for Parenteral and Enteral Nutrition; 2012:116.

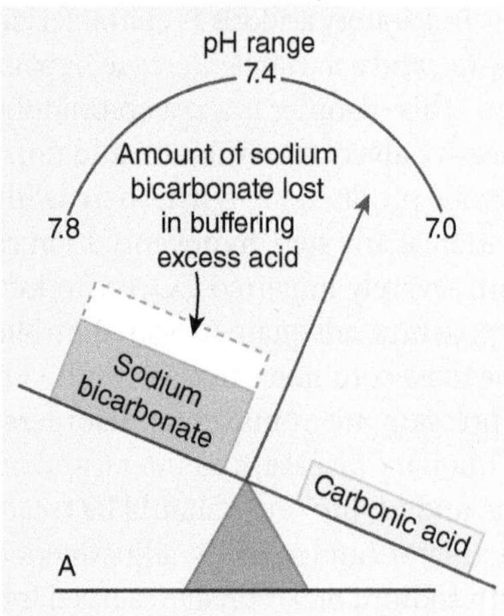

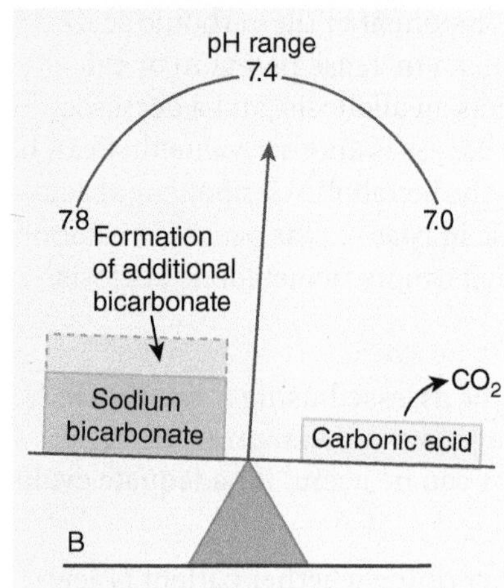

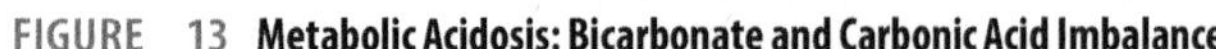

FIGURE 13 **Metabolic Acidosis: Bicarbonate and Carbonic Acid Imbalance**

causes of respiratory acid–base imbalances.

Metabolic acidosis is characterized by a low pH, a low HCO_3^- concentration, and a compensatory hyperventilation that contributes to a decreased $PaCO_2$. Figure 13 illustrates bicarbonate and carbonic acid imbalance in metabolic acidosis and compensation. This condition can result from either the inability of kidneys to excrete the dietary hydrogen ion load or an increase in hydrogen ion generation due to an addition of hydrogen ions or a loss of bicarbonate. Calculating the anion gap with the equation listed above can assist in the diagnosis of metabolic acidosis. The anion gap (approximately 8-16 mEq/L) represents the unmeasured serum ions including proteins, phosphate, sulfate, and organic ions.[28] In particular, albumin accounts for a large portion of unmeasured serum anions. For every decrease in 1 g/dL in serum albumin, the anion gap increases by approximately 2.5 mEq/L.[10] Calculating the anion gap allows clinicians to differentiate between normal anion gap acidosis or elevated anion gap acidosis.

Normal anion-gap acidosis (anion gap 8-16 mEq/L) occurs when there is milliequivalent-for-milliequivalent replacement of extracellular bicarbonate by chloride. As a result, there is a normal anion gap because the sum remains constant for the major measured anions. The most common causes of this disorder, also known as hypercholeremic metabolic acidosis, include increased GI or renal bicarbonate loss. *High anion-gap metabolic acidosis* (anion gap >25 mEq/L) is a result of metabolic acidosis associated with accumulation of unmeasured anions. This condition is most commonly caused by renal failure to excrete acid, diabetic ketoacidosis, and lactic acidosis from shock. Hypovolemia must be addressed with expansion of extracellular volume and IV insulin infusion should be administered to stop production of ketoacids. Once volume is replenished and insulin is administered, potassium should be replaced. Table 7 outlines the causes of normal and increased anion gap metabolic acidosis.

TABLE 7 CAUSES OF METABOLIC ACIDOSIS

Normal Anion Gap	Increased Anion Gap
Gastrointestinal loss of HCO_3^- • Anion-exchange resins • Diarrhea • Ingestion of calcium or magnesium chloride • Obstructed ileal loop • Pancreatic fistula	Increased production of endogenous acid
Ingestions • Ammonium chloride • Parenteral nutrition (chloride salts) • Sulfur	Inborn errors of metabolism • Ketoacidosis • Lactic acidosis
Renal loss of HCO_3^- • Carbonic anhydrase inhibitors • Hypoaldosteronism • Hyperparathyroidism • Renal tubular acidosis	Failure to excrete acids • Ingestion of exogenous acid • Salicyclates, methanol, ethanol • Renal failure

Modified from Langley G, Tajchman S. *A.S.P.E.N. Adult Nutrition Support Core Curriculum Chapter 7: Fluids, Electrolytes, and Acid-Base Disorders*. 2nd ed. Washington DC: American Society for Parenteral and Enteral Nutrition; 2012:116.

Metabolic alkalosis is characterized by a high pH, a high bicarbonate concentration, and compensatory hypoventilation that contribute to an increased $PaCO_2$. This disorder is reported in approximately 33% to 55% of hospitalized patients with acid–base disturbances.[29] The most common causes of this disorder include loss of gastric acid from vomiting or nasogastric suction and loss of intravascular volume and chloride from diuretic use. In the clinical setting, the most common cause is overtreatment of metabolic acidosis with bicarbonate or an excess of acetate in PN, which becomes metabolized to bicarbonate. Hypokalemia in patients can cause a transcellular shift of hydrogen ions, which can also contribute to the development of metabolic alkalosis. Normally, the kidneys can correct this disorder by excreting the excess bicarbonate in urine. Therefore, maintenance of metabolic alkalosis indicates that patients may have some degree of impairment in renal bicarbonate excretion. Urine chloride concentration can be used to classify metabolic alkalosis into volume mediated (saline responsive) and volume independent (saline resistant) and predict which patients will respond to volume replacement.

Saline-responsive metabolic alkalosis (urine chloride <10 mEq/L) is the most common metabolic alkalosis. To treat this disorder, administration of normal saline is recommended to reverse the increase in bicarbonate reabsorption that maintains alkalosis. While sufficient repletion of sodium chloride can typically normalize bicarbonate concentration, metabolic alkalosis will not be reversed if associated with hypokalemia. Potassium chloride is required to correct this underlying disorder. *Saline resistant metabolic alkalosis* (urine chloride >10 mEq/L) is most frequently associated with hyperaldosteronism. Treatment of this disorder requires first addressing the underlying cause of mineralocorticoid excess. When hypokalemia is present with this disorder in primary hyperaldosteronism, clinicians should treat this deficiency with aggressive potassium repletion. Table 8 outlines common causes of saline-responsive and saline-resistant metabolic alkalosis.

Mixed acid–base disorders occur when patients have more than one acid–base disturbance occurring simultaneously. To diagnose a mixed acid–base disorder, clinicians must have an understanding of the extent of renal and respiratory compensations for each of the acid–base disturbances. When a set of blood gases does not fall within the range of expected responses for a simple acid–base disturbance, then clinicians should suspect that a mixed disorder exists. The most common mixed disorders include mixed respiratory acidosis and metabolic acidosis; mixed respiratory alkalosis and metabolic alkalosis; mixed metabolic acidosis and respiratory alkalosis; and mixed metabolic alkalosis and respiratory acidosis. If patients present with normal pH and alterations in pCO_2 and plasma bicarbonate, then clinicians should expect that a mixed acid–base disorder is present.

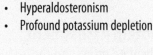

CORE CONCEPT 4

Fluid, electrolyte, and acid–base imbalances can lead to serious complications ranging from metabolic and gastrointestinal problems to cardiovascular, respiratory, and neurological concerns, each requiring careful evaluation, monitoring, and treatment.

Endocrine Function: Glucose and Glycosylated Hemoglobin

Glucose values are important in screening and diagnosing endocrine disorders and in monitoring patients with acute stress and critical illness. Evaluating trends in glucose measures is essential to determine glucose tolerance and to prevent adverse and potentially fatal consequences that may occur in patients experiencing abnormal glucose values.

Blood glucose, the measure of glucose in the plasma, is a short-term measure of glycemic response and glucose tolerance. Normal *fasting blood glucose* values range from 70 to 99 mg/dL or 3.9 to 5.5 mmol/L, while fasting blood glucose >100 mg/dL suggests impaired glucose metabolism. Diagnostic criteria for diabetes mellitus (DM) include the following: fasting plasma glucose ≥126 mg/dL (7.0 mmol/L), 2-hour postprandial plasma glucose ≥200 mg/dL (11.1 mmol/L), or classic symptoms of hyperglycemia or hyperglycemic crises with random plasma glucose ≥200 mg/dL.[30] Clinicians can use glucose testing to screen and diagnose patients, as well as to monitor patients receiving total PN. Figure 14 illustrates the comparison of blood glucose levels in nondiabetic and diabetic individuals after a glucose tolerance test.

Urine glucose, although not a diagnostic criteria, is also abnormal in patients with DM. Normal urine glucose tests should be negative, while patients with DM may present with

TABLE 8 CAUSES OF METABOLIC ALKALOSIS

Saline-Responsive (Urine Chloride <10 mEq/L)	Saline-Resistant (Urine Chloride >10 mEq/L)
• Diuretic therapy	• Cushing's syndrome
• Excessive bicarbonate administration	• Excess mineralocorticoids
• Gastrointestinal loss	• Excessive licorice ingestion
• Nasogastric suction	• Hyperaldosteronism
• Rapid correction of hypocapnia	• Profound potassium depletion
• Renal loss	
• Vomiting	

Modified from Langley G, Tajchman S. *A.S.P.E.N. Adult Nutrition Support Core Curriculum Chapter 7: Fluids, Electrolytes, and Acid-Base Disorders*. 2nd ed. Washington DC: American Society for Parenteral and Enteral Nutrition; 2012:116.

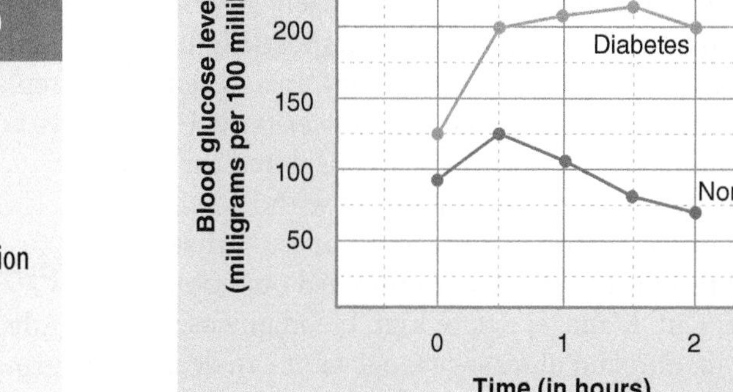

FIGURE 14 **Comparison of Blood Glucose levels of a Non-Diabetic and Diabetic After a Glucose Tolerance Test**

levels of 2 to 10 g/dL. A positive urine glucose result (glucosuria) is rarely found in benign conditions. Treatment includes managing DM and improving hydration status, due to the loss of water that follows when glucose is present in urine.

Urine ketones should be tested if glucose levels are elevated in patients during periods of illness or stress. For patients with DM, urine ketones should be tested if blood glucose is consistently greater than 300 mg/dL. In healthy nondiabetic patients, urine ketones should be negative. Uncontrolled DM is the most common cause of positive urine ketones. Other potential causes include fever, anorexia, certain GI disturbances, persistent vomiting, cachexia, fasting, and starvation. Positive urine ketones represent a condition that can lead to diabetic ketoacidosis, resulting in dehydration and electrolyte imbalances due to osmotic diuresis. Without immediate treatment of diabetic ketoacidosis, this condition can be fatal. Treatment includes assessment and treatment of severe hyperglycemia with IV fluids, insulin, and electrolytes. Doses of supplemental insulin are required until metabolic stability returns.

Glycosylated hemoglobin (HbA1c) is a measure of the percentage of glucose bound to hemoglobin in red blood cells. The subfraction of HbA1c in hemoglobin has a unique chemical structure that causes nonenzymatic glycation at the amino-terminal valines of the beta chains of hemoglobin A. As the lifespan of red blood cells is approximately 3 months, HbA1c is directly related to the average blood glucose levels during this length of time. A 1% change in HbA1c means a change in plasma glucose by approximately 35 mg/dL.[32] Unlike blood glucose levels, an HbA1c test does not reflect recent changes, making it a useful measure to differentiate between short-term hyperglycemia in individuals under stress or those with DM. HbA1c has been added to the diagnostic criteria for DM. In adults with normal blood glucose control, HbA1c values range from 4.3% to 5.8%.[33] **Table 9** correlates HbA1c with average blood glucose levels.

Diagnosis of DM is confirmed when an initial value is followed up with a repeat HbA1c ≥6.5% or plasma glucose ≥200 mg/dL. Because HbA1c is related to the lifespan of the erythrocyte, conditions that increase or decrease red blood cell turnover may alter results. For example, anemias which prolong erythrocyte turnover can lead to falsely elevated HbA1c levels. Conversely, conditions that increase erythrocyte production and turnover such as such as gestational diabetes can lead to falsely low HbA1c. Because of this, HbA1c is not a useful diagnostic indicator after the first few months of pregnancy. In addition to using HbA1c as a component of diagnostic criteria, HbA1c and trends in blood glucose levels are considered the best indicators of glycemic control in patients with DM. Clinicians can interpret trends in these levels and use these values to make recommendations for improved nutrition and DM management. Management of high blood glucose levels through insulin and glucose management can decrease HbA1c levels in people with DM and reduce risk of comorbidities associated with DM.

TABLE 9 HEMOGLOBIN A1C AND ESTIMATED EQUIVALENT AVERAGE BLOOD GLUCOSE[31]

Hemoglobin A1c	Mean Blood Glucose
6%	126 mg/dL
7%	154 mg/dL
8%	183 mg/dL
9%	212 mg/dL
10%	240 mg/dL
11%	269 mg/dL
12%	298 mg/dL

Data from Nathan DM, Kuenen J, Borg R, Zheng H, Schoenfeld D, Heine RJ. A1c-Derived Average Glucose Study Group. Translating the A1C assay into estimated average glucose values. *Diabetes Care*. 2008;31:1473–1478.

Hypoglycemia or low blood glucose can be caused by glycogen storage disease, liver disease, renal insufficiency, alcohol, abrupt PN cessation, cancer, or prolonged exercise. HbA1c is frequently used to assess for hypoglycemia, with values of 4.3% to 5.8% defining hypoglycemia for nondiabetic patients. Target HbA1c values for patients with DM range from 6.5% to 8% according to a patient's history of diabetes, hypoglycemia episodes, and diabetes-related health complications.[30]

Hyperglycemia is defined as blood glucose levels higher than the normal range. Mild hyperglycemia can result from uncontrolled diabetes, pancreatitis/pancreatic insufficiency, obesity, acute stress, or cirrhosis. Medications including thiazide and loop diuretics can cause mild hyperglycemia. Severe hyperglycemia (>400 mg/dL) is more commonly caused by diabetic ketoacidosis due to insulin deficiency and hyperosmolar hyperglycemic nonketotic dehydration. Common symptoms of severe hyperglycemia include increased urine output, glucosuria, hypernatremia, and headaches. Treatment of severe hyperglycemia requires replacement of fluids and electrolytes and insulin administration.

Protein Assessment

Adequate protein in the body is essential for cellular growth and metabolism. Despite the large amount of protein in muscle and viscera, the body strives to protect it from being used as an energy source by drawing primarily

CASE STUDY REVISITED

It is now postoperative day 6/HD 12 and Adam remains in the ICU. He is currently receiving enteral nutrition support since postop day 3, which provides him with 1,700 calories and 100 g protein.

Anthropometric Data:

Weight: 76 kg (167 lbs)
Last Weight: 77 kg (169 lbs) postop day 1/HD 7
Admit weight 75 kg (165 lbs)

Biochemical Data:

Albumin 2.1 g/dL (3.5-5.0 g/dL)
Prealbumin 14 g/dL (17-36 g/dL)
Urine urea nitrogen (UUN) 10 g/24 hours

Questions

1. **How do you interpret Adam's current albumin and prealbumin levels? What information does this provide to your assessment of Adam's nutritional status?**
2. **Calculate Adam's nitrogen balance. Is he in positive or negative nitrogen balance?**
3. **Based on this information, how would you assess Adam's current nutrition plan?**
4. **What biochemical indices can you monitor to further assess nutritional adequacy?**

from fat and glycogen stores. When the body experiences acute or chronic metabolic stress, protein from muscle may be drawn to meet energy needs. Although no single laboratory value can determine the precise protein status of a patient, a combination of measures can provide a more complete picture of protein status, including anthropometric, dietary, physical, and biochemical findings. Clinicians must interpret these measures in combination to adequately assess protein status and monitor and treat patients according to the etiology and severity of illness. Biochemical assessment of protein focuses on evaluation from two compartments: visceral and somatic proteins. Visceral proteins consist of approximately 25% of total body protein and include non-muscular protein in organs, structural components, serum proteins, and blood cells. Somatic proteins make up the other 75% of total body protein within skeletal muscle.

Total serum protein measures the total amount of protein in the blood, including albumin and globulin (alpha-1, alpha-2, and beta) levels. Normal total serum protein levels range from 6.4 to 8.3 g/dL, while abnormalities are likely due to change in volume of plasma fluid or change in concentration of one or more plasma proteins. A low total serum protein level can result from decreased production or increased protein loss. Some common causes of hypoproteinemia include liver disorders, kidney disorders, and GI malabsorption disorders (such as celiac disease or inflammatory bowel disease). Low total protein levels are also found in patients with severe malnutrition, but clinicians must assess other possible factors contributing to low protein levels before determining appropriate treatment. In contrast, high total protein levels or hyperproteinemia can result from chronic inflammation or infection including viral hepatitis or human immunodeficiency virus (HIV). Bone marrow disorders such as multiple myeloma may cause hyperproteinemia. Medications, inflammation, infection, prolonged bed rest, chronic illness, and pregnancy can also impact total serum protein levels. If patients have abnormal total serum protein levels, clinicians must further assess serum globulin and serum albumin levels to evaluate etiology and determine appropriate nutrition therapy.

Visceral Proteins

Visceral protein indirectly measures protein stores by assessing the proteins made by the viscera, namely, organs (primarily the liver). Because serum protein is affected by the amount of amino acids needed for protein synthesis in the liver, a change in serum proteins is consistent with a change in visceral protein status. When acute illness or trauma causes inflammatory and/or metabolic stress, hormones and cell-mediated responses trigger muscle breakdown. In response to inflammation, **acute-phase proteins** respond by either increasing (positive acute-phase proteins) or decreasing (negative acute-phase proteins). As a result, protein status can be difficult to assess in acutely ill patients because these acute-phase proteins do not accurately reflect changes in protein status. Inflammation identified by serum visceral protein can contribute to several nutrition-related issues as inflammation contributes to net protein loss from catabolism and can induce anorexia. Clinicians must take into account the differences in specificity, sensitivity, and reliability of each visceral protein measurement when assessing and treating patients with acute, stress-related illnesses.

Positive acute-phase proteins such as C-reactive protein, ferritin, and ceruloplasmin increase during inflammation. *C-reactive protein (CRP)* is a nonspecific inflammatory biomarker and a normal serum CRP level is less than 1 mg/dL. CRP increases as transport protein levels (such as prealbumin and albumin) decrease. Although the exact function of CRP is unclear, it increases during the initial stage of acute hypermetabolic stress, which is usually within 4 to 6 hours of surgery or other trauma. Generally, a higher CRP indicates increased nutritional risk.

Negative acute-phase proteins include serum albumin, prealbumin, retinal binding protein, and transferrin. These **constitutive** (or constantly active) transport proteins are synthesized in the liver and decrease during acute-inflammatory stress, injury, or illness.

Albumin accounts for approximately 60% of total serum proteins, and is mostly found in skin, muscle, and organs. Normal serum albumin levels range from 3.5 to 5.0 g/dL. Albumin serves many important functions in the body, including transport and vascular fluid and electrolyte balance. Major blood constituents, hormones, enzymes, medications, minerals, ions, fatty acids, and metabolites are all transported via albumin. Maintenance of colloidal osmotic pressure also requires albumin, with albumin making up approximately 80% of colloidal osmotic pressure of the plasma. Serum albumin is a biomarker that has been widely used in hospital settings and is often correlated with outcomes and mortality.[34,35] However, albumin has been found to be a poor indicator of nutrition support adequacy because proteolysis occurs despite nutrition provision. The half-life of albumin is 18 to 21 days, which decreases albumin's sensitivity to short-term changes in protein status or short-term nutrition therapy to improve protein status.

Several non-dietary factors can alter serum albumin levels, with decreased levels commonly due to changes in fluid distribution, decreased synthesis, or increased degradation of albumin. Acute stress and inflammatory response decrease serum albumin levels by altering at least one of the factors listed above. Specifically, albumin loss occurs with trauma such as burn injuries, nephritic syndrome, protein-losing enteropathy, and cirrhosis. Hypoalbuminemia may also occur with surgery, infection, multiple myeloma, acute or chronic inflammation, rheumatoid arthritis, and aging. Liver disease, cancer, and malabsorption can also decrease albumin levels. Hydration status also affects serum albumin levels because water in the plasma shifts between the interstitial compartment if patients are overhydrated (leading to decreased albumin) or dehydrated (leading to increased albumin).

Albumin levels also vary according to the specific types of malnutrition, **kwashiorkor** or **marasmus**. In patients with marasmus, associated with severe caloric depletion, the body conserves visceral protein levels. In this condition, weight may be less than or equal to 80% of normal body weight, while albumin levels remain within reference range.[36] In contrast, in patients with kwashiorkor, which is associated with protein degradation with or without caloric deficit, visceral protein stores become depleted. As a result, low albumin levels may be present, but weight may be normal or elevated due to edema (**Figure 15**).

Increased albumin levels (hyperalbuminemia) can result from dehydration and exogenous albumin administration. Anabolic hormones and corticoid steroids can also raise albumin levels higher than normal. Clinicians must interpret changes in albumin level with caution, recognizing that low albumin is likely an indicator of stress or inflammation and not overall protein status.

Prealbumin (PAB), also called transthyretin, is a hepatic protein transported in the serum bound to retinol-binding protein and vitamin A. Normal PAB levels range from 17 to 36 g/dL (177-363 mg/L). Prealbumin is responsible for transporting the thyroid hormones (triiodothyronine and thyroxine) and T_4-binding globulin. It is synthesized in the liver and is renally excreted, although it is not influenced by hydration status. Because PAB has a relatively short half-life of 2 to 3 days, clinicians may use levels as a possible indicator of protein status. As with albumin, serum PAB levels decrease with illness, infection, trauma, burns, surgery, and metabolic stress. Liver disorders such as hepatitis or cirrhosis, malabsorption, and hyperthyroidism may also cause low PAB levels. Serum PAB also decreases in the presence of zinc

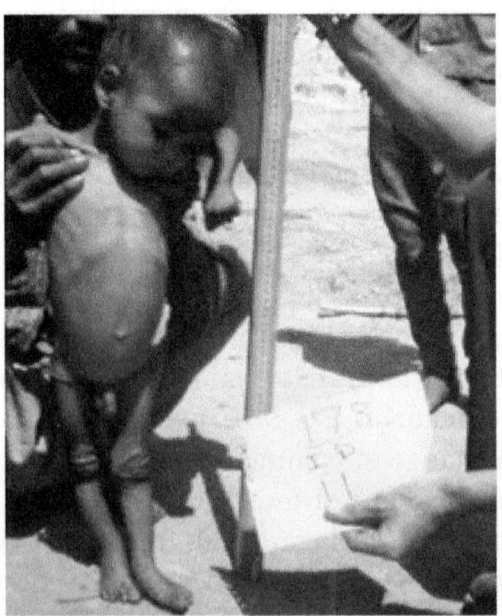

FIGURE 15 **Kwashiorkor** Extremity edema and a bloated abdomen are common in kwashiorkor.

deficiency because zinc is needed for synthesis and secretion of PAB in the liver. Clinicians must consider zinc status from diet intake and medical history and inflammation when interpreting low serum PAB levels.

PAB levels can be maintained in uncomplicated malnutrition and decreased in well-nourished individuals who have undergone recent stress or trauma. Also, when inflammatory stress causes a large drop in levels of PAB, its use as an indicator of nutritional status despite aggressive nutrition support is compromised. As a result, PAB may be assessed simultaneously with CRP. If CRP is also high, then PAB is not a reliable indicator of nutrition status. Other conditions can also increase PAB levels. Pregnancy may increase serum levels because changes in estrogen levels may stimulate PAB synthesis. Nephrotic syndrome can also increase PAB levels because proteinuria and hypoproteinemia may be present. With increased PAB synthesis, a disproportionate percentage of PAB exists in blood while other proteins take longer to produce. Hodgkin's disease and high doses of steroids can also increase serum PAB by stimulating PAB synthesis. Clinicians must take into account the etiology of PAB levels to assess and monitor the condition appropriately.

Retinol-binding protein (RBP) is an acute-phase protein produced in the liver whose main function is to transport vitamin A in the blood. RBP, whose normal levels range from 2.7 to 7.6 mg/dL, is considered one of the most sensitive indicators of protein status because of its short half-life (10-12 hours). RBP is a small protein that does not pass through the renal glomerulus because it circulates bound to PAB. Once RBP releases retinol in peripheral tissue, its affinity to PAB decreases and causes the PAB-RBP complex to dissociate. RBP is then filtered by the glomerulus and catabolized in the renal tubule.

As with the other negative acute-phase proteins, RBP decreases in the presence of inflammatory stress. Although a low RBP concentration is common in uncomplicated calorie malnutrition, RBP levels are not as affected by inflammatory stress as albumin, transferrin, or PAB in acutely stressed patients. Serum RBP is also low in patients with hyperthyroidism, liver failure, cystic fibrosis, vitamin A deficiency, and zinc deficiency. Therefore, when a patient has vitamin A deficiency, RBP cannot reliably assess protein status until the deficiency is addressed. Patients with renal failure are likely to have high serum RBP because it is not catabolized by the renal tubules. Therefore, RBP cannot accurately measure protein-energy status in patients with renal insufficiency.

Transferrin is a globulin protein that transports iron in blood to bone marrow for hemoglobin production. Normal serum transferrin levels range from 200 to 400 mg/dL. Serum transferrin can be measured directly or derived from total iron binding capacity (TIBC):

$$\text{Transferrin} = 0.8\ (\text{TIBC}) - 43$$

Serum transferrin levels are most strongly affected by the size of the iron storage pool. Transferrin levels increase when iron stores are depleted to accommodate the need for increased levels of transport. High transferrin levels are common in iron-deficiency anemia and dehydration. In contrast, serum transferrin levels can decrease due to impaired synthesis, which is often caused by infection, fever, malignancies, collagen vascular disease, liver disease, cirrhosis, and malnutrition. Although transferrin has a shorter half-life (8-10 days) than albumin, it does not respond fast enough to changes in intake to be a useful indicator of protein status in acute care patients. Transferrin is therefore not a specific indicator for malnutrition and not a valid measure for iron-deficiency anemia in acute illness.

CORE CONCEPT 5

Visceral proteins can be altered by acute and chronic metabolic stress, making them more accurate indicators of inflammation than indicators of nutritional status.

PRACTICE POINT

During acute stress, exogenous protein alone will not attenuate loss of endogenous protein.

Somatic Proteins

Similar to assessment of visceral proteins, assessment of somatic proteins (in skeletal muscle) can provide clinicians with a more in-depth understanding of protein status and requirements, while recognizing how certain conditions may influence interpretation of these values.

Nitrogen balance occurs when nitrogen input (Nin) or intake (oral, enteral, or parenteral) is equal to nitrogen output (Nout) or excretion (urinary, fecal, or wound drainage). Because nitrogen is a key component of protein, its measure is used to assess protein status in patients. Urine urea nitrogen (UUN) is the primary biochemical measure used to calculate Nout. It is the end product of protein breakdown in the body and signifies protein catabolism. One gram (g) of nitrogen loss is thought to equal about 30 g of lean tissue loss. The extent of protein breakdown can be categorized into mild catabolism (5-10 g UUN), moderate catabolism (10-15 g UUN), and severe catabolism (>15 g UUN).[36] To calculate nitrogen balance (Nbal) a 24 hour urine collection is needed for analysis of UUN. Because urea nitrogen only represents 85% of total urine nitrogen (TUN), with ammonia being the other significant contributor of nitrogen in the urine, a correction factor of 0.85 is applied. In addition, a factor of 2-4 g of nitrogen is added to Nout to represent non-urinary nitrogen losses that occur in sweat, stool, and wound exudate, which can also vary based on the output of these variables. To calculate Nin, a 24-hour dietary intake of protein is determined.

Total protein intake is converted to g of nitrogen using a factor of 6.25 (1 g nitrogen = 6.25 g protein). The following equation is used to calculate Nbal:

$$\text{Nbal} = \text{Nin–Nout}$$

$$\text{Nbal} = \text{Dietary protein intake/6.25 g Nitrogen} - [(\text{UUN}/0.85) + 2]$$

Sample Calculation: Protein intake = 94 g protein; UUN = 13 g/24 hours; Non-urinary nitrogen losses = 2 g/24 hours

$$\text{Nbal} = 94/6.25 - [(13/0.85) + 2]$$

$$\text{Nbal} = 15 - 17$$

$$\text{Nbal} = -2 \text{ g nitrogen}$$

For patients with a dietary intake of 94 g protein and a UUN of 13 g/24 hours, the Nbal would be negative by 2 g, meaning they are in negative nitrogen balance. Protein intake would have to be increased by 2 g nitrogen (or 12.5 g protein) to reach balance. Because the goal for anabolism requires the patient be positive by 2-4 g nitrogen an additional 12-25 g of protein may be added to their protein intake goal.

Nitrogen balance can be used for critically ill patients receiving nutrition support. If patients have a negative nitrogen balance, recommendations typically include increasing protein and caloric intake via diet, enteral, or parenteral nutrition. Nitrogen balance is imprecise as an indicator of protein status in acute care patients because it cannot accurately reflect protein anabolism and catabolism. True protein status can be better described by protein turnover or flux, which requires labeled protein (stable isotope) to measure protein synthesis and breakdown. This is done primarily as part of a research protocol as opposed to routine protein assessment. A valid 24-hour urine collection can be inconvenient and tedious to collect unless a patient has a catheter. Urine collection also fails to take into account nitrogen losses from wounds, burns, diarrhea, and vomiting. Equally confounding is the use of a factor of 0.85 to determine TUN from UUN, which is flawed in patients with variable excretion of ammonia, as is true during trauma, renal disease, and liver failure. If nitrogen balance is used to estimate protein status in critically ill patients or those with conditions that alter the nitrogen content of urine, clinicians must recognize the limitations of this UUN as a measure of nitrogen output. When possible, TUN should be measured; however, this is often not available in a clinical setting.

Creatinine is another value used to assess somatic protein status in patients. It is formed from muscle creatine phosphate at a constant daily rate. Creatine is formed from amino acids glycine and arginine with addition of a methyl group from the folate and vitamin B_{12}–dependent methionine-S-adenosylmethionine (SAM)-homocysteine cycle. Creatine phosphate, which is found almost exclusively in muscle, works as a high-energy phosphate buffer by providing a constant supply of ATP for muscle contractions. Through an irreversible, nonenzymatic reaction, some creatine phosphate is converted to creatinine during dephosphorylation. While creatinine is not stored in muscle and has no specific biologic function, it is continuously cleared from muscle and excreted by the kidneys. As a result, daily urine output of creatinine has been found to correlate with total muscle mass.

Although urinary creatinine can be effective in assessing somatic protein status in some patients, this indicator is confounded by many variables. First, dietary creatinine cannot be distinguished from endogenously produced creatinine in the body. As a result, the size of the somatic muscle protein pool is directly proportional to the amount of creatinine excreted only when a patient is following a meat-restricted diet. This factor accounts for the higher serum levels and larger amounts of creatinine excreted in men in comparison to women and among those with greater muscular development than those with less muscle.

Creatinine height index (CHI) is often calculated to take into account height and sex, by expressing creatinine excretion rate as a percentage of a standard value. A calculated CHI >80% is considered normal; 60% to 80% suggests mild skeletal muscle depletion; 40% to 60% suggests moderate skeletal muscle depletion; and <40% suggests severe skeletal muscle depletion.[37] CHI is calculated using the following equation:

$$\text{CHI} = \text{Actual 24-hour urine creatinine (mg)} / \text{Expected 24-hour urine creatinine (mg)}$$

where expected creatinine excretion is:

Female: 18 mg/kg

Male: 23 mg/kg

Sample Calculation: 66 kg female; 24-hour creatinine excretion: 890 mg

$$890 \text{ mg} / (18 \text{ mg/kg} \times 66 \text{ kg})$$

$$890/1188 \times 100 = 75\%$$

Therefore, a female weighing 66 kg with a 24 creatinine excretion of 890 mg/24 hours has CHI of 75% suggesting mild depletion.

CHI has limitations in measurement that clinicians must consider. As with UUN excretion, a test of urine creatinine excretion can be difficult to obtain. Furthermore, standards in the calculations for urinary creatinine do not account for variations in age, disease, physical training, body frame size, or weight status. Many conditions have been found to increase or decrease creatinine excretion. Sepsis, trauma, fever, strenuous exercise, and the second half of menstruation can also increase creatinine excretion. In contrast, renal function, low urine output, aging, and muscle atrophy unrelated to malnutrition can decrease creatinine excretion. Clinicians must account for these factors, beyond protein intake, that can alter urine creatinine laboratory values when evaluating and determining appropriate nutrition therapy.

While urinary creatinine has been used to assess somatic proteins status, *serum creatinine* is more commonly used in addition to BUN to assess renal function. Normal serum creatinine levels range from 0.4 to 1.3 mg/dL. Since serum creatinine is maintained within a relatively narrow range by the kidneys, elevated levels are most commonly a result of impaired renal function due to poor clearance of creatinine from the blood. In contrast, low serum creatinine levels can result from protein catabolism, which is common in patients with protein-energy malnutrition and muscular dystrophy, or in aging. Clinicians need to evaluate serum creatinine among other measures before determining etiology and treatment of abnormal values.

Blood urea nitrogen (BUN) is primarily used to assess renal function in addition to serum creatinine, but many other conditions can also alter BUN values. Normal BUN levels are 6 to 24 mg/dL. Urea is the metabolic byproduct of protein metabolism that is formed in the liver. Dietary protein is also broken down into amino acids, which are then catabolized to form free ammonia. Ammonia is then converted to urea and renally cleared. The kidneys filter urea out of the blood and into the urine, effectively eliminating excess nitrogen in the body. As a result, blood urea nitrogen consists of the normal waste products from endogenous protein metabolism and exogenous protein intake. In healthy individuals, there is usually a small amount of urea nitrogen in the blood, although many factors can alter BUN levels.

High BUN levels can often result from altered urea excretion rate due to renal insufficiency or dehydration. Altered protein metabolic rate from excessive protein intake, GI bleeding, and catabolism can also increase BUN levels. BUN should be interpreted in conjunction with creatinine to assess kidney function. In kidney and liver disease, BUN levels may rise and then return to normal. Clinicians should be careful in interpreting this drop because it does not suggest improved renal excretory function, but rather may reflect the inability of the liver to form urea. While BUN may remain normal or only slightly elevated, blood ammonia levels will increase as the liver continues to decline in these patients. Dehydration can also temporarily increase BUN levels and can be important in assessing hydration status in patients. Starvation, excessive protein intake, GI bleeding, and excessive protein catabolism (fever, burns, stress) can also increase BUN levels. Increased BUN levels is also common in patients with acute myocardial infarction because a decrease in cardiac function decreases renal blood flow, reducing renal excretion of BUN and consequently increasing serum BUN.

In contrast, low BUN levels are much less common and found in only a few conditions. Low BUN levels may result in patients with negative nitrogen balance, low protein intake, protein-energy malnutrition, increased protein synthesis (such as in pregnant women and in infancy), severe liver damage, impaired absorption, nephritic syndrome, and overhydration. However, low BUN levels are rarely used to diagnose or monitor the conditions described above.

A BUN:creatinine ratio can be used to help clinicians determine the etiology of abnormal BUN levels. A normal BUN:creatinine ratio ranges from 12 to 20, with most individuals ranging from 12 to 16. A normal BUN/high creatinine is usually indicative of muscle wasting, steroid administration, acute tubular necrosis, low protein intake, or severe liver disease. A high BUN/normal creatinine (BUN/creatinine >15:1) is common in dehydration, protein-energy malnutrition (catabolic state of tissue breakdown), excessive protein intake, GI bleeding, and catabolism. However, a ratio may be found to be normal in patients with renal insufficiency because both BUN and creatinine levels are higher than normal. Both BUN and BUN:creatinine values must be interpreted cautiously. Treatment of abnormal BUN levels will vary depending on the etiology and should take into account other protein assessment measures in addition to BUN.

Enzymes

A biochemical assessment of specific serum enzymes can provide clinicians with a more comprehensive evaluation of conditions affecting various organ systems. Aspartate transaminase, alanine transaminase, alkaline phosphatase, and lactate dehydrogenase are among the most common enzymes found within the blood in abnormal levels when patients have a variety of health conditions such as liver, kidney, cardiac, and bone disorders. Clinicians must evaluate these serum enzyme values in conjunction with the other serum proteins listed above to assess and treat patients according to the etiology and symptoms presented in patients.

Aspartate transaminase (AST) is an enzyme found primarily in the heart, liver, skeletal muscle cells, and to a lesser extent in the kidneys and pancreas. Normal serum AST values range from 10 to 35 IU/L. High serum AST values can be found in hepatocellular disease and coronary occlusive heart disease. An increase in AST is directly correlated to the number of cells affected by the disease or injury, with levels peaking about 8 hours after cell injury. In patients having a myocardial infarction, AST typically rises within 6 to 10 hours, peaking at 12 to 48 hours, and then returning to normal levels in 3 to 7 days unless another cardiac injury occurs.[39] Therefore, AST levels are often evaluated to estimate the time of myocardial infarction. Despite therapy, a second rise of AST may indicate additional cardiac injury. AST does not rise in angina, pericarditis, or rheumatic carditis. Liver damage also increases AST levels, peaking at up to 20 times the normal value then falling. As with myocardial infarction, the rise in AST is directly related to the degree of active inflammation. In chronic liver disease, high AST levels persist. Other conditions that may increase AST levels include hypothyroidism, acute pancreatitis, pulmonary emboli, Reye's syndrome, and skeletal muscle diseases.

Low serum AST is common in patients with vitamin B_6 deficiency, beriberi (thiamin deficiency), diabetic ketoacidosis, kidney disorders (acute, renal dialysis, uremia), chronic liver disease, and pregnancy. Treatment of abnormal AST values will vary based on the underlying cause. Monitoring AST levels and comparing values to other serum enzymes tests is important in determining etiology and appropriate treatment.

Alanine transaminase (ALT) is an enzyme found mostly in the liver and to a lesser extent in the kidneys, heart, and skeletal muscle. Normal serum ALT levels range from 4 to 36 units/L. High ALT levels are most commonly found in liver disorders (cholestasis, hepatitis, hepatic ischemia, cirrhosis or necrosis, liver cancer, obstructive jaundice). Very high ALT levels (10 times normal) are often due to acute hepatitis and may remain high for months before returning to normal. Drugs or other substances toxic to the liver and decreased blood flow to the liver (hepatic ischemia) also result in extremely high ALT levels (up to 100 times normal). In comparison, chronic hepatitis, cholestasis, cirrhosis, heart damage, alcohol abuse, and malignancies in the liver cause a more moderate increase in ALT levels (less than 4 times normal). Myocardial infarction, myositis, pancreatitis, infectious mononucleosis, severe burns, and shock may also cause elevated ALT levels. Strenuous exercise, medications injected into muscle tissue, and other medications including statins, antibiotics, aspirin, and chemotherapy can also increase ALT levels. Although ALT is more specific to the liver, AST:ALT ratio is frequently used to determine the etiology of abnormal ALT values and recognize heart or muscle injury in patients. In most types of liver diseases, ALT level is higher than AST (AST:ALT <1.0), with a few exceptions. An AST:ALT ratio >1.0 is commonly seen in patients with alcoholic hepatitis, cirrhosis, and heart or muscle injury for a few days after the onset of acute hepatitis.[39] Although AST and ALT are often referred to as "liver function tests," they are a better measure of hepatocellular damage instead of function, which makes the designation confusing. Note that certain proteins, such as albumin and clotting factors, which can reflect the liver's synthetic function, may be better indicators of actual liver function.

While low AST levels are not typically a concern, low ALT can be correlated to malnutrition and urinary tract infection. Treatment of abnormal ALT values will depend upon the underlying cause and severity. Clinicians must look to other markers for a comprehensive assessment and appropriate treatment.

Alkaline phosphatase (ALP) is an enzyme found in the liver and bones. Normal serum ALP values range from 30 to 120 units/L. High ALP levels are common in patients with liver disorders and can be useful in detecting blocked bile ducts and tumors (leukemia and lymphoma) if one or more bile ducts are obstructed. ALP levels are elevated as much as AST and ALT in hepatitis, while bile duct obstruction (gallstones, scars, surgery, previous gallstones, cancer) usually results in increased ALP more than AST or ALT. Because ALP is also present in bone, high levels of ALP can result from conditions affecting bone growth or increased activity of bone cells including osteomalacia, osteoblastic tumors, rickets, Paget's disease, and hyperparathyroidism. In cases of bone cancer or Paget's disease, where bones become enlarged and deformed, ALP levels will increase initially and then decrease, returning to normal over time in response to treatment. Moderately elevated ALP levels can also result from congestive heart failure, ulcerative colitis, and certain bacterial infections. ALP levels may also be temporarily elevated in women during pregnancy, in children and adolescents during large growth spurts, and with some medications such as anti-epileptics.

In contrast, ALP levels may decrease temporarily after blood transfusions or heart bypass surgery. Malnutrition, protein deficiency, zinc deficiency, vitamin B_{12} deficiency, hypothyroidism, hypophosphatemia, and Wilson's disease can also cause low ALP levels. Hypophosphatasia is a rare genetic disorder caused by a mutation in the gene producing ALP, while Wilson's disease is another genetic disorder causing copper to accumulate, leading to low ALP levels as a result of severe liver failure. Some medications including oral contraceptives and estrogen replacement therapy can also lower ALP levels. Treatment of abnormal ALP values varies based on the etiology and must address underlying cause and symptoms, such as vitamin D deficiency in bone disorders or zinc deficiency. Monitoring ALP can provide clinicians with important insight on progression and treatment of certain diseases.

Lactate dehydrogenase (LDH) is an enzyme present in the heart, liver, skeletal muscle, brain, red blood cells, and lung cells. LDH is released when a disease of injury affects cells and causes cell lysis. Normal serum LDH values range from 208 to 378 IU/L. LDH is not considered an indicator of any one disease affecting one organ. In contrast, five isoenzymes of LDH differentiate LDH among different organs: LDH-1 is mainly from the heart and blood vessels; LDH-2 is mostly from the reticuloendothelial system; LDH-3 is primarily from the lungs; LDH-4 is from the kidney, placenta, and pancreas; and LDH-5 is primarily from striated muscle and the liver.

In healthy individuals, LDH-2 is typically higher than the other isoenzymes. An elevated LDH-1 above LDH-2 (LDH flip) most often results from hemolytic anemia, megaloblastic anemia and/or sickle cell anemia. By assessing the time elapsed to peak values, clinicians can differentiate among these conditions. The LDH flip is also common in patients with myocardial infarction, although this is not the primary measure used for this diagnosis. An elevated LDH-5 in isolation most often suggests hepatocellular injury or disease, while elevated LDH-2 and LDH-3 suggest pulmonary injury or disease. When all LDH isoenzymes are high, the cause is likely multi-organ failure, advanced malignancy, or diffuse autoimmune inflammatory disease. Clinicians must treat abnormal LDH levels according to etiology. Patients with abnormal LDH levels should be monitored closely to monitor effectiveness of treatment and evaluate potential progression of certain diseases.

Troponin is a complex of three regulatory proteins—troponin C, troponin I, and troponin T—that are critical for muscle contraction in skeletal and cardiac muscle cells. A troponin test is most commonly performed to assess cardiac conditions because troponin is released into the blood when the heart muscle is damaged. In a healthy individual, troponin will not be detected in a blood sample. In contrast, a slight increase in troponin is often an indication of some damage to the heart, with very high levels most often indicating that a myocardial infarction has occurred. Typically patients who have had a myocardial infarction have raised troponin levels within 6 to 12 hours after the episode.[40] Other causes of high troponin levels include abnormally fast heartbeat, hypertension in lung arteries, congestive heart failure, long-term kidney disease, and cardiomyopathy. Medical nutrition therapy will vary according to the patient's cardiac condition and will require close monitoring to assess patient's needs.

Lipid Profile

As with proteins, lipids also serve many critical functions in the body. Triglycerides are an important source of stored energy in the body and cholesterol is the building block of hormones and cell membranes. When cholesterol is bound to protein (apolipoproteins) in the blood, it also plays an important role in transporting lipids throughout the body. Several health conditions can alter lipid metabolism, reflected in a lipid profile consisting of serum total cholesterol, very-low-density lipoprotein cholesterol (VLDL), low-density lipoprotein cholesterol (LDL), high-density lipoprotein cholesterol (HDL), and triglycerides. Both low and high lipid values are correlated to serious health conditions, impacting many organs in the body. The term *hyperlipidemia* or *dyslipidemia* is often used to refer to a condition of abnormal blood lipid levels, which may include total cholesterol, VLDL, LDL, HDL, and/or triglycerides. Clinicians must become skilled at interpreting abnormal blood lipid values as part of the nutrition care process because adequate medical nutrition therapy can play an important role in prevention, treatment, and symptom management of various disease states.

Lipoproteins transport endogenous lipids from the liver to the rest of the body and are characterized by their density. The density of lipoproteins varies according to the lipid-to-protein ratio and lipid composition (cholesterol, triglyceride, and phospholipids). VLDL cholesterol have the least amount of protein and the highest amount of triglycerides compared to LDL and HDL. VLDLs are produced in the liver and travel in the blood, converted to intermediate-density lipoprotein (IDL), and then to LDL as they lose triglycerides.

Currently, there is no simple way to measure VLDL cholesterol in the blood. However, this value can be estimated based on triglyceride values because VLDL cholesterol contains most of the circulating triglycerides and the composition of the different particles is relatively constant. To estimate VLDL cholesterol, divide fasting triglyceride value (in mg/dL) by five. This is not accurate for triglyceride levels higher than 400 mg/dL or in patients who have not fasted. An elevated VLDL cholesterol level (>30 mg/dL) increases an individual's risk of heart disease and stroke because high VLDL cholesterol suggests that conversion to LDL cholesterol is slowed, causing an accumulation of intermediate particles in the blood and contributing to atherosclerosis and coronary heart disease. VLDL cholesterol levels must be assessed in conjunction with other lipid values before determining appropriate nutrition therapy. Low VLDL cholesterol levels are generally not of concern and do not require nutrition therapy.

LDL cholesterol which are higher in protein and cholesterol, are considered the end point of forward transport of lipids to tissues. LDL particles are removed from circulation and taken up by tissues in need of cholesterol for structural support. If there is too much LDL cholesterol in the blood, these particles can adhere to the walls of arteries, forming plaque. Plaque can narrow arteries, contribute to high blood pressure, and initiate the process of atherosclerosis, or the buildup of fatty deposits in artery walls. Oxidized LDL cholesterol is more likely to be taken up by atherosclerotic plaque and continue development of existing plaque, increasing risk for myocardial infarction and stroke. For these reasons, LDL cholesterol is commonly known as the "bad" cholesterol.

As with the other lipid values, patients ideally fast 12 hours for an accurate laboratory result. Elevated LDL cholesterol (>100 mg/dL) is the lipid biomarker most closely associated with increased risk of heart disease and is commonly found in patients with preexisting coronary heart disease.[41] There is strong evidence that dietary saturated fat and trans fat are positively associated with LDL cholesterol, while dietary cholesterol is not as strongly correlated with LDL levels or risk of cardiovascular disease.[42] The source of saturated fat may differ in its effect on LDL cholesterol and risk of cardiovascular disease. Genetics (family history of premature heart disease), age and sex (>45 years for men and >55 years for women), cigarette smoking, high blood pressure, diabetes mellitus, and pregnancy can also raise LDL cholesterol levels. Nutrition therapy will vary depending on the underlying cause. For instance, management of DM with carbohydrate control, blood pressure with sodium restriction, or cardiovascular risk factors with limited trans fat and saturated fat may be recommended. Depending on the severity and comorbidities, cholesterol-lowering medications may be prescribed in conjunction to a dietary intervention.

Low LDL cholesterol (<60 mg/dL) is rarely seen, but can occur in a few conditions. Acute illness, immediately following a myocardial infarction, and stress from surgery or trauma can lower LDL cholesterol temporarily.[43] In addition, malnutrition, cancer, infection, inflammation, hyperthyroidism, cirrhosis, and people with inherited lipid disorders may have low LDL cholesterol. Low LDL is not generally a concern and should be evaluated with other measures to determine effective nutrition therapy. Malnutrition should be further assessed with other protein biomarkers to determine etiology and treatment with continuous monitoring.

HDL cholesterol is involved in the reverse cholesterol transport, taking cholesterol from tissues and other lipoproteins and transporting it back to the liver. HDL cholesterol is considered the "good" or protective cholesterol because of its role in returning cholesterol to the liver reduces cholesterol in plaque, which is associated with cardiovascular problems. Normal blood HDL cholesterol levels range from 40 to 59 mg/dL, while patients with HDL cholesterol levels less than 40 mg/dL are at increased risk of heart disease, independent of other risk factors such as LDL cholesterol levels. As with LDL cholesterol, HDL cholesterol levels may also be altered during acute illness, immediately increasing after an myocardial infarction, during stress, and during pregnancy.[43] To address low HDL cholesterol, treatment should focus on addressing the underlying cause, with treatment ranging from smoking cessation and increasing physical activity to nutrition therapy, with similar recommendations to that of LDL cholesterol. Figure 16 illustrates the composition of LDL and HDL cholesterol.

Total cholesterol is a calculated value representing the total amount of cholesterol found within the blood. It equals the sum of HDL cholesterol, LDL cholesterol, and 20% of triglycerides levels in mg/dL during 12 hours of fasting. Normal total cholesterol levels range from 140 to 200 mg/dL. Borderline high is considered in the range of 200 to 239 mg/dL, and high cholesterol or hypercholesterolemia is classified as greater than 240 mg/dL for adults and greater than 170 mg/dL for children and adolescents.[43] As with LDL and HDL cholesterol, several factors can increase total cholesterol levels including age, smoking, hypertension, family history, myocardial infarction, DM, obesity, and pregnancy. A diet high in saturated fat and trans fat is also directly correlated to high total cholesterol levels and increased risk of cardiovascular disease. Medications, including anabolic steroids, beta-blockers, epinephrine, oral contraceptives, and vitamin D, can also increase total cholesterol levels.

Low total cholesterol (<100 mg/dL) is commonly found in patients with malnutrition, liver disease, and cancer. Although there is no evidence that low cholesterol causes any of these issues, low total cholesterol values can be assessed with other protein biomarkers to determine underlying cause and appropriate treatment.

Total/HDL cholesterol is considered to be a more accurate measure of heart disease risk than total cholesterol and LDL cholesterol because this ratio takes into account HDL relative to total cholesterol. An optimal ratio of total cholesterol to HDL cholesterol is less than 3.5:1, while a ratio greater than 3.5:1 is associated with increased risk of heart disease.[43] Clinicians should treat elevated total/HDL ratio and elevated total cholesterol similar to elevated LDL cholesterol; restrict trans fats and limit saturated fats, depending on the underlying cause.

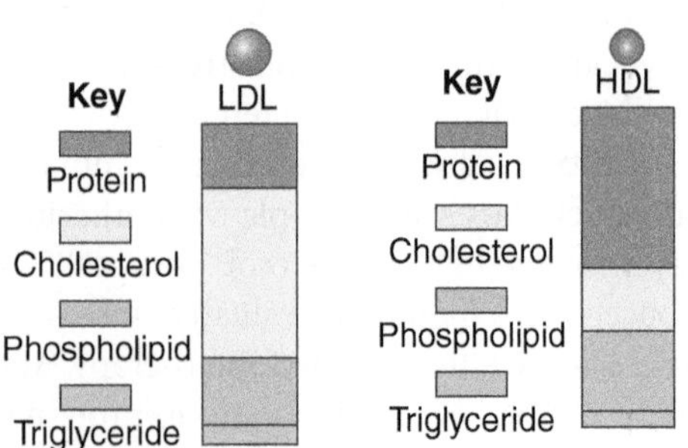

FIGURE 16 **Composition of LDL and HDL Cholesterol**

PRACTICE POINT

Interpreting LDL and HDL cholesterol levels in the context of total cholesterol provides more clinical significance than any one lipid value alone. A patient with an elevated HDL with an elevated total cholesterol will likely be at lower risk of health complications than a patient with both elevated LDL and elevated total cholesterol.

Triglycerides make up the largest percentage of fat in the body and are an important source of energy. As a component of lipoproteins, triglycerides are also important in transporting fat to cells. Normal triglyceride levels range from 40 to 150 mg/dL.[43] Borderline high triglyceride levels are 150 to 199 mg/dL and high triglyceride levels or hypertriglyceridemia are defined as values greater than 200 mg/dL. Hypertriglyceridemia is often found in patients who are overweight or obese, and those who have DM, kidney disease, and thyroid or liver disease. In addition, extremely high triglyceride levels greater than 1,000 mg/dL, known as severe hypertriglyceridemia, is associated with hypertriglyceridemic pancreatitis and cardiovascular disease.[44]

Dietary intake (high in refined grains, saturated fat, and trans fats), lack of exercise, smoking, and excess alcohol consumption can also increase triglyceride levels. Patients with hypertriglyceridemia combined with either low or high HDL are also considered at increased risk of atherosclerosis. Patients receiving PN who have combined hypertriglyceridemia are also at increased risk of glucose intolerance. Triglycerides levels should be closely monitored in patients at risk for these conditions. Nutrition therapy should focus on treating the underlying cause and reducing symptoms with a diet low in saturated fat, added sugar, refined grains, and alcohol.

CORE CONCEPT 6

Lipid profile results can be used to assess risk of cardiovascular (elevated low-density lipoprotein, decreased high-density/low-density lipoprotein ratio) and metabolic (elevated triglycerides) disorders, as well as risk of malnutrition (decreased cholesterol) in patients.

Hematology

A hematological assessment is another important component of biochemical assessment that is key to diagnosis and treatment for patients with all types of anemia and other blood disorders impacting nutrition needs. **Anemia** is defined as a reduction in erythrocytes per unit of blood

Clinical Roundtable

Topic: Use of LDL Cholesterol Particle Size in Assessing Cardiovascular Disease Risk

Background: An addition to the blood lipid test assessing the size and density of LDL particles has been studied but is not a standard measurement used in healthcare settings. Researchers are finding that the role of LDL cholesterol in cardiovascular disease risk may depend on the size and density of particles. As with other lipid values, composition of LDL particles, ranging from large, buoyant particles to small, dense particles, can be influenced by diet, genetics, and body weight.

Studies have found that high LDL particle size (LDL-P), which contains small, dense particles, may be associated with cardiovascular disease and metabolic syndrome more than low LDL-P, regardless of LDL cholesterol levels. High LDL-P can be seen with elevated LDL cholesterol levels as well as in individuals with normal and low LDL cholesterol levels.

Roundtable Discussion

1. How might these findings influence the way clinicians assess and diagnose risk of cardiovascular disease or metabolic syndrome?
2. Discuss whether you would use composition of LDL particle size to interpret a patient's risk of cardiovascular disease. Why or why not?

References

1. Kathiresan S, Otvos JD, Sullivan LM, et al. Increased small low-density lipoprotein particle number: A prominent feature of the metabolic syndrome in the Framingham heart study. *Circulation*. 2006;113(1):20-29.
2. Davidson MH, Ballantyne CM, Jacobson TA, et al. Clinical utility of inflammatory markers and advanced lipoprotein testing: Advice from an expert panel of lipid specialists. *J Clin Lipidol.* 2011;5(5):338-367.

CASE STUDY

It is now HD 15 and Adam is recovering well. He has been moved out of the ICU to the medical ward and is preparing for discharge home. His appetite and oral intake are improving. Based on his labs and symptom of fatigue, an iron supplement is ordered.

Biochemical Data (HD 15):

Hemoglobin 12.0 (13.5-17.5 g/dL)
Hematocrit 34 (42-52%)
Mean corpuscular volume 98 (80–100 fL)
Red cell distribution width (RDW-SD) 50 (39-46 fL)

Clinical Data:

Medications: iron, protonix, lipitor, captopril

Dietary Data:

Diet Prescription: Regular

Questions

1. **Describe the abnormalities in Adam's biochemical data.**
2. **What type of anemia or anemias might Adam have? What are his risk factors?**
3. **What additional biochemical measures would be required to make a more accurate assessment?**

volume or a decrease in hemoglobin of blood to below level of physiological needs. Although anemia is not a disease, it is a symptom of various conditions and the cause of anemia is usually multifactorial. Anemia can result from extensive blood loss (acute or chronic bleeding), excessive blood cell destruction (hemolytic anemia), or decreased red blood cell formation/production (bone marrow failure, micronutrient deficiency, erythropoietin deficiency). Figure 17 compares healthy and anemic red blood cells. The causes of anemia are not mutually exclusive, as many patients have multiple causes leading to anemia. Anemia is observed in many hospitalized patients, varying in micro-

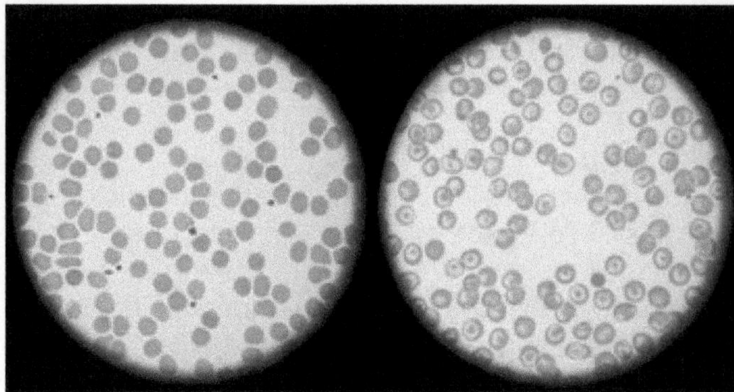

FIGURE 17 **Comparison of a Image of a Healthy Red Blood Cell (left) and an Anemic Red Blood Cell (right)**

nutrients involved (iron, folate, vitamin B_{12}, copper, zinc) and etiology (nutritional inadequacy, acute or chronic disease). See Table 10 for a summary of the key roles of iron, folate, copper, vitamin B_{12}, and zinc in red blood cell synthesis. Malnourished patients; young children; pregnant women; older adults; and patients with kidney disease, uncontrolled chronic illness, cancer, and extensive GI surgeries are considered at higher risk of anemia. Table 11 outlines the primary sites of GI absorption of macronutrients associated with anemia.

The size, shape, and color of erythrocytes (red blood cells) and a CBC can help clinicians evaluate etiology, severity, and appropriate treatment of these conditions. A CBC provides a count of cells in the blood and description of red blood cells including serum red blood cells, white blood cells, hemoglobin concentration, hematocrit, mean

TABLE 10 KEY MINERALS INVOLVED IN RED BLOOD CELL SYNTHESIS

Micronutrient	Major Physiological Role
Iron	Key component of hemoglobin
Vitamin B_{12}	Cofactor for amino acid synthesis and tricarboxylic acid cycle, facilitated in maturation and differentiation of erythroid lining
Folate	Key component of 1-carbon transfer system for protein and DNA synthesis and cell division
Copper	Key for regulation of iron transport from intestine and release into circulation
Zinc	Cofactor required for protein synthesis, and regulation for cell differentiation

Data from from Chan LN, Mike LA. The science and practice of micronutrient supplementations in nutritional anemia: An evidence-based review. *JPEN J Parenter Enteral Nutr*. 2014;38(6):656-672.

TABLE 11 PRIMARY GI ABSORPTION SITES OF MICRONUTRIENTS ASSOCIATED WITH ANEMIA

Micronutrient	Primary Site of Absorption
Non-heme iron	Duodenum (transporter also has affinity for lead, cobalt, manganese, copper, and zinc)
Heme iron	Duodenum and proximal jejunum
Vitamin B_{12}	Terminal ileum
Folate	Duodenum and proximal jejunum (transporter enhanced by vitamin D and inhibited by alcohol)
Copper	Most of small intestine
Zinc	Duodenum and jejunum

Modified from Chan LN, Mike LA. The science and practice of micronutrient supplementations in nutritional anemia: An evidence-based review. *JPEN J Parenter Enteral Nutr*. 2014;38(6):656-672.

corpuscular volume, red cell distribution width, and mean corpuscular hemoglobin concentration. Laboratory assessment of several of these blood parameters should be evaluated to distinguish between nutrition adequacies and other factors contributing to anemia. Biochemical assessment in addition to clinical signs and symptoms (Table 12) and medical status should be used to help clinicians evaluate etiology, severity, and appropriate treatment of anemia and other blood-related conditions.

Hemoglobin (Hgb) concentration is a measure of the total amount of hemoglobin in peripheral blood. Hemoglobin is the protein in erythrocytes that delivers oxygen to cells and picks up CO_2 for expiration by the lungs. Figure 18 depicts the structure of hemoglobin. Hgb concentration is considered the primary biochemical marker for diagnosis of anemia, defined as a hemoglobin concentration <95th percentile for healthy reference populations. According to World Health Organization recommendations, the cutoff of hemoglobin concentrations in defining anemia varies by age and sex: adult males (older than 15 years) <13.0 g/dL, adult females (older than 15 years) <12.0 g/dL, and pregnant adult females (older than 15 years) <11.0 g/dL.[44]

Low hemoglobin levels can be found in patients with four different types of nutritional anemias. However, Hgb concentration is not a sensitive or specific test for differentiating between nutritional anemias. Therefore, other laboratory values and a recent medical history need to be evaluated to determine appropriate nutrition therapy for patients with signs and symptoms of anemia. Hyperthyroidism,

TABLE 12 CLINICAL SIGNS AND SYMPTOMS OF ANEMIA

Fatigue, lethargy
Irritability
Difficulty concentrating, sleepiness
Pallor, pale sclera
Cold extremities
Muscle aches
GI distress (nausea, vomiting, diarrhea, cramping)
Reproductive dysfunction (amenorrhea, loss of libido)
Paresthesia
Cheilosis, glossitis
Spoon-shaped fingernails
Clubbing of joints in the digits
Cardiovascular sequelae (heart palpitation, tachycardia, dyspnea, angina)

Data from Pirker R. Symptoms of anemia. In: Recombinant Human Erythropoietin (rhEPO) in Clinical Oncology. New York, NY: Springer;2008:307-315

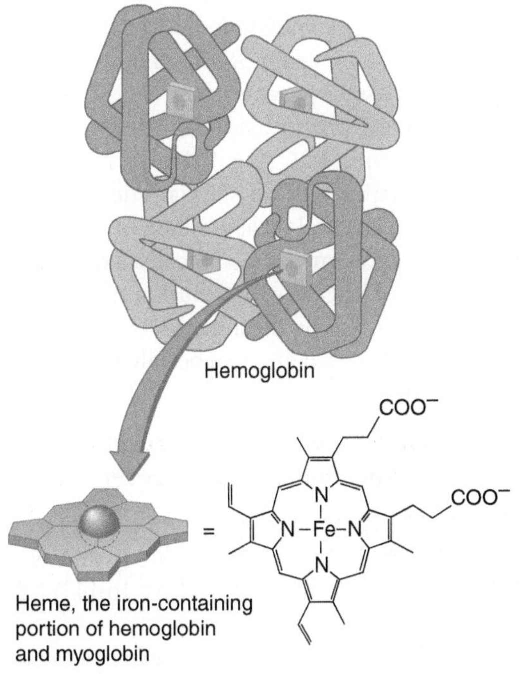

FIGURE 18 **Structure of Hemoglobin**

cirrhosis, leukemia, chronic infection, hemolysis, marrow failure, and kidney disease can lower Hgb levels. Genetic aberrations, aging, lead poisoning, pregnancy, and overhydration can also cause low Hgb levels. In contrast, high Hgb concentration is found in patients with blood transfusions and in patients at higher altitudes.

Red blood cell (RBC) count is a component of the CBC that measures the volume of red blood cells in the blood in femoliters (fL), which is one-quadrillionth of a liter. Red blood cells contain hemoglobin and make up the largest percentage of blood volume. They are regenerated approximately every 4 months with production, development, and function dependent on nutritional status, genetics, and environmental influences. Normal serum RBC values range from 4.7 to $6.1 \times 10^6/\mu L$ in males and 4.2 to $5.4 \times 10^6/\mu L$ in females. As with low hemoglobin concentrations, low RBC values may result from nutritional deficits or in patients with hemorrhage, hemolysis, genetic aberrations, marrow failure, renal disease, or consumption of certain medications. As with Hgb, RBC values are not sensitive to nutritional causes of anemia.

Hematocrit (Hct) percentage is also used with Hgb concentration to evaluate anemia. Hematocrit is the measure of the percentage of red blood cells in total blood volume and is often referred to as packed RBC volume. In healthy individuals, hematocrit percentage is typically three times the Hgb concentration in grams per deciliter. Normal serum Hct percentage values range from 42% to 52% in males, 35% to 47% in females, 33% in pregnant women, and 44% to 64% in newborns.[45] Hct percentage values are lower than normal under the same conditions that cause low Hgb and RBCs. Anemia, leukemia, hyperthyroidism, cirrhosis, massive blood loss, pregnancy, and poor iron intake can decrease Hct levels. On the other hand, high Hct levels may result from COPD, dehydration, or shock. As with Hgb, Hct is also not a sensitive or specific test for anemia. For example, Hct value is affected by an extremely high white blood cell count and hydration status. Also, high altitudes can increase Hct values during the first 72 hours in a high altitude because adaptations are made to lower arterial oxygen partial pressure due to diminished barometric pressure.[46] In addition, patients older than 50 years have slightly lower Hct values than younger adults, which can be caused by several factors including decreased production of intrinsic factor, physiological changes postmenarche, and chronic disease. As a result of the variation among individuals, other laboratory values and a recent medical history should be evaluated to determine appropriate nutrition therapy for patients with abnormal Hct values.

Mean corpuscular volume (MCV) or mean cell volume is the average size or volume of red blood cells. Normal serum MCV ranges from 80 to 99 fL in adults and 96 to 108 fL in newborns. MCV can be a helpful biomarker to characterize anemia by red blood cell size and can provide clinicians with a better understanding of the cause of dysregulation. High levels of MCV are associated with macrocytic anemia, pernicious anemia, and vitamin B_{12} (cyanocabalamin) and/or folate deficiency. In contrast, low MCV values are associated with microcytic anemia, iron-deficiency anemia, and anemia of chronic disease. **Microcytic anemia** (small cell size) is defined as MCV less than 80 fL, **macrocytic anemia** (large cell size) is MCV greater than 100 fL, and **normocytic anemia** (normal cell size) occurs when MCV is between 80 and 99 fL. This

TABLE 13 DIETARY SOURCES OF IRON

Food Sources	Iron (mg)
Heme Iron:	
Clams (3 oz)	14
Beef (3 oz)	4
Sardines (3 oz)	3
Poultry (3 oz)	1
Nonheme Iron:	
Fortified cereal (1 cup)	9
Spinach (1 cup)	6
Kidney beans (1 cup)	5
Pumpkin seeds (1 oz)	3

Data from US Department of Agriculture, Agricultural Research Service, USDA Food Composition Databases. USDA National Nutrient Database for Standard Reference, Release 28. Version Current: September 2015. Internet: https//ndb.nal.usda.gov/ndb/nutrients/report/.

categorization can provide clinicians with a better understanding of the cause of dysregulation.

Microcytic anemia can result from impaired heme synthesis (inability to absorb, transport, store, or utilize iron) or impaired synthetic abilities (protein, iron, ascorbate, vitamin A, pyridoxine, copper, or manganese deficiency). The most common conditions associated with microcytic anemia are iron deficiency, thalassemia (genetic blood disorder), and inflammation from chronic disease. Copper, zinc, lead, cadmium, and other heavy metals can also impair heme synthesis. Table 13 provides examples of common dietary sources of iron.

Macrocytic anemia results from the decreased ability of the red blood cell to divide appropriately or to synthesize new cells and DNA, leading to larger than normal red blood cells. Macrocytic anemia may be due to deficiency or impaired utilization of vitamin B_{12}, folate, thiamin, or pyroxidine. Dietary intake, genetic disorders in DNA synthesis, alcoholism, and liver disease are common causes of macrocytic anemia. Further evaluation of folate and vitamin B_{12} status is needed to determine etiology of anemia.

Normocytic anemia is associated with several chronic and inflammatory diseases including rheumatic disease, chronic heart failure, chronic infection, cancer, severe tissue injury, multiple fractures, and Hodgkin's disease. These conditions cannot be treated effectively with iron supplementation. MCV may appear within normal range if iron deficiency is concurrent with vitamin B_{12} and/or folate deficiency because the large size cell volume of the macrocytosis is masked by the small size cell volume of the microcytosis in the MCV value. MCV may also appear within normal range in the early stages of iron deficiency. In these cases, vitamin B_{12} and folate deficiency must be ruled out before iron-deficiency anemia is diagnosed and treated. Microcytosis and macrocytosis are not sensitive to marginal nutrient deficiencies. Additional laboratory values are needed to distinguish between various nutritional and non-nutritional causes of anemia and to determine appropriate treatment.

PRACTICE POINT

Evaluation of a patient's mean corpuscular volume (MCV) is an important in determining a patient's type of anemia (microcytic, macrocytic, normocytic) and developing appropriate nutrition therapy for the patient.

Mean corpuscular hemoglobin concentration (MCHC), or mean cellular hemoglobin concentration, is another one of the RBC indices that make up the CBC test. MCHC is the average concentration of hemoglobin within red blood cells presented as a ratio of hemoglobin mass to volume of red blood cells. It is calculated from the Hgb concentration and Hct using the following formula:

$$\text{MCHC} = \text{Hgb (g/dL)/Hct (\%)}$$

Normal serum MCHC levels range from 32 to 36 g/dL for children and adults and 32 to 33 g/dL for newborns. Abnormal MCHC values are evaluated similarly to MCV values; decreased MCHC is common in patients with iron deficiency and thalassemia trait. As with MCV, MCHC is not sensitive to marginal nutrient deficiencies.

Red cell distribution width (RDW) and MCV have become the most useful parameters in classifying anemias in clinical settings. RDW measures the degree of anisocytosis, or variation in RBC size variation or volume, as a coefficient of variation (CV) or standard deviation (SD). RDW-SD (fL) is the actual measurement of the width of RBC size distribution, measured by calculating the width at 20% height level of RBC size distribution range. Therefore, RDW-SD is not affected by the average RBC size (MCV). RDW-CV (%) is also used and can be calculated with the following equation:

$$\text{RDW} - \text{CV} = 1 \text{ standard deviation of RBC volume/MCV} \times 100\%$$

Unlike RDW-SD, RDW-CV is affected by the average RBC size (MCV). Normal serum RDW values in adults range from 39 to 46 fL for RDW-SD and 11.6% to 14.6% for RDW-CV.

Because RDW becomes elevated earlier than other blood measures, high RDW can be important in diagnosing early nutritional deficiencies, including iron, folate, or vitamin B_{12}. In addition, evaluation of RDW in conjunction with MCV can help clinicians determine the etiology of anemia by differentiating among microcytic, macrocytic, and normocytic anemia. Normal MCV and elevated RDW are common in patients with early iron, vitamin B_{12}, or folate deficiency; sickle cell disease; and chronic liver disease. Low MCV and normal RDW are associated with heterozygous thalassemia and anemia of inflammation and chronic disease, while low MCV and high RDW are associated with iron deficiency and sickle cell-β-thalassemia. In patients with high MCV and normal RDW, aplastic anemia, liver disease, chemotherapy, or alcohol is likely the cause. High MCV and high RDW is also associated with chronic liver disease, in addition to folate or vitamin B_{12} deficiency. If patients have normal RDW and normal MCV, anemia is likely associated with chronic disease, acute blood loss or hemolysis, or renal disease. While RDW and MCV values can further evaluate etiology of blood disorders, these measures must be assessed with other blood measures and clinical signs and symptoms before diagnosis and treatment of anemia or blood disorder. Treatment of blood disorders should focus on addressing the underlying causes and addressing protein and/or micronutrient deficiencies when appropriate.

White blood cell (WBC) count is another component of CBC that can help differentiate non-nutritional causes of anemia. White blood cells, also called leukocytes, are produced in bone marrow and play an important role in immune functioning, fighting infection or inflammation.

Normal serum WBC values are 5 to 10×10^9/L for adults, 6 to 17×10^9/L for children, and 9 to 30×10^9/L for newborns. Increased WBC count (leukocytosis) may be caused by infection, inflammation (rheumatoid arthritis, irritable bowel disease), leukemia, neoplasm, allergic response, or stress (trauma, burns, surgery). Decreased WBC count (leucopenia) may result from bone marrow damage or disorder, lymphoma or other cancer spreading to bone marrow, autoimmune disease, protein-energy malnutrition, overwhelming infection (e.g., sepsis), or effects chemotherapy or radiation therapy. Abnormal WBC values often require further assessment when symptoms are nonspecific and inflammatory autoimmune disease is expected. Reticulocyte (immature red blood cells) and platelet (components of red blood cells that function to clot blood) counts can help clinicians determine etiology and appropriate treatment of the underlying condition and anemia. Monitoring WBC levels can be useful for clinicians to assess whether the condition is generally worsening or improving if WBC counts are decreasing or increasing, respectively.

In addition to WBC count, differential WBC measures can be assessed to evaluate the levels of different types of leukocytes and related infections. These WBC measures include neutrophils (pyogenic infection), eosinophils (allergy and parasitic infection), basophils (parasitic infection), lymphocytes (viral infection), monocytes (severe infection), polymorphonuclear leukocytosis or PMNs (circulating mature cells), and bands (circulating immature cells).

Interpretation of Anemia

Iron Studies (Microcytic Anemia from Iron Deficiency)

Iron-deficiency anemia is the most prevalent of all types of anemia worldwide and one of the most common nutritional deficiencies. Suboptimal iron stores can have significant detrimental effects on biochemical processes of cellular metabolism including impaired growth and mental status in children, and depressed immune and cognitive function in adults. Figure 19 shows the major functions of iron. In contrast, iron overload can lead to cell destruction, tissue injury, and organ failure. Clinicians must understand the etiology of iron-deficiency anemia and interpret lab values appropriately to determine effective nutrition therapy with careful monitoring.

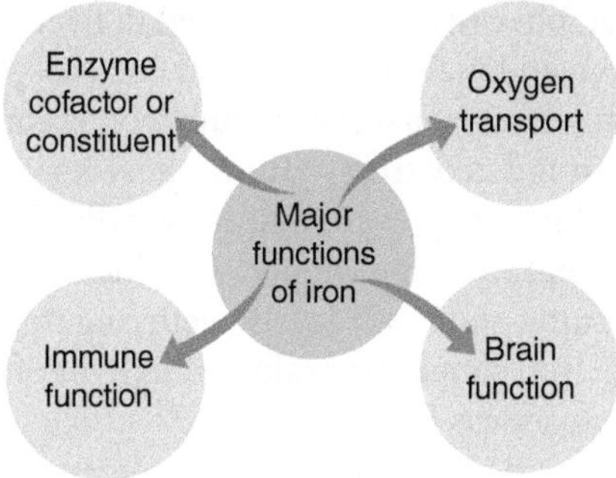

FIGURE 19 **Major Functions of Iron**

Iron-deficiency anemia can result from blood loss, decreased iron intake or absorption, or increased iron requirements. Infants, young children, adolescents, women, and patients with renal insufficiency or undergoing gastric bypass surgery are at risk of iron-deficiency anemia. The most common symptoms are fatigue, anorexia, growth abnormalities, koilonychia (spoon-shaped nails), and glossitis. Typically, patients with iron-deficiency anemia have low Hgb, low Hct, and low MCV.

While these are the primary indicators of iron-deficiency anemia, folate and vitamin B_{12} deficiency can both mask iron deficiency by keeping MCV levels within a normal range. In addition, these tests are not sensitive to marginal deficiencies so they cannot detect early stages of anemia. If abnormal results are found with a CBC test, iron studies are often used to further assess presence of iron-deficiency anemia, including tests of serum iron, ferritin, transferrin, and total iron binding capacity. Clinical signs and symptoms should also be compared to results from iron studies to differentiate among iron-deficiency anemia, anemia of inflammation and chronic disease (described in detail below), and anemia of acute infection, because iron stores can be heavily influenced by many medical conditions causing inflammation and infection.

Serum iron measures the amount of circulating iron that is bound to transferrin, the iron transport protein in the blood. Normal serum iron levels range from 50 to 170 μg/dL. Levels less than 15 μg/dL reflect absent or reduced iron stores. Low serum iron levels are common in patients with gastric surgery due to peptic ulcer disease or obesity, GI bleed, malabsorption, leukemia, end-stage renal disease, and infection. Levels greater than 170 μg/dL may reflect iron overload, but can also be increased in liver disease, inflammation, and malignancies. Oral contraceptives may also increase serum iron levels. Serum iron is considered a relatively poor index of iron status because its value varies greatly from day to day, even in healthy individuals. In addition, diurnal variation occurs, with higher levels occurring midmorning and lower levels occurring in midafternoon. Serum iron should be evaluated in light of other iron study values to assess iron status.

Serum ferritin is a more accurate indicator of iron stores in patients. Normal ferritin levels are 20 to 500 ng/mL in males and 20 to 200 ng/mL in females. Ferritin is a storage protein that holds iron inside hepatocytes and other iron storage cells for later use. In healthy individuals, as iron supply increases, ferritin levels increase intracellularly to accommodate iron storage. Serum ferritin less than 12 to 15 ng/mL indicates that iron stores are depleted. Decreased serum ferritin can result from iron deficiency and malnutrition, with 1 ng/mL decrease of serum ferritin equal to approximately 8 mg decrease of stored iron.[47] During conditions of acute inflammation and some chronic diseases, serum ferritin is not an accurate indicator of serum ferritin status. Inflammatory disease, renal failure, malignancy, hepatitis, and iron overload can increase serum ferritin levels.

As a positive acute-phase protein, ferritin levels rise during stress and inflammation with increased synthesis and ferritin leakage from cells. Increased ferritin is often associated with acute inflammation, uremia, metastatic cancer, or alcohol-related liver disease, with elevated ferritin evident 1 to 2 days after onset of acute illness peaking at 3 to 5 days after injury or illness.[48] Under these conditions, other iron biomarkers must be used to evaluate the presence of iron deficiency.

Ferritin also fails to correlate with iron stores in **anemia of inflammation and chronic disease (AICD)**, a common form of anemia in hospitalized patients. In patients with AICD, cytokines such as interleukin-1 and tumor necrosis factor are released during inflammation due to inadequate mobilization of iron stores, which decreases red blood cell production. Low Hgb and Hct are the common indicators of AICD, and can occur in normocytic–hypochromic, microcytic-hypochromic, and normocytic-normochromic anemias due to failure of compensatory erythropoiesis.

AICD often occurs in patients with cancer or chronic inflammatory or infectious disorders, such as rheumatoid arthritis. Iron stores may also become depleted in arthritis from reduced absorption and in patients with regular use of nonsteroidal anti-inflammatory drugs or with GI blood loss. In patients with microcytic anemia, serum ferritin may remain normal or increase while serum iron levels are low. In this case, inflammatory mediators may also cause ferritin levels to remain normal, although iron stores can be depleted. Clinicians must distinguish the many forms of AICD from iron-deficiency anemia by comparing iron laboratory measures so that iron supplementation is not initiated when anemia is not caused by iron deficiency.

Transferrin is a globulin protein synthesized in the liver that transports iron to bone marrow for production of hemoglobin. The size of the iron storage pool controls the level of plasma transferrin. In healthy individuals, when iron stores are depleted, transferrin synthesis increases. Normal serum transferrin levels range from 170 to 370 mg/dL.[48] Increased transferrin levels are associated with iron-deficiency anemia, while low transferrin levels are common in liver disease, cirrhosis, malnutrition, infection, and fever. Like albumin, transferrin is a negative acute-phase protein, which means that decreased transferrin is found in patients with acute inflammation, malignancies, collagen vascular diseases, and liver diseases. Protein energy malnutrition and fluid overload can also decrease serum transferrin levels. As a result, low iron stores may not be reflected in transferrin measures when these conditions are present because transferrin levels may be falsely increased or remain within a normal range. Other iron biomarkers are needed to further assess the underlying cause of anemia and develop appropriate treatment. Clinicians may use transferrin as a measure of severity of illness and to monitor for progress if patients have these conditions.

Total iron binding capacity (TIBC) measures the saturation ability of transferrin, or the potential for plasma transferrin to bind to ferric acid (Fe^{3+}). Under normal conditions, approximately 30% of iron-binding sites on transferrin molecules are saturated. Each transferrin molecule binds to ferric ions at two or more binding sites and two bicarbonate ions at different sites. TIBC can be calculated using the following equation:

Transferrin Saturation (%) = (serum iron level / TIBC) × 100

Sample Calculation: serum iron 48 μg/dL; TIBC 352 μg/dL

Transferrin Saturation % = (48/352) × 100

Transferrin Saturation % = 14%

Therefore, an individual with a serum iron of 48 and TIBC of 352 has a total iron binding capacity of 14%, which suggests iron deficiency.

Under most conditions, as the body's requirements for iron and overall iron status changes, transferrin saturation changes in response. Normal TIBC values range from 300 to 360 μg/dL. Generally, decreased transferrin saturation and increased TIBC values are associated with iron-deficiency anemia. Increased TIBC can also result from hypoxia, pregnancy, and medications including oral contraceptives and estrogen replacement therapy. TIBC decreases in patients with malignancies, nephritis, hemolytic anemia, and iron overload. As with serum transferrin, TIBC will remain normal or decrease in response to chronic or acute

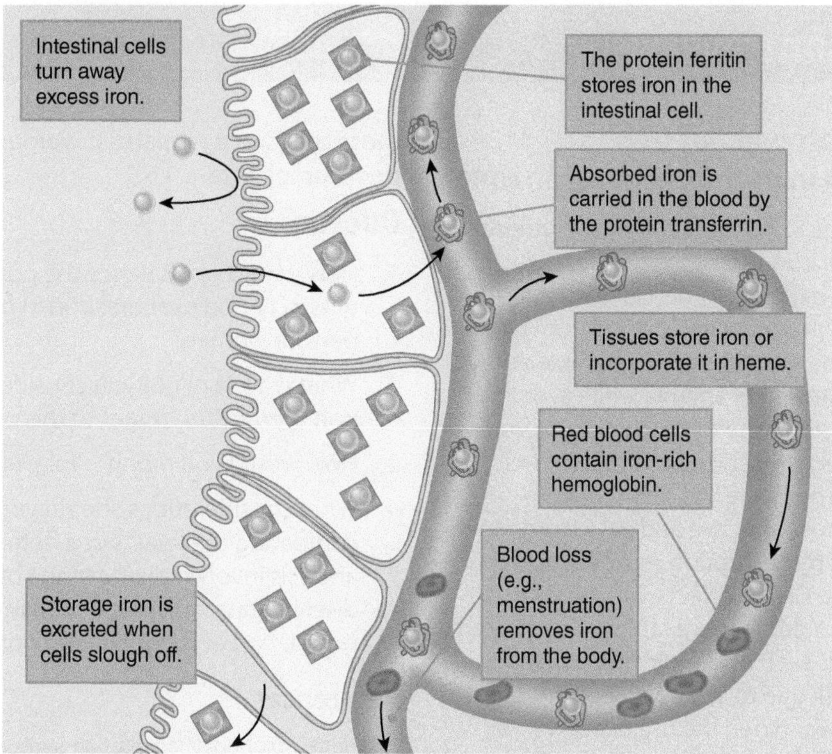
Intestinal cells turn away excess iron.
The protein ferritin stores iron in the intestinal cell.
Absorbed iron is carried in the blood by the protein transferrin.
Tissues store iron or incorporate it in heme.
Red blood cells contain iron-rich hemoglobin.
Blood loss (e.g., menstruation) removes iron from the body.
Storage iron is excreted when cells slough off.

FIGURE 20 **Iron Absorption in the Gastrointestinal Tract**

inflammation. TIBC and transferrin saturation values persist until severe deficiency develops. Other biomarkers of iron status are necessary to accurately assess iron stores and detect early signs of anemia in patients.

Treatment of iron-deficiency anemia involves managing the underlying cause(s) of deficiency, restoring Hgb concentrations, and replenishing iron stores. Supplemental iron should increase serum reticulocyte count within a few days, although an increase in Hgb concentrations will not be evident for 2 to 3 weeks because iron utilization by bone marrow takes longer. Repletion of iron stores, measured by normalization of ferritin, will take even longer to improve. As a result, treatment duration should be at least 3 months to fully restore serum ferritin concentration. Iron supplementation can be administered orally (enterally) or intravenously. Figure 20 illustrates iron absorption. Oral iron supplementation is preferred, as ferric salt, with amounts of elemental iron varying depending on salt form of product (ferrous calcium citrate, ferrous gluconate, ferrous ammonium citrate, ferrous dextran, and ferrous sucrose). After iron levels are restored, clinicians are recommended to recheck levels every 3 to 4 months for up to 1 year.[48]

Parenteral iron administration has historically been reserved for patients in whom oral iron therapy is ineffective or for those with malabsorptive disorders. Certain parenteral iron supplements such as iron dextran come with the risk of anaphylactic reactions. As a result, patients receiving iron dextran may benefit from a small test dose in a facility equipped for resuscitation with close monitoring for adverse reactions prior to receiving the full infusion. Other IV iron formulations such as iron sucrose have lower risk of anaphylaxis and may be better tolerated.

Macrocytic Anemias from B-Vitamin Deficiencies

Iron, vitamin B_{12}, and folate are the most important micronutrients for generation of erythrocytes. While iron deficiency alters production of hemoglobin, resulting in microcytic anemia, vitamin B_{12}, and folate deficiency impair synthesis of DNA and proteins and cell division, resulting in macrocytic anemia (large, nucleated red blood cells). Clinicians must assess patients further for vitamin B_{12} and folate deficiencies if abnormal CBC results (high MCV, low Hgb) indicate that macrocytic anemia may be present. Because MCV and Hgb are nonspecific measures and MCV value may be masked if iron deficiency is present, further assessment is needed to evaluate for vitamin B_{12} and folate deficiencies. As the clinical symptoms of vitamin B_{12} and folate deficiency are similar, a biochemical assessment of these vitamin levels is necessary to distinguish between B deficiencies. A static measurement of folate and vitamin B_{12} deficiency in the blood is used, testing the ability of a patient's blood specimen to support growth of microbes requiring folate or vitamin B_{12}.

Serum cobalamin was most commonly used to measure vitamin B_{12} status. Vitamin B_{12} is absorbed in the

⚠ Clinical Controversy

Oral Iron versus Intravenous Iron Supplementation in Iron-Deficiency Anemia

Iron-deficiency anemia is the most common nutrient deficiency worldwide. Iron supplementation is crucial in the treatment of iron-deficiency anemia, particularly in at-risk groups such as pregnant and postpartum women. Because anemia can be associated with adverse outcomes, adequate treatment of anemia while avoiding red blood cell transfusions due to increased infectious risk, possibility of allergic reactions, cost, and scarcity is critical. Use of oral iron in the treatment of iron-deficiency anemia is cost effective and easy to administer but can be limited by absorption as well as noncompliance due to adverse GI side effects. Intravenous (IV) iron may replete hemoglobin more rapidly, but concern exists with side effects such as allergic reactions and increased infection risk due to iron's pro-oxidant nature. Various studies have examined the use of oral versus IV iron to ascertain the preferred treatment route in pre- and postpartum women. Many studies have identified that IV iron is an effective mode of therapy over oral iron in the treatment of iron deficiency in pregnant and postpartum women. However, Litton et al. examined the use of IV iron through a meta-analysis of 75 randomized clinical trials (across many conditions and disease states) and found that IV iron administration was associated with increased hemoglobin and reduced risk of blood transfusion, but was also associated with an increased risk of infection when compared to oral or no iron supplementation. As oral iron is a common treatment for the prevention and treatment of iron deficiency in pregnant and postpartum women, IV iron may warrant consideration as an alternate iron delivery method for those pre- and post-partum women with anemia or poor compliance.

Questions

1. How would you balance the potential risks and benefits of IV iron over oral iron in pregnant and post-partum women?
2. What criteria might you consider in recommending iron therapy treatment to this population?
3. How would you monitor for potential risks?
4. What considerations should you be mindful of when comparing the results of a heterogeneous meta-analysis involving wide range of conditions and disease states to clinical trails involving the target population of pregnant and post-partum women?

References

1. Rudra S, Chandna A, Nath J. Comparison of intravenous iron sucrose with oral iron in pregnant women with iron deficiency anaemia. *Int J Reprod Contracept Obstet Gynecol.* 2016;5(3):747-751.
2. Neeru S, Sreekumaran Nair N, Rai L. Iron sucrose versus oral iron therapy in pregnancy anemia. *Indian J Community Med.* 2012; 37(4):214–218. doi: 10.4103/0970-0218.103467
3. Verma S, Inamdar SA, Malhotra N. Intravenous iron therapy versus oral iron in postpartum patients in rural area. *JSAFOG.* 2011;3(2):67-70.
4. Litton E, Xiao J, Ho KM. Safety and efficacy of intravenous iron therapy in reducing requirement for allogeneic blood transfusion: systematic review and meta-analysis of randomized clinical trials. *BMJ.* 2013;347:f4822. doi: https://doi.org/10.1136/bmj.f4822

ileum and stored in the liver and plays an important role in DNA synthesis and myelin synthesis. Normal values of serum cobalamin range from 200 to 900 pg/mL[49]. However, serum cobalamin has low sensitivity except in extremely deficient states, making its wide reference range for deficiency difficult to detect accurately. Serum levels may be elevated if patients receive IV minerals and vitamin infusions. Generally, low serum levels indicate macrocytosis and are associated with high MCV, high RDW, and low Hgb.

Vitamin B_{12} deficiency is now more accurately assessed using parameters in the metabolic pathways of *homocysteine (Hcy)* and *methylmalonic acid (MMA)*. This represents a functional assay as it describes the physiologic functioning of vitamin B_{12} as opposed to simply its quantity in the blood. Vitamin B_{12} plays a key role in converting homocysteine into methionine, one of the building blocks needed for protein synthesis. Vitamin B_{12} is a coenzyme in the reaction of MMA to succinyl coA. Therefore, high levels of serum MMA and Hcy are strongly associated with vitamin B_{12} deficiency. For patients with renal insufficiency, MMA is considered to be a more specific marker than Hcy because Hcy may be elevated due to decreased renal function, with or without the presence of vitamin B_{12} deficiency.

Subclinical vitamin B_{12} deficiency, defined as low serum vitamin B_{12} concentration and/or elevated MMA or Hcy that is responsive to vitamin B_{12} therapy, is commonly found in geriatric and vegan patients. Elderly patients and patients taking proton pump inhibitors are at higher risk of vitamin B_{12} deficiency due to decreased production of gastric acid, which is necessary for vitamin B_{12} absorption. For these patients, chronic supplementation of vitamin B_{12} may not be necessary. Oral cyanocobalamin, the synthetic form of vitamin B_{12}, is considered an effective treatment approach for vitamin B_{12} deficiency, but only if a significant portion of ileum is present and functional. For the first week, doses should range from 250 to 2,000 µg/day. This treatment should be followed by a maintenance period with at least 125 µg/day until symptoms have resolved in patients.[50] If treatment is taking several months for repletion of vitamin B_{12} stores and if clinical symptoms are not improving, a more intense therapy is needed. If neurological symptoms are present with deficiency, parenteral therapy is the preferred approach. Clinicians can use both MMA and Hcy to monitor progress and evaluate effectiveness of treatment.

Folate is absorbed in the small intestine and required for DNA synthesis. *Red blood cell folate (RBC folate)* is considered the most accurate measure of folate status in patients. Normal serum folate levels vary by age and are: 2-20 ng/mL in adults; and 5-21 ng/mL in children. In comparison to serum folate, RBC folate is more concentrated and more closely reflects tissue stores despite fluctuations in dietary intake. Normal RBC folate is 140-628 ng/mL in adults and >160 ng/mL in children. Low RBC folate is associated with folate deficiency and macrocytosis (high MCV, high RDW). Because folate is absorbed in the jejunum, folate deficiency may be caused by malabsorption in patients with celiac disease and those who have had bariatric surgery. Chronic alcohol consumption and long-term use of folate antagonists or antifolate medications including anticonvulsants and sulfasalazine can also cause folate deficiency. **Table 14** outlines common biochemical measures in iron-deficiency anemia, AICD, and folate and vitamin B_{12} deficiency anemias.

Before treating folate deficiency, vitamin B_{12} status must be assessed because treatment of folate deficiency can mask the symptoms of untreated vitamin B_{12} deficiency such as neuropathy. Once vitamin B_{12} status is sufficient or corrected, treatment of folate deficiency should focus on correcting anemia and replenishing folate stores as reflected by

TABLE 14 LABORATORY MEASURES IN IRON DEFICIENCY ANEMIA, ANEMIA OF INFLAMMATION AND CHRONIC DISEASE, FOLATE DEFICIENCY AND VITAMIN B_{12} DEFICIENCY

Laboratory Measure	IDA	AICD	Folate Deficiency	B_{12} Deficiency
Hemoglobin (Hgb)	↓	↓	↓	↓
Hematocrit (Hct)	↓	↓	↓	↓
Mean Corpuscular Volume (MCV)*	↓	↓	↑	↑
Red Cell Distribution Width (RDW)*	↑	WNL	↑	↑
Serum Ferritin	↓	WNL/↑	WNL	WNL
Serum Iron	↓	↓	WNL	WNL
Serum Transferrin	↑	↓/WNL	WNL	WNL
Transferrin Saturation	↓	↓	WNL	WNL
Red Blood Cell Folate	WNL	WNL	↓	WNL
Methylmalonic acid (MMA)	WNL	WNL	WNL	↑

*Expected levels may vary if more than one anemia or deficiency is present
↓= reduced
↑= increased
WNL=within normal limits
Modified from Clark, S. F. Iron deficiency anemia. *Nutr Clin Pract*. 2008; 23(2):128-141.

normal RBC folate concentration. Although the appropriate dose of folate to prevent anemia in nonpregnant individuals is not well established by clinical trials, current data suggest that oral folic acid supplementation of 5 to 10 mg/day is well tolerated.[51] Treatment duration should be at least 3 to 4 months depending on patients' RBC folate levels. If RBC folate levels remain low due to increased demand or malabsorptive disorders, a daily folic acid supplementation may be recommended to prevent recurrent anemia. In these circumstances, 500 to 800 µg daily may be a reasonable dose, although the most effective dose remains unclear.[52] **Table 15** differentiates microcytic and macrocytic anemia classifications.

Supplemental doses should take into account dietary intake of folate and RBC folate concentrations. Although folate-deficiency anemia can be prevented in most patients by optimizing diet intake, including foods fortified with folic acid, patients with suboptimal dietary folate intake may benefit from a weekly supplement of 500 µg of folic acid to prevent folate deficiency anemia. Because folate deficiency during pregnancy increases risk of neural tube defects, the U.S. Public Health Service and Centers for Disease Control and Prevention recommend that all women of childbearing age consume 400 µg of folic acid supplements before and during early pregnancy.[53] Women at high risk of neural tube defects are recommended to consume an extra 4 mg of synthetic folic acid supplements.[52] Unlike most supplement forms of vitamins and minerals, synthetic folic acid has been found to be more bioavailable than food sources of folate,[54] which supports the use of synthetic folic acid supplementation for primary treatment of folate deficiency. **Table 16** outlines the different types of anemias and associated nutrition deficiencies and toxicities.

TABLE 15 CLASSIFYING NUTRITIONAL ANEMIA (MICROCYTIC VERSUS MACROCYTIC)

Macrocytic	Deficiencies: • Vitamin B_{12}, folate, thiamin, pyridoxine
Microcytic	Deficiencies: • Protein, iron, ascorbate, vitamin A, pyridoxine, copper, manganese Toxicities: • Copper, zinc, lead, cadmium, other heavy metals

Data from Chulilla, J. A. M., Colás, M. S. R., & Martín, M. G. (2009). Classification of anemia for gastroenterologists. *World journal of gastroenterology*: WJG, 15(37), 4627.

TABLE 16 TYPES OF ANEMIAS AND RELATED NUTRITION DEFICIENCIES/TOXICITIES

Micronutrient Deficiency	Laboratory Values	Factors Affecting Laboratory Values
Iron	Low serum iron Low transferrin saturation or high TIBC Low ferritin Low MCV High Zinc protoporphyrin	Ferritin increases with inflammation (not accurate indicator in critically ill patient, or patients with acute inflammation) MCV may appear normal if concurrent deficiency in vitamin B_{12} and/or folate
Vitamin B_{12}	High MMA High serum homocysteine High MCV	Homocysteine can increase in presence of renal dysfunction (not an accurate indicator in these patients) MCV may appear normal if concurrent with iron deficiency
Folate	Low erythrocyte folate Low serum folate (fasting) High MCV	Serum folate can increase for up to 5 hours after meal, so measures made during fasting are most accurate MCV may appear normal if concurrent with iron deficiency
Copper	Low plasma copper Low ceruloplasmin	Plasma copper and ceruloplasmin increase with inflammation (not accurate indicators if inflammation present)
Zinc	Low 24-hour urine zinc excretion Low plasma/serum zinc	Plasma zinc decreases with inflammation (do not check in critically ill, consider checking C-reactive protein instead)

Modified from Chan LN, Mike LA. The science and practice of micronutrient supplementations in nutritional anemia: An evidence-based review. *JPEN J Parenter Enteral Nutr*. 2014;38(6):656-67.

CORE CONCEPT 7

Deficiencies in iron, vitamin B_{12}, and folate, and toxicities of copper and zinc, can all compromise red blood cell functioning and contribute to anemia.

Chapter Summary

Biochemical assessment is a critical component of the nutrition care process, providing important information regarding an individual's nutritional status as it relates to pertinent underlying health conditions. Interpreting trends in electrolyte, fluid, and acid–base levels can provide critical information about the progression or treatment of health conditions and about the most appropriate nutrition therapy plan. Consideration of these values in the context of other assessment measures (anthropometrics, functional assessment, and diet history) is crucial to accurately evaluate a patient's condition and nutritional needs. A collective evaluation of endocrine biomarkers, liver enzymes, lipid levels, and visceral proteins can help clinicians evaluate endocrine, liver, and cardiovascular function, as was a level of inflammatory stress, because these conditions can have a significant impact on a patient's nutritional status and needs. By assessing trends in these values, a clinician can determine whether a patient's health condition is progressing or improving, having important nutritional implications. Several biochemical values are also used to assess iron status and anemia and understanding how values can differentiate between types of anemia and treatment methods is critical. Prioritizing a patient's most severe and pertinent abnormal laboratory values in the context of nutritional status and needs is important in order for clinicians to provide the most effective nutrition therapy to patients.

Key Terms

static assay, functional assay, hemodilution, hemoconcentration, electrolytes, basic metabolic panel, comprehensive metabolic panel, complete blood count, differential count, osmotic pressure, isotonic, hypertonic, hypotonic, third spacing, hypervolemia, hypovolemia, hyponatremia, osmotic demyelination syndrome (ODS), hypernatremia, hypokalemia, hyperkalemia, hypocalcemia, hypercalcemia, hypophosphatemia, hyperphosphatemia, hypomagnesemia, hypermagnesemia, refeeding syndrome, hypochloremia, hyperchloremia, acidemia, alkalemia, acidosis, alkalosis, arterial blood gases (ABGs), respiratory acidosis, respiratory alkalosis, metabolic acidosis, metabolic alkalosis, hypoglycemia, hyperglycemia, visceral protein, acute-phase proteins, positive acute-phase proteins, negative acute-phase proteins, constitutive, marasmus, kwashiorkor, nitrogen balance, creatinine height index (CHI), anemia, microcytic anemia, macrocytic anemia, normocytic anemia, iron-deficiency anemia, anemia of inflammation and chronic disease (AICD)

References

1. Litchford MD. *Laboratory Assessment of Nutritional Status: Bridging Theory and Practice*. Greensboro, NC: CASE Software; 2010.
2. Oh MS: Evaluation of renal function, water, electrolyte and acid-base balance. In: McPherson RA, Pincus MR, eds. *Henry's Clinical Diagnosis and Management by Laboratory Methods*. 22nd ed. Philadelphia: W.B. Saunders; 2011:169-192.
3. Holcombe B. Parenteral nutrition product shortages. Impact on safety. *JPEN J Parenter Enteral Nutr*. 2012;36(2 suppl):44S-47S.
4. Hawkins RC. Age and gender as risk factors for hyponatremia and hypernatremia. *Clinica Chimica Acta*. 2003;337(1):169-172.
5. Verbalis JG, Goldsmith SR, Greenberg A, et al. Diagnosis, evaluation, and treatment of hyponatremia: expert panel recommendations. *Am J Med*. 2013;126(10):S1-S42.
6. Elhassan EA, Schrier RW. Hyponatremia: Diagnosis, complications, and management including V2 receptor antagonists. *Curr Opin Nephrol Hypertens*. 2011;20(2):161-168.
7. Sterns RH, Nigwekar SU, Hix JK. The treatment of hyponatremia. *Semin Nephrol*. 2009;29(3):282-299.
8. Snyder NA, Feigal DW, Arief AI. Hypernatremia in elderly patients: a heterogeneous, morbid, and iatrogenic entity. *Ann Intern Med*. 1987;107(3):309-319.
9. Burton D, Theodore P. *Clinical Physiology of Acid-Base and Electrolyte Disorders*. 5th ed. New York: McGraw-Hill; 2001.
10. Rose BD. *Clinical Physiology of Acid-Base and Electrolyte Disorders*. New York: McGraw-Hill; 1977.
11. Paice BJ, Paterson KR, Onyanga-Omara F, Donnelly T, Gray JM, Lawson DH. Record linkage study of hypokalaemia in hospitalized patients. *Postgrad Med J*. 1986;62(725):187-191.
12. Kraft MD, Btaiche IF, Sacks GS, Kudsk KA. Treatment of electrolyte disorders in adult patients in the intensive care unit. *AJHP*. 2005;62(16):1663.
13. Kruse JA, Clark VL, Carlson RW, Geheb MA. Concentrated potassium chloride infusions in critically ill patients with hypokalemia. *J Pharmacol Clin Toxicol*. 1994;34(11):1077-1082.
14. Mandal AK. Hypokalemia and hyperkalemia. *Med Clin North Am*. 1997;81(3):611-639.
15. Bushinsky DA, Monk RD. Calcium. *The Lancet*. 1998;352(9124):306-311.
16. Hanzlik RP, Fowler SC, Fisher DH. Relative bioavailability of calcium from calcium formate, calcium citrate, and calcium carbonate. *J Pharmacol Exp Ther*. 2005;313(3):1217-1222.
17. French S, Subauste J, Geraci S. Calcium abnormalities in hospitalized patients. *South Med J*. 2012;105:231-237.
18. Semple P, Both C. Calcium chloride: a reminder. *Anaesthesia*. 1996;51(1):93-93.
19. Davis KD, Attie MF. Management of severe hypercalcemia. *Crit Care Clin*. 1991;7(1):175-190.
20. Mundy GR, Guise TA. Hypercalcemia of malignancy. *Am J Med*. 1997;103(2):134-145.
21. Brunelli SM, Goldfarb S. Hypophosphatemia: clinical consequences and management. *J Am Soc Nephrol*. 2007;18(7):1999-2003.
22. Rude RK. Magnesium metabolism and deficiency. *Endocrinol Metab Clin North Am*. 1993;22(2):377-395
23. Whang R, Oei TO, Aikawa JK, et al. Predictors of clinical hypomagnesemia: hypokalemia, hypophosphatemia, hyponatremia, and hypocalcemia. *Arch Intern Med*. 1984;144(9):1794-1796.
24. Skipper A. Refeeding syndrome or refeeding hypophosphatemia: a systematic review of cases. *Nutr Clin Pract*. 2012;27(1):34-40.

25. Mehanna HM, Moledina J, Travis J. Refeeding syndrome: what it is, and how to prevent and treat it. *BMJ*. 2008;336(7659):1495-1498.
26. Sherwood L. *Human Physiology: From Cells to Systems*. 8th ed. Boston, MA: Cengage Learning; 2015.
27. Kurtz I, Maher T, Hulter HN, Schambelan M, Sebastian A. Effect of diet on plasma acid-base composition in normal humans. *Kidney Int*. 1983;24(5):670-680.
28. Winter SD, Pearson JR, Gabow PA, Schultz AL, Lepoff RB. The fall of the serum anion gap. *Arch Intern Med*. 1990;150(2):311-313.
29. Hodgkin JE, Soeprono FF, Chan DM. Incidence of metabolic alkalemia in hospitalized patients. *Crit Care Med*. 1980;8(12):725-728.
30. American Diabetes Association. Standards of medical care in Diabetes—2018. *Diabetes Care*. 2018;41(1):S1–S159.
31. Nathan, DM, Kuenen J, Borg R, Zheng H, Schoenfeld D, Heine RJ. Translating the A1C assay into estimated average glucose values. *Diabetes Care*. 2008; 31(8):1473-1478.
32. Rahbar S. The discovery of glycated hemoglobin: a major event in the study of nonenzymatic chemistry in biological systems. *Ann N Y Acad Sci*. 2005;1043(1):9-19.
33. American Diabetes Association. (6) glycemic targets. *Diabetes Care*. 2015;38(suppl):S33-40.
34. Keys A. Caloric undernutrition and starvation, with notes on protein deficiency. *J Am Med Assoc*. 1948;138(7):500-511.
35. Jensen GL, Bistrian B, Roubenoff R, Heimburger DC. Malnutrition syndromes: a conundrum vs continuum. *JPEN J Parenter Enteral Nutr*. 2009;33(6):710-716.
36. Dickerson RN, Tidwell AC, Minard G, Croce MA, Brown RO. Predicting total urinary nitrogen excretion from urinary urea nitrogen excretion in multiple-trauma patients receiving specialized nutritional support. *Nutrition*. 2005;21(3):332-338.
37. Blackburn GL, Bistrian BR, Maini BS, Schlamm HT, Smith MF. Nutritional and metabolic assessment of the hospitalized patient. *JPEN J Parenter Enteral Nutr*. 1977;1(1):11-22.
38. Fuhrman MP, Charney P, Mueller CM. Hepatic proteins and nutrition assessment. *J Am Diet Assoc*. 2004;104(8):1258-1264.
39. Chalasani N, Younossi Z, Lavine JE, et al. The diagnosis and management of non-alcoholic fatty liver disease: practice guideline by the American Association for the Study of Liver Diseases, American College of Gastroenterology, and the American Gastroenterological Association. *Hepatology*. 2012;55(6):2005-2023.
40. Patil H, Vaidya O, Bogart D. A review of causes and systemic approach to cardiac troponin elevation. *Clin Cardiol*. 2011;34(12):723-728.
41. Sharrett AR, Ballantyne CM, Coady SA, et al. Coronary heart disease prediction from lipoprotein cholesterol levels, triglycerides, lipoprotein(a), apolipoproteins A-I and B, and HDL density subfractions: the atherosclerosis risk in communities (ARIC) study. *Circulation*. 2001;104(10):1108-1113.
42. Wilson PW, D'Agostino RB, Levy D, Belanger AM, Silbershatz H, Kannel WB. Prediction of coronary heart disease using risk factor categories. *Circulation*. 1998;97(18):1837-1847.
43. Ewald PDN, Kloer H. Treatment options for severe hypertriglyceridemia (SHTG): the role of apheresis. *Clin Res Cardiol Suppl*. 2012;7(1):31-35.
44. World Health Organization. Haemoglobin concentrations for the diagnosis of anaemia and assessment of severity. Vitamin and Mineral Nutrition Information System. Geneva, 2011 (WHO/NMH/NHD/MNM/11.1) http://www.who.int/vmnis/indicators/haemoglobin.pdf Accessed November 5, 2017.
45. Clark SF. Iron deficiency anemia. *Nutr Clin Pract*. 2008;23(2):128-141.
46. Zubieta-Calleja G, Paulev P, Zubieta-Calleja L, Zubieta-Castillo G. Altitude adaptation through hematocrit changes. *J Physiol Pharmacol*. 2007;58(5):811-818.
47. Chan LN, Mike LA. The science and practice of micronutrient supplementations in nutritional anemia: an evidence-based review. *JPEN J Parenter Enteral Nutr*. 2014;38(6):656-672.
48. Taylor P. Martinez-Torres C, Leets I, Ramirez J, Garcia-Casal MN, Layrisse M. Relationships among Iron Absorption, percent saturation of plasma transferrin and serum ferritin concentration in humans. *J Nutr*. 1988;118:1110-1115.
49. Stabler SP. Vitamin B_{12} deficiency. *N Engl J Med*. 2013;368(2):149-160.
50. Solomon LR. Disorders of cobalamin (vitamin B_{12}) metabolism: emerging concepts in pathophysiology, diagnosis, and treatment. *Blood Rev*. 2007;21(3):113-130.
51. Butterworth CE Jr, Tamura T. Folic acid safety and toxicity: a brief review. *Am J Clin Nutr*. 1989;50(2):353-358.
52. Joseph B, Ramesh N. Weekly dose of iron-folate supplementation with vitamin-C in the workplace can prevent anaemia in women employees. *Pak J Med Sci*. 2013;29(1):47-52.
53. Folic acid recommendations. Centers for Disease Control and Prevention website. https://www.cdc.gov/ncbddd/folicacid/recommendations.html Updated December 28, 2016. Accessed November 9, 2017.
54. Suitor CW, Bailey LB. Dietary folate equivalents: interpretation and application. *J Am Diet Assoc*. 2000;100(1):88-94.

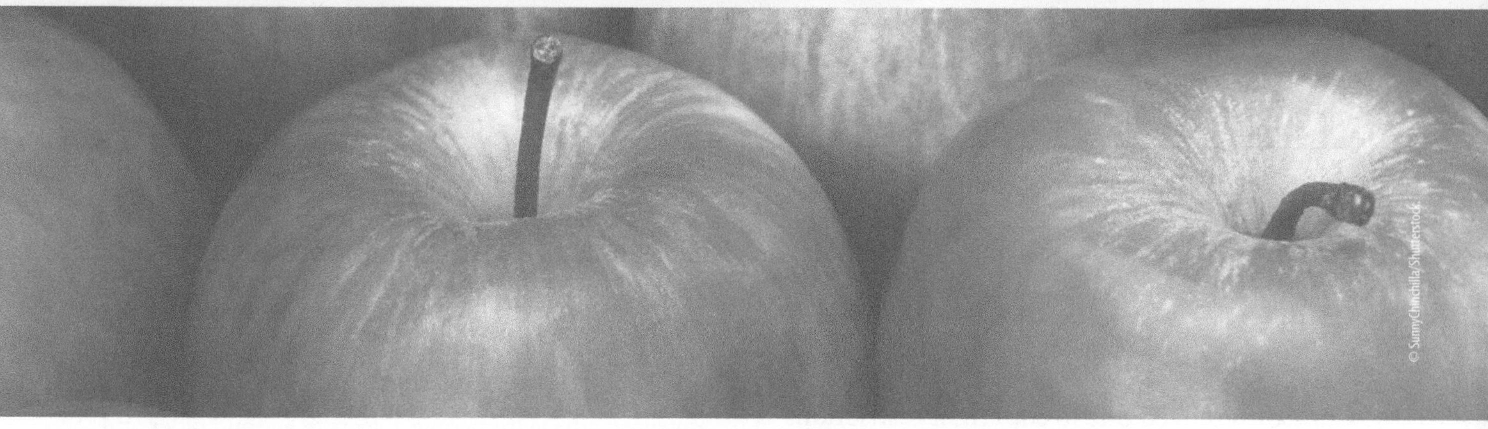

Standards for Desirable Nutrient Intake

Jessica Pearl, MS, RD, CSSD, CSCS, CLT, CDN, FAND

CHAPTER OUTLINE

- Introduction
- Historical Perspective for Dietary Standards and Recommendations
- Dietary Reference Intake (DRI)
- Tolerable Upper Intake Level (UL)
- Energy Requirements
- Macronutrient Recommendations
- Nutrient Density and Nutritional Rating
- Diet Quality Indicators
- *Dietary Guidelines for Americans 2015*
- Food Labeling and Nutrition
- Food Guides (MyPlate Food Exchange)
- Chapter Summary

LEARNING OBJECTIVES

After reading this chapter, the learner will be able to:

1. Describe the process that led to the formation of the *Dietary Guidelines* and the Dietary Reference Intakes (DRIs).
2. Identify the main USDA food guides.
3. Explain why the DRIs were developed and what purpose each value is intended to serve.
4. Identify the components of total energy expenditure and the methods used to measure energy expenditure.
5. Summarize the intake recommendations for protein, fat, and carbohydrates as established by the Recommended Dietary Allowance (RDA), Estimated Average Requirement (EAR), tolerable upper intake level (UL), and Acceptable Macronutrient Distribution Range (AMDR).
6. Explain the profiling tools most commonly used to guide consumer food choices.
7. Summarize the purpose of the Healthy Eating Index and food pattern modeling analysis.
8. Summarize the process for developing the *Dietary Guidelines for Americans* and MyPlate, including the key recommendations of the *Dietary Guidelines for Americans 2015*.
9. Explain the reasoning for the major changes to the Nutrition Facts Label.

Content removed due to copyright restrictions

Introduction

Throughout the past century, as our understanding of the relationship between food intake and health evolved, so did the eating habits of individuals. As a result, the standards of desirable nutrient intake and eating patterns also transitioned. These standards, established by government agencies including the United States Department of Agriculture (USDA) and the Department of Health and Human Services (HHS), are meant to encourage optimal eating behaviors throughout the population. The first USDA food guide was developed in 1916 with "Food for Young Children" and "How to Select Food" using food groups and household measures to encourage proper intake. Today the food guide has taken the form of MyPlate, a graphic image created to support conformance to the *Dietary Guidelines for Americans* (*Dietary Guidelines*). Since it was first issued in 1980, the *Dietary Guidelines* has served as the basis for the USDA food guides. The guidelines are updated every five years to reflect current scientific data, and food guides are revised as necessary to best reflect the message of the *Dietary Guidelines* and most effectively resonate with the public.

Historical Perspective for Dietary Standards and Recommendations

Preview The *Dietary Guidelines for Americans*, Dietary Reference Intakes, and USDA food guides have collectively evolved over the past century to guide the intake of the American population.

History of the *Dietary Guidelines*

In 1977, the US Senate Select Committee on Nutrition and Human Needs recommended that dietary goals be established for the American people. The goals consisted of complementary nutrient based and food-based recommendations. Since 1980, the *Dietary Guidelines for Americans* has been the authoritative source of nutrition advice for people 2 years of age and older and serve as the basis for federal food and nutrition education programs.[1] The *Dietary Guidelines* are revised and published every five years by the HHS Office of Disease Prevention and Health Promotion and the USDA's Center for Nutrition Science and Policy, along with the Agriculture Research Service (**TABLE 1**). Since the first dietary goals were established, the *Dietary Guidelines* has changed in important ways to reflect available scientific evidence, but the guidelines have also been consistent in their recommendations of the components needed to follow a healthy diet (**TABLE 2**).

Development of the *Dietary Guidelines*

Table 2 summarizes the key recommendations of the *Dietary Guidelines* for each year they have been issued.

Many landmark changes have been added to each edition of the *Dietary Guidelines*[1]:

- First edition (1980): *Dietary Guidelines* recommendations are developed and released by the federal government.
- Second edition (1985): For the first time, the *Dietary Guidelines* advisory committee presented a report of recommendations to the federal government based on nutrition science evidence. This report was then used to inform the *Dietary Guidelines 1985*.
- Third edition (1990): The definition of "healthy" weight considers body mass index, waist-to-hip ratio, and weight-related health problems. Numerical goals are suggested for total fat and saturated fat in the diets of adults.
- Fourth edition (1995): Estimated Average Requirement (EAR), Recommended Dietary Allowance (RDA), and Estimated Energy Requirement (EER) are defined by specific criteria of nutrient adequacy. Tolerable upper intake level (UL) is set according to a specific endpoint.
- Fifth edition (2000): Ten key messages are established and split into three groups instead of seven key messages. The emphasis of this issue was "nutrition and your health."
- Sixth edition (2005): This was the first time a policy document intended primarily for policy

TABLE 1	Historical Timeline: *The Dietary Guidelines for Americans*
1977	*Dietary Goals for the United States* is issued. Shift in focus from ensuring adequate nutrient intake to avoiding excessive intake of nutrients potentially linked to chronic disease. Goals were met with controversy from nutrition professionals and others who had concerns.
1979	*Healthy People: The Surgeon General's Report on Health Promotion and Disease Prevention* is released. Reports findings from a panel assembled by the American Society for Clinical Nutrition to study the relationship between dietary practice and health outcomes.
1980	*Nutrition and Your Health: Dietary Guidelines for Americans* released by the USDA and HHS. Contained seven principles for a healthy diet. US Senate Committee on Appropriations report calls for establishment of a committee to review scientific evidence and recommend revisions to the 1980 nutrition guidelines.
1983	*The Dietary Guidelines* reviewed by federal advisory committee. A federal advisory committee composed of nine nutrition scientists is formed to review the guidelines and report recommendations to the HHS and USDA.
1985	*The Dietary Guidelines for Americans* (2nd ed.) released by the HHS and USDA. Main amendments made were for clarification and modification of scientific knowledge to reflect new findings of relationship between diet and chronic disease.
1987	*Conference Report of the House Committee on Appropriations* specifies that the *Dietary Guidelines* are to be reviewed periodically.
1989	Federal advisory group reviews *1985 Dietary Guidelines* to assess need for modifications or updates.
1990	*The Dietary Guidelines for Americans* (3rd ed.) released by the HHS and the USDA. Focus on total diet and specifics on food selection. First edition containing numerical recommendations for dietary fat and saturated fat intake. National Nutrition Monitoring and Related Research Act requires that the *Dietary Guidelines for Americans* be published every five years.
1993	The 1995 *Dietary Guidelines* committee is established by the HHS and the USDA.
1994	The secretaries of the HHS and USDA appoint an 11-member *Dietary Guidelines* advisory committee to review the third edition of the *Dietary Guidelines for Americans* and assess the need for changes and make recommendations as necessary.
1995	The report of the *Dietary Guidelines* advisory committee was published, serving as the basis for the fourth edition of *Nutrition and Your Health: Dietary Guidelines for Americans*. The *Dietary Guidelines for Americans* (4th ed.) released by the HHS and the USDA. Changes to this edition were inclusion of the Food Guide Pyramid, Nutrition Facts Label boxes highlighting good food sources of key nutrients, and a chart representing three weight ranges in relation to height.
1997	The 2000 *Dietary Guidelines* advisory committee is established by the USDA charter.
1998	The secretaries of the HHS and the USDA appoint an 11-member *Dietary Guidelines* advisory committee to again review the latest edition of the *Dietary Guidelines for Americans* and recommend any needed changes.
2000	The *Dietary Guidelines for Americans* (5th ed.) is issued by the president, the HHS, and the USDA. Changes to this document include 10 statements instead of seven; this was accomplished by separating physical activity from weight guidelines, separating grains from fruits and vegetables, and adding a new guideline on safe food handling.

(*continues*)

TABLE 1 *(continued)*

2003	The 2005 *Dietary Guidelines* advisory committee is established by the HHS charter. The secretaries of the HHS and the USDA appoint a 13-member *Dietary Guidelines* advisory committee to once again review the latest edition of the *Dietary Guidelines for Americans* and make recommendations for revisions.
2003–2004	Committee members systematically reviewed the scientific literature to address issues include the relationship between diet and physical activity and health promotion and chronic disease prevention. Resources consulted include reports from the Institute of Medicine (Dietary Reference Intake), the Agency for Healthcare Research and Quality, and the World Health Organization. The USDA completed food intake pattern modeling analyses and the Committee analyzed national data sets as well as the input of experts.
2004	The committee submits its report to the secretaries of the HHS and the USDA; the report serves as the basis for the *Nutrition and Your Health: Dietary Guidelines for Americans* (6th ed.).
2005	The *Dietary Guidelines for Americans* (6th ed.) released by the HHS and the USDA. Intended for use primarily by policy makers, healthcare providers, nutritionists, and nutrition educators. Composed of nine main messages that specified 41 key recommendations; 23 for the general public and 18 for special populations. Examples of eating patterns used to exemplify the *Dietary Guidelines* include the USDA food guide and DASH eating plan. A supplementary brochure, *Finding Your Way to a Healthier You*, was provided to advise consumers in their food choices. The USDA released the MyPyramid food-guidance system, an update of the Food Guide Pyramid containing additional advice for consumers.
2008	The 2010 Dietary Guidelines advisory committee is established by the USDA charter. The secretaries of HHS and USDA appoint a 13-member *Dietary Guidelines* advisory committee to review the sixth edition of the *Dietary Guidelines for Americans* and make recommendations for revisions.
2009	The Nutrition Evidence Library is established by the USDA to review scientific literature.
2010	The committee submits its report to the secretaries of the HHS and the USDA, and it serves as the basis for the seventh edition of the *Dietary Guidelines for Americans*.

Data from Dietary Guidelines Advisory Committee. (2010). Report of the Dietary Guidelines Advisory Committee on the *Dietary Guidelines for Americans*, 2010, to the Secretary of Agriculture and the Secretary of Health and Human Services. Appendix E-4: History of the Dietary Guidelines for Americans. Pages 434-437. https://www.cnpp.usda.gov/sites/default/files/dietary_guidelines_for_americans/2010DGACReport-camera-ready-Jan11-11.pdf.

makers, healthcare professionals, nutritionists, and nutrition educators was prepared. The *Dietary Guidelines* included 41 key recommendations, 23 of which were for the general population and 18 for specific populations. The USDA food guide and the Dietary Approaches to Stop Hypertension (DASH) were used as examples of eating patterns consistent with the *Dietary Guidelines*. The USDA MyPyramid Food Guidance System replaced the Food Guide Pyramid.

- Seventh edition (2011): This version encompassed the overarching concepts of consuming nutrient-dense foods and beverages and maintaining calorie balance to achieve and sustain a healthy weight. For this edition, the eating patterns were updated to assist individuals in building healthful diets based on the *Dietary Guidelines*. MyPlate was released to serve as a visual icon to help consumers follow the *Dietary Guidelines*.
- Eighth edition (2015): The most recent version of the guidelines is designed to help Americans eat a healthier diet. This issue of the *Dietary Guidelines* emphasizes the importance of following an overall healthy eating pattern to reduce the risk of diseases and maintain health by making favorable shifts in food choices.

TABLE 2 Evolution of the *Dietary Guidelines for Americans*

	1980	1985	1990	1995	2000	
1	Eat a variety of foods.	Eat a variety of foods.	Eat a variety of foods.	Eat a variety of foods.	Aim for a healthy weight.	Aim for fitness.
2	Maintain ideal weight.	Maintain desirable weight.	Maintain healthy weight.	Balance the food you eat with physical activity.	Be physical active every day.	
3	Avoid fat, saturated fat, and cholesterol.	Avoid fat, saturated fat, and cholesterol.	Choose a diet low in fat, saturated fat, and cholesterol.	Choose a diet with plenty of grain products, vegetables, and fruits.	Let the Food Pyramid guide your food choices.	Build a healthy base.
4	Eat foods with adequate starch and fiber.	Eat foods with adequate starch and fiber.	Choose a diet with plenty of vegetables, fruits, and grain products.	Choose a diet low in fat, saturated fat, and cholesterol.	Choose a variety of grains daily, especially whole grains.	
5	Avoid sugar.	Avoid sugar.	Use sugars only in moderation.	Choose a diet moderate in sugars.	Choose a variety of fruits and vegetables daily.	
6	Avoid sodium.	Avoid sodium.	Use salt and sodium only in moderation.	Choose a diet moderate in salt and sodium.	Keep food safe to eat.	
7	If you drink alcohol, do so in moderation.	If you drink alcoholic beverages, do so in moderation.	If you drink alcoholic beverages, do so in moderation.	If you drink alcoholic beverages, do so in moderation.	Choose a diet low in saturated fat and cholesterol and moderate in total fat.	Choose sensibly.
8					Choose beverages and foods to moderate your intake of sugars.	
9					Choose and prepare foods with less salt.	
10					If you drink alcoholic beverages, do so in moderation.	

(*continues*)

TABLE 2 *(continued)*

	2005	2010	2015
1	Consume a variety of foods within and among the basic food groups while staying within energy needs	Maintain calorie balance over time to achieve and sustain a healthy weight	Follow a healthy eating pattern across the life span
2	Control calorie intake to manage body weight	Focus on consuming nutrient-dense foods and beverages	Focus on variety, nutrient density, and amount
3	Be physically active every day		Limit calories from added sugars and saturated fat and reduce sodium intake
4	Increase daily intake of fruits and vegetables, whole grains, and nonfat or low-fat milk and milk products		Shift to healthier food and beverage choices
5	Choose fats wisely for good health		Support healthy eating patterns for all
6	Choose carbohydrates wisely for good health		
7	Choose and prepare foods with little salt		
8	If you drink alcohol, do so in moderation		
9	Keep food safe to eat		

Data from US Department of Agriculture (USDA), US Department of Health and Human Services (HHS). Dietary Guidelines for Americans 1980–2015. Retrieved from: https://health.gov/dietaryguidelines.
USDA, HHS. *Nutrition and Your Health: Dietary Guidelines for Americans*. Washington, DC: US Government Printing Office; 1980.
USDA, HHS. *Nutrition and Your Health: Dietary Guidelines for Americans* 2nd ed. Washington, DC: U. S. Government Printing Office, 1985.
USDA, HHS. *Dietary Guidelines for Americans* 3rd ed. Washington, DC: US Government Printing Office; 1990.
USDA, HHS. *Dietary Guidelines for Americans* 4th ed. Washington, DC: US Government Printing Office; 1995.
USDA, HHS. *Dietary Guidelines for Americans* 5th ed. Washington, DC: US Government Printing Office; 2000.
USDA, HHS. *Dietary Guidelines for Americans* 6th ed. Washington, DC: US Government Printing Office; 2005.
USDA, HHS. *Dietary Guidelines for Americans, 2010* 7th ed. Washington, DC: US Government Printing Office; 2010.
USDA, HHS. *2015-2020 Dietary Guidelines For Americans* 8th ed. Washington, DC: US Government Printing Office; 2015.

History of the Dietary Reference Intakes

The **Dietary Reference Intakes (DRIs)** are the reference values used to guide nutrient assessment and planning in the United States and Canada. The DRIs replace the Recommended Dietary Allowances that were issued periodically from 1941 to 1989 by the National Academy of Sciences and the Recommended Nutrient Intakes (RNIs) published by the Canadian government. The Dietary Reference Intakes are a set of reference values for specific nutrients established in 1994; each DRI category has a special use. Since the RDAs were originally established, there has been significant growth in the research basis relevant to the defining and understanding of nutrient requirements and food constituents and the relationship to various aspects of health. There was a need for developing DRIs for diet planning, nutrition assessment, food labeling, and nutrition policy development.[2] The historical timeline of the establishment of DRIs is shown in **TABLE 3**. From 1997 to 2004, the first DRI reports were based on the work of nutrient expert committees to define and set the DRI values, set chronic disease endpoints, review available data on requirements for children, and assess the health benefits of nonessential substances in foods.[3] Many applications such as the *Dietary Guidelines for Americans* and other food-guidance programs are based on the DRI nutrient values necessitating current and accurate evidence for their ongoing utility and application.

Historical Timeline of USDA Food Guides

As early as 1916 and into the 1930s, *Food for Young Children* and *How to Select Food* established guidance for Americans based on food groups and household measures and focused on "protective foods."

In the 1940s, *A Guide to Good Eating (Basic Seven)* highlighted the foundation diet for nutrient adequacy. It included the daily number of servings

TABLE 3 Historical timeline: Dietary reference intakes

1941	Recommended Dietary Allowances (RDAs) are published by the National Academy of Medicine. They serve as the primary components for nutrition policy in the United States, with the Dietary Standards/Recommended Nutrient Intakes (RNIs) serving that role in Canada. As nutrition science continues to advance in the coming years, the RDIs and RDAs continually change to reflect the progressive increase in knowledge and transition in consumer eating behaviors.
1990s	Scientific knowledge of the link between diet, health, and chronic disease increases. Additional advancements made in technology allow for measurement of small changes in individual adaptations to several nutrients. Eating behaviors shift to include increased consumption of nutrients in their pure form as well as fortified and enriched products. The risk for excess nutrient intake warrants investigation of possible effects.
1994	The Food and Nutrition Board of the National Academies' Institute of Medicine is supported by the American and Canadian governments in their quest to develop a new, broader set of dietary reference values. This become the Dietary Reference Intakes (DRIs).
1997–2005	The *Dietary Reference Intakes* report is published. RDAs and RNIs have been replaced with four values of categories aimed at helping individuals optimize health, prevent disease, and avoid overconsumption of any nutrients.
2005–Present	The Food and Nutrition Board and Health Canada jointly release *Dietary Reference Intakes: The Essential Guide to Nutrient Requirements.* Rooted in the key concepts and primary recommendations introduced by the DRI series, this resource provides a practical, hands-on reference to facilitate in the education of individuals, groups, and students by health care professionals.

Data from Institute of Medicine of the National Academies (2006). *Dietary Reference Intakes: The Essential Guide to Nutrient Requirements*. Otten, J. J., Hellwig, J. P., Meyers, L. D. Pages 1, 5. https://www.nap.edu/catalog/11537/dietary-reference-intakes-the-essential-guide-to-nutrient-requirements. Accessed July 27, 2016.

needed from each of seven food groups, but it lacked serving sizes and was considered too complex. *Food for Fitness, A Daily Food Guide (Basic Four)* from 1956 to the 1970s continued with the foundation diet approach and gave goals for nutrient adequacy, with specified amounts from four food groups. It did not provide guidance on appropriate amounts of fat, sugar, and calories. The *Hassle-Free Daily Food Guide* was developed in 1979 after the 1977 dietary goals for the United States were released. They were again based on the basic four but included an additional fifth group to impress the need for Americans to moderate their intake of fat, sweets, and alcohol. In 1984, the *Food Wheel: A Pattern for Daily Food Choices* was created to give a total diet approach, including goals for both nutrient adequacy and moderation. Five food groups formed the basis for the Food Guide Pyramid, with daily amounts of food specified at three calorie levels. It was originally illustrated as a food wheel for an American Red Cross nutrition course. The Food Guide Pyramid, which was developed in 1992, again provided a graphic illustration of the total diet approach, with goals for both nutrient adequacy and moderation. It was developed using consumer research for the purpose of bringing awareness about the new food patterns. The visual focused on variety, moderation, and proportion by depicting images of added fats and sugars and a range for daily amounts of food for three calorie levels. The Food Guide Pyramid is shown in **FIGURE 1**.

In 2005, the MyPyramid food guidance system was introduced again with an update to the Food Guide Pyramid food patterns for the *2005*

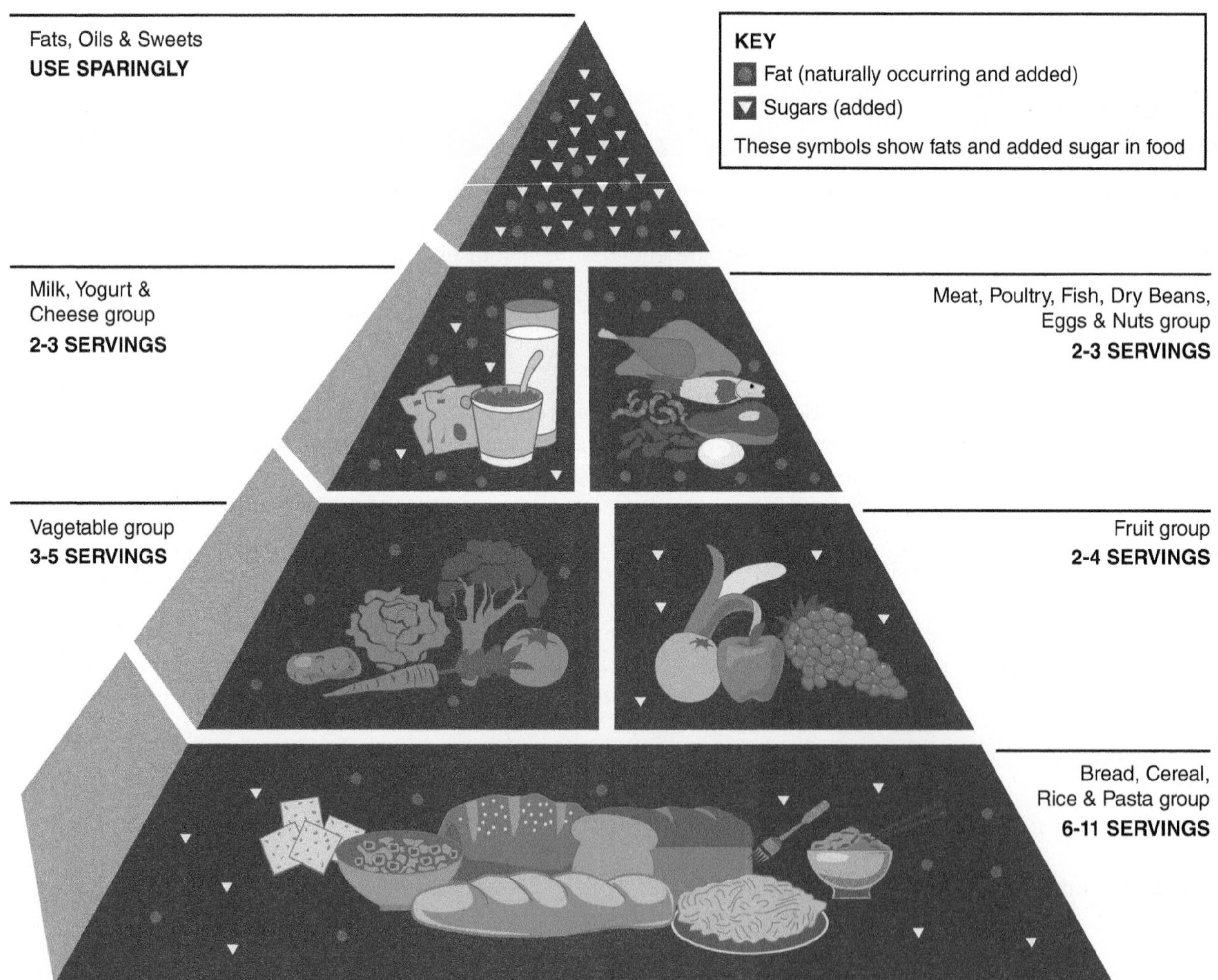

FIGURE 1 Food Guide Pyramid 1992

Reproduced from U.S. Department of Agriculture, U.S. Department of Health and Human Services (1992). Food Guide Pyramid. https://www.cnpp.usda.gov/sites/default/files/archived_projects/FGPLargeGIF.gif.

Dietary Guidelines for Americans, and included daily amounts of food at 12 calorie levels. The information remained in a pyramid shape but with simplified illustrations and a band added for oils and physical activity. Further details are made available on MyPyramid.gov. Concepts represented include variety, moderation, and proportion. The MyPyramid visual is represented in **FIGURE 2**.

MyPlate was introduced in 2011 along with an update of the USDA food patterns for the *2010 Dietary Guidelines*. The shape was changed, with icons serving as reminders for healthy eating but without any specific messages provided. The plate visual is meant to be a familiar mealtime symbol for consumers and links to food.[4] A historical review of USDA food guides is summarized in **TABLE 4**. The MyPlate graphic can be seen in **FIGURE 3**.

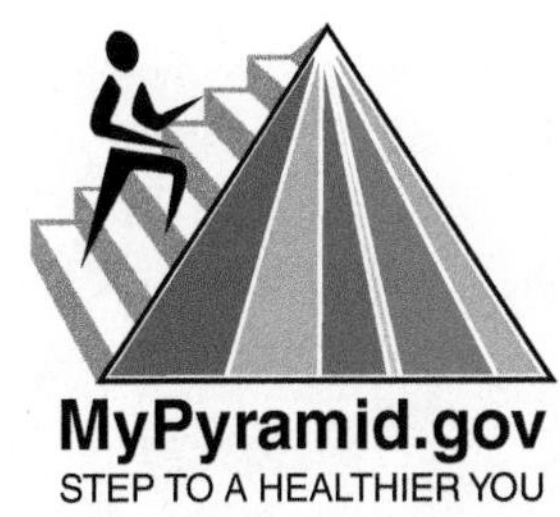

FIGURE 2 MyPyramid food-guidance system

Reproduced from U.S. Department of Agriculture, U.S. Department of Health and Human Services (1995). MyPyramid. https://www.cnpp.usda.gov/sites/default/files/archived_projects/MyPyramid.psd.

TABLE 4 Historical timeline: Summary of USDA food guides

1916–1930s	*Food for Young Children* and *How to Select Food* establish guidance based on food groups and household measures. They are focused on "protective foods."
1940s	*A Guide to Good Eating (Basic Seven)* highlights the foundation diet for nutrient adequacy. It included the daily number of servings needed from each of seven food groups, but it lacked serving sizes and was considered too complex.
1956–1970s	*Food for Fitness, A Daily Food Guide (Basic Four)* continues with the foundation diet approach and gives goals for nutrient adequacy with specified amounts from four food groups. It did not provide guidance on appropriate amounts of fat, sugar, and calories.
1979	*Hassle-Free Daily Food Guide* was developed after the 1977 Dietary Goals for the United States were released. They were again based on the basic four but included an additional fifth group to impress the need to moderate intake of fats, sweets, and alcohol.
1984	*Food Wheel: A Pattern for Daily Food Choices* gives a total diet approach, including goals for both nutrient adequacy and moderation. Five food groups and amounts formed the basis for the Food Guide Pyramid, with daily amounts of food specified at three calorie levels. It was originally illustrated as a food wheel for an American Red Cross nutrition course.
1992	Food Guide Pyramid again gives a total diet approach with goals included for both nutrient adequacy and moderation. It was developed using consumer research for the purpose of bringing awareness to the new USDA Food Patterns. The visual focused on variety, moderation, and proportion, depicting images of added fats and sugars and a range for daily amounts of food for three calorie levels.
2005	MyPyramid food-guidance system is introduced again with an update of the Food Guide Pyramid Food Patterns for the *2005 Dietary Guidelines for Americans*, which includes daily amounts of food at 12 calorie levels. Information is again presented in a "pyramid" shape but with simplified illustration and a band added for oils and physical activity. Further details are made available on MyPyramid.gov. Concepts represented include variety, moderation, and proportion.
2011	MyPlate is introduced along with an update of the USDA Food Patterns for the *2010 Dietary Guidelines for Americans*. The shape is changed, with icons serving as reminders for healthy eating, not providing specific messages. The plate visual is meant to be a familiar mealtime symbol for consumers and links to food.

Modified from U.S. Department of Agriculture. A Brief History of USDA Food Guides. USDA Choose MyPlate. https://www.choosemyplate.gov/content/brief-history-usda-food-guides. Updated January 25, 2017. Accessed September 28, 2016.

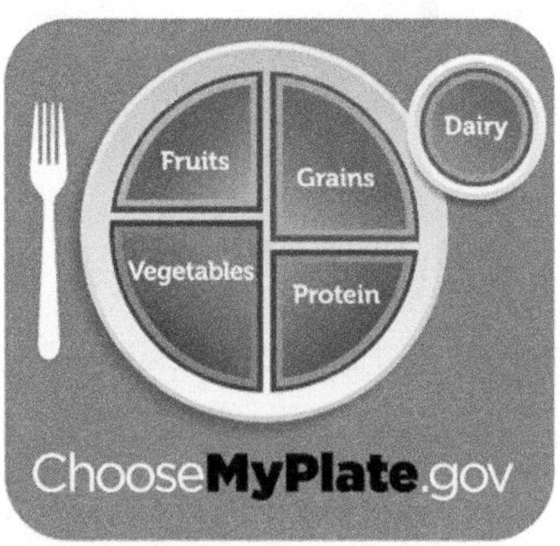

FIGURE 3 Choose MyPlate

Reproduced from United States Department of Agriculture. Choose MyPlate. choosemyplate.gov. https://choosemyplate-prod.azureedge.net/sites/default/files/printablematerials/myplate_green.jpg

Recap The progression of dietary standards since the first food guides were established in 1916 have led to a current nutritional guidance landscape consisting of *Dietary Guidelines* that are updated and issued every five years. Current nutrient guidance includes four nutrient standard values known as the Dietary Reference Intakes and the MyPlate food guide, which was established to show healthy eating choices.

Dietary Reference Intake

Preview The Dietary Reference Intakes are a widely applicable and complete set of nutrient intake standards that have been set to guide the population's intake according to the most accurate scientific information available.

The DRIs are a nutrient-based reference values that have replaced the former Recommended Dietary Allowances in the United States and the RNIs in Canada. The DRIs encompass a more complete set of values that were developed in response to the increasingly widespread use of quantitative reference values as well as the development of more advanced approaches to dietary planning and assessment. Four nutrient-based values are included in the DRI: (1) the Estimated Average Requirement, the Recommended Dietary Allowance, Adequate Intake, and Tolerable Upper Intake Level (UL).

The DRIs represented a shift from the focus of the RDAs and RNIs to reduce the incidence of diseases of deficiency to help people optimize their health and prevent disease as well as avoid overconsuming any nutrient. There are other key ways in which the DRIs differ from the previous intake standards. Data on a nutrient's safety and role in health are considered in the formulation of a recommendation—specifically, the potential reduction in risk of chronic disease. Probability and risk are assessed in the process of determining the DRIs. Emphasis is on the distribution of nutrient requirements within a population rather than on just a single value. ULs of nutrient intake are established to addresses the risk of adverse effects. And components of food that are not natural but may introduce health risks or benefits are reviewed, and standards are established for those with available data.

The primary purposes served by these standards are to assess the intakes of individuals and population groups, as well as plan diets for individuals and groups. In addition, the DRIs are used in dietary-planning activities such as dietary guidance, institutional food planning, military food and nutrition planning, planning for food assistance programs, food labeling, food fortification, developing new or modified food products, and food safety assurance.[5]

DRI Review and Update Process

The American and Canadian governments have both established federal DRI committees that collaborate to identify DRI needs and procure government sponsorship of DRI reviews and related activities. The DRIs have been developed under the sponsorship of the Institute of Medicine with financial support from the American and Canadian governments. The DRIs represent nutrient reference values that are fundamental to national nutrition policies and important to professionals working in nutrition and health.

Nutrients nominated for review must be submitted with a cover letter and literature search. The cover letter contains the rationale and description of why a review is warranted as well as how it would address a current public health concern. The literature search gives a description of the search strategy and lists new, relevant literature published since the last DRI review. The two government DRI committees prioritize nutrients for government-funded reviews and commission expert reviews to establish reference values. New reviews are established based on current public health concerns along with significant, new, and relevant data since the previous DRI review. The DRI committees also determine whether any methodological issues identified as possible impedances to a new review have been resolved. Procuring funds also plays a factor in the initiation of new reviews.

Significant, new, and relevant data are defined by the following criteria:

- *Significant*: The overall scientific quality of the evidence, the number of new studies, the consistency of the results, and whether the new study results expand the DRI-related information

available to the original DRI expert panel. Randomized controlled trials of high scientific quality are of particular interest.
- *New*: Research that was unlikely to have been available to the previous DRI expert panel.
- *Relevant*: Study results are generalizable to the North American population and to DRI development.

The DRI committees consider input from both individuals and organizations within and outside the government when making future prioritization decisions. The committees established a nomination process to assist in planning for new DRI reviews of nutrition and related substances to be renewed from previous DRI reports. Nominations have been made for various nutrients including: arachidonic acid, choline, chromium, docosahexaenoic acid (DHA), eicosapentaenoic acid (EPA), fiber, magnesium, niacin, potassium, protein, saturated fat, sodium, stearic acid, vitamin B_6, vitamin E, and zinc. The DRI committee for each country is prompted to select its top three priority nutrients based on public health or public policy. Omega-3 fatty acids, sodium, magnesium, and vitamin E were selected for further consideration based on these submissions. Nutrient-assessment working groups were established with staff from the United States and Canada. Each group was to determine if any new science had been published since the last DRI review. Government agencies jointly prioritized the nutrients and came to the conclusion that a workshop on the potential use of chronic disease endpoints in setting DRI values was necessary before a proper nutrient DRI review would be conducted. A workshop commissioned by the federal government took place in March 2015 to address if and how chronic disease outcomes can be incorporated into setting DRI values. This is expected to be the foundation for an expert report on this facet of public health.[5]

The Panel on Micronutrients, Panel on the Definition of Dietary Fiber, Subcommittee on Upper Reference Levels of Nutrients (UL Subcommittee), Subcommittee on Interpretation and Uses of Dietary Reference Intakes (Uses Subcommittee), and the Standing Committee on the Scientific Evaluation of Dietary Reference Intakes (DRI committee) analyzed evidence on the risks and benefits of nutrients and other components to determine the appropriate reference levels. DRI values were determined primarily from scientific data from observational and experimental studies in peer-reviewed journals.[6]

Estimated Average Requirement

The **Estimated Average Requirement (EAR)** is the average daily nutrient-intake level estimated to meet the requirements of half of the healthy individuals in a particular life stage or gender group. It represents an estimated median requirement. This means the EAR exceeds the needs of half of the group and is unable to meet the needs of the other half.[5] The main purposes of the EAR are to assess the adequacy of population intakes and to be used as the basis for calculating Recommended Dietary Allowances. It was not itself designed to be used as a goal for daily intake by individuals.[6] **TABLE 5** shows the EAR for all nutrients. EARs have not been established for vitamin D, vitamin K, pantothenic acid, biotin, choline, calcium, chromium, fluoride, manganese, and other nutrients not yet evaluated by the DRI committee.[5] For further detail on the EAR for macronutrients, see the section titled "Macronutrient Recommendations."

Recommended Dietary Allowance and Adequate Intake

The **Recommended Dietary Allowance (RDA)** is the average daily dietary nutrient-intake level sufficient to meet the nutrient requirements of nearly all (approximately 98%) of healthy individuals in a particular life stage and gender group. The RDA therefore exceeds the requirements of almost all members of the group. The RDA serves as a guide for daily intake by individuals and it is not intended to be used to assess the intake of groups. Because it exceeds the requirements for almost all individuals, intake at RDA levels is unlikely to be inadequate.[5]

If an EAR cannot be set because of data limitations, no RDA will be established. For those nutrients with a statistically normal requirement distribution, the RDA is set by adding two standard deviations (SDs) to the EAR:

$$\text{RDA} = \text{EAR} + 2 \times \text{SD}$$

In the event an RDA cannot be determined, the **adequate intake (AI)** value is used to set the reference level. AI is a recommended average daily intake level based on observed or experimentally determined approximations or estimates of nutrient intake by a group of individuals who appear to be healthy and are assumed to be in adequate nutritional state. It is expected to at least meet the needs of most individuals in a specific life stage and gender group. For healthy breastfed infants, the AI is the mean intake. As for other life stages and gender groups, although AIs are assumed to cover the needs of all healthy individuals, the limited data available prevent definitive determination of what percentage it actually covers. The AI is ultimately not particularly useful in assessments.[5]

The RDAs for macronutrients can be found in **TABLE 6**; see "Macronutrient Recommendations" for more information on these RDAs. RDAs for micronutrients are presented in **TABLE 7**.

TABLE 5 Estimated average requirement

	Infants (Months)		Children (Years)		Males (Years)						Females (Years)					Pregnancy (Years)			Lactation (Years)		
	7–12	1–3	4–8	9–13	14–18	19–30	31–50	50–70	>70	9–13	14–18	19–30	31–50	50–70	>70	14–18	19–30	31–50	14–18	19–30	31–50
Carbohydrate (g/d)		100	100	100	100	100	100	100	100	100	100	100	100	100	100	135	135	135	160	160	160
Protein (g/kg/d)	1.0	0.87	0.76	0.76	0.73	0.66	0.66	0.66	0.66	0.76	0.71	0.66	0.66	0.66	0.66	0.88	0.88	0.88	1.05	1.05	1.05
Vitamin A (μg/d)		210	275	445	630	625	625	625	625	420	485	500	500	500	500	530	550	550	885	900	900
Vitamin C (mg/d)		13	22	39	63	75	75	75	75	39	56	60	60	60	60	66	70	70	96	100	100
Vitamin E (mg/d)		5	6	9	12	12	12	12	12	9	12	12	12	12	12	12	12	12	16	16	16
Thiamin (mg/d)		0.4	0.5	0.7	1.0	1.0	1.0	1.0	1.0	0.7	0.9	0.9	0.9	0.9	0.9	1.2	1.2	1.2	1.2	1.2	1.2
Riboflavin (mg/d)		0.4	0.5	0.8	1.1	1.1	1.1	1.1	1.1	0.8	0.9	0.9	0.9	0.9	0.9	1.2	1.2	1.2	1.3	1.3	1.3
Niacin (mg/d)		5	6	9	12	12	12	12	12	9	11	11	11	11	11	1.6	1.6	1.6	1.7	1.7	1.7
Vitamin B_6 (mg/d)		0.4	0.5	0.8	1.1	1.1	1.1	1.4	1.4	0.8	1.0	1.1	1.1	1.3	1.3	2.2	2.2	2.2	2.4	2.4	2.4
Folate (μg/d)		120	160	250	330	320	320	320	320	250	330	320	320	320	320	520	520	520	450	450	450
Vitamin B_{12} (μg/d)		0.7	1.0	1.5	2.0	2.0	2.0	2.0	2.0	1.5	2.0	2.0	2.0	2.0	2.0	2.2	2.2	2.2	2.4	2.4	2.4
Copper (μg/d)		260	340	540	685	700	700	700	700	540	685	700	700	700	700	785	800	800	985	1000	1000
Iodine (μg/d)		65	65	73	95	95	95	95	95	73	95	95	95	95	95	160	160	160	209	209	209
Iron (mg/d)	6.9	3.0	4.1	5.9	7.7	6	6	6	6	5.7	7.9	8.1	8.1	5	5	23	22	22	7	6.5	6.5
Magnesium (mg/d)		65	110	200	340	330	350	350	350	200	300	255	265	265	265	335	290	300	300	255	265
Molybdenum (μg/d)		13	17	26	33	34	34	34	34	26	33	34	34	34	34	40	40	40	35	36	36
Phosphorus (mg/d)		380	405	1055	1055	580	580	580	580	1055	1055	580	580	580	580	1055	580	580	1055	580	580
Selenium (μg/d)		17	23	35	45	45	45	45	45	35	45	45	45	45	45	49	49	49	59	59	59
Zinc (mg/d)	2.5	2.5	4.0	7.0	8.5	9.4	9.4	9.4	9.4	7.0	7.3	6.8	6.8	6.8	6.8	10.5	9.5	9.5	10.9	10.4	10.4

Adapted from Institute of Medicine of the National Academies (2006). *Dietary Reference Intakes: The Essential Guide to Nutrient Requirements*. Otten, J. J., Hellwig, J. P., Meyers, L. D. Pages 530-531. https://www.nap.edu/catalog/11537/dietary-reference-intakes-the-essential-guide-to-nutrient-requirements. Accessed July 27, 2016.

TABLE 6 Recommended Dietary Allowances (RDAs) for macronutrients

	Infant (Months)		Children (Years)			Males (Years)					Females (Years)					
	0–6	7–12	1–3	4–8	9–13	14–18	19–30	31–50	50–70	>70	9–13	14–18	19–30	31–50	50–70	>70
Carbohydrate (g/d)	60	95	130	130	130	130	130	130	130	130	130	130	130	130	130	130
Fiber (g/d)	ND	ND	19	25	31	38	38	38	30	30	26	26	25	5	21	21
Fat (g/d)	31	30	ND	ND	ND	ND	ND	ND	ND	ND	ND	ND	ND	ND	ND	ND
Linoleic Acid (g/d)	4.4	4.6	7	10	12	16	17	17	14	14	10	11	12	12	11	11
α-Linoleic Acid (g/d)	0.5	0.5	0.7	0.9	1.2	1.6	1.6	1.6	1.6	1.6	1/0	1.1	1.1	1.1	1.1	1.1
Protein	9.1	11.0	13	19	34	52	56	56	56	56	34	46	46	46	46	46

	Pregnancy (Years)			Lactation (Years)		
	≤18	19–30	31–50	≤18	19–30	31–50
Carbohydrate (g/d)	175	175	175	210	210	210
Fiber (g/d)	28	28	28	29	29	29
Fat (g/d)	ND	ND	ND	ND	ND	ND
Linoleic Acid (g/d)	13	13	13	13	13	13
α-Linoleic Acid (g/d)	1.4	1.4	1.4	1.3	1.3	1.3
Protein (g/d)	71	71	71	71	71	71

AI

RDA

Adapted from Institute of Medicine of the National Academies (2002/2005). Dietary Reference Intakes for Energy, Carbohydrate, Fiber, Fat, Fatty Acids, Cholesterol, Protein, and Amino Acids (Macronutrients). Panel on Micronutrients, Panel on the Definition of Dietary Fiber, Subcommittee on Upper Reference Levels of Nutrients, Subcommittee on Interpretation and Uses of Dietary Reference Intakes, and the Standing Committee on the Scientific Evaluation of Dietary Reference Intakes. Page 1324. https://www.nap.edu/catalog/10490/dietary-reference-intakes-for-energy-carbohydrate-fiber-fat-fatty-acids-cholesterol-protein-and-amino-acids-macronutrients. Accessed July 27, 2016.

TABLE 7 Recommended Dietary Allowances (RDAs) for micronutrients

	Infant (Months)		Children (Years)			Males (Years)					Females (Years)						Pregnancy (Years)			Lactation (Years)		
	0–6	7–12	1–3	4–8	9–13	14–18	19–30	31–50	50–70	>70	9–13	14–18	19–30	31–50	50–70	>70	≤18	19–30	31–50	≤18	19–30	31–50
Vitamin A (µg/d)	400	500	300	400	600	900	900	900	900	900	600	700	700	700	700	700	750	770	770	1200	1300	1300
Vitamin C (mg/d)	40	50	15	25	45	75	90	90	90	90	45	65	75	75	75	75	80	85	85	115	120	120
Vitamin D (µg/d)	5	5	5	5	5	5	5	5	10	15	5	5	5	5	10	15	5	5	5	5	5	5
Vitamin E (mg/d)	4	5	6	7	11	15	15	15	15	15	11	15	15	15	15	15	15	15	15	19	19	19
Vitamin K (µg/d)	2.0	2.5	30	55	60	75	120	120	120	120	60	75	90	90	90	90	75	90	90	75	90	90
Thiamin (mg/d)	0.2	0.3	0.5	0.6	0.9	1,2	1,2	1,2	1,2	1,2	0.9	1.0	1.1	1.1	1.1	1.1	1.4	1.4	1.4	1.4	1.4	1.4
Riboflavin (mg/d)	0.3	0.4	0.5	0.6	0.9	1.3	1.3	1.3	1.3	1.3	0.9	1.0	1.1	1.1	1.1	1.1	1.4	1.4	1.4	1.6	1.6	1.6
Niacin (mg/d)	2	4	6	8	12	16	16	16	16	16	12	14	14	14	14	14	18	18	18	17	17	17
Vitamin B_6 (mg/d)	0.1	0.3	0.5	0.6	1.0	1.3	1.3	1.3	1.7	1.7	1.0	1.2	1.3	1.3	1.5	1.5	1.9	1.9	1.9	2.0	2.0	2.0
Folate (µg/d)	65	80	150	200	300	400	400	400	400	400	300	400	400	400	400	400	600	600	600	500	500	500
Vitamin B_{12} (µg/d)	0.4	0.5	0.9	1.2	1.8	2.4	2.4	2.4	2.4	2.4	1.8	2.4	2.4	2.4	2.4	2.4	2.6	2.6	2.6	2.8	2.8	2.8
Pantothenic Acid \ (mg/d)	1.7	1.8	2	3	4	5	5	5	5	5	4	5	5	5	5	5	6	6	6	7	7	7
Biotin (µg/d)	5	6	8	12	20	25	30	30	30	30	20	25	30	30	30	30	30	30	30	35	35	35
Choline (mg/d)	125	150	200	250	375	550	550	550	550	550	375	400	425	425	425	425	450	450	450	550	550	550
Calcium (mg/d)	210	270	500	800	1300	1300	1000	1000	1200	1200	1300	1300	1000	1000	1200	1200	1300	1000	1000	1300	1000	1000
Chromium (µg/d)	0.2	5.5	11	15	25	35	35	35	30	30	21	24	25	25	20	20	29	30	30	44	45	45
Copper (µg/d)	200	220		440	700	890	900	900	900	900	700	890	900	900	900	900	1000	1000	1000	1300	1300	1300
Fluoride (mg/d)	0.01	0.5	0.7	1	2	3	4	4	4	4	2	3	3	3	3	3	3	3	3	3	3	3
Iodine (µg/d)	110	130	90	90	120	150	150	150	150	150	120	150	150	150	150	150	220	220	220	290	290	290
Iron (mg/d)	0.27	11	7	10	8	11	8	8	8	8	8	15	18	18	8	8	27	27	27	10	9	9
Magnesium (mg/d)	30	75	80	130	240	410	400	420	420	420	240	360	310	320	320	320	400	350	360	360	310	320
Manganese (mg/d)	0.0003	0.6	1.2	1.5	1.9	2.2	2.3	2.3	2.3	2.3	1.6	1.6	1.8	1.8	1.8	1.8	2.0	2.0	2.0	2.6	2.6	2.6
Molybdenum (µg/d)	2	3	17	22	34	43	45	45	45	45	34	43	45	45	45	45	50	50	50	50	50	50
Phosphorus (mg/d)	100	275	460	500	1250	1250	700	700	700	700	1250	1250	700	700	700	700	1250	700	700	1250	700	700
Selenium (µg/d)	12	20	20	30	40	55	55	55	55	55	40	55	55	55	55	55	60	60	60	70	70	70
Zinc (mg/d)	2	3	3	5	8	11	11	11	11	11	8	9	8	8	8	8	12	11	11	13	12	12
Potassium (g/d)	0.4	0.7	3.0	3.8	4.5	4.7	4.7	4.7	4.7	4.7	4.5	4.7	4.7	4.7	4.7	4.7	4.7	4.7	4.7	5.1	5.1	5.1
Sodium (g/d)	0.12	0.37	1.0	1.2	1.5	1.5	1.5	1.5	1.3	1.2	1.5	1.5	1.5	1.5	1.3	1.2	1.5	1.5	1.5	1.5	1.5	1.5
Chloride (g/d)	0.18	0.57	1.5	1.9	2.3	2.3	2.3	2.3	2.0	1.8	2.3	2.3	2.3	2.3	2.0	1.8	2.3	2.3	2.3	2.3	2.3	2.3

AI RDA

Adapted from Institute of Medicine of the National Academies (2002/2005). Dietary Reference Intakes for Energy, Carbohydrate, Fiber, Fat, Fatty Acids, Cholesterol, Protein, and Amino Acids (Macronutrients). Panel on Micronutrients, Panel on the Definition of Dietary Fiber, Subcommittee on Upper Reference Levels of Nutrients, Subcommittee on Interpretation and Uses of Dietary Reference Intakes, and the Standing Committee on the Scientific Evaluation of Dietary Reference Intakes. Page 1320-1323. https://www.nap.edu/catalog/10490/dietary-reference-intakes-for-energy-carbohydrate-fiber-fat-fatty-acids-cholesterol-protein-and-amino-acids-macronutrients. Accessed July 27, 2016.

Recap The DRIs were established to replace the RNIs and RDAs, and they consist of four nutrient categories developed to promote health, prevent disease, and discourage nutrient overconsumption. The process for developing the DRIs involves committees from the United States and Canada reviewing scientific data for nominated nutrients to determine if evidence exists to warrant a DRI. Of particular concern is the nutrient's relationship to chronic diseases.

Tolerable Upper Intake Level

The **tolerable upper intake level (UL)** is the highest average daily nutrient-intake level likely to pose no risk of adverse health effects for almost all individuals in a particular group. It represents the highest intake level that can be tolerated without the possibility of undesirable health effects and was established in response to the growing number of foods with nutrient fortification and increased amount of dietary supplementation usage. In groups, it is used to estimate the percentage of the population at risk for adverse effects from excessive nutrient intake. As intake increases above the UL, the risk increases for potential adverse events.

The tolerable upper level is derived using a risk-assessment model consisting of a systematic series of scientific considerations and judgments. The UL value represents the total daily intake of a nutrient from all available sources (food, water, supplements) if potential harmful effects have been identified.[5] **TABLE 8** shows the UL for micronutrients. Macronutrient standards were unable to be established because of insufficient data.

Recap The EAR is used as the basis for establishing the RDA. It assesses the adequacy of population intakes and is not used to evaluate individual dietary consumption. The RDA is an average intake level adequate to meet the needs of nearly every member of a population. Intake at this level is unlikely to be inadequate. When the RDA is indeterminable, adequate intake (AI)—an average based on observed or estimated nutrient intake of individuals in a group—is used in its place. The UL represents the highest average daily nutrient intake that can be safely consumed without the risk of detrimental health consequences. The impetus for establishment of the UL was the rising concern of nutrient overconsumption introduced by the increased availability of fortified foods and dietary supplements on the market.

Energy Requirements

Preview Energy requirements determined for an individual are based on several factors, including energy expended at rest, after eating, during physical activity; and age and gender; weight and weight goals; and medical conditions, among others.

The **Estimated Energy Requirement (EER)** is the average dietary energy intake predicted to maintain energy balance in a healthy adult of a defined age, gender, weight, height, and level of physical activity consistent with good health. For children and pregnant or lactating women, the EER includes energy needs required for the deposition of tissue or secretion of milk at rates consistent with good health.[5] Because the variability of measured energy intake between individuals is greater than that of energy expenditure, there is an impedance to measuring energy intake without accounting for intake behaviors. Therefore, energy requirement is more precisely estimated from energy expenditure than from energy intake.

Components of Total Energy Expenditure

Energy is expended in the body in the form of Basal Energy Expenditure (Resting Energy Expenditure), Thermic Effect of Food, and Activity Thermogenesis (physical activity and activities of daily living). These three factors make up an individual's total daily energy expenditure. The percent contribution of each to total energy expenditure is depicted in **FIGURE 4**.

Basal Energy Expenditure (BEE) is the minimum amount of energy expended that is compatible with life. It typically represents 60% to 70% total energy

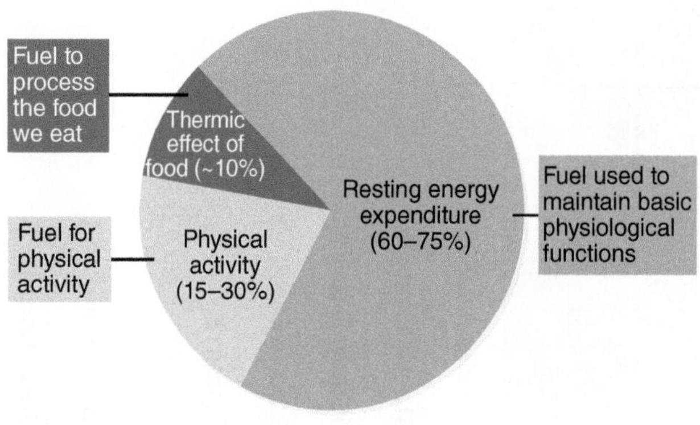

FIGURE 4 Components of total energy expenditure

TABLE 8 The UL for certain micronutrients

	Infant (Months)		Children (Years)		Males/Females (Years)				Pregnancy (Years)		Lactation (Years)	
	0–6	7–12	1–3	4–8	9–13	14–18	19–70	>70	14–18	19–50	14–18	19–50
Vitamin A (μg/d)	600	600	600	900	1700	2800	3000	3000	2800	3000	2800	3000
Vitamin C (mg/d)	ND	ND	400	650	1200	1800	2000	2000	1800	2000	1800	2000
Vitamin D (μg/d)	25	25	50	50	50	50	50	50	50	50	50	50
Vitamin E (mg/d)	ND	ND	200	300	600	800	1000	1000	800	1000	800	1000
Vitamin K	ND	ND	ND	ND	ND	ND	ND	ND	ND	ND	ND	ND
Thiamin	ND	ND	ND	ND	ND	ND	ND	ND	ND	ND	ND	ND
Riboflavin	ND	ND	ND	ND	ND	ND	ND	ND	ND	ND	ND	ND
Niacin (mg/d)	ND	ND	10	15	20	30	35	35	30	35	30	35
Vitamin B_6 (mg/d)	ND	ND	30	40	60	80	100	100	80	100	80	100
Folate (μg/d)	ND	ND	300	400	600	800	1000	1000	800	1000	800	1000
Vitamin B_{12}	ND	ND	ND	ND	ND	ND	ND	ND	ND	ND	ND	ND
Pantothenic Acid	ND	ND	ND	ND	ND	ND	ND	ND	ND	ND	ND	ND
Biotin	ND	ND	ND	ND	ND	ND	ND	ND	ND	ND	ND	ND
Choline (g/d)	ND	ND	1.0	1.0	2.0	3.0	3.5	3.5	3.0	3.5	3.0	3.5
Carotenoids	ND	ND	ND	ND	ND	ND	ND	ND	ND	ND	ND	ND
Arsenic	ND	ND	ND	ND	ND	ND	ND	ND	ND	ND	ND	ND
Boron (mg/d)	ND	ND	3	6	11	17	20	20	17	20	17	20
Calcium (g/d)	ND	ND	2.5	2.5	2.5	2.5	2.5	2.5	2.5	2.5	2.5	2.5
Chromium	ND	ND	ND	ND	ND	ND	ND	ND	ND	ND	ND	ND

TABLE 8 *(continued)*

	Infant (Months)		Children (Years)		Males/Females (Years)				Pregnancy (Years)		Lactation (Years)	
	0–6	7–12	1–3	4–8	9–13	14–18	19–70	>70	14–18	19–50	14–18	19–50
Copper (µg/d)	ND	ND	1000	3000	5000	8000	10,000	10,000	8000	10,000	8000	10,000
Fluoride (mg/d)	0.7	0.9	1.3	2.2	10	10	10	10	10	10	10	10
Iodine (µg/d)	ND	ND	200	300	600	900	1100	1100	900	1100	900	1100
Iron (mg/d)	40	40	40	40	40	45	45	45	45	45	45	45
Magnesium (mg/d)	ND	ND	65	110	350	350	350	350	350	350	350	350
Manganese (mg/d)	ND	ND	2	3	6	9	11	11	9	11	9	11
Molybdenum (µg/d)	ND	ND	300	600	1100	1700	2000	2000	1700	2000	1700	2000
Nickel (mg/d)	ND	ND	0.2	0.3	0.6	1.0	1.0	1.0	1.0	1.0	1.0	1.0
Phosphorus (g/d)	ND	ND	3.0	3.0	4.0	4.0	4.0	3.0	3.5	3.5	4.0	4.0
Potassium	ND	ND	ND	ND	ND	ND	ND	ND	ND	ND	ND	ND
Selenium (µg/d)	45	60	90	150	280	400	400	400	400	400	400	400
Silicon	ND	ND	ND	ND	ND	ND	ND	ND	ND	ND	ND	ND
Sulfate	ND	ND	ND	ND	ND	ND	ND	ND	ND	ND	ND	ND
Vanadium (mg/d)	ND	ND	ND	ND	ND	ND	1.8	1.8	ND	ND	ND	ND
Zinc (mg/d)	4	5	7	12	23	34	40	40	34	40	34	40
Sodium (g/d)	ND	ND	1.5	1.9	2.2	2.3	2.3	2.3	2.3	2.3	2.3	2.3
Chloride (g/d)	ND	ND	2.3	2.9	3.4	3.6	3.6	3.6	3.6	3.6	3.6	3.6

ND: Not determinable as limited data exists on adverse effects in regards to inability to handle excess amounts for this age group

Adapted from Institute of Medicine of the National Academies (2002/2005). Dietary Reference Intakes for Energy, Carbohydrate, Fiber, Fat, Fatty Acids, Cholesterol, Protein, and Amino Acids (Macronutrients). Panel on Micronutrients, Panel on the Definition of Dietary Fiber, Subcommittee on Upper Reference Levels of Nutrients, Subcommittee on Interpretation and Uses of Dietary Reference Intakes, and the Standing Committee on the Scientific Evaluation of Dietary Reference Intakes. Page 1320-1323. https://www.nap.edu/catalog/10490/dietary-reference-intakes-for-energy-carbohydrate-fiber-fat-fatty-acids-cholesterol-protein-and-amino-acids-macronutrients. Accessed July 27, 2016.

expenditure. **Resting Energy Expenditure (REE)** is the amount of energy expended by a resting individual in a thermoneutral environment without the effects of meal consumption, physical activity, or other physiological or mental stress. The value can be as much as 10% to 20% higher than the true basal metabolic rate, which is measured in the morning after 12–18 hours of rest. Interindividual variations exist between individuals with regard to REE, depending on age, gender, height, and weight within the range of 7.5% to 17.9%. Energy expended at rest is generated from many sources including maintaining the biochemical and structural integrity of the body and the cost of cellular work, ion pumps, synthesis and degradation of cell constituents, and biochemical cycles.

To measure energy adequately, several conditions must be met. Subjects should be awake but at rest, lying in a supine position in a physically comfortable test site (thermoneutral) that is quiet and not brightly lit. The subjects should be fasting and not consume food, energy-containing beverages, or drugs that artificially increase energy expenditure (such as ethanol or nicotine) for at least four hours before the energy assessment. The assessment should be performed at least two hours after meal consumption, with the exemption of those patients who are receiving continuous nutritional support. Subjects should be given adequate time to recover from activities of daily living such as getting dressed and traveling to the testing location; at least 20 minutes is recommended. Individuals should not engage in physical activity in the previous four to six hours before testing. Medically strenuous activities such as a wound dressing change, chest physiotherapy, or physical therapy should be avoided for 60 minutes prior to measuring energy expenditure. The procedure should not be performed within 24 hours of a hemodialysis session. During the test, subjects should lay motionless and refrain from talking or engaging in any other stimulating distractions. The measurement period should last until a steady state is achieved—which is characterized by five consecutive minute measurements of VO_2 within 10% of each other and corresponding respiratory quotients within 5% of each other). The measurement period should be no longer than 20 to 30 minutes.

The **thermic effect of food (TEF)** is the increase in energy expenditure immediately following meal digestion. It is also referred to as *diet-induced thermogenesis* and *specific dynamic action*. The primary determinants of TEF are the nutrient composition and energy content of the food consumed. Protein has been found to elicit the greatest increase in metabolic rate, followed by a mixed-nutrient meal, glucose, and then fat. The magnitude of the TEF is found to closely reflect the energy load contained in the test meal. The components of TEF include obligatory and facultative thermogenesis. Obligatory thermogenesis is the energy expended absorbing, processing, and storing nutrients. Facultative thermogenesis involves sympathetic nervous system activation and is otherwise not as well understood.

The **thermic effect of activity (TEA)** is the energy expended above the resting level both during and after physical activity. Activity thermogenesis is divided into exercise and nonexercise activity thermogenesis. Exercise activity thermogenesis contributes approximately 15% to 30% of total daily energy expenditure for those who exercise regularly. The intensity and duration of activity determine the contribution of exercise to total energy expenditure. The rate of energy expenditure for the duration of activity may be from 1.5 × resting metabolic rate (RMR) (such as with clerical work) to 15 × RMR (such as with running). Research has found that exercise has no effect on RMR unless it is prolonged or severe. The contribution of exercise to energy balance is demonstrated in several ways. First, thermogenesis is retained by maintaining fat-free mass. Second, energy expenditure is increased by exercise. Finally, excess postexercise oxygen consumption may increase energy expenditure in relation to the duration and intensity of activity.

Nonexercise activity thermogenesis (NEAT) is the energy expenditure of spontaneous physical activity, including the combined energy costs of the physical activities of daily living, fidgeting, spontaneous muscle contraction, and maintaining posture when not recumbent. NEAT accounts for the remainder of the total daily energy expenditure and explains the variation in activity thermogenesis in adults of similar size. Its major determinants include occupation and leisure time, which varies from 15% to more than 50% of total daily energy expenditures. Occupational NEAT can vary from 700 to 2,300 kcal/day, depending on strenuous level of work activities. Variation in leisure activities may reach 1,000 kcal/day. Altering energy balance in individuals is possible by changing the factor of NEAT to become more active. NEAT may also be influenced by biological, genetic, and environmental changes attributed to the human population over the last century and a half, primarily as a decrease.[7]

Methods of Measuring Energy Expenditure

The methods of measuring energy expenditure are summarized in **FIGURE 5** and include calorimetric and noncalorimetric techniques. Calorimetric techniques include direct and indirect calorimetry.

Approach and type of calorimeter	Indirect calorimeter					Direct calorimeter	Non-calorimetric methods
	Room open-air circuit	Hood/canopy open-circuit	Open-circuit expiratory collection	Doubly labelled water	Total collection Douglas bag		
Basal metabolic rate and resting metabolic rate	Y	Y	Y*	N	Y	Y	N
Thermic effect of food	Y	Y	Y*	N	Y*	Y	N
Activity related energy expenditure	Y	Y	Y	N	Y	Y	N
Total daily energy expenditure	Y#	N	Y*	Y	N	Y#	E

Y= "yes" a technique can be used to perform the measurement
N= 'No" it cannot be used to perform the measurement
E= estimated
* indicates that precision maybe unreliable
# indicates a confined subject

FIGURE 5 Techniques used to measure energy expenditure in humans

Data from Academy of Nutrition and Dietetics. Measurement of Energy Expenditure. Nutrition Care Manual. https://www.nutritioncaremanual.org/topic.cfm?ncm_category_id=11&lv1=144882&lv2=144900&ncm_toc_id=144900&ncm_heading=&. Accessed July 27, 2016.

Noncalorimetric techniques include the isotope-dilution method (doubly labeled water) DLW, kinematics recordings (mechanical activity meters), human observations and records (time and motion studies), and physiologic measurements (heart rate, energy intake, and electromyography).[8]

Direct Calorimetry

Direct measurement of metabolic rate is performed by assessing heat loss. The sum of convective, conductive, and evaporative heat transfer and radiant heat exchange are measured, with the total heat loss equaling the rate of energy use when body temperature is constant. This method is based purely on conservation of energy and does not involve any assumptions made about the physiology of energy metabolism. The subject is placed in a thermically isolated chamber, and the heat dissipated by the individual is collected and measured.

Several limitations exist that prevent direct calorimetry from being widely used. These include the confining nature of the testing environment, the inability to use calorimetry in measuring short-term effects of thermogenic stimuli (i.e., food) on heat exchange because of the body's large heat-storage capacity, and the costly nature of the instruments required.[9]

Indirect Calorimetry

Indirect calorimetry involves estimating the metabolic rate from measurements of oxygen consumption and carbon dioxide production using a set of assumptions and equations. It is assumed that all oxygen consumed (VO_2) is used to oxidize degradable fuels and that all carbon dioxide expended (VCO_2) is recovered. Eventually, all energy is converted into heat, so direct and indirect calorimetry provide identical rates of energy expenditure within steady-state conditions. The percentage of error for indirect calorimetry (respiratory gas exchange) is 2% compared to direct calorimetry.[9]

Energy expenditure from VO_2 and VCO_2 is calculated using the Weir equation:

$$\text{Energy expenditure} = (3.94 \times VO_2) + (1.11 \times VCO_2)$$

Use of indirect calorimetry is indicated under the following conditions:

- Clinical disorders that significantly alter REE
- Failure of an individual to respond to adequate nutrition support
- Individualizing nutrition support in an intensive care unit
- Individualizing nutrition program for healthy or ambulatory individuals receiving nutrition therapy for a disease such as diabetes

Estimating an individual's energy needs involves three steps. First, determine whether REE should be estimated or measured. Second, use critical thinking skills to evaluate REE. Third, determine when REE should be reevaluated.

Doubly Labeled Water

The DLW method of measuring energy expenditure assumes that the oxygen in respiratory CO_2 is in isotopic-exchange equilibrium with the oxygen contained in body water. Two isotopes of water are given, and their disappearance rates from the body (through urine and other bodily fluids) are monitored for one to three half-lives for isotope disappearance.[9]

Estimating Calorie Needs

The total number of calories a person needs daily varies by age, gender, weight, and level of physical activity. A need or desire to lose, maintain, or gain weight, among other factors, affects the total number of calories that should be consumed.[10,11] The estimated amounts of calories needed to maintain caloric balances for different age and gender groups across three levels of physical activity are provided in **TABLE 9**.

The estimates in Table 9 are based on the EER equations, using reference average heights and healthy weights for the different age and gender groups. Reference height and weight vary for children and adolescents. The adult reference height and weights are 5′10″ and 154 pounds for men and 5′4″ and 126 pounds for women. Estimates range from 1,600–2,400 calories per day for adult women and 2,000–3,000 calories per day for adult men. The lower end is of each range is designated for those individuals who are more sedentary, and the higher end is for those who are more active. Calorie needs decrease for adults with age, as basal metabolic rate steadily declines, therefore necessitating a lower energy intake.

Estimates range from 1,000–2,000 calories per day for young children and 1,400–3,200 calories per day for older children and adolescents. In general, boys have higher calorie needs than girls. Approximations of calorie needs can be determined on a more individual basis at www.supertracker.usda.gov.[10,11]

Predictive Equations

Energy requirements are traditionally estimated based on multiples of REE, which are known as *physical activity levels* (PALs). More recently, the regression approach, which is based on data of total energy expenditure from DLW studies, has formed the basis for the Dietary Reference Intakes for energy.[5,12] The Dietary Reference Intake EERs can be found in **Table 10.** Several predictive equations have been developed for estimating resting energy expenditure with applications for multiple settings. RDNs working with the healthcare team complete a full nutrition assessment that includes an estimate of energy expenditure using the appropriate predictive formula based on clinical and individual considerations. The equation most commonly used in the clinical setting is Mifflin St.-Jeor because it is the most accurate.

Recap Energy requirements vary based on age, gender, and level of physical activity, among other factors. Individual requirements are typically calculated using energy expenditure based on a series of estimates and reference equations.

▸ Macronutrient Recommendations

Preview The recommendations for carbohydrate, protein, and fat are each determined by different means and are dependent on availability and their metabolic functions within the body.

Estimated Average Requirement for Macronutrients

The EAR for carbohydrates is established based on the average amount of glucose used by the brain. No EAR is set for fat because the percent of energy derived from fat varies, yet it still can meet daily energy needs. Furthermore, no EAR exists for saturated fatty acids, monounsaturated fatty acids, or cholesterol because they are produced by the body and pose no benefit in the prevention of chronic disease.[13] For energy, an EER is provided.[5] (See the previous section titled "Energy Requirements.") The EAR and other DRIs for macronutrients are summarized in **TABLE 11**.

Recommended Dietary Allowance (RDA) for Macronutrients

The RDA for carbohydrates is 130 grams per day for adults and children. No RDA exists for fats, including saturated fatty acids, monounsaturated fatty acids, or cholesterol, because they are produced by the body and pose no benefit in preventing chronic disease. The RDA for protein is 0.8 grams per kilogram body weight per day for both men and women. It is established based on meta-analysis of nitrogen balance studies.[6] The RDAs for macronutrients can be found in Table 6.

Research has shown that consuming an imbalance of macronutrients may increase the risk of chronic disease. In response to this, the **acceptable macronutrient distribution range (AMDR)** for

TABLE 9 Estimated calorie needs per day by age, sex, and physical activity level

	Males			Females		
Age	**Sedentary**	**Moderately Active**	**Active**	**Sedentary**	**Moderately Active**	**Active**
2	1000	1000	1000	1000	1000	1000
3	1000	1400	1400	1000	1200	1400
4	1200	1400	1600	1200	1400	1400
5	1200	1400	1600	1200	1400	1600
6	1400	1600	1800	1200	1400	1600
7	1400	1600	1800	1200	1600	1800
8	1400	1600	2000	1400	1600	1800
9	1600	1800	2000	1400	1600	1800
10	1600	1800	2200	1400	1800	2000
11	1800	2000	2200	1600	1800	2000
12	1800	2200	2400	1600	2000	2200
13	2000	2200	2600	1600	2000	2200
14	2000	2400	2800	1800	2000	2400
15	2200	2600	3000	1800	2000	2400
16–18	2400	2800	3200	1800	2000	2400
19–20	2600	2800	3000	2000	2200	2400
21–25	2400	2800	3000	2000	2200	2400
26–30	2400	2600	3000	1800	2000	2400
31–35	2400	2600	3000	1800	2000	2200
36–40	2400	2600	2800	1800	2000	2200
41–45	2200	2600	2800	1800	2000	2200
46–50	2200	2400	2800	1800	2000	2200
51–55	2200	2400	2800	1600	1800	2200
56–60	2200	2400	2600	1600	1800	2200
61–65	2000	2400	2600	1600	1800	2000
66–70	2000	2200	2600	1600	1800	2000
71–75	2000	2200	2600	1600	1800	2000
76+	2000	2200	2400	1600	1800	2000

Sedentary: a lifestyle that includes only the physical activity of independent living.

Moderately active: a lifestyle that includes physical activity equivalent to walking 1.5–3 miles per day at 3–4 miles per hour in addition to activities of independent living.

Active: a lifestyle that includes physical activity equivalent to walking more than 3 miles per day at 3–4 miles per hour in addition to the activities of independent living.

Estimates for females do not include women who are pregnant or breastfeeding.

Reproduced from U.S. Department of Health and Human Services and U.S. Department of Agriculture (2015). 2015-2020 *Dietary Guidelines For Americans* 8th Edition. Appendix 2. Estimated Calorie Needs per Day, by Age, Sex and Physical Activity Level. Pages 77-78/ https://health.gov/dietaryguidelines/2015/guidelines/appendix-2/. Accessed July 27, 2016.

TABLE 10A Equations used to predict EER: Dietary Reference Intake Estimated Energy Requirements		
Infants and Children	**Months**	EER = Total Energy Expenditure + Energy Deposition
	0–3	EER = (89 x weight – 100) + 175
	4–6	EER = (89 x weight – 100) + 56
	7–12	EER = (89 x weight – 100) + 22
	13–35	EER = (89 x weight – 100) + 20
Children and Adolescents	**Years**	EER = Total Energy Expenditure + Energy Deposition
	Boys 3–8	EER = 88.5 – (61.9 x age) + PA x [(26.7 x weight) + (903 x height)] + 20
	Boys 9–18	EER = 88.5 – (61.9 x age) + PA x [(26.7 x weight) + (903 x height)] + 25
	Girls 3–8	EER = 135.3 – (30.8 x age) + PA x [(10.0 x weight) + (934 x height)] + 20
	Girls 9–18	EER = 135.3 – (30.8 x age) + PA x [(10.0 x weight) + (934 x height)] + 25
Adults 19+	**Gender**	EER = Total Energy Expenditure
	Men	EER = 662 – (9.53 x age) + PA x [(15.91 x weight) + (539.6 x height)]
	Women	EER = 354 – (6.91 x age) + PA x [(9.36 x weight) + (726 x height)]
Pregnancy	**Trimester**	EER = Nonpregnant EER + Pregnancy Energy Deposition
	First	EER = Nonpregnant EER + 0
	Second	EER = Nonpregnant EER + 340
	Third	EER = Nonpregnant EER + 452
Lactation	**Months Postpartum**	EER = Nonpregnant EER + Milk Energy Output – Weight Loss
	0–6	EER = Nonpregnant EER + 500 – 170
	7–12	EER = Nonpregnant EER + 400 – 0

TABLE 10B Equations used to predict EER: Physical Activity Coefficients for EER Equations					
	Males (Years)		**Females (Years)**		
	3–18	**19+**	**3–18**	**19+**	
Sedentary (PAL 1.0–1.39)	1.00	1.00	1.00	1.00	Typical ADL (activities of daily living)
Low Active (PAL 1.4–1.59)	1.13	1.11	1.16	1.12	Typical ADL + 30–60 minutes daily moderate activity (e.g., walking at 5–7 km/h)
Active (PAL 1.6–1.89)	1.26	1.25	1.31	1.27	Typical ADL + ≥ 60 minutes daily moderate activity
Very Active (PAL 1.9–2.5)	1.42	1.48	1.56	1.45	Typical ADL + ≥ 60 minutes daily moderate activity + 60 minutes vigorous activity or 120 minutes moderate activity

TABLE 10C Equations used to predict EER: Predictive Equations for Estimating REE

Harris-Benedict	Men	RMR = 66.47 + (13.75 x weight) + (5 x height) – (6.76 x age)
	Women	RMR = 655.1 + (9.56 x weight) + (1.7 x height) – (4.7 x age)
Mifflin-St Jeor	Men	RMR = (9.99 x weight) + (6.25 x height) – (4.92 x age) + 5
	Women	RMR = (9.99 x weight) + (6.25 x height) – (4.92 x age) – 161
Owen	Men	RMR = 879 + (10.2 x weight)
	Women	RMR = 795 + (7.18 x weight)
Ireton-Jones Energy Equation	Breathing	(s) = 629 – (11 x age) + (25 x weight) – (609 x O)
	Ventilator	(v) = 1925 – 10(A) + 5(W) + 281(S) + 292(T) + 851(B)
World Health Organization	Age: 18–30 years old	
	Men	RMR = 15.3 × weight + 679
		RMR = 15.4 × weight – 27 × height + 717
	Women	RMR = 14.7 × weight + 496
		RMR = 13.3 × weight + 334 × height + 35
	Age: 31–60 years old	
	Men	RMR = 11.6 × weight + 879
		RMR = 11.3 × weight + 16 × height + 901
	Women	RMR = 8.7 × weight + 829
		RMR = 8.7 × weight – 25 × height + 865
	Age: 60+ years old	
	Men	RMR = 13.5 × weight + 487
		RMR = 8.8 × weight + 1128 × height + 1071
	Women	RMR = 10.5 × weight + 596
		RMR = 9.2 × weight + 637 × height – 302

Adapted from Institute of Medicine of the National Academies (2006). *Dietary Reference Intakes: The Essential Guide to Nutrient Requirements*. Otten, J. J., Hellwig, J. P., Meyers, L. D. Page 82. https://www.nap.edu/catalog/11537/dietary-reference-intakes-the-essential-guide-to-nutrient-requirements. Accessed July 27, 2016.

Note: Weight in kilograms, height in centimeters, age in years for equations below unless otherwise indicated.
Adapted from Institute of Medicine of the National Academies (2006). *Dietary Reference Intakes: The Essential Guide to Nutrient Requirements*. Otten, J. J., Hellwig, J. P., Meyers, L. D. Page 84. https://www.nap.edu/catalog/11537/dietary-reference-intakes-the-essential-guide-to-nutrient-requirements. Accessed July 27, 2016.

Adapted from Academy of Nutrition and Dietetics. Equations. Nutrition Care Manual. https://www.nutritioncaremanual.org/topic.cfm?ncm_category_id=11&lv1=255519&ncm_toc_id=255519&ncm_heading=&. Accessed July 27, 2016.

TABLE 11 Standards of nutrient intake for macronutrients

	Recommended Dietary Allowance (RDA)	Estimated Average Requirement (EAR)	Upper Tolerable Intake Level (UL)
Carbohydrate	130 g/kg for adults	Established based on average amount of glucose used by the brain	Insufficient data to set for added sugars Recommended maximum level ≤25% total energy
Fat	No RDA for saturated, monounsaturated fatty acids, or cholesterol; these nutrients are produced by the body and do not play any role in the prevention of chronic disease	Not set; % energy derived from fat varies yet can still meet daily energy needs	Insufficient data for fat, monounsaturated fatty acids, *n*-6 and *n*-3 polyunsaturated fatty acids
Protein	0.8 g/kg body weight for men and women		Insufficient data for protein and amino acids

Data from Dietary Reference Intakes for Energy, Carbohydrate, Fiber, Fat, Fatty Acids, Cholesterol, Protein, and Amino Acids (Macronutrients), www.nap.edu.

macronutrients has been established (**TABLE 12**). AMDR is the range of intake of an energy source that correlates to a reduced risk of chronic disease and is able to provide adequate amounts of essential nutrients. It is presented as a percentage of total energy intake, giving a range; numbers below or above that percentage represent an elevated risk of chronic disease.[5]

TABLE 13 lists additional macronutrient recommendations.

TABLE 12 Acceptable macronutrient distribution ranges

	Children, 1–3 yo (%)	Children, 4–18 yo (%)	Adults (%)
Fat	30–40	25–35	20–35
n-6 polyunsaturated fatty acids* (linoleic acid)	5–10	5–10	5–10
n-3 polyunsaturated fatty acids* (α-linoleic acid)	0.6–1.2	0.6–1.2	0.6–1.2
Carbohydrate	45–65	45–65	45–65
Protein	5–20	10–30	10–35

*Approximately 10% of the total can come from longer-chain *n*-3 or *n*-6 fatty acids.

Adapted from Institute of Medicine of the National Academies (2002/2005). Dietary Reference Intakes for Energy, Carbohydrate, Fiber, Fat, Fatty Acids, Cholesterol, Protein, and Amino Acids (Macronutrients). Panel on Micronutrients, Panel on the Definition of Dietary Fiber, Subcommittee on Upper Reference Levels of Nutrients, Subcommittee on Interpretation and Uses of Dietary Reference Intakes, and the Standing Committee on the Scientific Evaluation of Dietary Reference Intakes. Page 1325. https://www.nap.edu/catalog/10490/dietary-reference-intakes-for-energy-carbohydrate-fiber-fat-fatty-acids-cholesterol-protein-and-amino-acids-macronutrients. Accessed July 27, 2016.

TABLE 13 Additional macronutrient recommendations

Macronutrient	Recommendation
Dietary cholesterol	As low as possible while consuming a nutritionally adequate diet
Trans fatty acids	As low as possible while consuming a nutritionally adequate diet
Saturated fatty acids	As low as possible while consuming a nutritionally adequate diet
Added sugars*	Limit to no more than 25% of total energy

*Not a recommended intake. A daily intake of added sugars that individuals should aim for to achieve a healthful diet was not set.

Adapted from Institute of Medicine of the National Academies (2002/2005). Dietary Reference Intakes for Energy, Carbohydrate, Fiber, Fat, Fatty Acids, Cholesterol, Protein, and Amino Acids (Macronutrients). Panel on Micronutrients, Panel on the Definition of Dietary Fiber, Subcommittee on Upper Reference Levels of Nutrients, Subcommittee on Interpretation and Uses of Dietary Reference Intakes, and the Standing Committee on the Scientific Evaluation of Dietary Reference Intakes. Page 1325. https://www.nap.edu/catalog/10490/dietary-reference-intakes-for-energy-carbohydrate-fiber-fat-fatty-acids-cholesterol-protein-and-amino-acids-macronutrients. Accessed July 27, 2016.

Tolerable Upper Intake Level for Macronutrients

The data for UL typically proves insufficient to set the levels for macronutrients. For carbohydrates, a maximal level of ≤25% total energy is suggested. This amount is deemed adequate to avoid displacement of foods that serve as major sources of essential micronutrients. As for fat, the data were not sufficient enough for total fat, monounsaturated fatty acids, and omega polyunsaturated fatty acids to use the model of risk assessment to set values for these nutrients. As for saturated fatty acids, trans fatty acids and cholesterol, the level at which risk increases is relatively low and unlikely to be achieved by usual diets that still have adequate intakes of other required nutrients. The consumption of these nutrients is recommended to be as low as possible when consuming a nutritionally adequate diet. Data was insufficient for protein to establish any UL.[6]

Recap The amount of dietary intake recommended per day for each macronutrient is primarily based on its chronic disease prevention qualities and the optimal level known to reduce risk.

▶ Nutrient Density and Nutritional Rating

Preview Nutrient-dense foods have a high nutrient value per amount of food, whereas energy-dense foods have a high calorie content per amount of food. An eating pattern that contains more nutrient-dense foods is more nutritious, promotes health, is better at reducing the risk of chronic degenerative conditions, and supports a healthy body weight.

Nutrient density is a characteristic of foods and beverages that provide vitamins, minerals, and other substances that contribute to adequate nutrient intake or otherwise have positive health effects. Nutrient-dense food items contain little or no solid fats, added sugars, refined starches, or sodium. They are ideally in forms that retain naturally occurring components such as dietary fiber.[10] The underlying concept of nutrient density is the concentration of nutrients per amount of food or caloric contribution of that food.[14] All vegetables, fruits, whole grains, seafood, eggs, beans and peas, unsalted nuts and seeds, fat-free and low-fat dairy products, and lean meats and poultry are nutrient dense—granted they are prepared with little or no added solid fats, sugars, refined starches, or sodium.[10]

Nutrient-dense items contribute to meeting food group recommendations within calorie and sodium limits. Nutrients and other beneficial substances in a nutrient-dense food have not been "diluted" by extra calories from added solid fats, sugars, or refined starches or by solid fats naturally present in the food. Foods in nutrient-dense forms contain essential vitamins and minerals as well as dietary fiber and other naturally occurring substances with positive health effects.[10] A diet consisting of nutrient-dense items includes whole grains, low-fat dairy products, fruits and vegetables. Regular intake of all these foods promotes the prevention of chronic disease.[14]

Adopting Nutrient-Dense Eating Patterns

The *Dietary Guidelines* emphasize substituting less healthy options with nutrient-dense foods and beverages. To increase dietary intake of these foods, the *Dietary Guidelines* suggests shifting common food and beverage choices from those containing solid fats, added sugars, refined starches, or sodium to foods that are more nutrient dense.[10] **FIGURE 6** includes examples of nutrient-dense foods and beverages.

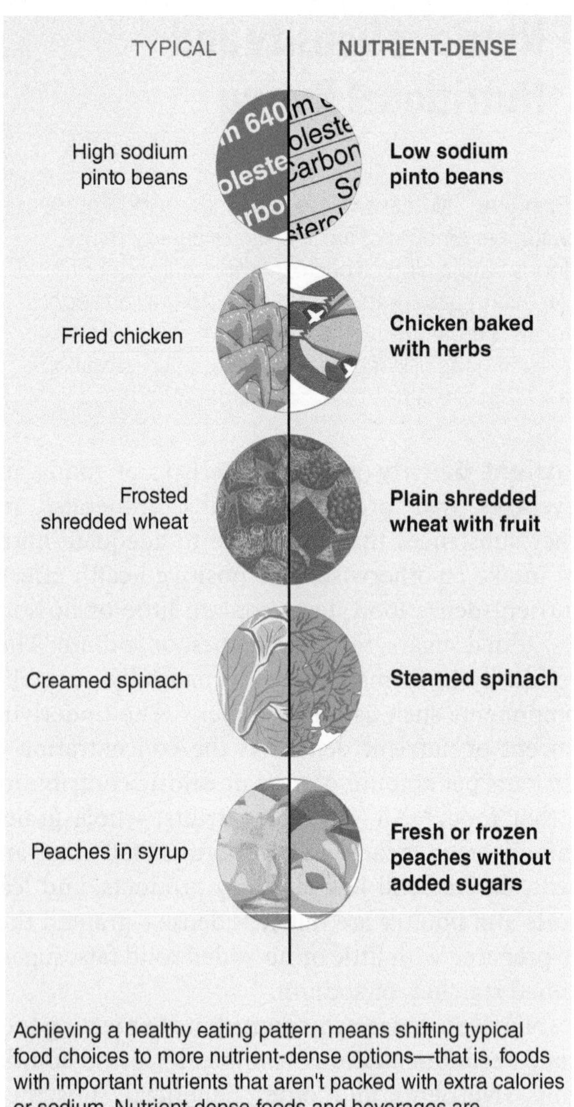

TYPICAL
NUTRIENT-DENSE
High sodium pinto beans
Low sodium pinto beans
Fried chicken
Chicken baked with herbs
Frosted shredded wheat
Plain shredded wheat with fruit
Creamed spinach
Steamed spinach
Peaches in syrup
Fresh or frozen peaches without added sugars
Achieving a healthy eating pattern means shifting typical food choices to more nutrient-dense options—that is, foods with important nutrients that aren't packed with extra calories or sodium. Nutrient-dense foods and beverages are naturally lean or low in solid fats and have little or no **added** solid fats, sugars, refined starches, or sodium.

FIGURE 6 Typical versus nutrient-dense foods and beverages

Reproduced from U.S. Department of Health and Human Services and U.S. Department of Agriculture (2015). 2015-2020 *Dietary Guidelines For Americans* 8th Edition. Figure 2-8 Typical Versus Nutrient–Dense Foods & Beverages. Page 53. https://health.gov/dietaryguidelines/2015/guidelines. Accessed July 27, 2016.

Rating Nutrient Density of Foods

Systematic ranking and classification structures have been developed to rate the nutrient density of food. Established algorithms are used to assign each food a score based on the presence or absence of specific nutrients, using specific criteria. The resulting score is converted into a practical tool for consumers to use in choosing foods with a balance of essential nutrients versus those foods considered less healthy and linked to poor health outcomes—for example, those containing added sugars, saturated fat, trans fat, and sodium. More than a dozen nutrient-density rating tools have been developed for and tested with the public to help consumers differentiate between similar, less-healthful products and make smart, nutrient-dense choices.[14] The tools created in both the United States and internationally are summarized in **TABLES 14** and **15**.

Although the tools are useful they have limitations. Nutrient-density profiling tools tend to consider both beneficial nutrients as well as those identified as having negative effects on health when consumed in excessive amounts. Certain tools are more specific to essential nutrients. In addition, several nutrient-density ranking tools highlight nutrients based on their known influences on primary health outcomes. For instance, scores in the NuVal system reflect what is known about relationships between saturated fatty acids, *n*-3 fatty acids, and cardiovascular disease, and therefore, they promote *n*-3 fatty acids as beneficial for preventing cardiovascular disease. Each nutrition-profiling system uses different methods to present similarly directed information. The Guiding Stars program, for example, assigns foods one to three stars to denote how nutrient dense they are, whereas the NuVal scale ranges from 1 to 100.

Front-of-package (FOP) labeling presents a symbol or logo on food packaging to indicate the nutritional quality of the food and communicate any health claims. It restates facts already included on the Nutrition Facts Panel such as calories, nutrients, and their percentage Daily Value (DV) per serving. Foods are ranked as high or low in certain nutrients based on predetermined criteria, and this ranking is communicated to consumers through logos, symbols, or colors. This tool is effective because consumers have been shown to respond to visuals on packaging. The US Facts Up Front campaign is one example of FOP labeling. The Grocery Manufacturers Association and Food Marketing Institute joined together to direct consumers' attention to calories per serving; saturated fat, sodium, and sugar (which have specified limits); and fiber, potassium, calcium, iron, protein, vitamin C, vitamin A, and vitamin D (which people are encouraged to consume). The aforementioned nutrients would only appear on packaging when the product contained ≥10% of the daily value per serving. Facts Up Front packaging is not mandatory and carries a fee for manufacturers who choose to use this particular labeling. The Healthy Eating System is the most widely used FOP labeling tool and was found to resonate best with consumers. This nutrient-density profiling tool provides guidance to consumers on how frequently they should consume specific foods to meet dietary guidelines.

Content removed due to copyright restrictions

Research in the United States and Canada has found that more than 50% of consumers prefer government-regulated FOP labeling. It has been established as an effective way to help consumers select healthier foods. For food manufacturers to sell their products in the European Union, they must meet three criteria when it comes to FOP labeling: (1) it must help consumers meet dietary guidelines, (2) it must be used to guide or inform public policy, and (3) it must help prevent the development of chronic diseases for diverse populations throughout the life span. The nutrient-profile model has been proposed by the Pan American Health Organization to assess the nutrient density of foods and guide consumers to identify which products contain added sugars, sodium, total fat, saturated fat, and trans fat. The purpose is to promote less consumption of these undesirable nutrients and is geared toward promoting polices and regulations, including FOP labeling and nutrition guidelines, that will help the school food environment.

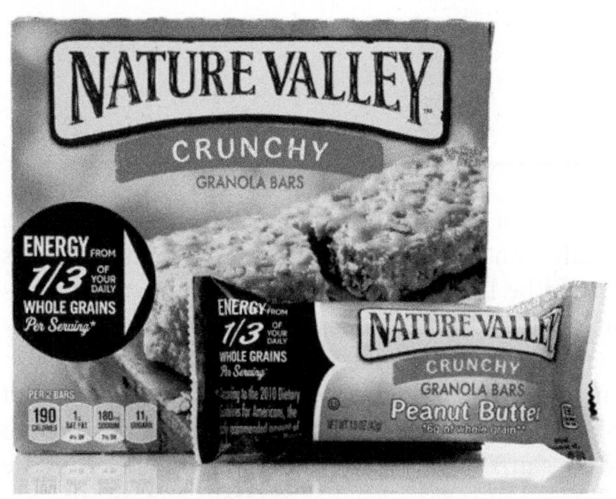

© Perry Correll/Shutterstock.

The underlying considerations of these nutrition tools is that they be grounded in science, be validated against objective measures of diet quality, and be able to effectively translate recommendations into actionable strategies. In short, they should be user-friendly and allow for easy identification of nutrient-dense foods. In terms of terminology, *nutrient rich* and *rich in nutrients* were found to resonate more with consumers than does *nutrient dense*.[14]

Energy Density

Energy density is the amount of energy per weight of food or beverage. Foods low in energy density have

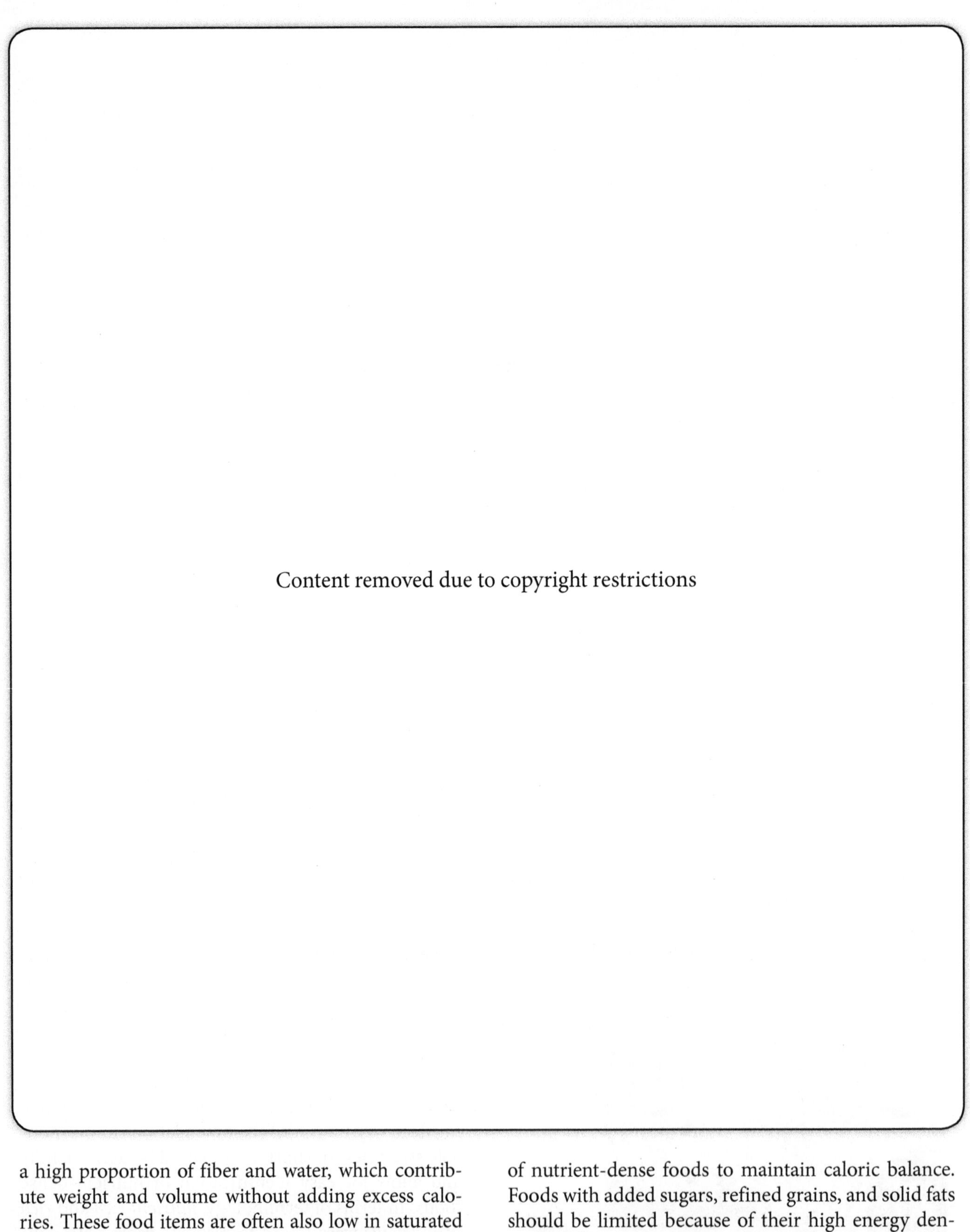

Content removed due to copyright restrictions

a high proportion of fiber and water, which contribute weight and volume without adding excess calories. These food items are often also low in saturated fat and added sugar, making them high in nutrient density. This supports the supposition that low energy-dense foods promote weight loss and weight maintenance in adults. The *Dietary Guidelines* advise staying within individual energy requirements and also suggest meeting nutrition needs from a selection of nutrient-dense foods to maintain caloric balance. Foods with added sugars, refined grains, and solid fats should be limited because of their high energy density and low nutrient density. One concern in recommending nutrient-dense foods is that some are also energy-dense foods—olive oil, avocado, nuts, and seeds, for example. Consumers are now being urged to make shifts within each food group to nutrient-dense choices and strike a balance of intake and calories.[14]

Recap The *Dietary Guidelines* aim to influence consumers to choose nutrient-dense items because they contain high quantities of nutrients per amount of calories. Nutrient-density profiling tools have been created to help the public identify optimal food options.

Diet Quality Indicators

Preview Measuring diet quality provides information about the nutritional adequacy of a population or a population group's dietary intake and identifies nutrients and groups to target for improvement.

Healthy Eating Index

The Healthy Eating Index (HEI) is a measure of diet quality that assesses adherence to the *Dietary Guidelines for Americans*.[15] Its primary use is in monitoring the diet quality of the American population and low-income subpopulations using data, specifically 24-hour dietary recalls, from the National Health and Nutrition Examination Survey (NHANES). The tool is also used to assess relationships between diet and health-related outcomes as well as the quality of food-assistance packages, menus, and the food supply.[15] The key features of the HEI are outlined in **FIGURE 7**.

HEI standards are based on the USDA food patterns, which translate key recommendations from the *Dietary Guidelines* into specific food types and amounts people should be eating per calorie level.

Content removed due to copyright restrictions

The HEI helps nutrition practitioners understand and keep tabs on public eating habits and discern which areas need improvement. Diet quality is scored on a 100-point scale. A score of 100 indicates complete fulfillment of the *Dietary Guidelines* recommendations.[16] An HEI score of >80 suggests a good diet, a score of 51–80 implies the quality of diet needs improvement, and a score <51 indicates the diet is poor.

Data from NHANES (2009–2010) determined that the HEI score the of the American population was 57, thus putting the nation's overall diet into the "needs improvement" range. Although better than the previous score of 52 from 2001–2002, diet quality did not improve significantly in the interim years. The conclusion was that Americans are "eating too little fruits, too few vegetables, not enough whole grains and not enough low-fat dairy and fish and seafood." Also noted was an "overconsumption of empty calories . . . such as refined grains." Dietitians and other healthcare professionals are tasked with supporting a score close to 80 and to help reverse the trend of diet-related diseases. The 2009–2010 HEI total and component scores for 2010 are shown in **FIGURE 8**.

The HEI was established by the USDA's Center for Nutrition Policy and Promotion (CNPP) in 1995 and is continually updated as revisions are made to the *Dietary Guidelines*.[14] The HEI has several important uses in public health and nutrition policy. Examining relationships between diet and outcomes of public health concern, evaluating the food environment, and determining the relationship between diet cost and diet quality are primary uses of HEI data. HEI findings can be used to assessing the quality of food-assistance packages, menus, and the American food supply, and evaluating intervention trials, and assessing dietary patterns.[16] The USDA's consumer website contains interactive tools to help individuals use the *Dietary Guidelines* to improve the quality of their diets.[16]

Food Pattern Modeling Analysis

The purpose of food pattern modeling analysis is to determine whether the USDA food patterns continue to meet nutritional goals for adequacy and moderation while staying within the established calorie targets. This type of analysis uses the food patterns presented in the 2010 *Dietary Guidelines*, with updated food group nutrient profiles based on the most recent food consumption and nutrient-composition data. As part of the assessment, all foods reported in the What We Eat in America/National Health and National Health and

HEI-2010 Dietary Component (maximum score)	Children 2–17 years (n = 2,990)	Adults 18–64 years (n = 4,673)	Older Adults ≥ 65 years (n = 1,379)
		Mean score (standard error)	
Total fruit (5)	3.82 (0.19)	2.93 (0.08)	4.40 (0.13)
Whole fruit (5)	4.77 (0.22)	3.92 (0.12)	5.00 (0.00)
Total vegetables (5)	2.10 (0.05)	3.49 (0.07)	4.21 (0.11)
Greens and beans (5)	0.56 (0.07)	2.92 (0.12)	3.37 (0.31)
Whole grains (10)	2.22 (0.08)	2.47 (0.13)	3.52 (0.16)
Dairy (10)	9.23 (0.19)	6.23 (0.12)	6.19 (0.20)
Total protein foods (5)	4.59 (0.14)	5.00 (0.00)	5.00 (0.00)
Seafood and plant proteins (5)	2.90 (0.23)	4.03 (0.23)	4.98 (0.06)
Fatty acids (10)	3.08 (0.10)	4.39 (0.14)	4.69 (0.15)
Refined grains (10)	4.54 (0.21)	6.35 (0.16)	7.29 (0.20)
Sodium (10)	4.50 (0.17)	3.57 (0.13)	3.30 (0.26)
Empty calories (20)	11.17 (0.23)	12.04 (0.26)	13.94 (0.33)
Total HEI score (100)	**53.47 (0.77)**	**57.34 (0.86)**	**65.90 (0.56)**

[1]Calculated using the population ratio method.

FIGURE 8 HEI-2010 total and component scores for children, adults, and older adults during 2009–2010

Reproduced from United States Department of Agriculture. Healthy Eating Index. USDA Center for Nutrition Policy and Promotion. https://www.cnpp.usda.gov/healthyeatingindex. Accessed September 28, 2016.

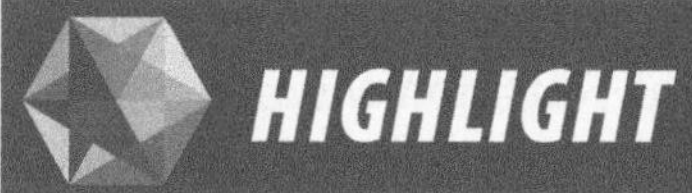

Applications of the Healthy Eating Index (HEI)

The Healthy Eating Index has been used for more than simply assessing diet quality. Applications of the HEI in literature encompass epidemiology, population monitoring, nutrition intervention, the relationship between diet quality and biomarkers, and diet quality of a specific set of foods in the food environment.

Diet and Chronic Disease

The HEI is effective in assessing diet quality and health outcomes in populations with existing diagnoses: for example, diet quality and risk for cardiovascular disease deaths and diet quality among cancer survivors. The impact of dietary intervention is also assessed for diet quality and glycemic index improvement in individuals with type 2 diabetes.

Population Estimates of Diet Quality

In addition to monitoring the diet quality of the entire American population, the HEI is also effective for analyzing subgroups, including children and adolescents, older adults, and specific races and ethnicities.

The National Healthy and Nutrition Examination Survey (NHANES) incorporates a section titled "What We Eat," a data set useful for assessing diet quality in the American population. NHANES data are frequently referenced to provide insight about diet quality—specifically its association with health outcomes, health behaviors, and biomarkers of disease risk.

Children

Research studies incorporating the HEI assess the diet quality of children and adolescents in regard to its association with television viewing time, dental caries, and food away from home. The diet quality of children enrolled in federal nutrition programs is also explored.

Federal Nutrition Programs

The HEI serves as a measuring tool to ascertain the diet quality of the foods made available by federal nutrition programs (guided by the *Dietary Guidelines for Americans*) and the diet quality of the groups assisted by the program. The Supplemental Nutrition Assistance Program, the National School Lunch Program, and the Supplemental Nutrition Program for Women, Infants, and Children were investigated. These programs generally are targeted toward food-insecure and vulnerable population groups, providing valuable data regarding disparities in diet quality among income groups, education levels, and additional sociodemographic indicators.

Food Environment

The HEI scores of restaurant menus, grocery store flyers, and the entire American supply are compared against the *Dietary Guidelines for Americans* to determine how well the food supply aligns with the recommendations. The analysis is effective in identifying which aspects of food availability require improvement.

Global Applications

The HEI lends support to other countries because its framework serves as a model on which they can base their own diet quality indexes; adjustments are made for their own specific populations. This is possible because the 12 components of the HEI represent basic food groups that are culturally neutral.

Further information on the HEI is available on the websites of the Center for Nutrition Policy and Promotion (cnpp.usda.gov) and the National Cancer Institute (www.epi.grants.cancer.gov/hei/). The sites include updated scores for population levels, research tools, and fact sheets.

Modified from Healthy Eating Index – beyond the score. *J Acad Nutr Diet*. 2017; 117(4):519-521.

Nutrition Examination Survey (WWEIA NHANES) 2009–2010 were assigned to appropriate item clusters. Then the nutrient profiles were calculated for each food group or subgroup using the nutrient data for representative foods and the proportional consumption of each item cluster from the group composite. The existing recommended intake amounts for each food group and energy levels for the patterns were compared to the usual intake distributions. The calories and nutrients provided by each pattern were calculated from the nutrient profile and recommended intake amounts. Then nutrients in each pattern were compared with nutrient recommendations, and then nutritional goals that were or were not met for age and gender groups were identified at each calorie level.[17]

Alternative Healthy Eating Index

The Alternative Healthy Eating Index (AHEI) incorporates some aspects of the original HEI as well as some components corresponding to the existing *Dietary Guidelines*. The AHEI's six components are (1) vegetables, (2) fruit, (3) nuts and soy, (4) cereal fiber, (5) polyunsaturated fatty acids and saturated fatty acids, and (6) white and red meat. Alcohol and trans fats are also assessed.[18] Other diet quality indicators that have been used include the Diet Quality Index, Programme National Nutrition Santé Guideline Score, DASH food group score, Mediterranean Diet Score, relative Med Diet Score, and Mediterranean-Style Pattern Score.

Recap The Healthy Eating Index and other indicators of diet quality serve to inform policy makers of the healthfulness of our population's diet and identify which aspects need improvement.

Dietary Guidelines for Americans 2015

Preview The *Dietary Guidelines for Americans* are reissued by the HHS and USDA every five years to reflect the most current nutrition science research and update the recommendations established to guide the population toward optimal health.

Purpose

The *Dietary Guidelines* are the evidence-based foundation for nutrition guidance created for the public by the federal government. The purpose is to direct professionals in their work with all individuals age 2 years and older and their families to support the consumption of healthy, nutritionally adequate diets. The *Dietary Guidelines* are published every five years as mandated by the National Nutrition Monitoring and Related Research Act (1990). Under the legislature, the Department of Health and Human Services and the Department of Agriculture must jointly publish a report consisting of nutrition and dietary guidelines and information for the general public. They strive to make recommendations regarding components of a healthy and nutritionally adequate diet that will both promote health and prevent chronic disease for current and future generations.[10]

The recommendations provided in the *Dietary Guidelines* aim to promote health, prevent chronic disease, and help people reach and maintain a healthy body weight. The *Dietary Guidelines* significantly affect nutrition in the United States because they form the basis of federal nutrition and policy programs; help local, state, and national health promotion and disease prevention initiatives; and inform numerous organizations and industries (i.e., products developed and marketed by the food and beverage industry). Public health agencies, healthcare providers, and educational institutions all base their fundamentals on the strategies, recommendations, and messages dictated in the *Dietary Guidelines*.[19]

Process

The main objective of the *Dietary Guidelines* is to help individuals maintain their overall health and reduce the prevalence of disease. The process for developing the *Dietary Guidelines* is summarized in **FIGURE 9** and includes a review of the science, development and implementation of the *Dietary Guidelines*.[20] The HHS and USDA assemble a *Dietary Guidelines* advisory

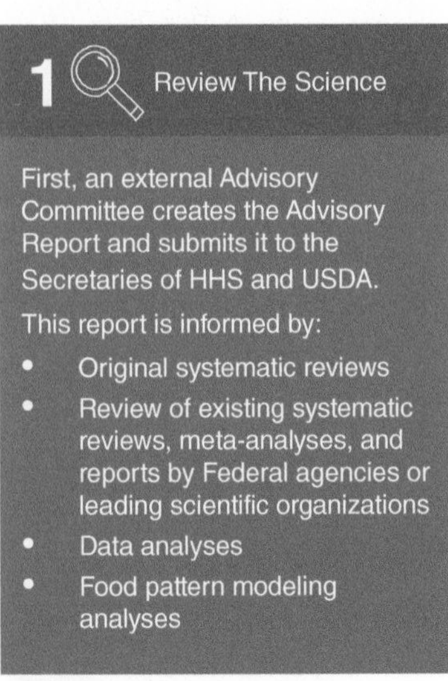

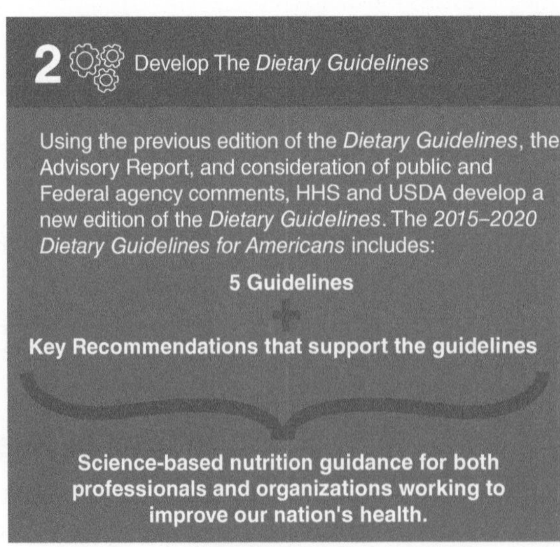

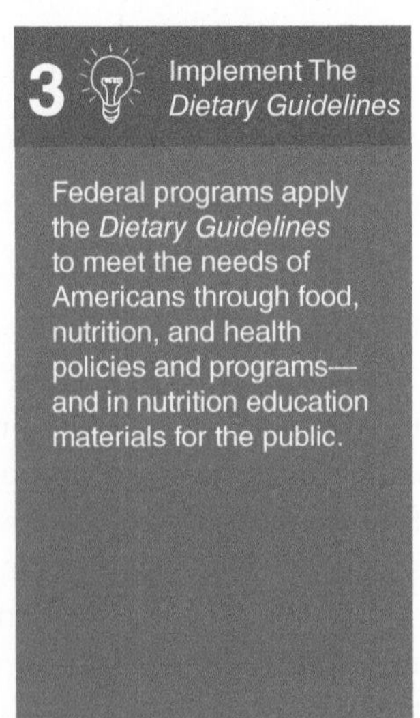

FIGURE 9 Process for reviewing, developing, and implementing the *Dietary Guidelines*

Reproduced from U.S. Department of Health and Human Services and U.S. Department of Agriculture (2015). 2015-2020 *Dietary Guidelines For Americans* 8th Edition. Figure I-3 Science, Policy, Implementation: Developing the 2015-2020 Dietary Guidelines for Americans. Page 6. https://health.gov/dietaryguidelines/2015/guidelines. Accessed July 27, 2016.

VIEWPOINT

Product Development Process

Lauren Grosskopf, MS

Ever wondered how much work goes into putting a new food product on the grocery shelf? To give you an overview, let's discuss the four-step process of product development used by a major food manufacturer.

1. Come up with an *idea* for a product.
   - During this phase, a few characteristics will be identified and defined: What is the product? What does the product look like? Does another manufacturer currently produce something like it? This is the blue-sky phase when the product has no limits.
2. Next comes *scoping*, which is background investigation.
   - After the idea is defined, it is time to shop grocery stores, natural food stores, convenience stores, and so on. Exploring a variety of stores allows developers to understand the competitive landscape. Using information from competitors will also allow developers to get an idea of the flavors, textures, and other thought starters to help execute the idea. Team tastings are typically used during this phase to get feedback from cross-functional teams and understand general preferences. Many questions will be asked during this phase to gain the appropriate knowledge to move the idea forward. At the end of this phase, a gold standard should be identified— the ideal product , flavor, or texture that the developer should be targeting.
3. The most involved part of the process is the product *development*.
   - This part of the process typically starts with benchtop development and then moves to small-scale development in a pilot plant setting before final large-scale development in a full plant trial. All raw materials, packaging, and manufacturing plants must be quality audited and approved. In between each phase of a trial, different levels of consumer research may be completed, ranging from concept testing to heat maps, central location tests, in-home use testing, and so on. Each phase gets the developer closer to the ideal product by learning more about what aspects of the product or packaging pleases consumers. After the product, package, and process have been finalized, several pieces need to fall in place. A shelf-life study should be implemented to understand the expected life span of the product under actual product storage conditions. In addition, regulatory, microbiological, quality, and legal groups will review the product as a whole. They will ensure that the product meets all quality and food safety standards and that Nutrition Fact Panels, ingredient line statements, and claims are all appropriately generated and substantiated with credible documentation.
4. Now it's time to get the product into the hands of consumers. This stage is called *execution*.
   - The product-development process is different for everyone. It can take anywhere from six months to several years to get a product on the shelf. Product approval requires alignment from many different business team partners, including research and development, marketing, operations, sales, and quality control. Once the business team is aligned with the product, then the team can move forward with first production. In this final step, products are manufactured to defined manufacturing and packaging specifications and established quality standards. The finished product is then shipped to distribution centers, where customers can begin to place orders to stock their store shelves. Ongoing quality reviews, confirmatory shelf-life studies, and consumer comment trackers are established and monitored for an extended period of time after initial production to ensure that the product continues to meet consumer expectations.

committee of nationally recognized nutrition and medical researchers, academics, and practitioners to review the current nutrition science. The committee holds a series of public meetings, one of them with the purpose of receiving oral comments from the public. Members of the public are also permitted to submit written comments to the advisory committee during the review process. The committee generates an advisory report comprising current scientific and medical evidence in nutrition. Within the report, science-based recommendations to the federal government are outlined for development of the new edition of the *Dietary Guidelines*.

First, an external advisory committee creates an advisory report that is submitted to the secretaries of the HHS and the USDA. Data and food pattern modeling are analyzed. The new edition is created by the HHS and the USDA with consideration of the previous *Dietary Guidelines* edition as well as input from the public and federal agencies. The guidelines are implemented by federal programs to meet the needs of Americans through food, health policies and programs, and nutrition education materials. A peer-review process is also completed, with nonfederal experts conducting a confidential review of the draft policy document. After the advisory report is completed, the public is again given the opportunity to respond orally or with written comments via the website. The information from the advisory report along with comments from the public and federal agents are used by the HHS and the USDA for the formation of the new edition of the *Dietary Guidelines*.[20]

Evolution

The *Dietary Guidelines* was first released in 1980. In 1990, Congress passed the National Nutrition Monitoring and Related Research Act, which required that the HHS and the USDA review, update, and jointly publish the *Dietary Guidelines* every five years. The guidelines have evolved to address shifting public health concerns and nutritional needs of specific populations. This is demonstrated in the fact that the *Dietary Guidelines* have typically focused on Americans ages 2 years and older, although newer science shows that dietary intake from birth—and even the mother's diet during gestation—may have lasting effects on a child's health and, therefore, should be included in the recommendations. In response, the federal government has pioneered a project to begin evaluating the scientific evidence available, with the potential to support dietary guidance in the future for infants and toddlers, from birth to 24 months of age, as well as women who are pregnant. The *Dietary Guidelines* are projected to include these special populations by 2020. Information on the Pregnancy and Birth to 24 Months Project is available at www.cnpp.usda.gov/birthto24months.[21]

The *Dietary Guidelines for Americans 2015*

In contrast to previous editions, which centered around individual dietary components including food groups and nutrients, the *Dietary Guidelines 2015* focuses on eating patterns and their food and nutrient characteristics. The DAG encourage a shift in eating behavior to patterns that promote the intake of foods that provide adequate nutrients to meet requirements and promote improved health overall. In summary, the key recommendations are to "consume a healthy eating pattern that accounts for all foods and beverages within the appropriate calorie level."[13] *The Dietary Guidelines for Americans 2015–2020* are summarized in **FIGURE 10.**

The Guidelines

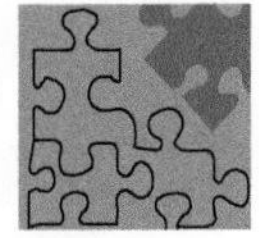

1. **Follow a healthy eating pattern across the lifespan.** All food and beverage choices matter. Choose a healthy eating pattern at an appropriate calorie level to help achieve and maintain a healthy body weight, support nutrient adequacy, and reduce the risk of chronic disease.
2. **Focus on variety, nutrient density, and amount.** To meet nutrient needs within calorie limits, choose a variety of nutrient-dense foods across and within all food groups in recommended amounts.
3. **Limit calories from added sugars and saturated fats and reduce sodium intake.** Consume an eating pattern low in added sugars, saturated fats, and sodium. Cut back on foods and beverages higher in these components to amounts that fit within healthy eating patterns.
4. **Shift to healthier food and beverage choices.** Choose nutrient-dense foods and beverages across and within all food groups in place of less healthy choices. Consider cultural and personal preferences to make these shifts easier to accomplish and maintain.
5. **Support healthy eating patterns for all.** Everyone has a role in helping to create and support healthy eating patterns in multiple settings nationwide, from home to school to work to communities.

FIGURE 10 The five guidelines of the 2015–2020 *Dietary Guidelines for Americans*

Reproduced from the 2015-2020 *Dietary Guidelines for Americans*. Dietary Guidelines available at: https://health.gov/dietaryguidelines/2015/guidelines/executive-summary/#the-guidelines

The *Dietary Guidelines 2015* emphasizes choosing nutrient-dense foods and beverages in favor of less healthy options. The main objective of the *Dietary Guidelines* is to help individuals maintain overall health and reduce the prevalence of disease. Described in the *Dietary Guidelines* are the healthy eating patterns that have been found to support overall health (including body weight and chronic disease risk) throughout the life span, in accordance with Key Recommendations, including:

- An eating pattern that represents the totality of all foods and beverages consumed
- Meeting nutritional needs primarily from foods
- Having adaptable healthy eating patterns

The healthy eating patterns are the result of a combination of three evaluative measures: systematic reviews

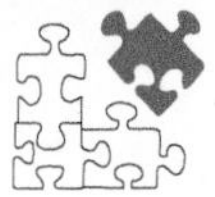

Consume a healthy eating pattern that accounts for all foods and beverages within an appropriate calorie level.

A healthy eating pattern includes:[1]

- A variety of vegetables from all of the subgroups—dark green, red and orange, legumes (beans and peas), starchy, and other
- Fruits, especially whole fruits
- Grains, at least half of which are whole grains
- Fat-free or low-fat dairy, including milk, yogurt, cheese, and/or fortified soy beverages
- A variety of protein foods, including seafood, lean meats and poultry, eggs, legumes (beans and peas), and nuts, seeds, and soy products
- Oils

A healthy eating pattern limits:

- Saturated fats and *trans* fats, added sugars, and sodium

Key Recommendations that are quantitative are provided for several components of the diet that should be limited. These components are of particular public health concern in the United States, and the specified limits can help individuals achieve healthy eating patterns within calorie limits:

- Consume less than 10 percent of calories per day from added sugars[2]
- Consume less than 10 percent of calories per day from saturated fats[3]
- Consume less than 2,300 milligrams (mg) per day of sodium[4]
- If alcohol is consumed, it should be consumed in moderation—up to one drink per day for women and up to two drinks per day for men—and only by adults of legal drinking age.[5]

In tandem with the recommendations above, Americans of all ages—children, adolescents, adults, and older adults—should meet the Physical Activity Guidelines for Americans to help promote health and reduce the risk of chronic disease. Americans should aim to achieve and maintain a healthy body weight. The relationship between diet and physical activity contributes to calorie balance and managing body weight. As such, the Dietary Guidelines includes a Key Recommendation to:

- Meet the *Physical Activity Guidelines for Americans*.[6]

[1] Definitions for each food group and subgroup are provided throughout the chapter and are compiled in Appendix 3. USDA Food Patterns: Healthy U.S.-Style Eating Pattern.

[2] The recommendation to limit intake of calories from added sugars to less than 10 percent per day is a target based on food pattern modeling and national data on intakes of calories from added sugars that demonstrate the public health need to limit calories from added sugars to meet food group and nutrient needs within calorie limits. The limit on calories from added sugars is not a Tolerable Upper Intake Level (UL) set by the Institute of Medicine (IOM). For most calorie levels, there are not enough calories available after meeting food group needs to consume 10 percent of calories from added sugars and 10 percent of calories from saturated fats and still stay within calorie limits.

[3] The recommendation to limit intake of calories from saturated fats to less than 10 percent per day is a target based on evidence that replacing saturated fats with unsaturated fats is associated with reduced risk of cardiovascular disease. The limit on calories from saturated fats is not a UL set by the IOM. For most calorie levels, there are not enough calories available after meeting food group needs to consume 10 percent of calories from added sugars and 10 percent of calories from saturated fats and still stay within calorie limits.

[4] The recommendation to limit intake of sodium to less than 2,300 mg per day is the UL for individuals ages 14 years and older set by the IOM. The recommendations for children younger than 14 years of age are the IOM age- and sex-appropriate ULs (see Appendix 7. Nutritional Goals for Age-Sex Groups Based on Dietary Reference Intakes and Dietary Guidelines Recommendations).

[5] It is not recommended that individuals begin drinking or drink more for any reason. The amount of alcohol and calories in beverages varies and should be accounted for within the limits of healthy eating patterns. Alcohol should be consumed only by adults of legal drinking age. There are many circumstances in which individuals should not drink, such as during pregnancy. See Appendix 9. Alcohol for additional information.

[6] U.S. Department of Health and Human Services. 2008 Physical Activity Guidelines for Americans. Washington (DC): U.S. Department of Health and Human Services; 2008. ODPHP Publication No. U0036. Available at: http://www.health.gov/paguidelines. Accessed August 6, 2015.

FIGURE 11 Key Recommendations provide further guidance on how individuals can follow the five Guidelines. The Dietary Guidelines' Key Recommendations for healthy eating patterns should be applied in their entirety, given the interconnected relationship that each dietary component can have with others.

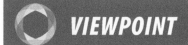

VIEWPOINT

Food Service Perspectives

Linda S. Eck Mills, MBA, RDN, LDN, FADA

At the center of the seal for the Academy of Nutrition and Dietetics (Figure 13) are three symbols that represent the profession's principal characteristics: a balance scale to represent science as the foundation and equality, a caduceus to represent the close relationship between dietetics and medicine, and a cooking vessel to represent cookery and food preparation.[1]

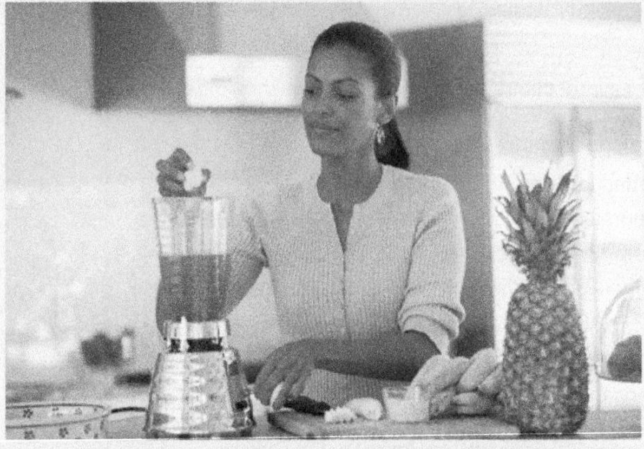

© Ariel Skelley/Getty Images.

During my career as a registered dietitian nutritionist, I have seen firsthand many changes to the "cooking vessel" and those who work in the food-service portion of the healthcare profession. My top-five list of changes in healthcare food service are the following:

1. *Dress of Dietitians.* We have gone from wearing white uniforms, white shoes, beige stockings, and a white nurses'-style cap in 1932 to wearing profession business attire and even position-appropriate clothing if working as a certified personal trainer. In 1932, dietitians wore dresses. Today, many dietitians wear pants.

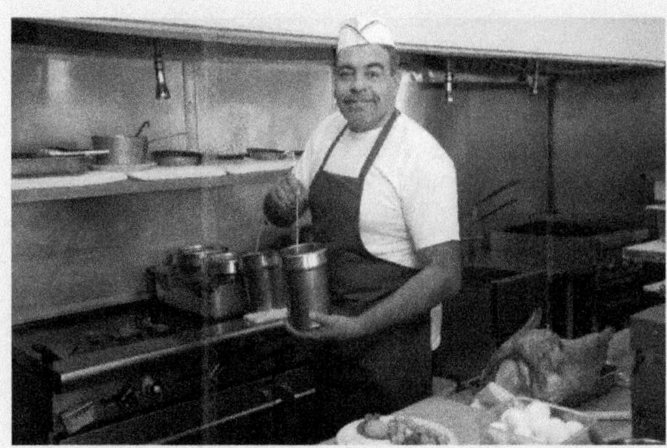

© Hill Street Studios/Blend Images/Thinkstock/Getty Images.

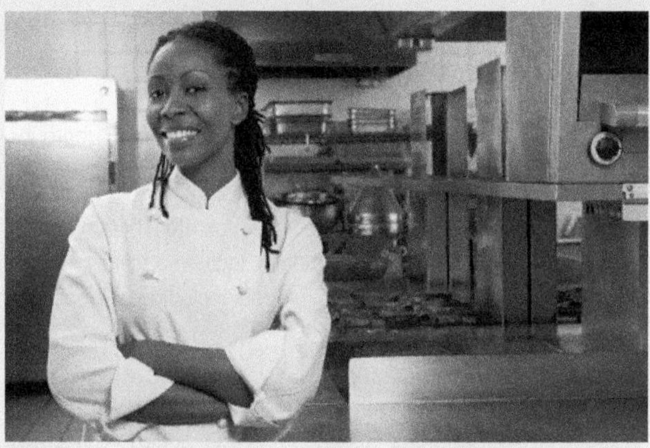

© sirtravelalot/Shutterstock.

2. *Tube Feedings.* In 1975, the *Simplified Diet Manual with Meal Patterns*, 4th ed., by the Nutrition Section of the Iowa State Department of Health in cooperation with the Iowa Dietetic Association, provided a nutritionally adequate formula for tube feeding.[2] Today, commercial products are able to meet the needs of a variety of medical complications requiring oral or tube feeding.

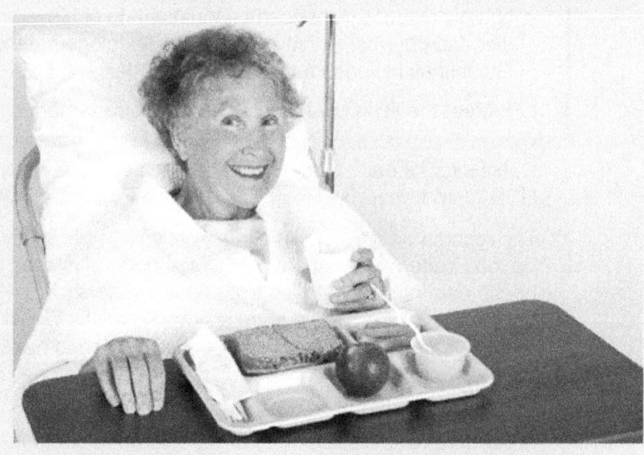

© Lisa F. Young/Shutterstock.

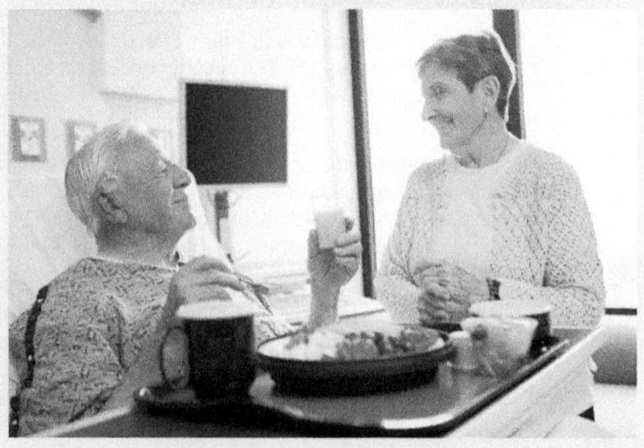

© Monkey Business Images/Shutterstock.

3. *Methods of Cooking and Production Equipment.* Naturally, cooking methods have changed over time. Cook-chill systems have been used in large facilities where foods are prepared as many as five days in advance and then rapidly chilled and held in refrigeration until they can be plated and rethermalized before serving.[3,4,5] Some facilities are now using short-order cooking with their room-service systems.

   For decades, the standard kitchen equipment was a stove top, an oven, and a steamer. Now when you walk into a kitchen, you might see convection and conduction ovens and multifunction pieces of equipment. The trade show of the North American Food Equipment Manufacturers (NAFEM) show held in odd-numbered years is one of the best places to see the latest in food-service equipment.[6,7]

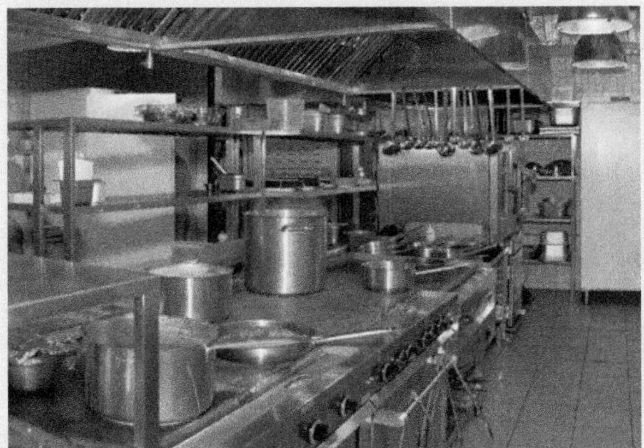

© Kondor83/Shutterstock.

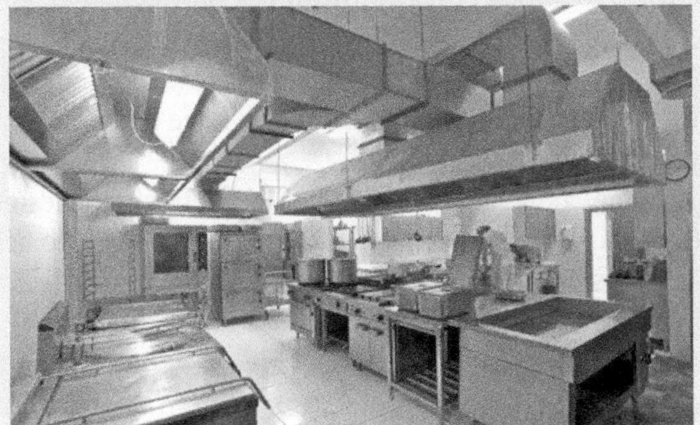

© Dalibor Sevaljevic/Shutterstock.

4. *Menus and Types of Meal Service.* As the length of stay and customer demands have changed over the years, menus have evolved from the nonselective menu, to a main meal with an alternate entrée, to restaurant-style items ordered from a menu.[8] Cultural change has transformed the institutional model for patient care in many ways, including meal service.[9] Restaurant-style menus are now common in health care.

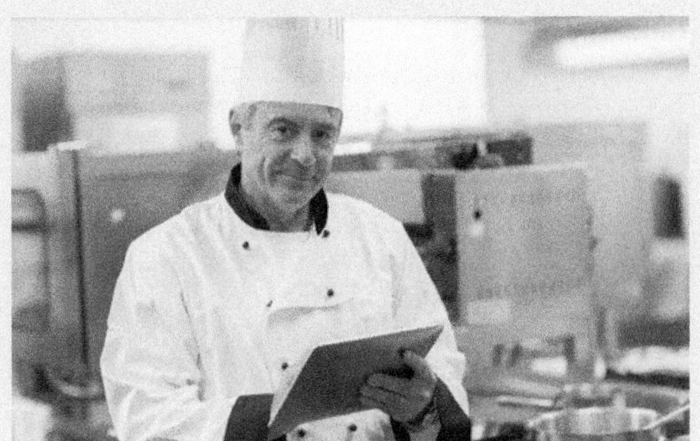

© ESB Professional/Shutterstock.

5. *Food-Service Management and Budgets.* Today's food-service management is increasingly being done by certified dietary managers instead of dietitians as we give up yet another piece of our scope of practice.[10]

   Change is inevitable in all aspects of our professional lives, and healthcare food service is no exception. Consumer demands and trends in this industry will continue to evolve, and as food and nutrition professionals we will need to keep up with these changes.[11]

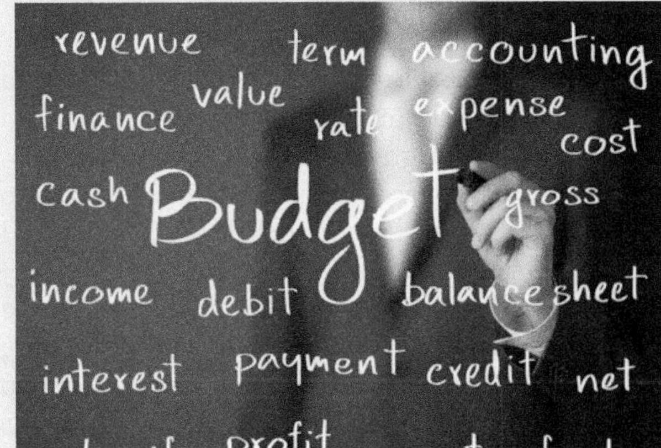

© Dusit/Shutterstock.

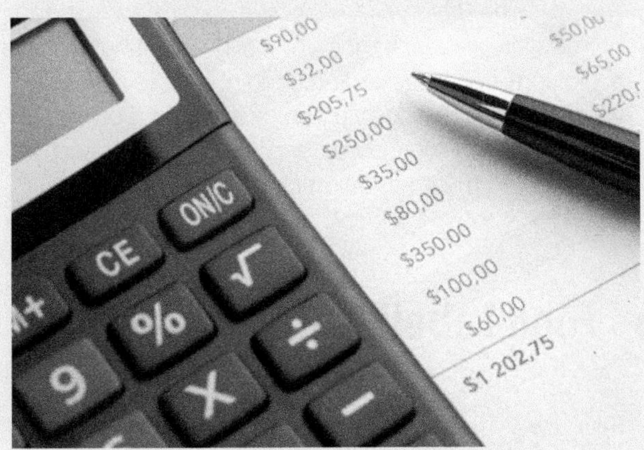

© Peter Kotoff/Shutterstock.

References

1. Academy of Nutrition and Dietetics. http://www.eatrightpro.org/. Accessed March 13, 2017.
2. Nutrition Section of the Iowa State Department of Health in cooperation with the Iowa Dietetic Association. *Simplified Diet Manual with Meal Patterns*. 4th ed. Ames, IA: Iowa State University Press; 1975.
3. Williams Refrigeration. Guide to Cook Chill. http://www.williams-refrigeration.com.hk/guides/the-cook-chill-process-explained. Accessed March 13, 2017.
4. Williams Refrigeration. Guide to Cook Chill. https://www.chefservicesgroup.com/services/cook-chill.html. Accessed March 13, 2017.
5. Nummer B. Cook-chill reduced-oxygen packaging in retail and foodservice operations. http://www.foodsafetymagazine.com/magazine-archive1/junejuly-2010/cook-chill-reduced-oxygen-packaging-in-retail-and-foodservice-operations/. Accessed March 13, 2017.
6. North American Food Equipment Manufacturers (NAFEM). https://www.nafem.org/. Accessed March 13, 2017.
7. NAFEM Show. https://www.thenafemshow.org/. Accessed March 13, 2017.
8. Hospitality School. Types of menus. http://www.hospitality-school.com/types-menus-restaurant. Accessed March 13, 2017.
9. Pioneer Network. Changing the culture of aging in the 21st century. https://www.pioneernetwork.net/. Accessed March 13, 2017.
10. Association of Nutrition and Foodservice Professionals. http://www.anfponline.org/
11. Keller M. That's progress—Advancements in hospital foodservice. *Today's Diet*. 2009; 11:28. http://www.todaysdietitian.com/newarchives/072709p28.shtm. Accessed March 13, 2017.

Publications

FoodService Director. http://www.foodservicedirector.com/.

Food-Service Equipment and Supplies. http://www.fesmag.com/.

Food Management. http://www.food-management.com/news-trends/business-industry.

of scientific research, food pattern modeling, and analysis of the food intake of the current American population. The integration of these three factors provides the evidence-based foundation for regulations to reduce the risk of diet-associated chronic disease and support nutrient adequacy.[10]

The *Dietary Guidelines* recommended food guides provide further information regarding healthy eating pattern as well as other tools to help the population meet its nutritional requirements through proper food choices.

Recap The *Dietary Guidelines* serve as a road map to help Americans reach their optimal health status and avoid common diseases and conditions associated with an unhealthy lifestyle. The development process is designed to ensure the information is current and relevant and the goals realistic and achievable.

Food Labeling and Nutrition

Preview The Nutrition Facts Label has been revised to more appropriately reflect consumer preferences as well as current nutrition sciences in relation to fats, sugar, fiber, and certain vitamins and minerals.

The New Food Label

The US Food and Drug Administration released the new Nutrition Facts Label in 2016, making it easier for consumers to make informed food choices. The changes were made to represent the most current scientific data, specifically the links between diet and chronic diseases such as obesity and heart disease. Manufacturers will need to use the new food label by July 26, 2018; small businesses will have an additional year to comply.

The new food label has a refreshed design (**FIGURE 12**).[22] The size of print showing calories, servings per container, and serving size has been increased. Bold type is used for calories and serving sizes. Manufacturers must provide the actual amounts and percentage daily values of vitamin D, calcium, iron, and potassium. They are given the option to declare the gram amount of other vitamins and minerals on a voluntary basis, and the footnote has been changed to clarify what percent daily value means. A footnote now states: "The % daily value tells you how much a nutrient in a serving of food contributes to a daily diet. 2,000 calories a day is used for general nutrition advice."[23] The changes to the Nutrition Facts Label are highlighted in **FIGURE 13**.

In addition, the new food label reflects updated information about nutrition science. Added sugars are included on the label in grams and percent daily

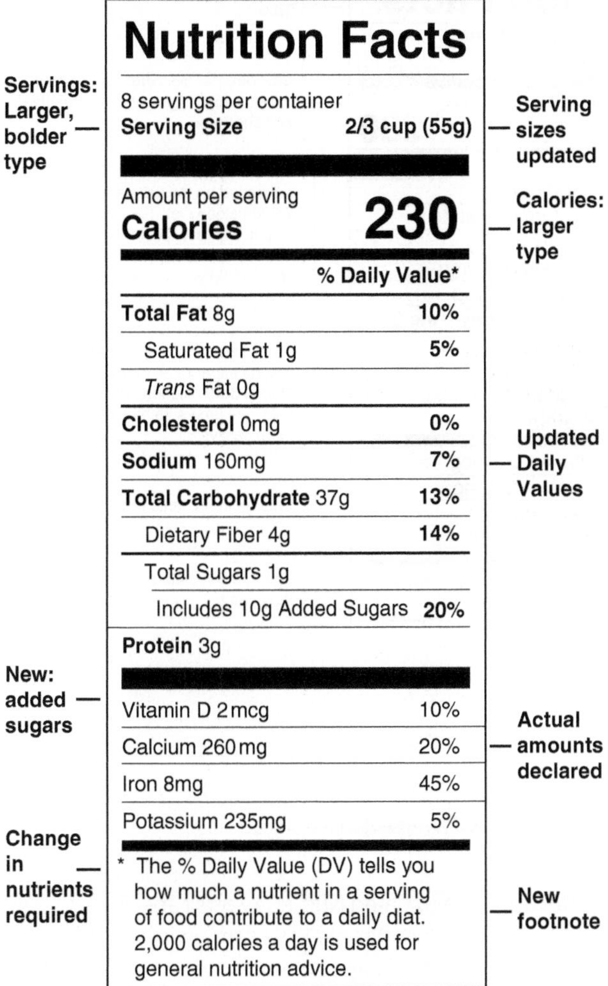

FIGURE 12 Changes to the Nutrition Facts Label

Reproduced from U. S. Food & Drug Administration. Changes to the Nutrition Facts Label. fda.gov. https://www.fda.gov/Food/GuidanceRegulation/GuidanceDocumentsRegulatoryInformation/LabelingNutrition/ucm385663.htm. Last updated 2/10/2017. Accessed September 6, 2016.

value. It is in accordance with the *Dietary Guidelines for Americans 2015–2020*, which notes the difficulty of meeting nutrient needs and staying within calorie limits if >10% of total daily calories are from added sugar. Additionally, the list of nutrients required to appear on the label has changed. Calcium and iron remain required, and vitamin D and potassium now mandated as well. Vitamins A and C are longer be required, and are now optional. Calories from fat will be removed because research has shown that the type of fat is more important than the amount. Therefore, total fat, saturated fat, and trans fat will remain on the label. Daily values for sodium, dietary fiber, and vitamin D are being updated based on newer scientific evidence from the National Academy of Medicine, the *Dietary Guidelines* advisory committee report, and other sources. Daily values are reference amounts of nutrients to consume or avoid overconsuming and are used to calculate the percent daily value—listed as "%DV"—that manufacturers put on labels. This reference value aids in consumer understanding of the nutrition information provided in the context of total daily diet.

Updated serving sizes and labeling requirements for certain package sizes are also required on the new label. Serving sizes are specified by law to be based on amounts of foods and beverages that people actually eat, not what they are recommended to be eating. The amounts people consume has changed, with a marked increase, since the previous serving size standards were established in 1993. Serving size references have changed from ½ cup to 1 cup of ice cream and 8 ounces to 12 ounces of soda, for example. For packages between one and two servings (e.g., a 20-ounce can of soda, a 15-ounce can of soup), the calories and other nutrients on the label will be indicated as one serving, because people typically consume the entire item in one sitting. It has been noted that package size affects how much people eat. Products that are more than one serving but could be consumed in one or multiple sittings will have a dual column label to address the amount of calories and nutrients per serving and per package or unit.

Compliance and Dates

As previously noted, manufacturers are required to transition to the new label by July 26, 2018. Those companies with less than $10 million in annual food sales are given an additional year to comply. Manufacturers also must ensure that by June 18, 2018, their products will contain no partially hydrogenated oils for uses other than those authorized by the Food and Drug Administration (FDA). Vending machine operators with glass-front vending machines must comply with all requirements of the vending machine labeling rule by July 26, 2018. The calorie declaration requirement has been delayed for certain food products sold in glass-front vending machines partly to maintain consistency with the compliance date for the new Nutrition Facts Label requirements. This allows manufacturers to make changes to FOP labeling for products they supply to vending operators at the same time they make changes to the Nutrition Facts Label. Food establishments covered by the menu-labeling rule must comply with menu labeling requirements by May 7, 2018. Targets for sodium reduction being developed by the FDA are voluntary and therefore do not have a compliance date. However, companies

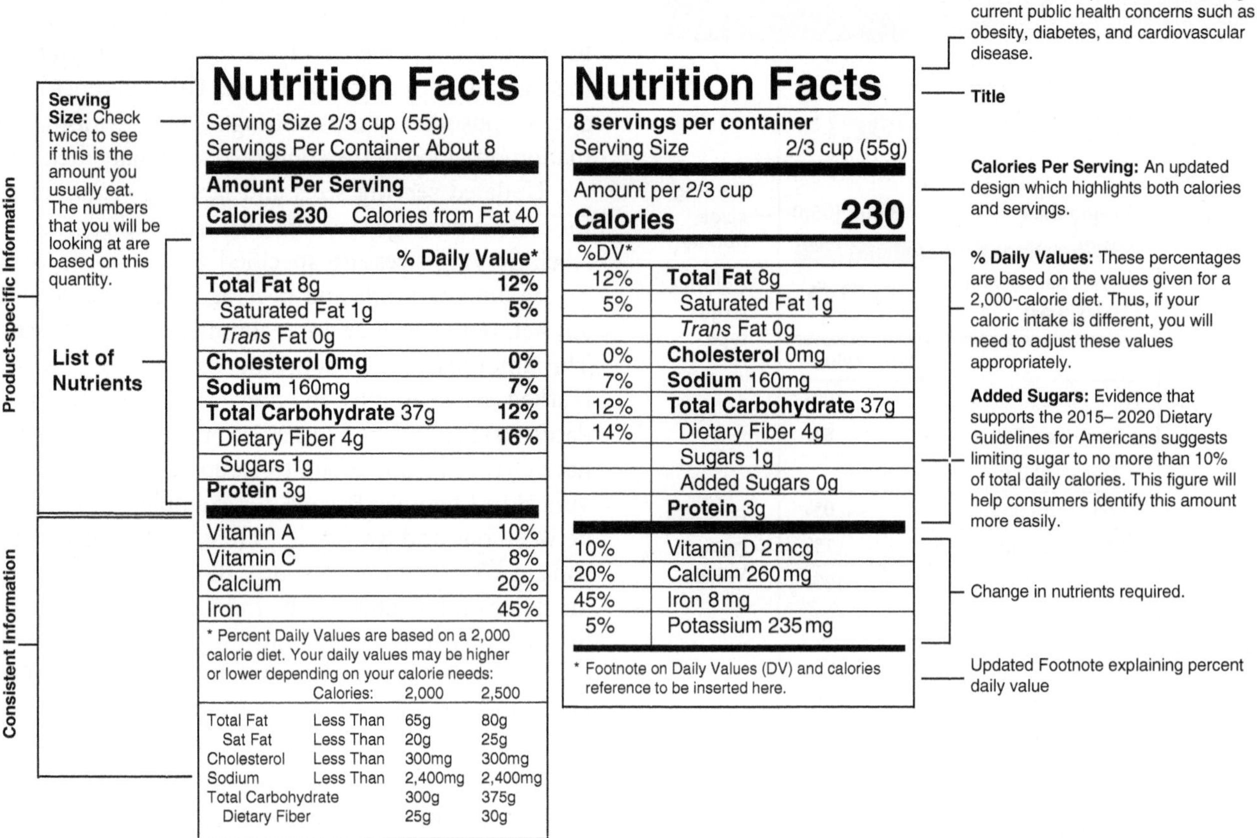

FIGURE 13 The New and Improved Nutrition Facts Label: Key Changes

Reproduced from U.S. Food and Drug Administration. The New and Improved Nutrition Facts Label- Key Changes https://www.fda.gov/downloads/food/ingredientspackaginglabeling/labelingnutrition/ucm511646.pdf

that choose to implement the targets do have recommended time frames by which to implement them. The FDA has published voluntary targets for reducing sodium in commercially produced and prepared foods for both the short and long terms (2 years and 10 years, respectively).[23]

Recap The updated Nutrition Facts Label is designed to highlight the key nutrition information consumers should pay attention to when considering food choices. With larger font, bold type, and revised requirements, the focus shifts to those parameters that have the largest effects on health.

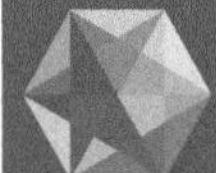

HIGHLIGHT

Best if Used By...

In addition to targeting the Nutrition Facts Label, the USDA, along with the Food Safety and Inspection Service (FSIS), have issued updated guidance regarding date labeling.

The Nutrition Facts Label is not the only packaging component to undergo review. The USDA and the FSIS have issued new guidance aimed at reducing food waste. As the new Nutrition Facts Label is designed to best resonate with the consumer, so too is the revised product dating. Product dating is not a federal requirement on any item other than infant formula. It turns out that the "Sell By" and "Use By" dates are confusing to consumers and result in perfectly usable and safe food products being thrown out. The USDA and FSIS thus recommend that manufacturers use "Best If Used By" to communicate quality to consumers. Adoption of this practice may help the USDA and EPA meet their 2015 goal of reducing national food waste 50% by 2030. The agencies have also taken steps to facilitate the donation of food, bringing about the allocation of 2.6 million pounds of products to establishments such as food banks in 2016.

Modified from USDA Food Safety and Inspection Service. USDA Revises Guidance on Date Labeling to Reduce Food Waste. fsis.usda.gov. https://www.fsis.usda.gov/wps/portal/fsis/newsroom/news-releases-statements-and-transcripts/news-release-archives-by-year/archive/2016/nr-121416-01. Accessed December 24, 2016.

HIGHLIGHT

Gluten-Free and Food Allergy Labeling

With continued updates in food-labeling requirements comes revised legislation regarding gluten-free claims. As of September 4, 2013, foods labeled as *gluten free*—including the variations *no gluten, free of gluten*, and *without gluten*—must either inherently not contain gluten or comply with all of the following requirements:

- They cannot contain any gluten-containing grain in any product ingredient.
- They cannot contain an ingredient derived from a gluten-containing grain that has not been processed to remove gluten.
- They cannot contain an ingredient that is derived from a gluten-containing grain that has been processed to remove gluten if that ingredient causes the final food product to contain 20 parts per million or more of gluten.

"May Contain" Statements

"May Contain" statements, referred to as allergy advisory statements, differ from "contains" statements. Of primary distinction is that "contains" statements are regulated under the Food Allergen Labeling and Consumer Protection Act, and "may contain" statements do not fall under any federal regulations.

"Manufactured in a facility that also contains wheat," another allergy advisory statement, provides information for consumers regarding food-processing procedures. However, these regulations are neither regulated nor mandatory, so they are not used by all manufacturers. Products were required to be in compliance with the gluten-free label ruling by August 5, 2014.

Modified from the gluten-free labeling rule: What registered dietitian nutritionists need to know to help clients with gluten-related disorders. *J Acad Nutr Diet*. 2015; 115(1):13-16.

Food Guides (MyPlate Food Exchange)

Preview In conjunction with the *Dietary Guidelines*, food guides serve as a tool to help Americans decide what types and amounts of foods to consume. The USDA has developed several food guides throughout the years to identify which patterns of eating would meet known nutrient needs at the time, as well as balance intake from various food groups. A timeline of these food guides was discussed previously in this chapter. Two of the contemporary remaining guides are MyPlate and the USDA Food Patterns.

MyPlate

MyPlate serves as a vehicle that reminds the public to create healthy eating patterns by making healthy choices in line with the *Dietary Guidelines*. MyPlate is used by federal and nonfederal programs to encourage Americans to make shifts in their daily food and beverage choices as dictated by the *Dietary Guidelines*.[10] MyPlate focuses on building the right mix of food to promote optimal health for the present and future.

Specifically, the main ideas focus on variety, amount, and nutrition. Individuals are encouraged to consume food from all five food groups—fruits, vegetables, grains, proteins, and dairy products—to receive adequate nutrients to meet their needs. Calories should be adequate based on their age, gender, height, weight, and level of physical activity. Adopting this healthy eating pattern should promote health, specifically with reduced risk of causing or exacerbating conditions such as heart disease, diabetes, cancer and obesity.

Americans are encouraged to choose foods and beverages with less saturated fat, sodium, and added sugars. Eating fewer calories from foods high in saturated fat and added sugars helps manage overall calorie intake and prevent overweight and obesity. Eating foods with less sodium reduces the risk of hypertension. To put these recommendations into practice, the guidelines emphasize starting with small changes to build healthier eating styles. These include covering half the plate with fruits and vegetables and half with whole grains and choosing fat-free dairy products in favor of low-fat, a variety of protein sources, and eating and drinking the appropriate amount per individual. Supporting healthy eating for everyone entails creating settings in which healthy choices are available and affordable for the community.[24]

Food Groups

Fruit for consumption is defined as fresh, canned, frozen, dried, whole, cut up, puréed, or 100% fruit juice. The specific amount needed per individual depends on age, gender, and level of physical activity. For recommended daily amounts of fruit as well as from other food groups, see **TABLE 16**. At least half the recommended amount of fruit should come from whole fruit because juice is lower in fiber and may contribute excess calories. If consumed, juices should be 100% whole juice. Canned fruit should contain no added sugars.[25]

Any vegetable—raw, cooked, fresh, frozen, canned, dried, whole, cut up, mashed, or as 100% vegetable juice—counts as a vegetable source. Vegetables are organized into five subgroups—dark green, starchy, red and orange, beans and peas, and other vegetables—based on nutrient content. As with fruit, the amount needed per individual depends on age, gender, and level of physical activity.[26] See Table 16 for recommended daily amounts of vegetables and the five other food groups. Recommended weekly amounts from each vegetable subgroup are found in **TABLE 17**.

The category of grains is characterized as food made from wheat, rice, oats, cornmeal, barley, or other cereal grains. The amount of grains needed depends on age, gender, and physical activity level. See Table 16 for specific recommendations per age group.[27] In addition to the daily recommendation, daily minimum amounts have also been established for whole grains.

Grains are divided into two subgroups: whole and refined. Whole grains contain the entire grain kernel—bran, germ, and endosperm. Examples include whole-wheat flour, bulgur, oatmeal, whole cornmeal, and brown rice. In contrast, refined grains have been milled, a process that removes the bran and germ and gives the resulting products finer texture and extended shelf life. Refining grains, however, removes dietary fiber, iron, and the B vitamins. Most refined grains are therefore enriched with some of the B vitamins (thiamin, riboflavin, niacin, folic acid) as well as iron, which is added after processing. Examples of refined grains include white flour, degermed cornmeal, white bread, and white rice. See **TABLE 18**.

The protein group constitutes foods made from meat, poultry, seafood, legumes, eggs, processed soy products, nuts, and seeds. Note that legumes, for example beans and peas, are classified in the vegetable group as well. A variety of protein foods intake is recommended for improved nutrient intake and overall health, including at least 8 ounces of cooked seafood per week. Young children need less, depending on age and calorie needs.[28] See Table 16 for protein recommendations based on age. With similar nutrient profiles to both proteins and vegetables, legumes can be counted toward the intake of either the protein or vegetable group.[10]

All fluid milk products and several foods made from milk are part of the dairy group. It is recommended that the majority of choices from the dairy group be fat-free or low-fat. Foods made from milk that retain their calcium are considered part of this group; foods made from milk that contains little to no calcium—cream cheese, cream, and butter—are not. Calcium-fortified soymilk and nut-milks are included in the dairy group. The amount of dairy needed depends on age.[29] See Table 16.

Fats that are liquid at room temperature count as oils. For example, vegetable oils used in cooking such as canola, olive, safflower, sunflower, and corn are considered oils. Although not considered a food group, oils provide essential nutrients and therefore are an integral part of the USDA Food Patterns. Nuts, olives, avocado, and certain fish are examples of foods naturally high in oils.[30]

USDA Food Patterns

The USDA Food Patterns are designed to meet food group and nutrient recommendations while remaining within calorie needs. Patterns are based on consuming foods in nutrient-dense forms. The Healthy US-Style Eating Pattern, the basis for the USDA Food Pattern, was created around the types and proportions of foods typically consumed by Americans, although in nutrient-dense forms and in appropriate amounts. The design focuses on consumers achieving nutrient needs without exceeding calorie requirements and staying within the limits for excessively consumed dietary components.

The Healthy US-Style Eating Pattern demonstrates the specific amounts and limits for food groups and other dietary components that form healthy eating patterns. It was formulated to comply with the RDA, AI, and AMDR established by the Food and Nutrition Board of the National Academy of Medicine. The guidance for healthy eating provided by the tool ensures success in meeting nutritional goals for almost all nutrients. Cup and ounce equivalents for foods with similar nutritional content are provided for each of the five food groups and allows consumers to easily identify which amount of food will be adequate to meet their goals. Amounts of each food group and subgroup are modified as needed to ensure they meet recommendations for nutrient intake and the *Dietary Guidelines* while staying within both the typical consumption range and the limits for calories and overconsumed dietary components. See **TABLE 19** for cup and ounce equivalents.

The standards for nutrient adequacy are set to reach the RDA, which is able to account for the needs

TABLE 16 MyPlate intake recommendations

	Children (Years)		Girls (Years)		Boys (Years)		Women (Years)			Men (Years)		
Food Group	**2–3**	**4–8**	**9–13**	**14–18**	**9–13**	**14–18**	**19–30**	**31–50**	**51+**	**19–30**	**31–50**	**51**
Fruit (cups)	1	1–1.5	1.5	1.5	1.5	2	2	1.5	1.5	2	2	2
Vegetables (cups)	1	0.5	2	2.5	2.5	3	2.5	2.5	2	3	3	2.5
Grains (oz. equiv)	3	5	5	6	6	8	6	6	5	8	7	6
Protein (oz. equiv)	2	4	5	5	5	6.5	5.5	5	5	6,5	6	5.5
Dairy (cups)	2	2.5	3	3	3	3	3	3	3	3	3	3
Oils (tsp)	3	4	5	5	5	6	6	5	5	7	6	6

Note: The amounts provided are specific to individuals with a physical activity level of <30 minutes per day of moderate activity, above activities of daily living (ADL). Those with increased activity may consume greater amounts, while staying within their estimated calorie needs. Adapted from USDA Choose MyPlate. choosemyplate.gov. https://www.choosemyplate.gov. Accessed September 28, 2016.

TABLE 17 Weekly vegetable subgroup recommendations

	Children (Years)		Girls (Years)		Boys (Years)		Women (Years)			Men (Years)		
Vegetable	**2–3**	**4–8**	**9–13**	**14–18**	**9–13**	**14–18**	**19–30**	**31–50**	**51+**	**19–30**	**31–50**	**51+**
Dark green (cups)	0.5	1	1.5	1.5	1.5	2	1.5	1.5	1.5	2	2	1.5
Red, orange (cups)	2.5	3	4	5.5	5.5	6	5.5	5.5	4	6	6	5.5
Beans, peas (cups)	0.5	0.5	1	1.5	1.5	2	1.5	1.5	1	2	2	1.5
Starchy (cups)	2	3.5	4	5	5	6	5	5	4	6	6	5
Other (cups)	1.5	2.5	3.5	4	4	5	4	4	3.5	5	5	4

Adapted from USDA Choose MyPlate. Vegetables. ChooseMyPlate.gov. https://www.choosemyplate.gov/vegetables. Last updated July 26, 2016. Accessed September 28, 2016.

TABLE 18 Daily minimum amount of whole grains (in oz. equivalents)

Children (Years)		Girls (Years)		Boys (Years)		Women (Years)			Men (Years)		
2–3	4–8	9–13	14–18	9–13	14–18	19–30	31–50	51+	19–30	31–50	51+
1.5	2.5	3	3	3	4	3	3	3	4	3.5	3

Modified from USDA Choose MyPlate. Grains. ChooseMyPlate.gov. https://www.choosemyplate.gov/grains. Last updated October 18, 2016. Accessed September 28, 2016.

of the majority of the population (approximately 98%), and adequate intake, the level used in the event average nutrient requirement is unable to be determined. Although the pattern does successfully cover the requirements for most nutrients, a few—vitamin D, vitamin E, potassium, and choline—have fallen marginally below the RDA or AI recommendations. However, inadequate intake for these nutrients has not been determined to be a public health concern. In addition to the Healthy US-Style Eating Pattern, the USDA has developed the Healthy Mediterranean-Style and Healthy Vegetarian Eating Patterns. The USDA Food Patterns are notably versatile, because they demonstrate healthy eating patterns that can be applied across the board to many cultures, many personal preferences, and varying dietary requirements. They are a

TABLE 19 Cup and ounce equivalents: USDA's Healthy US-Style Eating Pattern

	Vegetables	Fruits	Grains	Dairy	Protein
0.5 cup equivalent	0.5 cup green beans	0.5 cup strawberries	—	—	—
	1 cup raw spinach	0.25 cup raisins	—	—	—
0.75 cup equivalent	—	0.75 cup 100% OJ	—	6 oz. fat-free yogurt	
1 oz. equivalent	—	—	1 slice bread	—	1 large egg
	—	—	0.5 cup cooked brown rice	—	—
1 cup equivalent	—	—	—	1.5 oz. cheddar cheese	—
2 oz. equivalents	—	—	—	—	2 Tbsp peanut butter
	—	—	—	—	0.5 cup black beans
4 oz. equivalents	—	—	—	—	4 oz. pork

Modified from U.S. Department of Health and Human Services and U.S. Department of Agriculture (2015). 2015–2020 *Dietary Guidelines For Americans* 8th Edition. Figure 1-1 Cup-& Ounce-Equivalents. Page 19. https://health.gov/dietaryguidelines/2015/guidelines. Accessed July 27, 2016.

useful tool for planning and serving meals for home, school, work, and other everyday environments.[10]

Recap The MyPlate food guide was created as an interpretation of the *Dietary Guidelines* to help Americans apply the central ideas to their individual diets. The USDA Food Patterns summarize ways to meet these nutrient needs without consuming excessive calories.

Chapter Summary

The US Department of Agriculture, the Department of Health and Human Services, and other federal government agencies constantly assess the composition of foods and the quality of dietary intake among Americans in an effort to support consumption that meets recommended needs and reduces the risk of chronic disease. The *Dietary Guidelines for Americans* represent the ideal eating behaviors for optimal nutritional status. The *Dietary Guidelines* is the standard against which researchers compare population intake patterns and data collected through the use of dietary quality-assessment tools such as the Healthy Eating Index.

The USDA supplements the *Dietary Guidelines* with consumer education materials and infographics, the most current of which is MyPlate, the result of a 25-year evolution of the Food Guide Pyramid to accurately reflect the messages communicated by the latest *Dietary Guidelines*; its format is most likely to resonate with the American population. The concern of adequately communicating messages to consumers is also demonstrated in the newly revised Nutrition Facts Label. Changes were made to highlight key nutrients contributing to health status, with aesthetics designed to attract customer focus to the important components. Given the progressive change in our country's health status and eating behaviors, nutrition research, legislature, education, and recommendations will continue to adapt to keep up with current trends, knowledge, and needs.

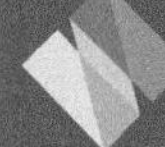

CASE STUDY

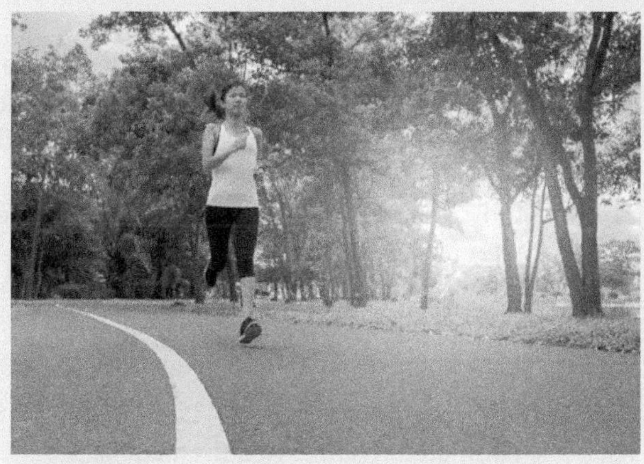

Providing dietary recommendations to an individual is a complex and involved process . Although these recommendations can be made for the broader population, it is often necessary to tailor them to a specific person's needs. Consider Joanne, for example.

Joanne is a 23-year-old woman who is 5′7″ and weighs 135 lbs. She currently works as a teaching assistant at a university, and spends 30 to 60 minutes a day walking around campus. She also jogs 60 minutes a day, six days a week. She has read on the Internet that in order to stay thin, she should limit her carbohydrate intake, and she is, therefore, currently consuming about 150 g of carbohydrate per day. Her daily energy intake is between 1,900 and 2,000 calories. She has been losing weight quite rapidly and is extremely fatigued, not only during her runs but also throughout the rest of the day.

Questions:

1. Calculate Joanne's estimated energy requirement (EER) using an equation from Table 9 and physical-activity coefficient from Table 10.
2. Is Joanne currently meeting her caloric requirements for the day?
3. Using the total energy expenditure (TEE) value that you calculate for Joanne, determine how many grams of carbohydrate, protein, and fat she should be consuming each day.
4. Assess Joanne's current carbohydrate intake compared to intake recommended for her. If she is not consuming enough carbohydrate, provide examples of healthy carbohydrate-containing foods that she can incorporate into her diet.
5. Using your calculations and Joanne's current diet and exercise regimen, provide possible reasons why Joanne is feeling fatigued and losing weight.

Learning Portfolio

Key Terms

Adequate intake (AI)
Acceptable macronutrient distribution range (AMDR)
Basal Energy Expenditure (BEE)
Dietary Reference Intakes (DRIs)
Energy density
Estimated Average Requirement (EAR)
Estimated Energy Requirement (EER)
Healthy Eating Index (HEI)
Nutrient density
Recommended Dietary Allowance (RDA)
Resting Energy Expenditure (REE)
Thermic effect of activity (TEA)
Thermic effect of food (TEF)
Tolerable upper intake level (UL)

Study Questions

1. What year were the first *Dietary Guidelines* released?
   a. 1985
   b. 1977
   c. 1980
   d. 1990
2. Who is responsible for issuing the *Dietary Guidelines*?
   a. USDA and HHS
   b. DHS and HHS
   c. USDA and FDA
   d. HHS and FDA
3. What year were the first USDA food guides issued?
   a. 1916
   b. 1956
   d. 1992
   d. 2011
4. Which food guide includes a visual representation for physical activity?
   a. MyPlate
   b. Food Guide Pyramid
   c. MyPyramid
   d. *Food for Fitness*
5. Which of the following is not one of the Dietary Reference Intakes?
   a. Recommended Dietary Allowance
   b. Adequate intake
   c. Acceptable macronutrient distribution range
   d. Estimated Average Requirement
6. The primary uses of the DRIs include all except:
   a. Assessing the intakes of individuals.
   b. Rating the intakes of individuals.
   c. Planning diets for individuals.
   d. Planning diets for groups.
7. The DRI committees have been established by governments of the United States and
   a. Australia.
   b. France.
   c. United Kingdom.
   d. Canada.
8. Which of the following pertains to *relevant* data:
   a. Study results are generalizable to the North American population and to DRI development.
   b. Study results are generalizable to the United States population and to DRI development.
   c. Research was unlikely to have been available to the previous DRI expert panel.
   d. Research has been conducted within the last two years.
9. The Estimated Average Requirement is:
   a. The average daily nutrient intake estimated to meet the needs of half of the healthy individuals in a group.
   b. The average daily nutrient intake level sufficient to meet the nutrient requirement of almost all healthy individuals in a group.
   c. The recommended average daily intake based on observed or experimentally determined approximations or estimations of nutrient intake by a group.
   d. A set of nutrient-based reference values that are quantitative estimates of nutrient intakes used for planning and assessing diets for healthy people.

10. The EAR has not been established for:
    a. Vitamin E
    b. Molybdenum
    c. Phosphorus
    d. Vitamin D
11. The EAR serves as the basis for calculating which other DRI standard?
    a. UL
    b. AI
    c. RDA
    d. EER
12. The main purpose of the EAR is to:
    a. Assess the adequacy of population intakes.
    b. Assess the adequacy of individual intakes.
    c. Be the goal for daily intake by individuals.
    d. Be the goal for daily intake by populations.
13. When the RDA cannot be determined, which other standard of nutrient intake is used?
    a. DRI
    b. EAR
    c. AMDR
    d. AI
14. The RDA is established based on which other standard of nutrient intake?
    a. AI
    b. EAR
    c. DRI
    d. UL
15. Which of the following is not true about the RDA?
    a. It is used to assess the intake of groups.
    b. It is used to assess the intake of individuals.
    c. It is determined from the EAR.
    d. It is sufficient to meet the requirements of 97% to 98% of healthy individuals in a group.
16. RDA is defined as:
    a. The average daily nutrient intake level sufficient to meet the nutrient requirement of half the individuals in a group.
    b. The average daily nutrient intake level sufficient to meet all of the individuals in a group.
    c. The average daily dietary nutrient intake level sufficient to meet the nutrient requirement of nearly all individuals in a group.
    d. The mean intake of a nutrient for individuals in a group.
17. Tolerable upper intake level is defined as:
    a. The recommended average daily intake based on observed or experimentally determined approximations or estimations of nutrient intake by a group.
    b. The highest average daily nutrient intake level likely to pose no risk of adverse health effects to almost all individuals in a group.
    c. A set of nutrient-based reference values that are quantitative estimates of nutrient intakes used for planning and assessing diets for healthy people.
    d. The average daily nutrient intake level sufficient to meet the nutrient requirement of almost all healthy individuals in a group.
18. Tolerable upper intake level has been established for:
    a. All micronutrients.
    b. All macronutrients.
    c. Some micronutrients.
    d. Some macronutrients.
19. Which of the following is true?
    a. As intake increases above the UL, the risk for potential adverse events decreases.
    b. As intake decreases below the UL, the risk for potential adverse events decreases.
    c. As intake decreases below the UL, the risk for potential adverse events increases.
    d. As intake increases above the UL, the risk for potential adverse events increases.
20. The UL was established in response to:
    a. Pressure by the federal government.
    b. The increase in fortified foods and dietary supplementation usage.
    c. The growing number of individuals with toxic levels of nutrients.
    d. The establishment of UL in Canada.
21. Energy requirement is most precisely measured from:
    a. Energy expenditure.
    b. Energy intake.
    c. Energy expenditure and energy intake.
    d. Energy intake and physical activity.
22. All of the following are methods used to measure energy expenditure in humans except:
    a. Indirect calorimetry.
    b. Direct calorimetry.
    c. Doubly labeled water.
    d. Double-blind water studies.
23. Which of the following is not a component of total energy expenditure?
    a. Resting Energy Expenditure
    b. Basal Energy Expenditure
    c. Exercise activity thermogenesis
    d. Resting activity thermogenesis

24. The total number of calories a person needs per day depends on which factors?
    i. Age
    ii. Sex
    iii. Physical activity level
    iv. Maximal oxygen consumption (VO_2max)
    v. Height
    vi. Weight
    vii. Medical condition
    a. i, ii, iii, v, vi
    b. i, ii, iii, iv, v, vi
    c. i, ii, v, vi
    d. i, ii, iii, v, vi, vii
25. The RDA for carbohydrates for adults and children is:
    a. 120 g/day.
    b. 100 g/day.
    c. 130 g/day.
    d. 140 g/day.
26. The EAR for carbohydrates is established based on:
    a. Amount of fat absorbed and stored as adipose tissue.
    b. Amount of protein able to be used by the body.
    c. Average amount of protein needed for physical activity.
    d. Average amount of glucose used by the brain.
27. Insufficient data exists for which standard of nutrient intake to establish any specific recommendations for macronutrients?
    a. EAR
    b. UL
    c. RDA
    d. AMDR
28. The AMDR was established in the interest of the risk for:
    a. Chronic disease.
    b. Obesity.
    c. Malnutrition.
    d. Fat overconsumption.
29. Nutrient-dense foods:
    a. Have a high concentration of nutrients per amount of food.
    b. Have a high concentration of fats and added sugars per amount of food.
    c. Contain a high number of individual vitamins and minerals.
    d. Contain a high number of vitamins, minerals, fats, and sugars.
30. All of the following are nutrient-density profiling tools except:
    a. The nutrient-dense foods index.
    b. The nutrient-rich foods index.
    c. The affordable nutrition index.
    d. The Guiding Stars program.
31. The most widely used front-of-packaging labeling tool is:
    a. Guiding Stars.
    b. Powerhouse Fruits and Vegetables.
    c. Healthy eating systems.
    d. Nutrient Density Climate Index.
32. Energy density is:
    a. The weight of a food or a beverage.
    b. The amount of calories in a food item.
    c. The amount of energy per weight of food or beverage.
    d. The amount of exercise required to burn off a food item.
33. The Healthy Eating Index (HEI) assesses conformance to:
    a. The *Dietary Guidelines for Americans*.
    b. Estimated Energy Requirement.
    c. Recommended Dietary Allowances.
    d. Macronutrient recommendations.
34. Which organization established the HEI?
    a. World Health Organization
    b. Centers for Disease Control and Prevention
    c. Center for Nutrition Policy and Promotion
    d. US Food and Drug Administration
35. Uses of the HEI include all except:
    a. Determining the relationship between diet cost and diet quality.
    b. Evaluating food environments.
    c. Evaluating personal food choices versus the food choices of others.
    d. Examining relationships between diet and outcomes of public health concern.
36. The components of the Alternative Healthy Eating Index (AHEI) include:
    a. Vegetables, fruit, nuts and soy, wheat, polyunsaturated and saturated fatty acids, red and white meat.
    b. Vegetables, fruit, nuts and soy, cereal fiber, monounsaturated fatty acids, red and white meat.
    c. Vegetables, fruit, nuts and soy, cereal fiber, saturated fatty acids, red and white meat.
    d. Vegetables, fruit, nuts and soy, cereal fiber, polyunsaturated and saturated fatty acids, red and white meat.

37. How often are the *Dietary Guidelines* published?
    a. Every 10 years
    b. Every five years
    c. Every year
    d. On an as-needed basis

38. The recommendations in the *Dietary Guidelines* are provided for the purpose of all of the following except:
    a. To promote health.
    b. To prevent chronic disease.
    c. To help people reach and maintain healthy weight.
    d. To help people maintain appropriate weight and manage their chronic diseases.

39. The process for developing the *Dietary Guidelines* includes all of the following except:
    a. Conducting the research.
    b. Reviewing the science.
    c. Developing the *Dietary Guidelines.*
    d. Implementing the *Dietary Guidelines.*

40. The *Dietary Guidelines 2015* recommend Americans:
    a. Consume <20% of their daily calories from added sugars.
    b. Consume <20% of their daily calories from total fat.
    c. Consume <2300 mg sodium per day.
    d. Consume <10% of their daily calories from saturated fats.

41. The size of print has been increased in the new Nutrition Facts Label for which three nutrition factors?
    a. Calories, servings per container, serving size
    b. Calories from fat, servings per container, serving size
    c. Calories, trans fat, serving size
    d. Calories, trans fat, saturated fat

42. Daily values for which three nutrients are being updated?
    a. Sodium, calcium, vitamin D
    b. Saturated fat, vitamin D, dietary fiber
    c. Sodium, dietary fiber, vitamin D
    d. Saturated fat, vitamin D, vitamin C

43. The % daily value is based on a diet of how many calories per day?
    a. 1500
    b. 2000
    c. 2200
    d. 1800

44. Which parameter has been removed from the new Nutrition Facts Label?
    a. Calories from fat
    b. Total fat
    c. Vitamin C
    d. Dietary fiber

45. The recommended daily amount of fruit intake for men and women ages 19 to 30 years old is:
    a. 1.5 cups
    b. 1–1.5 cups
    c. 2 cups
    d. 1 cup

46. The two subgroups of grains are:
    a. Unrefined and refined.
    b. Whole and refined.
    c. Gluten and gluten-free.
    d. White and whole wheat.

47. The healthy US-Style Eating Pattern was formulated to comply with which nutrient intake standards?
    i. DRI
    ii. RDA
    iii. EAR
    iv. UL
    v. AI
    vi. AMDR
    a. i, v, vi
    b. ii, iii, v, vi
    c. ii, v, vi
    d. ii, iiii, v

48. How many different calorie levels of Food Patterns are provided in the healthy US-Style Eating Pattern?
    a. 5
    b. 12
    c. 15
    d. 3

Discussion Questions

1. What standards and recommendations do you see being incorporated into future dietary guidelines and the USDA Food Guides?
2. Why might the progression of the USDA Food Guides have been geared toward giving consumers a visual representation of portion sizes, and how might the current MyPlate food guide be improved?
3. What are the main differences or improvements between the DRIs and the previous RDA and RNI standards?

4. Explain the key processes for creating and updating the DRIs. What is the basis for the DRI committees to review a nutrient?
5. Which nutrients do you think should be proposed for establishing an EAR in future reviews?
6. Explain why there is no EAR for saturated fat, monounsaturated fat. and cholesterol.
7. How does the RDA differ from the EAR in the way that it is determined, used, applied?
8. Do you think the UL is a useful or necessary DRI standard? Explain.
9. Compare and contrast indirect and direct calorimetry.
10. Consider a way in which an individual might increase total energy expenditure for the day without increasing amount of exercise (i.e. no change in the thermic effect of activity).
11. Discuss some of the ways in which variables such as age, gender, physical activity level, weight, and height contribute to the variation in estimated calorie needs per day (see Table 8) among different people.
12. What are some instances in which the AMDR would be useful?
13. What recommendation would you give someone about her daily allowance of saturated fat and cholesterol? Explain why there are no RDAs for these nutrients.
14. Provide examples of foods that are not nutrient dense and suggest preferred options.
15. Think of an example of a common energy-dense meal that is simultaneously low in nutrients. Consider how you might make substitutions to make it less energy dense while being *more* nutrient dense.
16. What initiatives or legislation would you suggest to improve the diet quality of the American population?
17. Describe a diet that would receive a Healthy Eating Index Score of 100. Refer to the *Dietary Guidelines for Americans.*
18. Do you think the *Dietary Guidelines* have been effective in influencing the eating habits of Americans?
19. Describe how new *Dietary Guidelines* would be developed, including the federal departments involved.
20. What other changes to the food label beyond those being implemented do you think would be beneficial and why?
21. Explain the reasoning behind the updates to the Nutrition Facts Label, including added sugars, calories from fat being removed, and daily values for sodium, dietary fiber, and Vitamin D.
22. Does the MyPlate visual adequately represent the food group recommendations specified in the literature?
23. Explain the four main focuses of MyPlate as well as examples of acceptable foods from each of the five food groups.

Activities

1. In a group of two or three students, write down what you ate for breakfast, lunch, and dinner yesterday. Distribute your food records among the group so that everyone is reading someone's record other than their own. Now identify which foods from your classmate's food record are nutrient dense and which are energy dense. Include the aspects of those foods that led you to label them as either nutrient or energy dense. Write down a suggestion on your classmate's paper about how they might substitute one or two of the foods they are eating with healthier, nutrient-dense options.
2. Review the *Dietary Guidelines for Americans 2015*, including the criteria for a healthy eating pattern. Then write a sample day of eating that follows the guidelines and consists of four different meals. Include food groups and types but not specific portion sizes.

   Example Meal
   One serving whole wheat bread
   Mashed avocado
   Two eggs, fried in olive oil
   One medium apple
   Glass of fat-free 2% milk

Online Resources

Center for Nutrition Policy and Promotion
www.cnpp.usda.gov

Department of Health and Human Services
www.hhs.gov

Food and Drug Administration
FDA.gov

MyPlate SuperTracker
supertracker.usda.gov

Nutrition Evidence Library
NEL.gov

Nutrition Facts Label
www.cfsan.fda.gov/~dms/foodlab.html

Nutrition Information
www.nutrition.gov

Office of Disease Prevention and Health Promotion
health.gov

United States Department of Agriculture
USDA.gov

References

1. US Department of Agriculture (USDA). 2015 Dietary Guidelines for Advisory Committee. DGAC Meeting 1: Materials and Presentations. https://health.gov/dietaryguidelines/2015-binder/meeting1/historycurrentuse.aspx.
2. Institute of Medicine (US), Committee on Use of Dietary Reference Intakes in Nutrition Labeling. Dietary Reference Intakes: Guiding Principles for Nutrition Labeling and Fortification. Washington, DC: National Academies Press; 2003: 4. https://www.ncbi.nlm.nih.gov/books/NBK208878/.
3. Murphy SP, Yates AA, Atkinson SA, Barr SI, Dwyer J. History of nutrition: The long road leading to the Dietary Reference Intakes for the United States and Canada. *Adv Nutr* 2016; 7:157-168.
4. USDA. Choose MyPlate. A brief history of USDA Food Guides. choosemyplate.gov. https://www.choosemyplate.gov/content/brief-history-usda-food-guides. Accessed September 28, 2016.
5. Institute of Medicine of the National Academies. *Dietary Reference Intakes: The Essential Guide to Nutrient Requirements.* Washington, DC: The National Academy Press; 2006.
6. National Academy of Sciences. *Dietary Reference Intakes for Energy, Carbohydrate, Fiber, Fat, Fatty Acids, Cholesterol, Protein, and Amino Acids (Macronutrients).* Washington, DC: National Academy Press; 2002/2005.
7. Academy of Nutrition and Dietetics. Definitions of energy expenditure. Nutrition Care Manual. https://www.nutritioncaremanual.org/topic.cfm?ncm_category_id=11&lv1=144882&lv2=144895&ncm_toc_id=144895&ncm_heading=&. Accessed July 27, 2016.
8. Academy of Nutrition and Dietetics. Energy metabolism. Nutrition Care Manual. https://www.nutritioncaremanual.org/topic.cfm?ncm_category_id=11&lv1=144882&ncm_toc_id=144882&ncm_heading=&. Accessed July 27, 2016.
9. Academy of Nutrition and Dietetics. Measurement of energy expenditure. Nutrition Care Manual. https://www.nutritioncaremanual.org/topic.cfm?ncm_category_id=11&lv1=144882&lv2=144900&ncm_toc_id=144900&ncm_heading=&. Accessed July 27, 2016.
10. US Department of Health and Human Services (HHS), USDA. *2015–2020 Dietary Guidelines For Americans.* 8th ed. Washington, DC: US Government Printing Office, 2015.
11. HHS, USDA. *2015–2020 Dietary Guidelines For Americans.* 8th ed. Appendix 2. Estimated calorie needs per day, by age, sex and physical activity level. Washington, DC: US Government Printing Office, 2015.
12. Academy of Nutrition and Dietetics. Predictive equations. Nutrition Care Manual. https://www.nutritioncaremanual.org/topic.cfm?ncm_category_id=11&lv1=144882&lv2=144904&ncm_toc_id=144905&ncm_heading=&.
13. Dietary Guidelines Advisory Committee. *Report of the Dietary Guidelines Advisory Committee on the Dietary Guidelines for Americans, 2010, to the Secretary of Agriculture and the Secretary of Health and Human Services.* Appendix E-4: History of the dietary guidelines for Americans. Washington, DC: USDA, Agricultural Research Service, 2010.
14. Hingle MD, Kandiah J, Maggi A. Practice paper of the Academy of Nutrition and Dietetics: Selecting nutrient-dense foods for good health. *J Acad Nutr Diet.* 2016; 116(9):1473-1479.
15. USDA Center for Nutrition Policy and Promotion. Healthy Eating Index (HEI). https://www.cnpp.usda.gov/healthyeatingindex. Accessed September 28, 2016.
16. Snetselaar L. Are Americans following US dietary guidelines? Elsevier.com. March 2, 2015. https://www.elsevier.com/connect/are-americans-following-us-dietary-guidelines-check-the-healthy-eating-index.
17. Scientific Report of the 2015 Dietary Guidelines Advisory Committee. Appendix E- 1. Adequacy of USDA Food Patterns. https://health.gov/dietaryguidelines/2015-scientific-report/PDFs/Appendix-E- 1.pdf. Accessed September 28, 2016.
18. USDA. *A Series of Systematic Reviews on the Relationship Between Dietary Patterns and Health Outcomes.* Alexandria, VA: USDA; 2014. http://www.nel.gov/vault/2440/web/files/DietaryPatterns/DPRptFullFinal.pdf.
19. Office of Disease Prevention and Health Promotion (ODPHP). Dietary Guidelines Purpose. health.gov. https://health.gov/dietaryguidelines/purpose.asp. Accessed July 27, 2016.
20. ODPHP. Dietary Guidelines Process. health.gov. https://health.gov/dietaryguidelines/process.asp. Accessed July 27, 2016.
21. ODPHP. Dietary Guidelines Evolution. health.gov. https://health.gov/dietaryguidelines/evolution.asp. Accessed July 27, 2016.
22. US Food and Drug Administration (FDA). How to understand and use the Nutrition Facts Label. fda.gov. http://www.fda.gov/Food/IngredientsPackagingLabeling/LabelingNutrition/ucm274593.htm. Accessed September 6, 2016.
23. FDA. Changes to the Nutrition Facts Label. fda.gov. http://www.fda.gov/Food/GuidanceRegulation/GuidanceDocumentsRegulatoryInformation/LabelingNutrition/ucm385663.htm. Accessed September 6, 2016.
24. USDA Choose MyPlate. Choose MyPlate. choosemyplate.gov. https://www.choosemyplate.gov. Accessed September 28, 2016.
25. USDA Choose MyPlate. Fruit. ChooseMyPlate.gov. https://www.choosemyplate.gov/fruit. Accessed September 28, 2016.
26. USDA Choose MyPlate. Vegetables. ChooseMyPlate.gov. https://www.choosemyplate.gov/vegetables. Accessed September 28, 2016.
27. USDA Choose MyPlate. Grains. ChooseMyPlate.gov. https://www.choosemyplate.gov/grains. Accessed September 28, 2016.
28. USDA Choose MyPlate. Protein. ChooseMyPlate.gov. https://www.choosemyplate.gov/protein-foods. Accessed September 28, 2016.
29. USDA Choose MyPlate. Dairy. ChooseMyPlate.gov. https://www.choosemyplate.gov/dairy. Accessed September 28, 2016.
30. USDA Choose MyPlate. Oils. ChooseMyPlate.gov. https://www.choosemyplate.gov/oils. Accessed September 28, 2016.

Enteral Nutrition

Nusheen Orandi
Kathy Prelack

Chapter Outline

CORE CONCEPTS

1. Enteral nutrition includes food, oral supplements, and formulas created specifically to prevent malnutrition and accommodate nutrient needs in various disease states.
2. A patient's specific disease state and anticipated length of feeding time determine the route of enteral nutrition.
3. Gastric feeding more closely mimics how the gastrointestinal tract functions physiologically, which offers a metabolic and lifestyle benefit.
4. Small-bowel feedings are recommended for patients with gastric complications, gastroparesis, or increased aspiration risk.
5. The feeding–fasting environment associated with bolus feeding induces a favorable hormonal and nutrient response that promotes protein synthesis and anabolism.
6. Enteral nutrition formulas include carbohydrates, fat, protein, vitamins and minerals, and fiber, and are nutritionally complete.
7. Disease specific formulas that deviate from standard formulations can be used in many disease states to aid patients in meeting their nutritional needs.
8. Patients must be monitored closely for complications related to enteral feeding or side effects to medical treatment. Feeding method and formula should be adjusted as needed.

Learning Objectives

1. **Explain the evolution of today's enteral nutrition.**
2. **Identify a patient's enteral nutrition route based on the current disease state and anticipated length of feeding time.**
3. **Explore the various short-term and long-term tube placements.**
4. **Describe the types of tubes and devices available for tube feeding.**
5. **State the advantages and disadvantages of gastric versus small-bowel feeding.**
6. **Identify three different formula delivery methods.**
7. **Describe the standard composition of enteral formulas.**
8. **Explain characteristics of specialty formulas and indications for their use.**
9. **Recognize complications associated with enteral nutrition and strategies to manage them.**

Introduction

Enteral nutrition (EN) refers to the delivery of nutrients into the gastrointestinal tract either by mouth or through a feeding tube. EN includes food, oral supplements, and formulas created specifically to prevent malnutrition and accommodate nutrient needs in various disease states.[1-2] The development of EN has transformed nutritional care in a hospital setting, where the inability to receive adequate nutrition by normal means is common. Obstacles to oral intake have many causes, including gastrointestinal disease, swallowing inabilities, or increased nutrient needs related to critical illness or wound healing.[3] The use of EN to target specific immune-related and physiologic processes and alter the course of disease is an exciting aspect of enteral nutrition support that is supported by a robust research platform.

The Evolution of Enteral Nutrition

Enteral nutrition has a long history that dates back to the early 20th century. The first nasoduodenal tube was placed in 1910 and had a formula of raw egg, milk, and lactose.[4] In 1918, the first reported jejunal feeding took place using a formula of peptonized milk, dextrose, and whiskey.[4] It was not until the 1950s that the first commercial formulas were used.[4] It was at this time that flexible polyethylene tubes were developed as well. The 1970s brought increased food technology, including the formulation of more synthetic tube feeds (TFs). Low-residue and lactose-free TFs were developed, as well as TFs with a range of osmolalities.

In the 1980s, EN resurged and became more clinically formalized to support nutrition and digestion, aid wound healing, help the immune system, and support the critically ill.[5] Around this time, the first **percutaneous endoscopic gastrostomy (PEG) tube** was placed.[6,7] Tube placement capabilities became more advanced and TF products proliferated. Formula began to be fortified with fiber, predigested to include di- and tri-peptides, and enhanced to be more calorically dense. Product developers soon began to create more specialized formulas specific to certain diseases.

EN technology continued to advance in the 1990s. The potential pharmacologic role of micronutrients in modulating cellular and systemic physiology demonstrated a clear connection among disease, inflammation, and nutrient metabolism. The era of **immunonutrition**, marked by the predominance of specialty formulas enhanced with glutamine, arginine, and omega-3 fatty acids, had arrived. Research on the safety and efficacy of these formulas in altering the progression of disease, at times lagging industrial gains, continues to help guide the appropriate use of these immune-enhancing enteral products.

CORE CONCEPT 1

Enteral nutrition includes food, oral supplements, and formulas created specifically to prevent malnutrition and accommodate nutrient needs in various disease states.

Determining the Route of Enteral Nutrition

Determination of the site and route of EN should consider an individual's anticipated length of feeding time; their medical condition or disease state, including anatomical barriers within the gastrointestinal tract; and the surgical options for that individual (Figure 1).

The timing of enteral delivery is determined according to several considerations. First is the anticipated duration of enteral support. If a person is expected to require short-term tube feeding, generally 4 weeks or fewer, then a **nasoenteric** or **oroenteric** tube may be used.[1,8] Nasoenteric or oroenteric feeds require that a tube be placed in the nose or mouth and advanced into the stomach or past the pylorus. Nasoenteric tubes are used more often than oroenteric tubes for short-term feeding because they are better tolerated by the patient. If a person is in need of long-term nutrition care, or nutrition care lasting for longer than 4 weeks, then a more permanent gastrostomy or jejunostomy method is used.[2,8,9] A patient's specific needs or gastrointestinal function determines the specific enteral route, as seen in Figure 2.

CORE CONCEPT 2

A patient's specific disease state and anticipated length of feeding time determine the route of enteral nutrition.

PRACTICE POINT

If a patient requires tube feeding for 4 weeks or fewer, utilize a nasoenteric tube. If a patient requires significantly more than 4 weeks of nutrition care, a gastric or postpyloric percutaneous tube placement can be considered.

CASE STUDY INTRODUCTION

Laura is a 58-year-old female admitted to the hospital due to severe epigastric distress. She has not been able to eat in the last 48 hours due to pain. A medical work up has identified a large lesion in the distal portion of her stomach. Laura now awaits gastric surgery for removal of the tumor. She will be unable to eat for the next 2 weeks. After surgery, she will require a 12-week course of radiation and chemotherapy. Laura lives alone at home. She has two adult children. Her oldest daughter is a nurse and lives nearby.

Anthropometric Data:

Height: 152 cm (60")
Weight: 74 kg (163 lb)
Body mass index: 32 kg/m^2
Weight History
Usual Weight: 79 kg (167 lb)

Biochemical Data:

Sodium 147 (135-145 mEq/L)
Potassium 4.7 (3.6-5.0 mEq/L)
Chloride 101 (98-110 mEq/L)
Carbon dioxide 23 (20-30 mEq/L)
Blood urea nitrogen 28 (6-24 mg/dL)
Creatinine 0.5 (0.4-1.3 mg/dL)
Glucose 101 (70-139 mg/dL)
Hemoglobin 11.1 (12.0-15.5 g/dL)
Hematocrit 30 (35%-42%)

Calcium 8.7 (8.5-10.5 mEq/L)
Phosphorus 4.7 (2.7-4.5 mg/dL)
Magnesium 1.6 (1.3-2.1 mEq/L)
Total protein 6.0 (6.4-8.3 g/dL)
Albumin 3.2 (3.5-5.0 g/dL)

Clinical Data:

Past Medical History: Hyperlipidemia, gastric reflux, migraines
Medications: Avorostatin, Prevacid
Vital Signs: Blood pressure 155/77 mm Hg; temperature 99.0°C; heart rate 98 beats/min
Nutrition-focused Physical Exam: Patient appears pale and tired. Abdominal exam reveals a distended, nontender abdomen. Skin, hair, nail and oral exam appear normal. Patient noted to have adequate fat and muscle stores. No edema noted.

Dietary Data:

Dietary History: Laura typically has a good appetite. "I tend to eat healthy, but for the last 2 days, I have had pain when eating foods, and have only had broth and water or cranberry juice."
24-hour Diet Recall:
Breakfast: Coffee (cream and sugar), oatmeal with honey, or fruit with yogurt
Lunch: Turkey on whole grain bread with mustard, chocolate chip cookies, diet soda
Dinner: Salmon, rice pilaf, garden salad, glass of wine
Diet Prescription: NPO (nothing by mouth) for surgery. Nutrition consult is placed for suggestion for enteral tube feeding recommendation.

Questions

1. **What are Laura's nutritional risk factors?**
2. **What labs are concerning? What additional labs might you ask for?**
3. **What type of enteral tube feeding placement do you recommend? Explain your rationale.**
4. **Provide recommendations for enteral feeding type and method of delivery.**

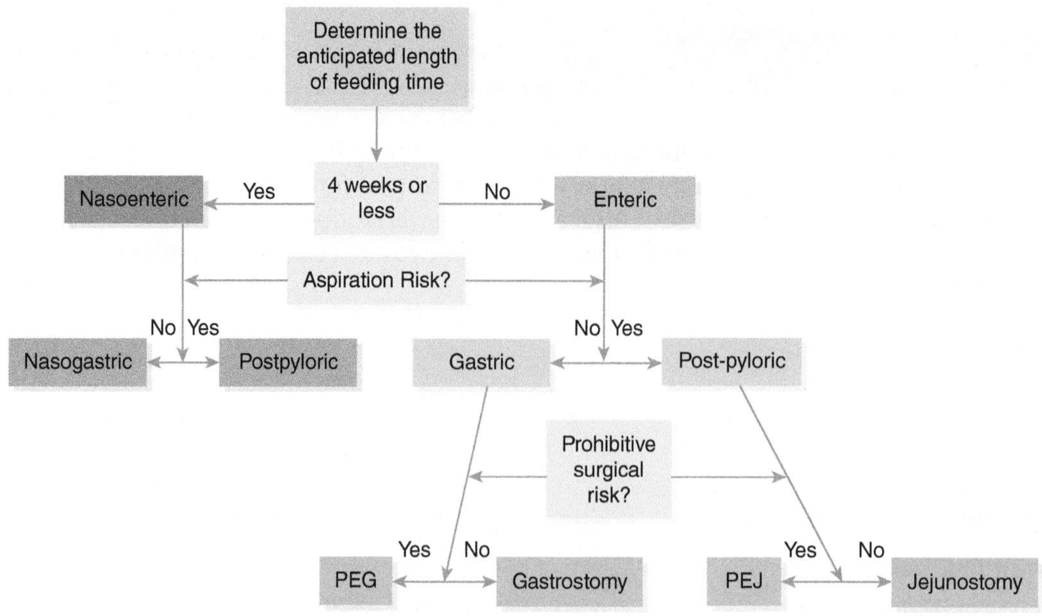

FIGURE 1 **Algorithm for Selection of Feeding Tube Placement**

Data from Gorman RC, Morris JB: Minimally invasive access to the gastrointestinal tract. In Rombeau JL, Rolandelli RH, eds. *Clinical nutrition: enteral and tube feeding*. 3rd ed. Philadelphia: WB Saunders; 1997.

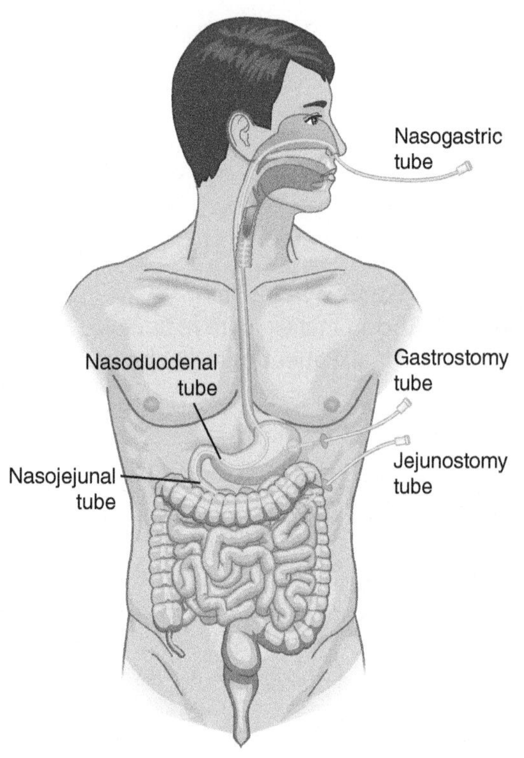

FIGURE 2 **Basic Tube Placement Options**

Short-term Placement

As mentioned, for patients who need short-term feeding, a nasoenteric or oroenteric method is used.[1,8,10-12] Nasoenteric tubes can be placed at the bedside, endoscopically, or fluoroscopically. **Nasogastric tube** placement is appropriate for patients who have normal gastric function. A tube is entered through the nose or mouth and is placed directly into the stomach. Postpyloric placement of nasoenteric tubes is used if a patient has gastric complications or aspiration risk but otherwise normal small intestine function. **Nasoduodenal tube** feeding requires the tube be placed from the nose, through the stomach, to the duodenum of the small intestine, and **nasojejunal tube** feedings require that the tube is placed from the nose and advanced to the jejunum of the small intestine. While nasogastric tubes can usually be placed at the bedside, nasojejunal tubes are better placed with endoscopic or fluoroscopic methods.[10,11]

Bedside Nasoenteral Technique

The bedside nasogastric tube placement begins by obtaining a small-bore tube, about 8 to 12 French (1 French [Fr] is equal to 0.33 mm in diameter).[13] A large-bore tube can also be used and is thought to prevent clogging; however, the small-bore tube can be more comfortable for the patient.[15] The length of the tube is determined by first measuring the distance from the patient's nose to the earlobe, and then from the earlobe to the xiphoid.[14] The patient lies on his or her right side and, as air is insufflated, the tube is bent and slowly enters through the patient's nose (Figure 3).[15,16] **Prokinetics**, which are medications that promote motility

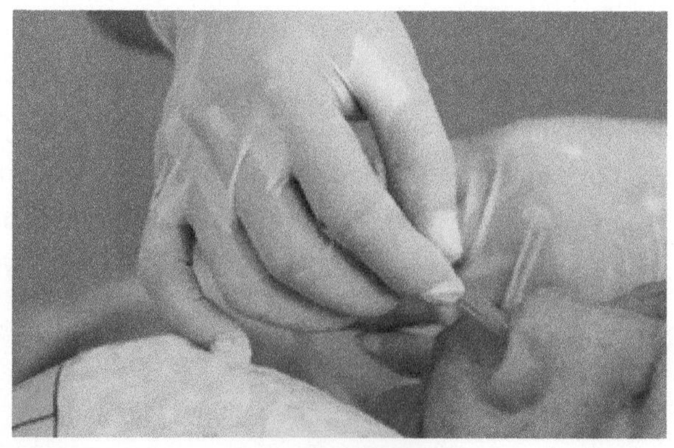

FIGURE 3 **Insertion of Nasoenteric Feeding Tube**

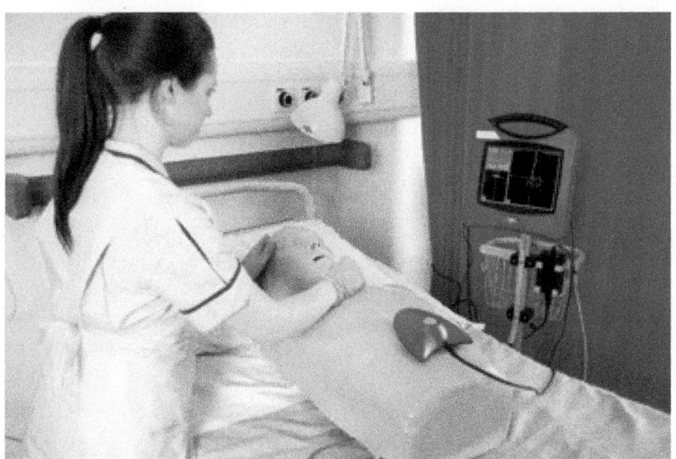

FIGURE 4 **Use of an Electromagnetically Guided Tube Placement Allows for Feedings to be Initiated Sooner and Without the Need for X-Ray**

Reproduced with permission Adam, Rouilly Limited.

by increasing small intestine contractions (such as metoclopramide and erythromycin) are often used to facilitate this technique.[14,16,17] Certain technologies are also used to ensure that the nasogastric tube is placed correctly; these include radiographs, typically a chest x-ray, as well as magnetically guided feeding tubes and electromagnetic imaging systems.[14,16,18-20] Electromagnetically guided feeding tubes have the advantage of being able to immediately confirm tube placement or identify tube misplacement so that the tube can be adjusted during placement. Not only does this alleviate the need for an additional chest x-ray, it also allows for feedings to be initiated sooner (Figure 4).[20]

Endoscopic Nasoenteral Technique

Nasoduodenal and nasojejunal tube placements are most easily done by endoscopic insertion.[16] A drag and pull technique is often utilized, where a suture is placed at the end of the nasoenteric tube and pushed with the tube from the patient's nostril to the stomach.[14,20] Meanwhile, an endoscope, with forceps, is advanced orally to the stomach.[16] In the stomach, the endoscopic forceps takes hold of the nasoenteric tube and suture, and the entire unit then enters the duodenum, or even the jejunum if possible.[14,16] In the small intestine, the forceps release the tube and the endoscope retracts.[14] Many studies suggest that there is greater placement success if the tube is placed after the ligament of Treitz.[11,14,16] With endoscopic aid, the nasoenteral tube is now properly placed in the small intestine.

Another endoscopic nasoenteral technique involves pushing an endoscope all the way to the small intestine with a guidewire to allow tube entry.[11,14,17] The guidewire is pushed through the transnasal channel with the endoscope and then remains in the small intestine while the endoscope is removed. The feeding tube is advanced over the guidewire to ultimately be placed in the small intestine through the same passage.

Fluoroscopic Nasoenteric Technique

Fluoroscopic nasoenteric tube placement involves using x-ray imaging as a guide when placing the feeding tube from the nose to the stomach or small intestine.[21] While there is success with this technique, it is not used as often as the bedside or endoscopic techniques because of radiation exposure or if the patient requires bedside attention due to critical illness.[11,17,21]

PRACTICE POINT

Nasogastric tube placement is commonly done on the patient at bedside. Nasoduodenal and nasojejunal tubes are more easily placed using endoscopic, and less commonly fluoroscopic, methods.

Long-term Placement

Percutaneous Endoscopic Gastrostomy Technique

Percutaneous endoscopic gastrostomy is the most common long-term tube placement method and can be performed at the bedside.[6,8,16,22,23] In what is called the pull technique, an endoscope is placed into the abdomen (Figure 5). Air is insufflated into the abdomen through the endoscope. The abdomen is then transilluminated to find the optimal spot for the tube placement and an indentation is placed on that spot.[16,23] After a small incision is made, a needle is placed through the abdominal wall and into the stomach so that a guidewire can be placed through the needle. An endoscopic snare is attached to the needle. The endoscope, needle, and snare are pulled back through the mouth, and the feeding tube is attached to the guidewire or placed over the guidewire.[20] The guidewire and tube are then pulled back through the esophagus and to the stomach. The tube is internally held in place by a bumper. An external bumper also ensures secure gastronomic placement.[16]

Percutaneous Endoscopic Jejunostomy Technique

If the patient has gastric complications, a **percutaneous endoscopic jejunostomy (PEJ)** can be performed. If there is an existing gastrostomy tube, a transpyloric feeding tube can be placed through the previously placed PEG tube and placed endoscopically into the jejunum.[16]

Another way of performing this procedure is to place the tube directly into the small bowel. The technique is similar to the PEG method, except the guidewire and tube are placed endoscopically into the jejunum.[6,16,22,24]

Surgical Methods

If a patient is in a traumatic condition or is undergoing surgery, a surgical means of tube placement may be used. This can be done in an open tube procedure or with laparoscopy under general anesthesia.[16,25] In **laparoscopy**, small ports are placed on the abdominal wall so that the peritoneal cavity can be accessed.[16] Once a camera and second port are placed, the stomach is attached to

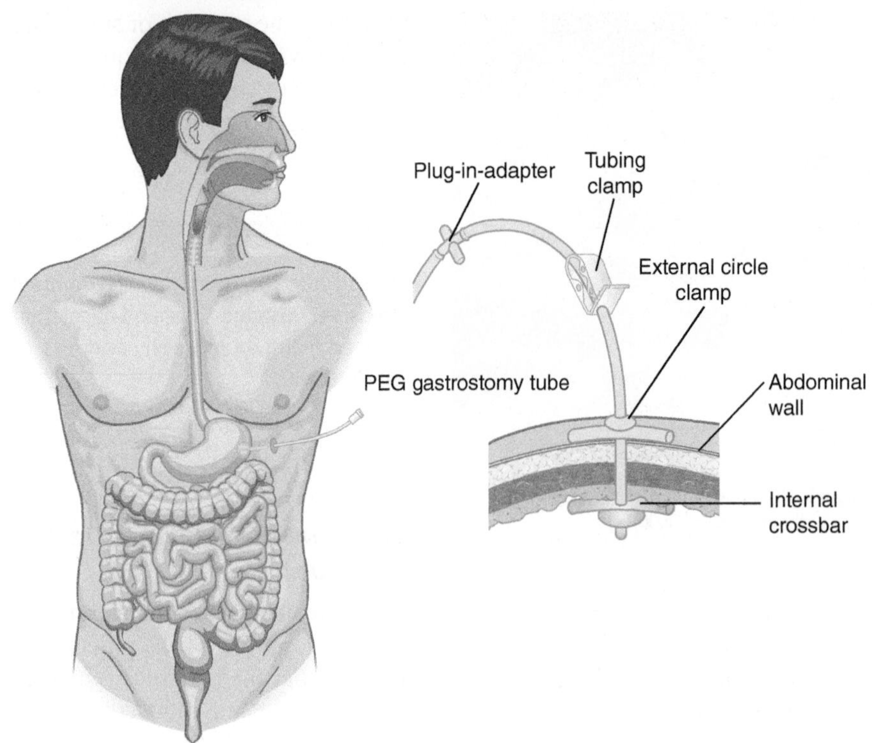

FIGURE 5 **Percutaneous Endoscopic Gastrostomy is the Most Common Long Term Tube Placement Method and can be Performed Bedside**

the abdominal wall by use of small structures called T-fasteners.[16,25] A needle and wire can then be placed into the stomach lumen so that a gastrostomy tube can finally be placed.

In the **open tube placement** technique, a small incision is made on the abdomen so that the gastrostomy tube can enter.[15,24] Sutures are placed to fasten the stomach around the feeding tube, as well as to fasten the stomach to the top of the abdomen wall.[15] Jejunostomy tubes can also be entered via open and laparoscopic techniques. A similar procedure is used in order to access the small bowel.

Types of Enteral Tubes

Feeding tubes have developed over time to become more comfortable for the patient and experience less clogging and other malfunctions. Nasogastric tubes made of polyvinyl chloride are more rigid and allow simple access. They can also be used for gastric suctioning and administering medications. Currently, most nasoenteric tubes are made out of polyurethane or silicone.[16,26,27,28] Polyurethane tubes are more pliable than polyvinyl chloride tubes and cause less nasopharyngeal erosion, which gives greater comfort to the patient. The structure of these tubes also makes it more difficult for a patient to aspirate, mitigating feeding complications. Silicone tubes are also flexible, more so than polyurethane, and therefore more comfortable to the patient. Nasoenteric tubes are generally sized 8 to 12 Fr.[16,27] For PEG tube placements, polyurethane and silicone tubes can be used, although silicone tubes tend to be used more often.[16] PEG tubes are generally sized 15 to 28 Fr in diameter.[27]

Gastric Versus Small-Bowel Feeding

There are certain indications that might prompt a clinician to initiate gastric versus postpyloric feeding in a patient. Both types have advantages and disadvantages that will be discussed further in this section.

Gastric Feeding

If normal gastric function is presumed, then gastric feedings are generally used. One advantage of gastric feedings is that they are more physiologic. The stomach acts as a natural reservoir for nutrients, so gastric placement of the feeding tube more closely mimics how the body receives nutrients.[12] It also allows for intermittent and bolus feeds, which have both metabolic and lifestyle benefits. Bolus intragastric feeding more closely resembles how the gastrointestinal tract functions physiologically, allowing contents to slowly empty into the small bowel.[12] The hydrochloric acid in the stomach also acts as bactericidal agent, providing less risk from any contaminants in the tube feeding. Also, certain nutrients require this acidification for proper absorption. Large-bore gastric tubes have less clogging than the small-bore tubes used in small-bowel feeding.[29,30] In addition, there is more ease to gastric tube placement; there are usually fewer attempts to place the tube correctly, and it can be done at bedside.[29,30] This usually makes gastric feeding more cost-effective than small-bowel feeding.[30] Lastly, the ease of bolus feedings has considerable lifestyle benefit. Incorporating bolus feedings on a routine schedule limits the amount of time the patient needs to be connected to a feeding pump, allowing more flexibility for the patient.

Clinical Roundtable

Background: One challenge to enteral feeding in a critical care setting is the need for interruption due to clinical interventions and procedures such as operating room visits, high-risk dressing changes, and extubation from a ventilator. Various strategies are employed to compensate for the energy and nutrient deficits associated with these procedures. Included among these are use of postpyloric feedings through the procedures, intermittent parenteral feedings during NPO phases, and volume-based feedings that increase the volume of feeding prior to and after procedures to assure adequate amount of feedings. Each of these strategies is associated with some degree of risk related to intolerance of feedings, aspiration, infection (in the case of PN), or hyperglycemia.

Roundtable Discussion

Discuss the pros and cons of these approaches. Are there certain patient populations that might benefit more from one approach or another? How does placement of feeding tube and central venous catheter access effect your decision?

References

1. McClave SA, Saad MA, Esterl M, et al. Volume-based feeding in the critically ill patient. *J Parenter Enteral Nutr.* 2015;39(6):707-712.
2. Varon DE, Freitas G, Goel N, et al. Intraoperative feeding improves calorie and protein delivery in acute burn patients. *J Burn Care Res.* 2017;38(5):299-303. doi: 10.1097/BCR.0000000000000514

Certain disadvantages also exist for gastric feeding. There can be several procedure-related feeding interruptions or other forms of intolerance.[29] A commonly cited risk is **aspiration**, or the movement of liquid into the patient's lungs.[29-31] Aspiration risk with continuous nasogastric feeding can lead to nosocomial (hospital-acquired) pneumonia.[12,29-31] Those who are at risk of aspiration include patients who are neurologically impaired, have experienced severe trauma, had a surgical operation, are heavily sedated, or have **gastroparesis** (delayed gastric emptying) due to a metabolic condition or operation.[29] In these cases, it may be more suitable to utilize small-bowel feeding.[29,30]

CORE CONCEPT 3

Gastric feeding more closely mimics how the gastrointestinal tract physiologically functions, which offers a metabolic and lifestyle benefit.

Small-bowel Feeding

Duodenal or jejunal feeding may be preferred if a patient has gastroparesis or reflux, or is diagnosed with aspiration risk.[29,31] It may also accommodate early satiety problems.

Small-bowel feedings afford an important advantage for patients who may have gastric complications or gastroparesis[29]. They decrease the risk of microaspiration, as well as of aspiration pneumonia.[29-31] Some studies demonstrate that small-bowel feedings allow patients to achieve a goal rate of infusion that may have not been attained with gastric feedings, providing a means of adequate nutrition.[29] It has also been shown that small-bowel feedings lead to decreased commencement of parenteral nutrition (PN). The benefit of being able to provide small-bowel feedings through clinical procedures has contributed to this decreased reliance on PN. Postpyloric feedings are now often continued during clinical interventions requiring anesthesia, either at the bedside or in the operating room. Major advancements in practice have led in some cases to intraoperative feedings, where EN is continuously provided throughout an operation. This practice has proven to be safe and effective in minimizing the energy and protein deficits that normally take place during planned surgeries.[32]

There is an increased cost associated with using small-bowel feedings, especially when using x-rays in fluoroscopy. Often, multiple attempts are needed to place the feeding tube correctly due to dislodgment of the feeding tube, and this can also be costly. Because it lacks holding capacity, the small intestine tends to be more sensitive to volume and osmotic load, so small-bowel feedings can lead to symptoms similar to **dumping syndrome**, a condition that causes rapid gastric emptying.[12] In this condition, food and liquid move from the stomach to the small intestine too quickly, causing abdominal pain and diarrhea shortly after a meal or feeding. Another disadvantage to small-bowel feedings is that bolus or large volume intermittent feeding cannot be provided.

CORE CONCEPT 4

Small-bowel feedings are recommended for patients with gastric complications, gastroparesis, or increased aspiration risk.

Formula Delivery Methods

There are several ways of delivering formula to make sure the patient is receiving adequate nutrition. Whether continuous, intermittent, or bolus feedings are used depends on the location of the feeding tube, the patient's gastrointestinal function and history of tolerance, and lifestyle considerations. Formula can be delivered to a patient via two systems. In a **closed tube feeding system**, a ready-to-use container or bag of formula is connected to the patient's feeding access.[26,33] In an **open tube feeding system**, formula from a can or package is poured into a separate container that is then attached to the patient's feeding access point.[26,33] A closed system product can safely be at room temperature for 24 to 48 hours, whereas an open system product should be at room temperature for 4 to 8 hours, depending upon the formula hanging.[26,33] This is known as the **hang time**. Reconstituted formulas should hang for no more than 4 hours while sterile decanted formula has an 8 hour hang time (except for neonates).[26,33] Clinicians may also wish to limit hang time for certain high risk populations, such as patients with burns or those who are immunocompromised. While closed tube feeding systems are preferred from an infection-control standpoint, at times open tube feeding systems are used when modular components are needed to enhance protein or calories specific to the patient's requirements.

Continuous

Continuous feeding is a common delivery method used for hospital patients. This method provides a slow infusion of feedings into the stomach or small intestine on an hourly basis. Using this method decreases risk for aspiration and gastric distention.[1] It tends to be the most easily tolerated because of its gradual delivery of feeding, and it allows for greater nutrient uptake in patients who may have marginal absorptive capacity. It also reduces the effect of thermogenesis. Most importantly, continuous feeding may be preferred for those patients with gastrointestinal complications or severe trauma because it has less risk of diarrhea and has been shown to reach nutrition goals more often.[34-36]

Despite a lack of evidence-based protocols for tube feeding advancement, conventional therapy consists of a moderate-to-low volume at initiation, followed by gradual advancement while continuously monitoring patient tolerance. Typically, continuous feeds begin at 20 to 55 mL/hour for adults and 0.5 to 1 mL/kg for children (depending on age). Once the patient can tolerate the tube feeding, the feeding rate advances incrementally. For adults, this rate increases by about 10 to 25 mL/hour every 4 to 24 hours until the goal rate is achieved. For children, this rate increases by 0.5 to 1 mL every 4 to 8 hours until the goal rate is achieved.

Intermittent

With **intermittent feeding**, feeding is delivered over a 20- to 60-minute interval, 4 to 6 times per day.[1] The duration and timing of intervals depend on the patient's formula need to attain adequate nutrition. Intermittent feeding can be administered using an infusion pump or by using the gravity drip method. Intermittent feeding provides the benefit of cyclic elevation of insulin levels. The rise in insulin in response to feeding creates an anabolic environment that promotes protein synthesis and improved protein nutritional status.[34]

Bolus Feedings

In **bolus feedings**, a specific volume of feeding is delivered over a short period of time a certain number of times per day.[1] An example feeding regimen would be rapid delivery of 200 to 400 mL of TF over approximately 5 to 20 minutes, 3 to 6 times per day.[1] Bolus feedings provide the benefit of mimicking normal eating.[1,12] Hormonal response to a feeding-fasting regimen is more anabolic than that seen with continuous feedings, resulting in increased amino acid and insulin levels and ultimately improved protein synthesis.[34] Often, a bolus regimen is preferable for stable patients because it does not rely on pumps and devices as much as the other methods, giving the patient an easier lifestyle.[1] While bolus feedings are less commonly used due to presumed risk of aspiration pneumonia and issues with tolerance, studies do not consistently support this notion, even in high-risk patients. This method of feeding, when compared to continuous feeding in critically ill adult patients, is shown to be equally well tolerated with no difference in gastroesophageal reflux, aspiration, aspiration pneumonia, glycemic variability, or time to reach calorie goal.[35-37]

CORE CONCEPT 5

The feeding–fasting environment associated with bolus feeding induces a favorable hormonal and nutrient response that promotes protein synthesis and anabolism.

CASE STUDY REVISITED

A percutaneous jejunostomy was successfully placed for enteral feedings. Laura is to remain NPO for 2 days. A nutrition consult is written for initiation of enteral feedings in 48 hours.

Her estimated energy and protein requirements based on your nutrition standard of care for surgical patients with mild stress/trauma are below:

Energy: 2,220 kcals per day (30 kcal/kg)

Protein: 111 g protein per day (1.5 g/kg)

Questions

1. **What general type of enteral feeding do you recommend (intact, semi-elemental, elemental)?**
2. **Do you recommend a standard or disease-specific enteral type of feeding?**
3. **Provide a recommendation for EN, including EN type, goal volume, method of delivery, and guidelines for initiation and advancement.**

Enteral Formula Compositions

A clinician must determine a formula that will meet a patient's nutrient needs. Many different standard formulas exist that are strategic compilations of carbohydrates, fat, protein, fiber, prebiotics and probiotics, vitamins, minerals, and water. Formulas for individuals with impaired digestion, also known as predigested; semi-elemental; or elemental formulas are available as well. Additionally, certain EN feedings are created for patients with specific diseases and conditions, such as diabetes; severe wounds; or complications with renal, pulmonary, or liver function. Lastly, immune-enhancing feedings are available for the critically ill and patients with altered metabolism. **Table 1** shows various EN products categorized by composition and indication for use.

TABLE 1 TYPES OF TUBE FEEDING FORMULAS FOR ADULTS

Formula	Indication	Examples
Standard	Normal gastrointestinal function and fluid needs, feeding well-tolerated	Osmolite Promote Nutren Replete
Standard with Fiber	Long-term need for tube feeding; diarrhea and/or constipation	Jevity Promote with fiber Nutren with fiber Replete with fiber
Standard-Nutrient Dense (high nitrogen or high calorie)	Increased wound healing	Osmolite 1 .2, 1.5 Jevity 1.2, 1.5 Isosource 1.5 Nutren 1.5
Fluid-Restricted	Restricted fluid allowance	Two Cal HN Nutren 2.0
Peptide-Based (partially hydrolyzed whey protein)	Impaired digestion	Peptamen, Peptamen 1.5 w/Prebio Vital Vital 1.5
Amino Acid Based (100% free amino acids)	Impaired digestion	Vivonex T.E.N
Immune-Enhanced	State of stress or trauma	Impact, Oxepa, Pivot
Renal	Kidney dysfunction and restrictions of potassium, phosphorus, and fluid	Nepro, Suplena Novosource Renal
Diabetes	Moderate carbohydrate, fiber enhanced	Glucerna Glytrol Diabetisource
Pulmonary	Moderate to low carbohydrate, higher fat content	Pulmocare Nutren Pulmonary
Hepatic	High branched-chain amino acids, low aromatic amino acids	Nutrihep

Tables 2 and 3 provide the nutrient composition of standard polymeric formulas and products used for patients with impaired digestion. The general nutritional content of these is similar; however, for those with impaired digestion, simpler or easier to digest forms of carbohydrate, protein, and fat are provided.

Carbohydrates

Carbohydrates are the primary energy source of enteral formula. They generally comprise 40%–90% of the formula.[38] Carbohydrate sources include monosaccharides such as glucose or fructose, and disaccharides including sucrose and maltose. Lactose is often omitted from enteral feeding products because it requires lactase, which is insufficient in some patients, leading to poor tolerance and symptoms of cramping, bloating and diarrhea.[38]

Other types of carbohydrates incorporated into formula include oligosaccharides and polysaccharides. Oligosaccharides are made of 2 to 10 glucose units. The most common oligosaccharide used in formula is maltodextrin, which is

TABLE 2 NUTRIENT COMPOSITION OF STANDARD ADULT POLYMERIC ENTERAL FORMULATIONS

Formula Name	Jevity Jevity 1.2 Jevity 1.5	Osmolite Osmolite 1.2 Osmolite 1.5	Promote Promote with Fiber	Replete Replete with Fiber	Nutren 1.0 Nutren 1.0 with Fiber Nutren 1.5	Two Cal HN Nutren 2.0
Concentration (kcal/mL)	1.06 1.2 1.5	1.06 1.2 1.5	1.0 1.0	1.0 1.0	1.0 1.0 1.5	2.0 2.0
Protein g/1,000 mL (% kcal)	44.3 (16.7) 55.5 (18.5) 63.8(17)	44.3 (16.7) 55.5 (18.5) 62.7 (16.7)	62.5 (25) 62.5 (25)	64 (25) 64 (25)	40 (16) 40 (16) 68 (18)	83.5 (16.7) 48 (16)
Carbohydrate g/1,000 mL (% kcal)	154.7 (58.3) 169.4 (56.4) 215.7 (57.5)	143.9 (54.3) 157.5 (52.5) 203.6 (54.3)	130 (52) 138.3 (55)	112 (45) 124 (45)	136 (54) 148 (54) 176 (47)	218.5 (43.2) 216 (43)
Fat g/1,000 mL (% kcal)	34.7 (29) 39.3 (29) 49.8 (30)	34.7 (29) 39.3 (29) 49.1 (29)	26 (23) 28.2 (25)	34 (30) 34 (30)	34 (30) 34 (30) 60 (35)	90.5 (40.1) 92 (41)
Sodium/ Potassium (mg/1000 mL)	930/1570 1,350/1850 1,400/2150	930/1570 1,340/1810 1,400/800	1,000/1,980 1,300/2,100	880/1,600 880/1,600	880/1,600 880/1,600 1,300/2,400	1,450/2,440 1,500/2,100
Calcium/ Phosphorus (mg/1000 mL)	910/760 1,200/1,200 1,200/1,200	760/760 1,200/1,200 1,000/1,000	1,200/1,200 1,200/1,200	800/800 800/800	800/800 800/800 1,200/1,200	1,050/1,050 1,600/1,400
Vitamin D (IU/1000 mL)	305 400 400	305 400 400	400 400	400 400	400 400 640	415 800
Zinc/Copper (mg/1000 mL)	18/1.6 23/2.0 23/2.0	18/1.6 23/2.0 23/2.0	24/2 24/2	16/1.6 16/1.6	14/1.6 14/1.6 20/2	24/2.1 24/2.4
Selenium (mcg/ 1000 mL)	54 70 70	54 70 70	70 70	60 60	60 60 80	74 100

TABLE 3 NUTRIENT COMPOSITION OF HYDROLYZED AND MONOMERIC ENTERAL FORMULATIONS

Formula Name	Vivonex TEN	Vital	Peptamen	Peptamen 1.5 with Prebio
Concentration (kcal/mL)	1.0	1.0	1.0	1.5
Protein g/1,000 mL (% kcal)	38.3 (14)	40 (16)	40 (16)	68 (18)
Carbohydrate g/1,000 mL (% kcal)	206 (83)	130 (52)	128 (51)	184 (48)
Fat g/1,000 mL (% kcal)	3 (3)	38.1 (34)	39.2 (33)	56 (34)
Sodium/Potassium (mg/1,000 mL)	617/937	1,050/1,400	560/1,500	1,020/1,860
Calcium/Phosphorus (mg/1,000 mL)	500/500	705/705	800/700	1,000/1,000
Vitamin D (IU/1,000 mL)	403	280	13.2 (mcg)	20 (mcg)
Zinc/Copper (mg/1,000 mL)	11/1.0	21/1.4	24/2.0	36/3.0
Selenium (mcg/1,000 mL)	37	56	50	76

more soluble than starch and contributes less to the osmolality of the formula than glucose alone. Polysaccharides are made of more than 10 glucose units and include corn syrup solids and cornstarch.

Fats

Fats, or triglycerides, are composed of glycerol and fatty acids. They consist of chains of carbons with a carboxyl group at the end. The chain length influences the feeding tolerance, and the type of chain (such as monounsaturated fatty acids, saturated fatty acids, or polyunsaturated fatty acids) influences a patient's physiology.[38] Lipids are a secondary energy source in formula composition. Common sources of lipids in formula include corn oil, safflower oil, and coconut oil.[38] In addition to providing energy, lipids are an important component of enteral formulas because they carry fat-soluble vitamins and essential fatty acids that are important for physiologic function. Lipids are also isotonic, which helps lower the osmolality of the formula.

Often, a mixture of long-chain and medium-chain fatty acids are used in enteral formulations. Long-chain fatty acids are carbon chains of 14 to 24 units. These are cleared slowly from the bloodstream and are preferentially re-esterified and stored as triglycerides. Long-chain fatty acids require carnitine, which aids in the transport of long-chain fatty acids across the mitochondrial membrane for energy production. Long-chain fatty acids are also a source of essential fatty acids, such as linoleic and linolenic fatty acids.

For patients with impaired digestion, absorption, and transport of fats, medium-chain fatty acids can be added to the formula.[35] Medium-chain fatty acids are carbon chains of 6 to 12 units. Common sources include palm kernel oil and coconut oil. Medium-chain fatty acids are easier to digest because they absorbed directly into portal circulation and are not re-esterified to triglycerides. They do not require pancreatic enzymes or bile salts for absorption. They also do not require carnitine for transport across the mitochondrial membrane. Therefore, medium-chain fatty acids are a rapid energy source. However, because medium-chain fatty acids do not provide any essential fatty acids, some long-chain fatty acids are usually concurrently added to make sure the patient meets nutrient needs.[35]

PRACTICE POINT

Medium-chain fatty acids are absorbed directly into the portal system and are easier to digest; however, they do not provide essential fatty acids and so long-chain fatty acids should be provided as well.

Protein

Protein in enteral formulas can come in different forms, depending on what is indicated by the patient's need and medical condition. These forms of protein include intact proteins, hydrolyzed protein, or free amino acids.[38] Intact proteins are large in size and have limited impact on the osmolality of a formula. They are the original, natural form of the protein, called an **isolate**.[38] Examples of intact proteins include soy isolates, casein or whey protein from milk, and the albumen from egg white. Intact proteins require normal levels of pancreatic enzymes for adequate digestion. For patients with gastrointestinal dysfunction or malabsorption issues, semi-elemental or elemental formulations may be used. These include hydrolyzed proteins such as di-peptides, tri-peptides, and free amino acids. These types of proteins are enzymatically broken down to smaller particles and increase the osmolality of the formula. The intestine can digest both smaller peptides and free amino acids because they use separate transport systems. Formulas may prefer smaller peptides because they are thought to more efficiently absorb nitrogen, but free amino acids and di- and tri-peptides cause less trophic stimulation on the bowel than intact protein.

Vitamins and Minerals

Vitamins and minerals are vital components in enteral formula. These micronutrients play an important role in the body as essential cofactors and coenzymes that are needed for metabolism and other physiologic functions. Formulas generally have 100% of the recommended dietary allowance (RDA) of each vitamin and mineral at specific volumes. Different metabolic stresses and disease states may require a higher or lower amount of certain micronutrients.

Fiber

Dietary fiber comes in soluble and insoluble forms and is added to some enteral formulas. Fiber is a plant polysaccharide that is indigestible by human digestive enzymes. The formulas that include fiber generally have about 4 to 14 g/L of total fiber.

Soluble fiber is viscous and found in legumes, oat bran, pectins, and gums. Anaerobic bacteria in the cecum rapidly ferment soluble fiber into short-chain fatty acids. Short-chain fatty acids offer the health benefits of maintaining colonic structure and function. This includes lowering the colonic pH to balance intestinal flora. It also enhances fluid and electrolyte absorption, which may help with diarrhea. Soluble fiber intake is also linked to lower serum cholesterol, as well as improved glucose tolerance. Soluble fiber is important to include in enteral formulas of patients who have glucose intolerance, have had bowel surgery, or are undergoing antibiotic therapy.

Insoluble fiber is nonviscous and found in the cellulose of plant foods. Insoluble fiber is beneficial because it holds water. This increases bulk in fecal mass and allows softer stools, which helps prevent constipation and is recommended for those undergoing long-term feeding. Insoluble fiber may also be beneficial for patients with diverticulosis, which is when pouches accumulate in the colon.

Pre- and Probiotics

Some formulas also include prebiotics and probiotics to promote gut health; however, the benefit of these additions is still under debate. Because outcomes differ per patient and condition, it is currently difficult to make any broad recommendation for prebiotics and probiotics in formula.

Prebiotics are energy sources for the beneficial bacteria in the colon, commonly provided in EN formulas as fiber, fructo-oligosaccharides, and inulin. Food sources include artichokes, banana, onions, garlic, and soy. Prebiotics are generally included with probiotics so that the microorganisms can flourish. **Probiotics** are ingested microorganisms thought to promote beneficial gut microflora and gastrointestinal function, as well as compete against pathogenic bacteria. A common form used in formula is lactic acid bacteria. Research suggests that prebiotics and probiotics in preterm infant formula have had successful outcomes, helping gut microbiota and gastrointestinal function, as well as decreasing mortality risk.[39,40] Use of probiotics also has been shown to reduce the risk of necrotizing enterocolitis in preterm infants, a condition in which damaged intestinal tissue cause bloating, diarrhea, inflammation, and infection.[39]

Because critical illness and its management alter the microflora, resulting in a loss of commensal flora and abundance of pathogenic flora, considerable interest in probiotic therapy exists.[41-43] Meta-analyses show a reduction in antibiotic-associated diarrhea with probiotic use, but the heterogeneity of the pooled data makes it difficult to draw conclusions to specific populations.[42] While favorable, the data have not been consistent with respect to risk and benefit of probiotics. Systematic reviews reveal no improvement in mortality, pneumonia, or length of intensive care unit stay with use of probiotics. Furthermore, safety concerns have been raised due to increased gut ischemia in probiotic treatment groups.[41,44] The risk of translocation and improper administration of probiotics, resulting in blood infection, has caused the U.S. Food and Drug Administration to issue a black box warning for probiotic use in hospitalized patients. Prebiotics and probiotics are not generally included in standard formula because evidence is still inconclusive on their health benefits for mortality risk or infectious complications. Research is also needed to clarify which strands are most beneficial to humans, especially because the microbiota in the gastrointestinal tract are so complex.

PRACTICE POINT

Enteral feedings can provide a mixture of soluble and insoluble fiber. Advancement of fiber-containing feeds should take into consideration the total amount of fiber provided based on EN goal rate as well as history of gastrointestinal function to assure adequate tolerance.

CORE CONCEPT 6

Enteral nutrition formulas include carbohydrates, fat, protein, vitamins and minerals, and fiber adequate for meeting full nutrient requirements in most patients.

Disease-Specific Formulas

Certain health conditions require specific enteral formulations to ensure a patient meets their nutrient needs. Selection of enteral formula takes into account a patient's fluid limitations, electrolyte imbalances, increased nutrient requirement, decreased ability to receive nutrients due to disease or condition, and ease of digestion (Table 4).

Renal Dysfunction

Patients with renal dysfunction may require a formula that is more calorically dense and lower in phosphorus and potassium than standard polymeric TFs. Renal formulas should also assure protein of high biological value to include proportionately more essential amino acids. Patients who have stage 3 or 4 chronic kidney disease and are not yet on dialysis may need less protein in their formula. Amounts of potassium, phosphorus, and sodium are also reduced. When on dialysis or renal replacement therapy, formula composition is higher in protein to reflect increased protein losses associated with these therapies. Supplementation with enteral feedings designed for renal patients or essential amino acids is associated with improved markers of nutritional status (as evidenced by body mass index, hand grip strength, and mid-arm circumference) as well as serum albumin and prealbumin.[45]

TABLE 4 DISEASE-SPECIFIC ENTERAL FORMULATIONS

Formula Name	Nutrihep	Nepro	Glucerna	Pulmocare
Concentration (kcal/mL)	1.5	1.8	1.0	1.5
Protein g/1,000 mL (% kcal)	40 (11)	81 (18)	41.8 (17)	62.6 (17)
Carbohydrate g/1,000 mL (% kcal)	290 (77)	161 (36)	95.6 (38)	105.7 (28)
Fat g/1,000 mL (% kcal)	21.2 (13)	96 (48)	54.4 (49)	93.3 (56)
Sodium/Potassium (mg/1,000 mL)	160/1,320	1,060/1,060	930/1,570	1,310/1,960
Calcium/Phosphorus (mg/1,000 mL)	956/1,000	1,060/720	705/705	1,060/1,060
Vitamin D (IU/1,000 mL)	400	85	285	425
Zinc/Copper (mg/1,000 mL)	15.2/2.0	27/2.1	16/1.5	24/2.2
Selenium (mcg/1,000 mL)	NA	74	50	74

Pulmonary Dysfunction

Formulas for patients with pulmonary dysfunction have a modified carbohydrate-to-fat ratio to decrease carbohydrate intake. Oxidation of carbohydrate results in greater carbon dioxide (CO_2) production than fat oxidation. This is considered especially useful in patients with **hypercapnia** (CO_2 retention). Clinically, use of high-fat, low-carbohydrate TF in patients with chronic obstructive pulmonary disease may improve pulmonary function (forced expiratory volume in 1 second, minute ventilation, oxygen consumption, and CO_2 production) as well as arterial blood gases.[46,47] Many formulas for pulmonary patients also incorporate immune-enhancing nutrients such omega-3 fatty acids and antioxidants. Omega-3 fatty acids are anti-inflammatory and signal pathways that complement therapeutic efforts to maximize lung function. Use of omega-3 fatty acids in patients with acute respiratory distress is associated with improved lung injury scores, fewer days on mechanical ventilation, and reduced stays on the intensive care unit.[48] The role of antioxidants in fighting free radicals and reducing lung cell injury remains a primary research interest.

Liver Dysfunction

Patients with advanced liver disease often have ascites, or fluid accumulation in the abdomen, which may cause them to not utilize nutrients efficiently. Because of this condition, formulas for these patients are often calorically dense, providing a high calorie-to-nitrogen ratio. Protein composition in formulations designed for patients with liver failure include a higher proportion of branched chain amino acids (BCAA) with lesser amounts of aromatic amino acids in attempt to minimize hepatic encephalophathy (a condition that is associated with liver disease). Levels of BCAA are often low in patients with liver disease due to their increased uptake in skeletal muscle to help detoxify and reduce ammonia.[49] While there is a lack of compelling evidence that nutritional support (enteral, parenteral, or oral) improves clinical outcomes in liver failure overall, use of BCAA-enhanced formulas during hepatic encephalopathy may be considered.[50]

Diabetes

Most patients with diabetes can be treated with standard polymeric TFs. Fiber-containing TFs by slowing gastric emptying and digestion of carbohydrates, can improve glycemic control. For better glycemic control, diabetes-specific feedings, which are higher in fructose and monounsaturated fatty acids, can be used.[51] These formulas generally have a carbohydrate content of about 35% to 40% of calories, approximately 10 to 15 g/L of soluble fiber, and fat (40%-50% of calories). In critically ill patients, where hyperglycemia can be exacerbated, diabetes-specific formulas improve glycemic control, lower insulin requirements, and decrease risk of acquired infections.[52] Because gastroparesis is common among diabetics, diabetes-specific formulas, given their higher fat and soluble fiber, may be poorly tolerated; postpyloric feedings can be used in these instances.

Trauma/Wound Healing

Specialty formulations are available for use in patients with trauma or increased wound healing requirements. EN solutions that are high in protein and include arginine and glutamine, as well as micronutrients zinc and vitamin C, should enhance the process of wound healing due to their effects on protein anabolism (arginine and glutamine) and collagen synthesis (zinc and vitamin C). Pressure injury healing time has been shown to decrease with use of these formulations.[53] Use of immune-enhancing formulas to promote wound healing in critically ill patients continues to be explored. These will be described in more detail in the immunonutrition section of this chapter.

CORE CONCEPT 7

Disease specific formulas that deviate from standard formulations can be used in many disease states to aid patients in meeting their nutritional needs.

Developing an EN Feeding Plan

Table 5 provides a step-wise procedure for developing an EN feeding plan for a patient. The first step is selection of EN type. Based on the plethora of EN products, a clinician must evaluate what formula to select based on a patient's nutrient requirements; clinical status, including fluid restrictions and electrolyte requirements; degree of metabolic stress; wound healing requirements; gastrointestinal function; cost; and supporting evidence of benefit and risk of specific nutrient components provided, particularly in disease-specific and immune-enhancing feeds. Figure 6 shows a mechanism for determining an optimal TF type.

Complication Monitoring

Patients who are receiving TF must be monitored routinely, because complications can arise. Clinicians must check for signs of nausea and vomiting, make note of the **gastric residuals** (volume of liquid that remains in stomach during enteral feeding), obtain a baseline of the abdominal girth with routine subsequent monitoring, and keep track of stool patterns. Certain complications can be associated with enteral feeding, as well as illness or treatment side effects that a patient may be experiencing. These include nausea and vomiting, aspiration, abdominal distention, delayed gastric emptying, constipation, and diarrhea.[54,55]

Aspiration

Aspiration is a common complication associated with tube feeding. It occurs when a patient inhales a substance, such as water or tube feed, into the airway, which causes dyspnea and coughing. Prolonged aspiration is dangerous because it can lead to pneumonia.[54]

TABLE 5	STEP-WISE PROCESS FOR DETERMINATION OF TUBE FEEDING VOLUME AND DELIVERY	
Step 1	Choose the EN formula type based on condition. Examples: Standard, Condition (Impaired Digestion, Stress/Trauma), Disease-Specific	Example: 58-year-old male with head injury due to motorcycle accident with a nasogastric feeding tube EN Formula: Replete
Step 2	Determine the amount of EN volume needed to meet the calorie goal.* 24-hour Calorie Goal/Formula Concentration (kcal/mL) = Total volume of EN needed over 24 hours *Consider: Stress level, malnourished vs. well nourished; clinical factors (intubated, sedated, sepsis); physical activity	Energy Goal: 2,000 kcal Protein Goal: 130 g protein Replete (1.0 kcal/mL) = 2,000 mL
Step 3	Calculate protein intake at that EN volume to assure protein is in range of patient's goal (Total EN volume/1000) × protein (g/L) = g protein/day OR (Total calorie intake at EN goal rate × % calories as protein)/4 = g protein/day	Replete has 62.5 g protein per 1,000 mL. 2,000/1000 = 2.000 × 62.5 g = 125 g protein on this regimen Protein intake is sufficient
Step 4	If both calorie and protein needs are met, determine hourly rate: EN volume/24 = hourly rate * Rounding numbers is preferred to make daily calculations of input/output and order writing simplified If protein needs are not met, consider a nutrient-dense feeding with higher nitrogen or adding modular protein	Hourly EN = ~2,000 mL/24 = 83.3 mL/hr Round up to 85 mL/hr
Step 5	Provide your TF type and hourly goal rate.	Full-strength Replete @ 85 mL/hr
Step 6	Document what the TF will actually provide. Note: This may be a little different from your initially established goal, due to rounding and fine-tuning	This regimen provides 2,040 kcal/128 g protein

CASE STUDY REVISITED

Laura was seen today in the clinic after completion of her first 6 weeks of chemotherapy. Treatment is going well for Laura; however, despite previously good tolerance, she is now experiencing diarrhea. It is unclear whether this is due to her treatment or the TF she is receiving.

Questions

1. **What factors might be contributing to her diarrhea?**
2. **How might you resolve antibiotic-induced diarrhea?**

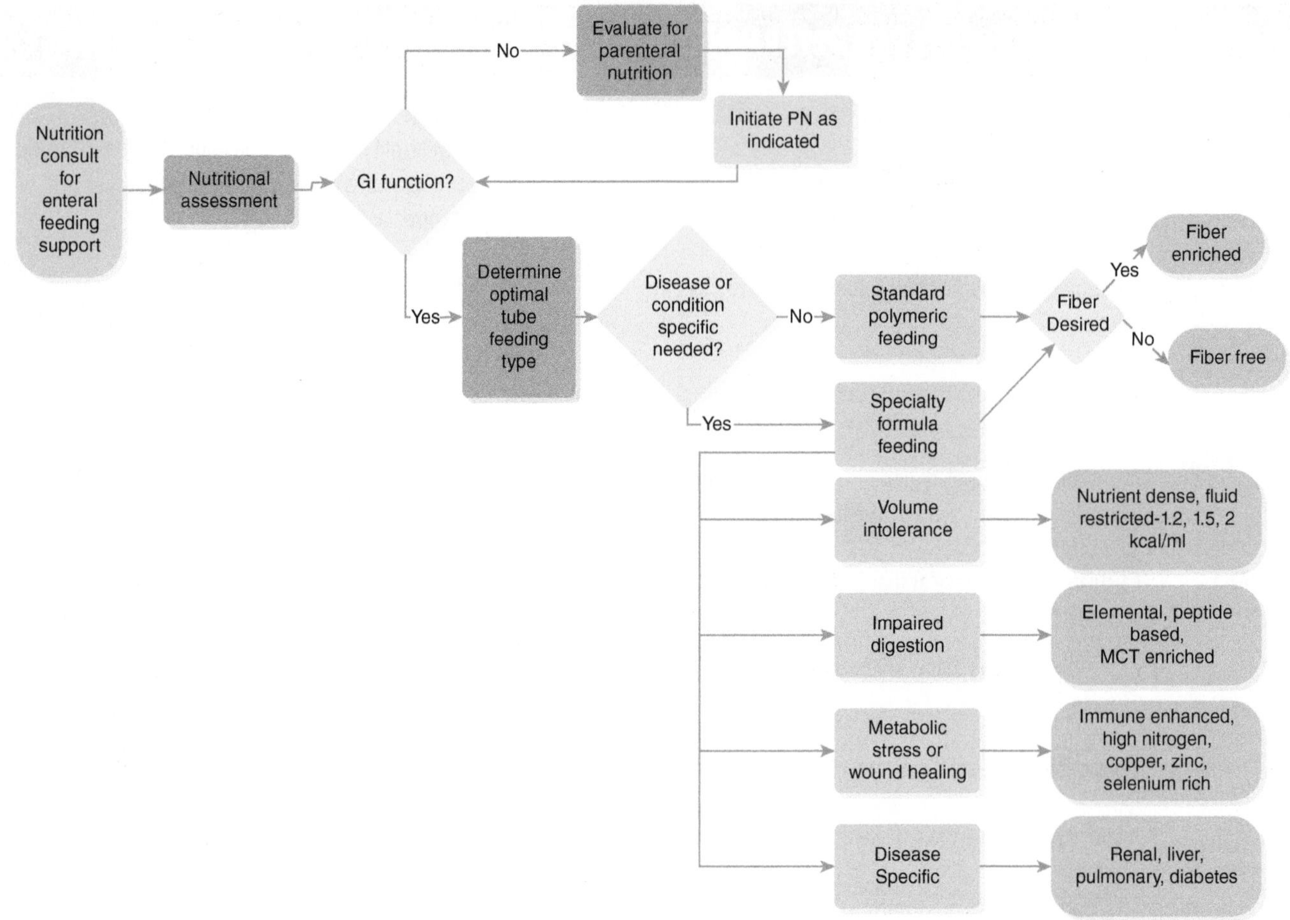

FIGURE 6 **Algorithm for Determining Tube Feeding Type**

Nausea/Vomiting

Nausea and vomiting are common complications to enteral feeding and increase the risk of aspiration and pneumonia.[54] There are many possible causes of nausea or vomiting. Both gastric retention and rapid infusion of hyperosmolar formula can cause nausea/vomiting. In these cases, a clinician must reduce the rate of feeding, but if the patient is vomiting, feedings should be held. The fat content of feeds also affects a patient's tolerance, with feedings that are lower in fat being generally better tolerated. The smell of the formula can affect the patient. Elemental formulas usually have a more unpleasant odor than polymeric formulas.

Abdominal Distention

Abdominal distention is the accumulation of air or liquid in a patient's abdomen and can cause major discomfort to the patient. Abdominal distention can be diagnosed by observing an increase in abdominal girth (about 8-10 cm) and/or palpating the abdomen.[54] A patient's report of symptoms such as bloating and cramping can also indicate abdominal distention.[54] Rapid bolus or intermittent feeds of cold formula can cause abdominal distention. Using continuous and room-temperature feeds can treat this. Abdominal distention can also be caused by nutrient malabsorption, delayed gastric emptying, or the onset of a septic episode.

PRACTICE POINT

Baseline and daily measurement of abdominal girth is useful for monitoring feeding tolerance and onset of sepsis. Sudden increases in abdominal girth may indicate the onset of a septic episode.

Gastroparesis (Delayed Gastric Emptying)

Many factors can delay the emptying of gastric contents into the small bowel. Gastroparesis can be induced by trauma or be caused by certain medications, such as opiates or paralytics. In order to mitigate the risk of gastroparesis, a clinician may check gastric residual volume (GRV) before initiating tube feeding, as well as every 4 hours after tube feeding. When monitoring gastric residuals, gastric fluid is suctioned. The amount of fluid collected is measured over 24 hours. Normal GRVs range from 250 to 500 mL.[56,57] Anything greater than 600 mL may indicate delayed gastric emptying, which puts a patient at risk for aspiration. Feeding tolerance, feeding administration rate, and duodeno-gastric reflux may also contribute to delayed gastric emptying and aspiration risk; therefore, certain adjustments may be instituted.[57] Continuous feeds may be preferred over intermittent or bolus feeds to normalize gastric emptying. A formula free of fiber and low in fat can also help. Prokinetic agents, such as metoclopramide and erythromycin, can mitigate delayed gastric emptying by increasing gastric motility.[14,16,17] Controversy exists about whether checking gastric residuals is truly necessary.[56,57] However, despite this controversy, it remains a common practice for patients in critical care.[57]

Constipation

Certain medications can cause constipation. It is therefore important to have a proactive bowel regime. Dehydration and lack of fiber are also frequent causes of constipation. Adding additional fluid to the formula in addition to fiber can prevent waste buildup.[45] Fecal impaction or obstruction is a type of stool accumulation that can be diagnosed by a rectal exam. Fecal implantation can be alleviated by rectal exam if it is close to the rectum, but surgical or endoscopic methods may have to be used if the impaction is higher in the colon.[45]

Diarrhea

Diarrhea is higher stool frequency, volume, and water content.[54] Most causes of diarrhea are not incidental to tube feeding. Certain medications, especially those containing magnesium, phosphorus, and sorbitol, can be hyperosmolar, causing diarrhea. Diarrhea can also be due to bacterial growth.[54] Prolonged antibiotic use creates an imbalance in gut microflora, resulting in antibiotic associated diarrhea. Despite the fact that *Clostridium difficile*, a bacteria that causes diarrhea, is only one of the possible causes, a stool culture is often done to confirm antibiotic-induced diarrhea. Use of pre- and probiotics promotes proliferation and can restore the patient's microbiota to resolve diarrhea associated with harmful bacterial overgrowth.[41,42]

Diarrhea can also be caused by aspects directly related to tube feeding. Included among these are rapid feed infusion, hyperosmolar formula, carbohydrate malabsorption, or intolerance to lactose in the formula. Additionally, patients can be exposed to bacterial growth on the tubing itself, leading to diarrhea. To prevent this, a closed tube feeding system can be used every 24 to 48 hours. Tubing should be changed every 24 hours. In an open system, formula hang time should be limited to 4 to 8 hours.[26,33] Tube feeding containers and tubing should be flushed frequently. Sterile water must always be used for reconstitution.

CORE CONCEPT 8

Patients must be monitored closely for complications related to enteral feeding or side effects to medical treatment. Feeding method and formula should be adjusted as needed.

Early Enteral Nutrition

Early enteral nutrition (EEN) generally refers to the initiation of EN within 48 hours of illness or a traumatic event. There are numerous proposed benefits to EEN, particularly in patients with systemic inflammation as is associated with multiple trauma, large burn injury, and acute pancreatitis. However, certain risks and complications associated with EEN mean that its use is controversial.[58-65] Evidence suggests that EEN reduces all-cause mortality,[59-62] shortens time needed to meet caloric and protein needs, and decreases hospital length of stay.[61,63,64] EEN also reduces cost of hospital-related expenses.[62] Many disease-related complications, including infections, are minimized with EEN.[61,63,64,66] There may be some benefit of EEN attenuating the postsurgical or trauma stress response.[64,67]

Although it is intuitive that enteral nutrition maintains gut integrity, EEN does so through increased **postprandial hyperemic response**.[68,69] With many diseases, blood flow to the intestine is diminished to accommodate other vital organs, complicating gastrointestinal function. However, enteral nutrients increase perfusion to the gastrointestinal tract; when cautiously delivered, EEN can be beneficial to gut integrity and prevention of ischemia.[70]

Although many benefits with EEN have been presented, EEN may not be indicated in certain scenarios. There are insufficient data to support whether EEN could be beneficial to respiratory-compromised or unstable hyperemic patients.[69-71] Because feedings can increase gut oxygen needs beyond what can be met, as well as induce gut ischemia or worsen an existing ischemic condition, EEN may be contraindicated. These findings underscore the delicate balance between promoting perfusion with judicious EEN and inducing gut ischemia through excessive nutrient provision.[70] Aspiration pneumonia is another concern because a patient may not be able to handle a substantial feeding load so early in treatment, depending on the disease or complication.[70] There are also inconsistencies in data supporting EEN reducing length of stay and infections.[70] Some studies also suggest that EEN alone may not be sufficient for a patient to meet nutritional needs.[70,71] These findings are a reminder that provision of EEN should be in conjunction with standardized criteria and close monitoring (Table 6).[59,71]

TABLE 6 CONTRAINDICATIONS FOR EARLY ENTERAL FEEDING[60]
Hemodynamically unstable; uncontrolled shock
Uncontrolled hypoxemia, hypercapnia, or acidosis
Overt bowel ischemia
High-output fistula if EEN cannot be safely provided distal to fistula
Abdominal compartment syndrome
Upper gastrointestinal bleed
Large gastrointestinal aspirates (>500 mL/24 hours)

Data from Reintam Blaser A, Starkopf J, Alhazzani W, et al. Early enteral nutrition in critically ill patients: ESICM clinical practice guidelines. *Intensive Care Medicine*. 2017;43(3):380-398. doi: 10.1007/s00134-016-4665-0.

Immunonutrition

Immunonutrition refers to the use of nutrients to alter or attenuate the inflammatory or immune response. This differs from conventional nutrition support therapy, where provision of nutrients is aimed at preventing deficiency or meeting requirements for increased utilization or losses. Nutrients such as the conditionally essential amino acids glutamine and arginine, omega-3 fatty acids, and antioxidants are considered to be beneficial in modulating inflammation and the course of disease. Today, numerous enteral formulations exist with these nutrients, either alone or in combination. These products often are used in critically ill patients in an attempt to counteract the inflammatory response to stress, both at the systemic and cellular levels. Research into the role of these select nutrients is ongoing and inconclusive despite the plethora of immune-enhancing specialty formulas. Scientific evidence of the potential benefit of these products, as well as possible harm, is ongoing.

Gastrointestinal Tract as an Immune Organ

Traditionally the gastrointestinal tract is viewed for its primary role in digestion and absorption (Figure 7). However, a better understanding of its morphology, structure, and mediatory response to stress clearly establishes the gut as having immunologic functions. First and foremost, the gut acts as a barrier to invasive organisms, preventing the spread of bacteria and toxins to other organs. This is accomplished through microbial, immunologic, and mechanical aspects of the gut. Increasing evidence confirms the role of the microbiome in immunology and health. Bacteria that are part of the normal intestinal flora inhibit colonization of invading bacteria, most basically by limiting the amount of space for bacteria to exist (Figure 8). Simply by virtue of their numbers, the normal gut bacteria can reduce the potential for bacterial invasion. In addition to space, the existing microbiome competes with foreign bacteria for nutrients, limiting the ability of pathogens to survive in the gut. This bacterial antagonism is essential for gut health and organ protection. Secondarily, the gut also contains immunologic factors, such as immunoglobulins that fight off foreign particles. Combined with the gut-associated lymphoid tissue (GALT), the gut is very effective at capturing and destroying invading bodies.[72]

From a mechanical perspective, the gut has a mucous gel layer, which prevents bacterial adhesion. Additionally, peristalsis protects against prolonged stasis, hindering the ability for bacteria to grow and multiply. The epithelial cell layer also plays a role in immunity by creating tight junctions and rearranging or shifting during -desquamation,

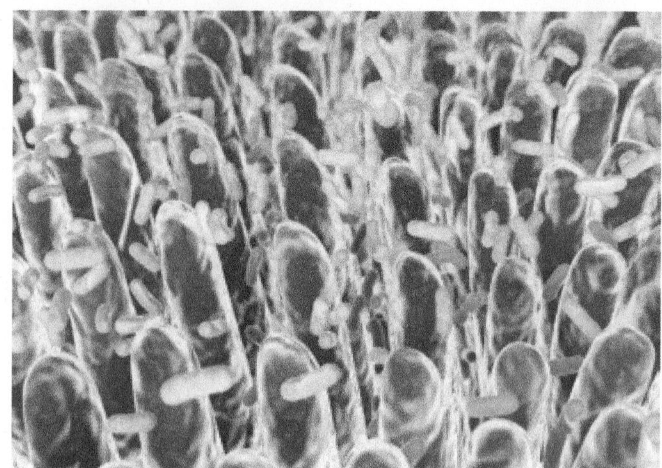

FIGURE 8 The Intestine is Home to the Microbiome

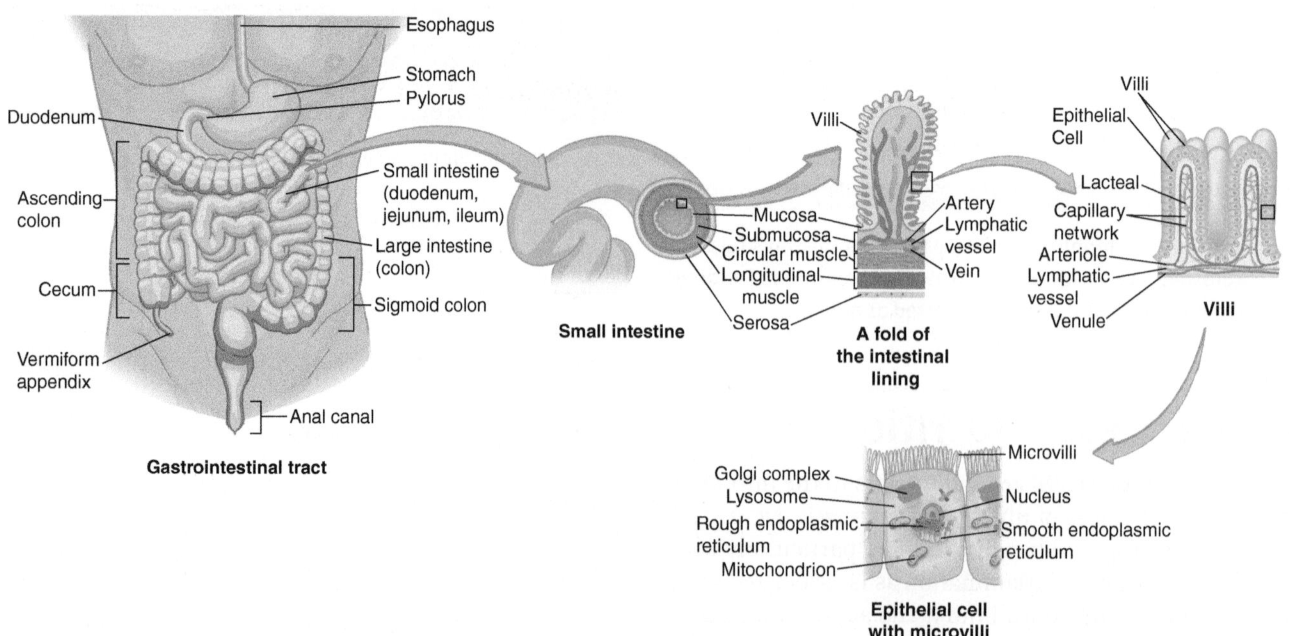

FIGURE 7 Morphology of the Intestinal Tract

making it difficult for foreign bacteria to enter from the lumen. Rearrangement of tight junctions prevents intestinal permeability. This aspect of the gut, combined with GALT, may explain why bacterial translocation in humans rarely progresses to the blood stream and other organs. Furthermore, the epithelial cells secrete cytokines that promote the synthesis of lymphocytes and immunity. By maintaining the epithelial layer and microbiome, EN facilitates the gut's immune function capacity.[72,73]

The Gut and Systemic Inflammatory Response System

The interaction between the gut and immunologic nutrients can be best seen in the context of the systemic inflammatory response. In systemic inflammatory response syndrome (SIRS), the intestine becomes a cytokine-generating organ due to ischemia (versus infection) as a result of certain conditions such as trauma, burns, obstructive gastrointestinal injury, hemorrhagic shock, or sepsis. Select nutrients can serve as substrates that mediate this cytokine-induced response. As shown in Figure 9, various nutritional substrates can induce immune activity both at the cellular and systemic level. For example, omega-3 fatty acids act as a substrate that systemically promotes anti-inflammatory eicosanoids and cytokines, as well as modulates smooth vascular muscle tone. The result is increased dilation of the vessels, improved platelet function, and reduction of bronchoconstriction. Similarly, the amino acids glutamine and arginine participate in macrophage activity at the cell-mediated immunity level.[74-76] The optimal dose and route of provision of these nutrients remain unknown, yet are imperative to achieving the beneficial aspects of these nutrients without posing harm. Table 7 provides examples of immune-enhancing EN formulas.

Conditionally Essential Amino Acids

Stress-induced depletion of glutamine and arginine in blood and tissue pools has earned these amino acids the title of conditionally essential amino acids. While they can be synthesized within the body, during stress, synthesis does not meet their requirement.

Glutamine

Glutamine is a gluconeogenic amino acid that is synthesized in all tissues, with skeletal muscle as the major site. It is an important fuel source for rapidly dividing cells such as the gut epithelium, macrophages, lymphocytes, and fibroblasts. It contains two amine groups, making it a useful nitrogen shuttle to other organs. Glutamine also donates nitrogen to purines and pyrimidines for DNA synthesis. Because it is a precursor to glutathione, a potent antioxidant, glutamine helps protect cells from free radical damage.[75] Due to its properties, glutamine is used therapeutically in patients with gastrointestinal disease and in patients with immune function disorders. It is also widely used among patients with metabolic stress, such as burn and trauma patients.

Arginine

Arginine plays a fundamental role in protein metabolism. As a precursor to insulin and growth hormone, it can play

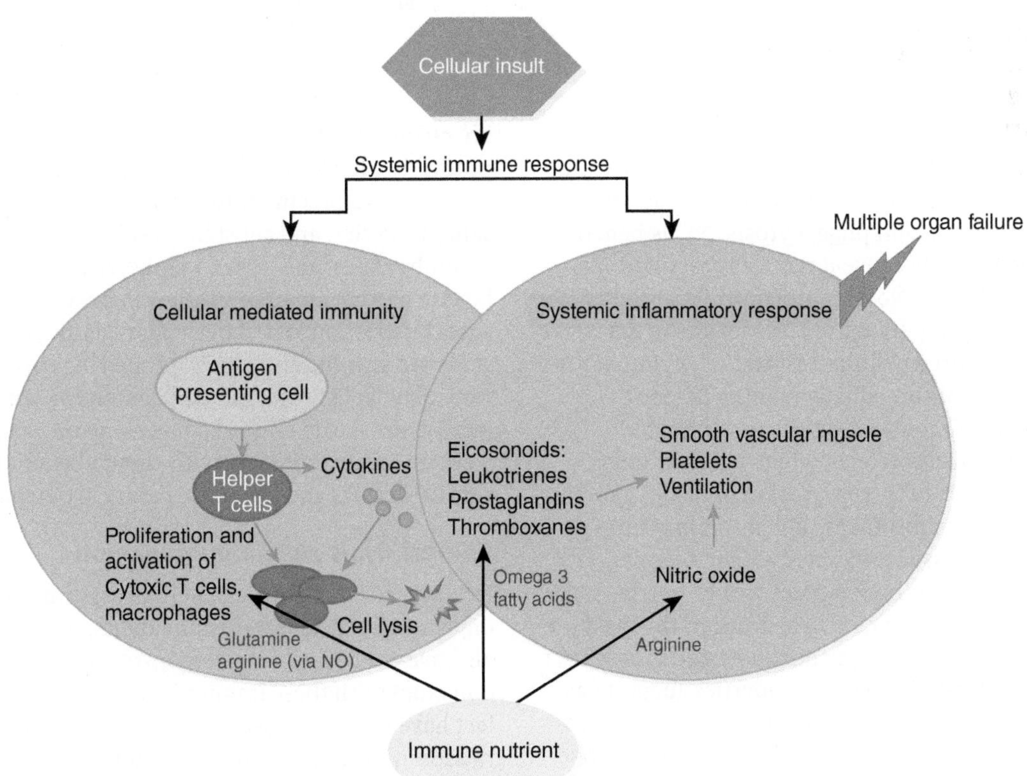

FIGURE 9 Immune Modulating Nutrients Act at Both the Cellular and Systemic Level

Data from Krauss H, Jablecka A, Sosnowski P, Bogdanski P. Influence of L-arginine on the nitric oxide concentration and level of oxidative stress during ischemia-reperfusion injury in a rat model. *J Clin Pharmacol Ther*. 2009 Aug;47(8):533-8; and 76. Gadek JE, DeMichele SJ, Karlstad MD. Enteral nutrition in ARDS study group. Effect of enteral feeding with eicosapentaenoic acid, gamma linolenic acid, and antioxidants in patients with acute respiratory distress syndrome. *Critical Care Medicine*. 1999; 27(8):1409-1420.

TABLE 7 NUTRIENT COMPOSITION OF IMMUNE-ENHANCING ENTERAL FORMULATIONS

Formula Name	Impact	Perative	Pivot 1.5	Oxepa
Concentration (kcal/mL)	1.0	1.3	1.5	1.5
Protein g/1,000 mL (% kcal)	56 (22)	66.7 (20.5)	93.8 (25)	62.7 (16.7)
Carbohydrate g/1,000 mL (% kcal)	132 (53)	180.3 (53)	172.4 (46)	105.3 (28)
Fat g/1,000 mL (% kcal)	28 (25)	35.2 (24)	50.8 (30)	93.8 (56)
Sodium/Potassium (mg/1,000 mL)	960/1,600	980/1,640	1,400/2,000	1,310/1,960
Calcium/Phosphorus (mg/1,000 mL)	800/800	840/840	1,000/1,000	1,060/1,060
Vitamin D (IU/1,000 mL)	13.2 (mcg)	332	400	425
Zinc/Copper (mg/1,000 mL)	15.2/1.7	18.8/1.68	25/2.0	24/2.2
Selenium (mcg/1,000 mL)	100	60	70	74

a major role in wound healing. Arginine is also a precursor to nitric oxide (NO), which provides cellular defense through the stimulus of increased lymphocyte activity, macrophage activation, and phagocytosis. NO is beneficial for tissue oxygenation because it reduces vascular tone, acting as a vasodilator.[74] Notably, uncontrolled production of NO can be damaging. Increased NO results in excessive inflammation, impaired cellular respiration, cytotoxicity, coagulation abnormalities, and worsening hemodynamic instability. NO is also a significant contributor in the ischemia reperfusion model, where a lack of oxygen and blood flow, followed by reperfusion of blood, generates powerful free radical substances such as perioxynitrate that can later cause tissue and microvascular damage.[77-79] Because NO can serve as both a precursor to free radical substances as well as a free radical scavenger, the need for the appropriate balance between adequate and excessive NO cannot be understated. These properties suggest caution when providing arginine in the diet. Figure 10 outlines the impact of NO in the systemic immune response.

Omega-3 Fatty Acids

Many specialty products will now provide information on their omega-6 to omega-3 fatty acid ratio. While both are essential fatty acids, they have unique and contrasting properties due to the physiologic pathways they undergo. Omega-6 is a precursor to arachidonic acid and the eicosanoid 2 series, and substances such as prostaglandin 2, thromboxanes, and series 4 leukotrienes (Figure 11). These factors participate in pro-inflammatory activities such as vasoconstriction and platelet aggregation. Omega-3 fatty acids are anti-inflammatory, promoting vasodilation, inhibiting platelet aggregation, and competing with omega-6 production. Early clinical trials using omega-3 fatty acids were initially promising, with shown benefit to decreasing ventilator days and improving clinical outcome.[76, 80,81]

Clinical Trials on Immunonutrition

Despite the mechanistic benefit of arginine, glutamine, omega-3 fatty acids, and antioxidants, recent clinical trials have not been able to demonstrate improved clinical outcomes with these immune-enhancing formulas, and in fact have raised the issue of adverse consequences.[82,83] One randomized trial providing immune-enhanced (glutamine, omega-3 fatty acid, and antioxidants), high-nitrogen formulas versus a simple high-nitrogen feeding failed to show a benefit with respect to infection rate and duration or length of stay. In fact, 6-month mortality was increased in the

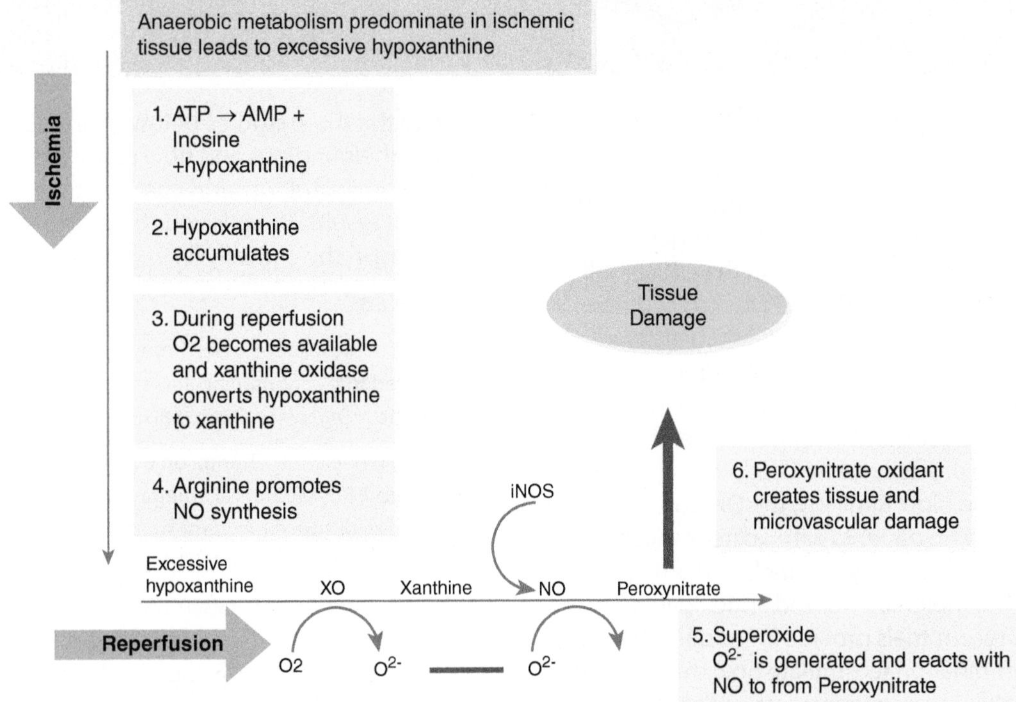

FIGURE 10 Nitric Oxide and the Ischemia-Reperfusion Model

Data from Yapca OE, Borekci B, Suleyman H. Ischemia-Reperfusion Damage. *The Eurasian Journal of Medicine.* 2013;45(2):126-127. doi: 0.5152/eajm.2013.24; and Beckman JS, Koppenol WH. Nitric oxide, superoxide, and peroxynitrite: the good, the bad, and ugly. *Am J Physiol.* 1996;271(5):C1424-C1437.

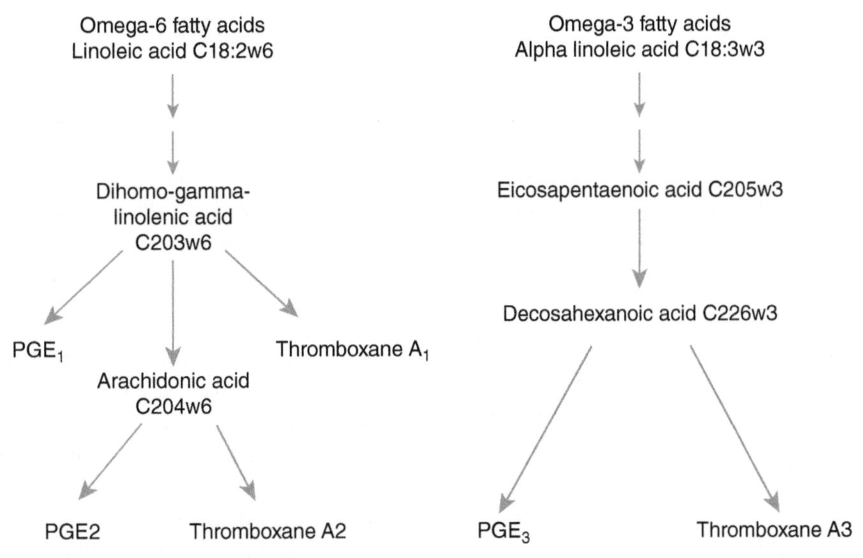

FIGURE 11 Omega-3 Versus 6 Fatty Acid Pathways

Data from Singer P, Theilla M, Fischer H, Gibstein L.Grozovski E, Cohen J. Benefit of an enteral diet enriched with eicosapentaenoic acid and gamma-linolenic acid in ventilated patients with acute lung injury. *Critical Care Medicine.* 2006;34(4):1033-1038.

immune-enhanced group by a hazard ratio of 1.57 (95% CI, 1.03 – 2.39; P = .04).[82] Meta-analysis of similar trials with glutamine showed no benefit in infectious complications or mortality.[83] Route of administration is considered particularly important in establishing glutamine as a beneficial immune nutrient. Unlike traditional practice and belief of enteral nutrient provision as superior, in the case of glutamine, parenteral delivery may be more advantageous in promoting protein synthesis during critical illness.[84] Intravenous glutamine results in a uniform uptake of glutamine in the splanchic region, which is more physiologic and typical of endogenous glutamine synthesis. This permits a more even distribution of glutamine throughout the body. Conversely, enteral glutamine undergoes a first-pass elimination at the gut level. Here, glutamine uptake by the enterocytes is substantial, reducing the amount of glutamine that enters the circulation.[85] Currently, IV glutamine is advocated over enteral for patients in the intensive care unit.[84] Finally, although initial studies with omega-3 fatty acids were promising, subsequent studies on omega-3 fatty acid–enriched diets with antioxidants added demonstrated no clinical benefit in ventilator-free days or ICU days.[86,87]

⚠ Clinical Controversy

Immunonutrition and Clinical Outcome

While meta-analyses demonstrate that immune-enhancing nutrients improve clinical outcomes, more recent clinical trials have raised questions regarding the general use of immunonutrition in the critically ill. The REDOX study (Reducing Deaths Due to Oxidative Stress) used selenium and found higher mortality in patients receiving enteral and parenteral glutamine. The detrimental effects were most profound in patients with multi-organ failure, and given that enteral and parenteral glutamine provision were used, overall dosing may have been too high. Similarly, the OMEGA found increased mortality in patients with acute respiratory distress syndrome. The study diet included omega-3 fatty acids, alpha-linolenic acid, and antioxidants. Notably, some recent trials provide immune-enhancing nutrients in combination to simulate how they interact in vivo. This makes interpretation somewhat obscured.

Read the three studies below on immunonutrition. Consider their findings and how study design, dosing, route of administration, and combination of nutrients may affect results. What is your opinion on use of immunonutrition in the critically ill?

References

1. Heyland D, Muscedere J, Wischmeyer PE, et al. A randomized controlled trial of glutamine and antioxidants in the critically ill patient. *N Engl J Med.* 2013;368(16):1489-1497.
2. Rice TW, Wheeler AP, Thompson BT, deBoiseblane BP, Steingrub J, Rock P. Enteral omega-3 fatty acid, gamma-linolenic acid, and antioxidant supplementation in acute lung injury. *JAMA.* 2011;306(14):1574-1582.
3. van Zanten AR, Sztark F, Kaisers UX, et al. High-protein enteral nutrition enriched with immune-modulating nutrients vs standard high-protein enteral nutrition and nosocomial infections in the ICU: a randomized clinical trial. *JAMA.* 2014;312(5):514-524.

Chapter Summary

Enteral nutrition is the preferred mode of feeding for most patients requiring nutrition support. Optimal outcome, however, depends on proper selection of feeding site, mode of delivery, and formula. Enteral feeding tube placement should take into consideration length of required support, gastric function, aspiration risk, and lifestyle needs of the patient. Formula selection is based on clinical and disease-related requirements of the patients. Over the past several decades, an abundance of specialized feeding products has become available. Choosing an appropriate formula can help support metabolic and disease-related needs in many patients. Disease- and condition-specific formulas are recognized for their unique nutrient characteristics, which can enhance provision of nitrogen and wound-healing nutrients. Differences in composition related to fiber, fluid, macronutrients, and micronutrients provide options to coincide with the medical management of the patient.

Key Terms

enteral nutrition (EN), percutaneous endoscopic gastrostomy (PEG) tube, immunonutrition, nasogastric tube, nasoenteric, oroenteric, nasoduodenal tube, nasojejunal tube, prokinetics, fluoroscopic tube placement, percutaneous endoscopic jejunostomy (PEJ), laparoscopy, open tube placement, aspiration, gastroparesis, dumping syndrome, closed tube feeding system, open tube feeding system, hang time, continuous feeding, intermittent feeding, bolus feeding, isolate, prebiotics, probiotics, hypercapnia, gastric residuals, early enteral nutrition (EEN), postprandial hyperemic response

References

1. Brantley S, Mills M. Overview of enteral nutrition. In: Mueller C, ed. *The A.S.P.E.N. Adult Nutrition Support Core Curriculum.* 2nd ed. Silver Spring, MD: American Society for Parenteral and Enteral Nutrition; 2012:170-184.
2. Volkert D, Berner YN, Berry E, et al. E.S.P.E.N guideline on enteral nutrition: geriatrics. *J Clin Nutr.* 2006;25(2):330-60.
3. White J, Guenter P, Jenson G, Malone A, Schofield M. Consensus Statement of the Academy of Nutrition and Dietetics/American Society for Parenteral and Enteral Nutrition: Characteristics Recommended for the Identification and Documentation of Adult Malnutrition (Undernutrition). *J Acad Nutr Diet.* 2012;112(5):730-738.
4. Harkness L. The history of enteral nutrition therapy: from raw eggs and nasal tubes to purified amino acids and early postoperative jejunal delivery. *J Am Diet Assoc.* 2002;102(3):399-404.
5. Bechtold ML, Mir FA, Boumitri C, et al. Long-term nutrition: a clinician's guide to successful long-term enteral access in adults. *Nutr Clin Pract.* 2016. [Epub ahead of print.] doi: 10.1177/0884533616670103
6. Dwolatzky T, Berezovski S, Friedmann R, et al. A prospective comparison of the use of nasogastric and percutaneous endoscopic gastrostomy tubes for long-term enteral feeding in older people. *Clin Nutr.* 2001;20(6):535-540.
7. Gauderer MW. Percutaneous endoscopic gastrostomy and the evolution of contemporary long-term enteral access. *Clin Nutr.* 2002;21(2):103-110.
8. Gopalan S, Khanna S. Enteral nutrition delivery technique. *Curr Opin Clin Nutr Metab Care.* 2003;6(3):313-317.
9. Nunes G, Santos CA, Santos C, Fonseca J. Percutaneous endoscopic gastrostomy for nutritional support in dementia patients. *Aging Clin Exp Res.* 2016;28(5):983-989.
10. Shastri YM, Shirodkar M, Mallath MK. Endoscopic feeding tube placement in patients with cancer: a prospective clinical audit of 2055 procedures in 1866 patients. *Aliment Pharmacol Ther.* 2008;27(8):649-658.

11. Fang JC, Hilden K, Holubkov R, Disario JA. Transnasal endoscopy vs. fluoroscopy for the placement of nasoenteric feeding tubes in critically ill patients. *Gastrointest Endosc.* 2005;62(5):661-666.
12. Jabbar A, McClave SA. Pre-pyloric versus post-pyloric feeding. *Clin Nutr.* 2005;24(5):719-726.
13. Nelms M, Sucher KP, Lacey K, Roth SL. *Nutrition therapy and pathophysiology.* 2nd ed. Boston, MA: Cengage Learning; 2010.
14. Vanek VW. Ins and outs of enteral access. Part 1: short-term enteral access. *Nutr Clin Pract.* 2002;17(5):275-283.
15. Haslam D, Fang J. Enteral access for nutrition in the intensive care unit. *Curr Opin Clin Nutr Metab Care.* 2006;9(2):155-159.
16. Fang John C, Bankhead R, and Kinikini M. Enteral access devices. In: Mueller C, Ed. *The A.S.P.E.N. Adult Nutrition Support Core Curriculum.* 2nd ed. Silver Spring, MD: American Society for Parenteral and Enteral Nutrition; 2012:206-217.
17. Niv E, Fireman Z, Vaisman N. Post-pyloric feeding. *World J Gastroenterol.* 2009;15(11):1281-1288.
18. Roberts S, Echeverria P, Gabriel SA. Devices and techniques for bedside enteral feeding tube placement. *Nutr Clin Pract.* 2007;22(4):412-420.
19. Disario JA. Endoscopic approaches to enteral nutritional support. *Best Pract Res Clin Gastroenterol.* 2006;20(3):605-630.
20. Bear DE, Champion A, Lei K, Smith J, Beale J, Camporota L, Barrett NA. Use of an electromagnetic device compared with chest x-ray to confirm nasogastric feeding tube position in critical care. *J Parenter Enteral Nutr.* 2016;40:581-586.
21. Kozin ED, Remenschneider AK, Cunnane ME, Deschler DG. Otolaryngologist-assisted fluoroscopic-guided nasogastric tube placement in the postoperative laryngectomy patient. *Laryngoscope.* 2014;124(4):916-920.
22. Ponsky JL. Percutaneous endoscopic gastrostomy. *J Gastrointest Surg.* 2004;8(7):901-904
23. Schrag SP, Sharma R, Jaik NP, et al. Complications related to percutaneous endoscopic gastrostomy (PEG) tubes. A comprehensive clinical review. *J Gastrointestin Liver Dis.* 2007;16(4):407-418.
24. Löser C, Aschl G, Hébuterne X, et al. ESPEN guidelines on artificial enteral nutrition-percutaneous endoscopic gastrostomy (PEG). *Clin Nutr.* 2005;24(5):848-861.
25. Bankhead RR, Fisher CA, Rolandelli RH. Gastrostomy tube placement outcomes: comparison of surgical, endoscopic, and laparoscopic methods. *Nutr Clin Pract.* 2005;20(6):607-612.
26. Bankhead R, Boullata J, Brantley S, et al. Enteral nutrition practice recommendations. *J Parenter Enteral Nutr.* 2009;33(2):122-167.
27. Kwon RS, Banerjee S, Desilets D, et al. Enteral nutrition access devices. *Gastrointest Endosc.* 2010;72(2):236-248.
28. Metheny NA, Titler MG. Assessing placement of feeding tubes. *Am J Nurs.* 2001;101(5):36-45.
29. Schlein K. Gastric versus small bowel feeding in critically ill adults. *Nutr Clin Pract.* 2016;31(4):514-522.
30. Marik PE, Zaloga GP. Gastric versus post-pyloric feeding: a systematic review. *Crit Care.* 2003;7(3):R46-51.
31. Jiyong J, Tiancha H, Huiqin W, Jingfen J. Effect of gastric versus post-pyloric feeding on the incidence of pneumonia in critically ill patients: observations from traditional and Bayesian random-effects meta-analysis. *Clin Nutr.* 2013;32(1):8-15.
32. Varon DE1, Freitas G, Goel N, et al. Intraoperative feeding improves calorie and protein delivery in acute burn patients. *J Burn Care Res.* 2017;38(5):299-303. doi: 10.1097/BCR.0000000000000514
33. Silva SMR, Silva de Assis MC, Rosane de Moraes Silveira C, Gomes M, Daniel de Mello E. Open versus closed enteral nutrition systems for critically ill adults: is there a difference? *Revista da Associação Médica Brasileira* (English Edition) 2012; 58(2): 229-233.
34. Davis TA, Fiorotto ML, Suryawan A. Bolus versus continuous feeding to optimize anabolism in neonates. *Curr Opin Clin Nutr Metab Care.* 2015;18(1):102-108.doi: 10.1097/MCO.0000000000000128
35. Bowling TE, Cliff B, Wright JW, Blackshaw PE, Perkins AC, Lobo DN. The effects of bolus and continuous nasogastric feeding on gastro-oesophageal reflux and gastric emptying in healthy volunteers: a randomised three-way crossover pilot study. *Clin Nutr.* 2008;27(4):608-613.
36. Evans DC, Forbes R, Jones C, et al. Continuous versus bolus tube feeds: Does the modality affect glycemic variability, tube feeding volume, caloric intake, or insulin utilization? *Int J Crit Illn Inj Sci.* 2016;6(1):9-15.
37. Kadamani I, Itani M, Zahran E, Taha N. Incidence of aspiration and gastrointestinal complications in critically ill patients using continuous versus bolus infusion of enteral nutrition: a pseudo-randomised controlled trial. *Aust Crit Care.* 2014;27(4):188-193. doi: 10.1016/j.aucc.2013.12.001.
38. Cresci G, Lefton J, Esper DH. Enteral formulations. In: Mueller C, ed. *The A.S.P.E.N. Adult Nutrition Support Core Curriculum.* 2nd ed. Silver Spring, MD: American Society for Parenteral and Enteral Nutrition; 2012:186-203.
39. Athalye-jape G, Deshpande G, Rao S, Patole S. Benefits of probiotics on enteral nutrition in preterm neonates: a systematic review. *Am J Clin Nutr.* 2014;100(6):1508-1519.
40. Dang S, Shook L, Garlitz K, Hanna M, Desai N. Nutritional outcomes with implementation of probiotics in preterm infants. *J Perinatol.* 2015;35(6):447-450.
41. Preiser J-C, van Zanten AR, Berger MM, et al. Metabolic and nutritional support of critically ill patients: consensus and controversies. *Crit Care.* 2015;19(1):35. doi: 10.1186/s13054-015-0737-8.
42. Hempel S, Newberry SJ, Maher AR, et al. Probiotics for the prevention and treatment of antibiotic-associated diarrhea: A systematic review and meta-analysis. *JAMA.* 2012;307 (18):1959-1969. doi: 10.1001/jama.2012.3507.
43. Barraud D, Bollaert PE, Gibot S. Impact of the administration of probiotics on mortality in critically ill adult patients: a meta-analysis of randomized controlled trials. *Chest.* 2013;143(3):646-655.
44. Besselink MG, van Santvoort HC, Buskens E, Boermeester MA, van Goor H, Timmerman HM, et al. Probiotic prophylaxis in predicted severe acute pancreatitis: a randomised, double-blind, placebo-controlled trial. *Lancet.* 2008;371:651-659.
45. Kalantar-Zadeh K, Cano NJ, Budde K, et al. Diets and enteral supplements for improving outcomes in chronic kidney disease. *Nature Rev Nephrol.* 2011;7(7):10.1038/nrneph.2011.60. doi: 10.1038/nrneph.2011.60.
46. Cai B1, Zhu Y, Ma Yi, et al. Effect of supplementing a high-fat, low-carbohydrate enteral formula in COPD patients. *Nutrition.* 2003;19(3):229-232.
47. Elamin EM, Miller AC, Ziad S. Immune enteral nutrition can improve outcomes in medical-surgical patients with ARDS: A prospective randomized controlled trial. *J Nutr Disord Ther.* 2012;2:109. doi: 10.4172/2161-0509.1000109.
48. Hsieh MJ, Yang TM, Tsai YH. Nutritional supplementation in patients with chronic obstructive pulmonary disease. *J Formos Med Assoc.* 2016;115(8):595-601. doi: 10.1016/j.jfma.2015.10.008.
49. Koretz RL, Avenell A, Lipman TO. Nutrition support for liver disease. *Cochrane Database Syst Rev.* 2012;(5):CD008344. doi: 10.1002/14651858.CD008344.pub2. Review.
50. Plauth M, Cabré E, Riggio O, et al. ESPEN Guidelines on enteral nutrition: liver disease. *Clin Nutr.* 2006;25(2):285-294.
51. Ojo O, Brooke J. Evaluation of the role of enteral nutrition in managing patients with diabetes: A systematic review. *Nutrients.* 2014;6(11):5142-5152. doi: 10.3390/nu6115142.

52. Mesejo A, Montejo-González JC, Vaquerizo-Alonso C, et al. Diabetes-specific enteral nutrition formula in hyperglycemic, mechanically ventilated, critically ill patients: a prospective, open-label, blind-randomized, multicenter study. *Crit Care.* 2015;19:390. doi: 10.1186/s13054-015-1108-1.
53. Ellinger S. Micronutrients, arginine, and glutamine: Does supplementation provide an efficient tool for prevention and treatment of different kinds of wounds? *Adv Wound Care.* 2014;3(11):691-707. doi: 10.1089/wound.2013.0482.
54. Malone A, Seres D, Lord L. Complications of enteral nutrition. In: Mueller C, ed. *The A.S.P.E.N. Adult Nutrition Support Core Curriculum.* 2nd ed. Silver Spring, MD: American Society for Parenteral and Enteral Nutrition; 2012:219-231.
55. Pancorbo-hidalgo PL, García-fernandez FP, Ramírez-Pérez C. Complications associated with enteral nutrition by nasogastric tube in an internal medicine unit. *J Clin Nurs.* 2001;10(4):482-90.
56. Montejo JC, Minambres E, Bordeje L, et al. Gastric residual volume during enteral nutrition in ICU patients: the REGANE study. *Intensive Care Med.* 2010;36(8):1386-1393.
57. Arabi YM, Casaer MP, Chapman M, et al. The intensive care medicine research agenda in nutrition and metabolism. *Intensive Care Med.* 2017. doi: 10.1007/s00134-017-4711-6.
58. Bistrian BR. The who, what, where, when, why, and how of early enteral feeding. *Am J Clin Nutr.* 2012;95(6):1303-1304.
59. Doig GS, Heighes PT, Simpson F, Sweetman EA. Early enteral nutrition reduces mortality in trauma patients requiring intensive care: a meta-analysis of randomized controlled trials. *Injury.* 2011;42:50-56.
60. Reintam Blaser A, Starkopf J, Alhazzani W, et al. Early enteral nutrition in critically ill patients: ESICM clinical practice guidelines. *Intensive Care Med.* 2017;43(3):380-398. doi: 10.1007/s00134-016-4665-0.
61. Li JY, Yu T, Chen GC, et al. Enteral nutrition within 48 hours of admission improves clinical outcomes of acute pancreatitis by reducing complications: a meta-analysis. *PLoS ONE.* 2013;8(6):e64926.
62. Mikhailov TA, Kuhn EM, Manzi J, et al. Early enteral nutrition is associated with lower mortality in critically ill children. *JPEN J Parenter Enteral Nutr.* 2014;38(4):459-466.
63. Szabo FK, Fei L, Cruz LA, Abu-el-haija M. Early enteral nutrition and aggressive fluid resuscitation are associated with improved clinical outcomes in acute pancreatitis. *J Pediatr.* 2015;167(2): 397-402.e1.
64. Liu J, Kong K, Tao Y, Cai W. Optimal timing for introducing enteral nutrition in the neonatal intensive care unit. *Asia Pac J Clin Nutr.* 2015;24(2):219-226.
65. Melis M, Fichera A, Ferguson MK. Bowel necrosis associated with early jejunal feeding: A complication of postoperative enteral nutrition. *Arch Surg.* 2006;141:701-704.
66. Bakiner O, Bozkirli E, Giray S, et al. Impact of early versus late enteral nutrition on cell mediated immunity and its relationship with glucagon like peptide-1 in intensive care unit patients: a prospective study. *Crit Care.* 2013;17(3):R123.
67. Chen W, Zhang Z, Xiong M, et al. Early enteral nutrition after total gastrectomy for gastric cancer. *Asia Pac J Clin Nutr.* 2014;23(4):607-611.
68. Martindale RG, Warren M. Should enteral nutrition be started in the first week of critical illness? *Curr Opin Clin Nutr Metab Care.* 2015;18(2):202-206.
69. Ibrahim EH, Mehringer L, Prentice D, et al. Early versus late enteral feeding of mechanically ventilated patients: results of a clinical trial. *JPEN J Parenter Enteral Nutr.* 2002;26(3):174-181.
70. Khalid I, Doshi P, Digiovine B. Early enteral nutrition and outcomes of critically ill patients treated with vasopressors and mechanical ventilation. *Am J Crit Care.* 2010;19(3):261-268.
71. Flordelís lasierra JL, Pérez-vela JL, Umezawa makikado LD, et al. Early enteral nutrition in patients with hemodynamic failure following cardiac surgery. *JPEN J Parenter Enteral Nutr.* 2015;39(2):154-162.
72. Hegazi RA, DeWitt T. Enteral nutrition and immune modulation of acute pancreatitis. *World J Gastroenterol.* 2014;20(43):16101-16105.
73. O'Hara AM, Shanahan F. The gut flora as a forgotten organ. *EMBO Reports.* 2006;7(7):688-693. doi: 10.1038/sj.embor.740073
74. Krauss H, Jablecka A, Sosnowski P, Bogdanski P. Influence of L-arginine on the nitric oxide concentration and level of oxidative stress during ischemia-reperfusion injury in a rat model. *Int J Clin Pharmacol Ther.* 2009;47(8):533-538.
75. Smith RJ. Glutamine metabolism and its physiologic importance. *JPEN J Parenter Enteral Nutr.* 1990;14(4 Suppl):40S-44S.
76. Gadek, JE, DeMichele SJ, Karlstad MD. Enteral nutrition in ARDS study group. Effect of enteral feeding with eicosapentaenoic acid, gamma linolenic acid, and antioxidants in patients with acute respiratory distress syndrome. *Crit Care Med.* 1999;27(8):1409-1420.
77. Grootjans J, Lenaerts K, Derikx JPM, et al. Human intestinal ischemia-reperfusion–induced inflammation characterized: Experiences from a new translational model. *Am J Pathol.* 2010;176(5):2283-2291. doi: 10.2353/ajpath.2010.091069.
78. Yapca OE, Borekci B, Suleyman H. Ischemia-reperfusion damage. *Eurasian J Med.* 2013;45(2):126-127. doi: 10.5152/eajm.2013.24.
79. Beckman JS, Koppenol WH. Nitric oxide, superoxide, and peroxynitrite: the good, the bad, and ugly. *Am J Physiol.* 1996;271(5):C1424-C1437.
80. Singer P, Theilla M, Fischer H, Gibstein L, Grozovski E, Cohen J. Benefit of an enteral diet enriched with eicosapentaenoic acid and gamma-linolenic acid in ventilated patients with acute lung injury. *Crit Care Med.* 2006;34(4):1033-1038.
81. Pontes-Arruda A, Aragao AM, Albequerque JD. Effects of enteral feeding with eicosapentaenoic acid, gamma-linolenic acid and antioxidants in mechanically ventilated patients with severe sepsis and septic shock. *Crit Care Med.* 2006;34(9):2325-2333.
82. van Zanten AR, Sztark F, Kaisers UX, et al. High-protein enteral nutrition enriched with immune-modulating nutrients vs standard high-protein enteral nutrition and nosocomial infections in the ICU: a randomized clinical trial. *JAMA.* 2014;6;312(5):514-24.
83. van Zanten ARH, Dhaliwal R, Garrel D, Heyland DH. Enteral glutamine supplementation in critically ill patients: A systematic review and meta-analysis. *Crit Care.* 2015;19:294-310.
84. Rodas PC, Rooyackers O, Hebert C, Norberg Å, Wernerman J. Glutamine and glutathione at ICU admission in relation to outcome. *Clin Sci.* 2012;122(Pt 12):591-597. doi: 10.1042/CS20110520.
85. Wernerman J. Glutamine supplementation. *Ann Intensive Care.* 2011;1:25. doi: 10.1186/2110-5820-1-25.
86. Li C, Bo L, Liu W, Lu X, Jin F. Enteral immunomodulatory diet (omega-3 fatty acid, gamma-linolenic acid and antioxidant supplementation) for acute lung injury and acute respiratory distress syndrome: An updated systematic review and analysis. *Nutrients.* 2015;7:5572-5585.
87. Rice TW, Wheeler AP, Thompson BT, deBoiseblane BP, Steingrub J, Rock P. Enteral omega-3 fatty acid, gamma-linolenic acid, and antioxidant supplementation in acute lung injury. *JAMA.* 2011;306(14):1574-1582.

Parenteral Nutrition Therapy

Katie Fort
Grace Ling
Kathy Prelack
Kelly Kane

Chapter Outline

CORE CONCEPTS

1. Parenteral nutrition is a low-volume, high-risk form of nutrition therapy that should only be used when clinically indicated. Enteral nutrition, if tolerated, is preferable to parenteral nutrition in patients who require nutrition support.
2. Venous access for parenteral nutrition is based on duration of therapy, desired concentration and solution type, and disease state/condition of the patient.
3. Candidates for parenteral nutrition must be fully evaluated for nutritional risk and nutritional status with adherence to standardized protocols for initiation of parenteral nutrition.
4. Parenteral nutrition is a hypertonic solution made up of, but not limited to, carbohydrate in the form of dextrose, crystalline amino acids, lipid emulsions, vitamins, minerals, and sterile water.
5. Many lipid emulsions are composed of primarily omega-6 fatty acids and should be provided judiciously given their role in inflammation.
6. Prescription of parenteral nutrition is based on energy and protein requirements with consideration of fluid specifications and substrate utilization of macronutrients.
7. Carbohydrate infusion from parenteral nutrition should not exceed 5 mg/kg/min in adults and children over the age of 2 years.
8. Parenteral nutrition formulations are customizable to the specific needs of each patient or patient population.
9. Monitoring of anthropometric, clinical, and biochemical indices such as electrolytes, acid–base balance, serum glucose, and liver function tests are critical to ensure the safety of the patient.
10. Parenteral nutrition may be a long-term or even life-long therapy for some patients.

Learning Objectives

1. **Understand the history of parenteral nutrition therapy and its importance as a form of nutrition support therapy.**
2. **Identify the various methods of central and peripheral venous access.**
3. **Assess whether a patient is a candidate for parenteral nutrition by critically evaluating their disease state and biochemical parameters.**
4. **Identify the nutrition components and additions that commonly comprise parenteral nutrition.**
5. **Calculate a sample parenteral nutrition prescription/order.**
6. **Identify the anthropometric, biochemical, and physical examination components that constitute effective monitoring of parenteral nutrition patients.**
7. **Describe the potential mechanical and metabolic complications of parenteral nutrition and strategies to prevent and/or resolve them.**

Introduction

Parenteral nutrition (PN) is a type of nutrition support that relies on the intravenous administration of nutrients to patients who are unable or unwilling to take adequate nutrition orally or enterally. PN may be used as an addition to an oral diet or enteral nutrition (EN) in order to meet needs, as the sole source of nutrition during recovery from illness or injury of the gastrointestinal (GI) tract, or as a long-term life-sustaining therapy for patients who have compromised ability to enterally absorb nutrients.

A **hypertonic** solution is a solution with increased osmotic pressure as compared to bodily fluid. It is administered intravenously and is customizable to the individual needs of the patient and may contain carbohydrates, amino acids, lipids, vitamins, minerals, and sterile water. There are potentially serious metabolic and mechanical dangers associated with PN. For this reason, PN is only utilized when nutrition support is necessary and enteral nutrition is inadequate and/or contraindicated.[1]

CORE CONCEPT 1

Parenteral nutrition is a low-volume, high-risk form of nutrition therapy that should only be used when clinically indicated. Enteral nutrition, if tolerated, is preferable to parenteral nutrition in patients who require nutrition support.

Brief History of Parenteral Nutrition

Since the 17th century, intravenous nutrition has been of interest to the medical and nutrition communities as a means to improve nutrition status; however, it was not until the 1960s that it was successfully utilized in a human model.[2] The pioneers of parenteral nutrition, Dr. George Blackburn, Dr. Stanley Dudrick, Dr. Harry Vars, and Dr. Douglas Wilmore, were most interested in treating protein-energy malnutrition in patients who were either unable to use the gastrointestinal tract or were experiencing failure to thrive despite sufficient oral consumption.[3]

Dudrick and his colleagues began their studies on the feasibility, efficacy, and safety of parenteral nutrition with a laboratory study. Six pedigreed beagle puppies were fed with parenteral nutrition for either 72, 100, 235, or 256 days after weaning from their mother at 8 weeks of age. The weight gain, skeletal growth, development, and activity of these puppies were compared to their orally fed littermates. At the end of the study period, the researchers found that each of the six intravenously fed puppies surpassed their controls in weight gain and matched them in skeletal growth, development, and activity. There were no significant differences between growth rates or weight gain between the experimental puppies.

The success of parenteral feeding with the beagles was encouraging for the researchers and prompted a clinical study in 30 human patients with chronic complicated gastrointestinal disease. The parenteral solution provided to these patients was customized by a clinician daily to meet individual needs and compounded by a pharmacist with 20% glucose, 5% fibrin hydrolysate, electrolytes, trace minerals, and vitamins. The infusion was administered through a central catheter placed percutaneously into the superior vena cava for 10 to 200 days, depending on the patient. In this clinical study, positive nitrogen balance was achieved in all patients. As a result, patients experienced improvements in wound healing, fistula closure, weight gain, and strength and activity.[4] These findings were groundbreaking, as the general consensus within the medical and nutrition communities during the 1960s was that feeding entirely by vein was not possible, practical, or affordable.

Despite its success in improving nutrition status of recipients, the research team encountered problems related to the preparation and administration of parenteral nutrition. Major challenges included formulating complete parenteral nutrient solutions, which did not exist at the time; concentrating hypertonic substrate components without precipitation; demonstrating utility and safety of long-term central venous catheterization; demonstrating efficacy and safety of long-term infusion of hypertonic nutrient solutions; maintaining **asepsis**, or the absence of bacteria throughout solution preparation and delivery; and anticipating, avoiding, and correcting metabolic imbalances or derangements.[2] Despite advances in medicine, many of these issues continue to be of concern with the preparation and administration of PN.

Parenteral Nutrition Administration

Venous Access

Depending on the type of venous access selected, PN may be referred to as **central parenteral nutrition** or

CASE STUDY INTRODUCTION

Alex is a 43-year-old male with a history of adenocarcinoma of the ileum and which has been in remission for 3 years. He now presents with intermittent abdominal cramping, abdominal distension, constipation, and loss of appetite and has not eaten for the past 4 days. The physician suspects that Alex's cancer treatment, including intensive radiation and two prior surgeries, has led to a small bowel obstruction. She orders a computerized tomography (CT) scan, which confirms that several intestinal adhesions have formed in the distal ileum, resulting in a complete bowel obstruction. Alex is scheduled for surgery in 5 days and is admitted to the hospital for management of his small bowel obstruction. Alex lives with his wife and 6-year-old daughter and works from home as a graphic designer.

Anthropometric Data:

Current weight: 64 kg (141 lbs)
Usual body weight (UBW): 70 kg (155 lbs)
Height: 175 cm (69 in)
Body mass index (BMI): 21kg/m^2

Biochemical Data:

Sodium 133 (135-145 mEq/L)
Potassium 3.5 (3.6-5.0 mEq/L)
Chloride 109 (98-110 mEq/L)
Carbon dioxide 20 (20-30 mEq/L)
Blood urea nitrogen 5 (6-24 mg/dL)
Creatinine 0.6 (0.4-1.3 mg/dL)
Glucose 88 (70-139 mg/dL)
Glomerular filtration rate 99 mL/min/1.73 m^2

Calcium 8.7 (8.5-10.5 mEq/L)
Phosphorus 2.9 (2.7-4.5 mg/dL)
Magnesium 1.5 (1.3-2.1 mEq/L)
Albumin 3.5 (3.5-5.0 g/dL)
Hemoglobin 12.7 (13.5-17.5 g/dL)
Hematocrit 35% (42%-52%)

Clinical Data:

Past Medical History: None
Medications: Imodium
Vitals: Blood pressure 110/77 mm Hg, Temperature 98.6°F
Nutrition-focused Physical Exam: Patient appears pale with decreased muscle tone and skin turgor. Abdomen is distended with minimal bowel sounds.

Dietary Data:

Dietary History: Alex states that he has experienced intermittent abdominal cramping and poor appetite for the past several weeks. As a result, he has been skipping meals or eating half-sized portions of his usual intake. He has not eaten for the past 4 days due to worsening cramping.
Diet Prescription: NPO

Questions

1. **How would you assess Alex's preoperative nutritional status?**
2. **Would you suggest initiating parenteral nutrition support to the medical team? Justify your answer. If you believe that parenteral nutrition support should be initiated prior to surgery, what type of venous access would you recommend?**

peripheral parenteral nutrition. In central PN, venous access is acquired in a central vessel, namely the superior or inferior vena cava or the right atrium.[5] In peripheral PN, access is obtained in a peripheral vessel, such as the vessels of the hand or forearm. Because catheters, also known as vascular access devices (VADs), may be advanced some distance through the vasculature, the distinction between central and peripheral PN is based solely on the location of the catheter tip. The location of the tip does not necessarily correspond with the site of **venipuncture** (the point where the catheter enters the vasculature) or the **exit site** (where the catheter exits the body).[5]

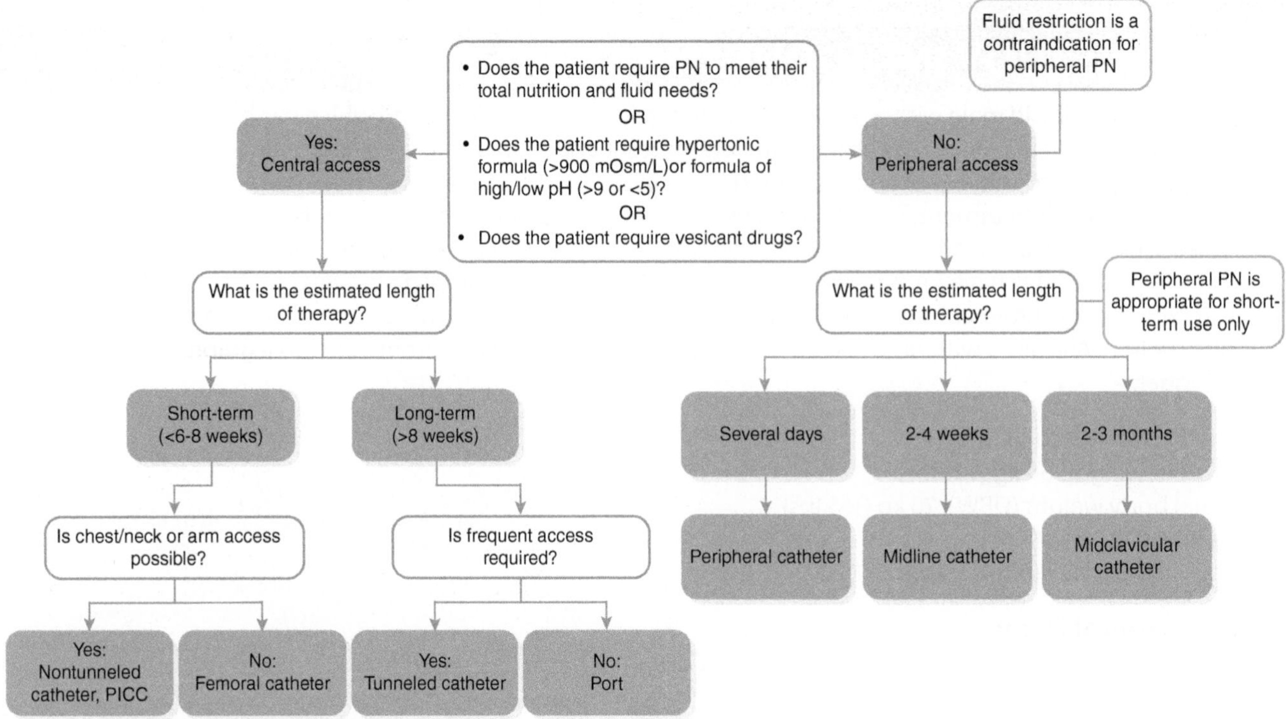

FIGURE 1 **Determining Type of Intravenous Access**

CORE CONCEPT 2

Several factors influence the decision to infuse centrally or peripherally, notably the type of PN formula. Because PN formulas are hypertonic to body fluids, the type of administration must be carefully considered to avoid complications.[3] Other considerations include the expected length of therapy; frequency of infusions; and patient characteristics such as medical history, preferences, and ability to care for the device.[6]

Figure 1 provides a basic algorithm for determining which form of access is appropriate for the patient.

Central Parenteral Nutrition

In central PN, the catheter tip is located in a large, high-flow vessel, typically the junction of the superior vena cava and right atrium. The vena cava and right atrium are sites of high blood flow that can quickly disperse PN solutions that might otherwise cause complications such as **thrombophlebitis**, or inflammation of a vein caused by a blood clot, and **extravasation**, or inadvertent administration or leakage of the PN into surrounding tissues instead of a vein.[5,7] The ideal tip location is the lower third of the superior vena cava or at the atrio-caval junction, as these locations are associated with the fewest mechanical and thrombotic complications.[7] However, the catheter tip should not be placed any deeper than this, as the risk of thrombotic complications increases when the catheter is inserted near the tricuspid valve or deeper.

The VAD may be centrally inserted and the location of the catheter tip is advanced from the site of venipuncture and threaded through the vasculature until the tip reaches the vena cava and/or right atrium.[5] There are two main types of central access: short-term and long-term **central venous catheters (CVCs)**. Short-term CVCs, often referred to as non-tunneled catheters, vary by insertion site and may be inserted in the subclavian, internal or external jugular, or femoral veins. Catheter insertion into the femoral vein is associated with a higher risk of infection and thrombosis, and is therefore not typically recommended for PN.[7] Alternately, short-term CVCs may be inserted in the arm via the cephalic or basilic vein. This form of access is considered a **peripherally inserted central catheter (PICC)** (Figures 2 and 3).[7]

Long-term central access seeks to separate the skin from the venous entry site in order to reduce infection risk. Long-term CVCs are often referred to as tunneled catheters (Figures 4 and 5) as they are tunneled under the skin to the venous site although the catheter exits through the

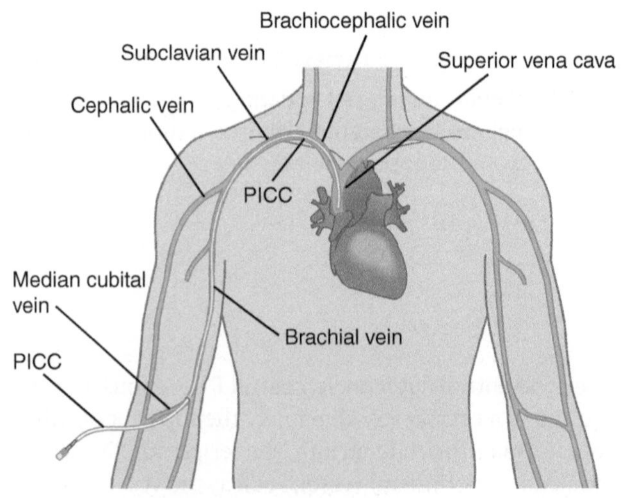

FIGURE 2 **Peripherally Inserted Central Catheter (PICC) Placement**

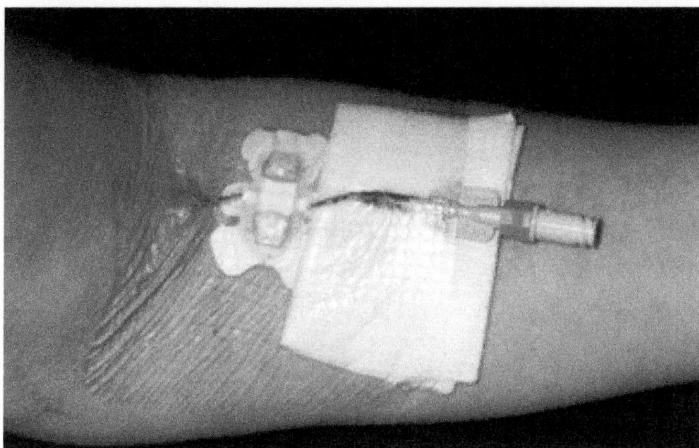

FIGURE 3 **Patient with a PICC Line**

© St Bartholomew's Hospital/Science Source.

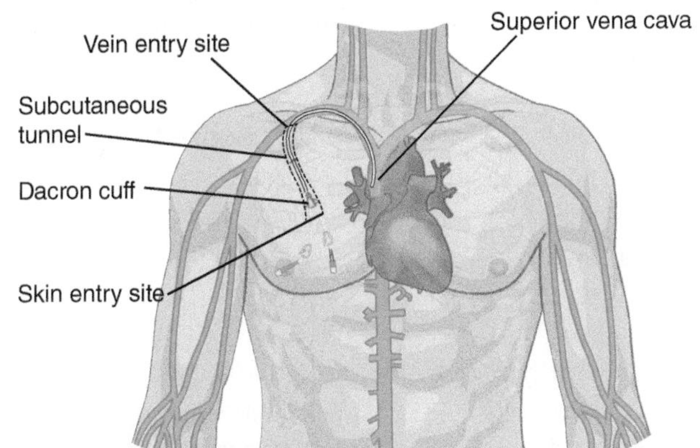

FIGURE 4 **Tunneled Catheter Placement**

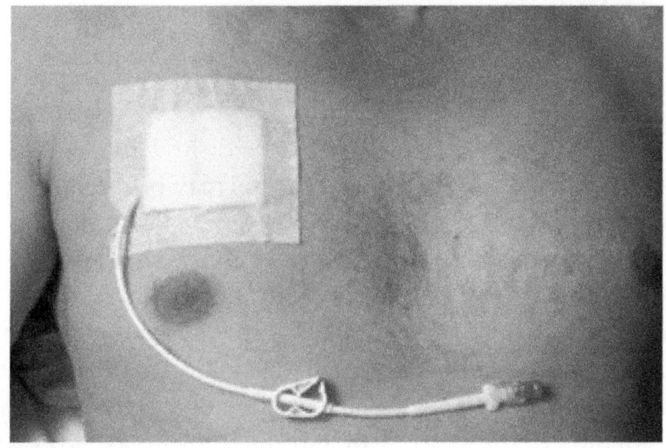

FIGURE 5 **Patient with a Tunneled Catheter**

© Dr P. Marazzi/Science Source.

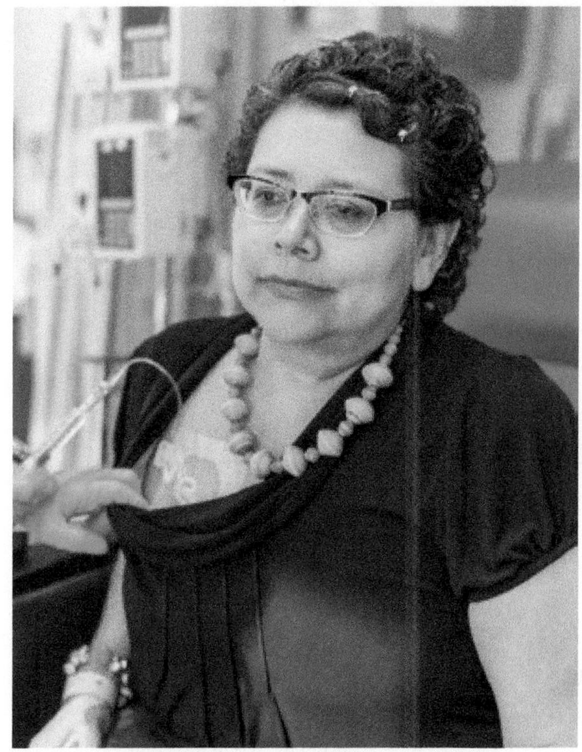

FIGURE 6 **Patient Receiving an Infusion Through Central Venous Port**

© Emerald Raindrops/Shutterstock.

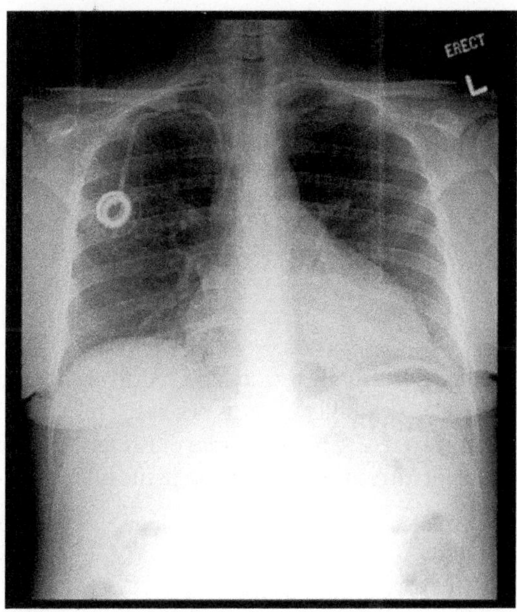

FIGURE 7 **X-Ray Indicating Placement of Central Venous Port**

© Living Art Enterprises / Science Source / Getty Images.

skin. Subcutaneously implanted ports are another form of long-term CVC where an entrance port is a device that exists under the skin with a catheter connecting the device to the vein. Implantable ports are different from tunneled catheters in that there is no catheter exiting the skin and access to the port requires puncturing the skin (**Figure 6**). Regardless of the entry site, the position of the tip should always be confirmed, whether through fluoroscopy or ultrasound during the procedure or through radiologic visualization after the procedure (**Figure 7**).[7]

There are advantages and disadvantages to both short-term and long-term CVCs. Short-term CVCs can typically be placed at the hospital bedside while long-term CVCs require surgical placement. Short-term CVCs, particularly those that are inserted through the subclavian, internal or external jugular, or femoral arteries, are more difficult to maintain sterile. Long-term CVCs are associated with lower infection risk and are preferred for use greater than 3 months.[7] **Table 1** describes various types of CVCs and their advantages and disadvantages.

TABLE 1 SUMMARY OF CENTRAL VENOUS CATHETERS[5]			
Type of Central Venous Catheter	**Description**	**Advantages**	**Disadvantages**
Percutaneous non-tunneled catheter	Typically used for short durations (days to weeks) in the acute care setting	• Less costly to place • Easy to remove • Can be exchanged over a guidewire	• High risk of catheter-related infection • Self-care can be difficult • Requires sutures to secure in place • Repair kits not readily available if catheter breaks
Peripherally inserted central catheter (PICC)	A type of percutaneous nontunneled catheter. Venipuncture occurs in a peripheral vein (e.g., basilic, cephalic, or brachial), but the tip is located in the vena cava. Can be used for weeks to months, including short term home PN.	• Low risk of placement-related complications • Can be placed at bedside or radiology suite	• Self-care can be difficult if placed in forearm • Repair kits not readily available • Cannot necessarily be used to sample blood
Tunneled catheter	The venipuncture site is removed from the catheter exit site, theoretically reducing the risk of infection. Appropriate for long-term use (months to years), including home PN.	• Easier for self-care • Dressings and sutures can be removed after 1 month • Repair kits are available	• Requires placement in operating room and a minor surgical procedure for removal
Implanted catheter	A subcutaneous port, usually placed in the chest. The port can be accessed 1000 to 2000 times and is ideal for patients who need infrequent IV therapy. Appropriate for long-term use, including home PN.	• Easier to care for (only requires care when accessed and a monthly heparin flush) • Is discrete, thus preserving body image • Difficult to break • Lowest rates of infection of all central venous access devices	• Requires a needle to access • Must be placed in operating room • Requires surgical procedure for removal

Central PN is usually the preferred form of access because it allows greater flexibility in the types of PN infusions that can be administered.[5] Characteristics of PN formulas that would necessitate central access include the following:

- Hyperosmolarity (≥10% glucose or ≥5% amino acids, or 900 mOsm/L)[7,8]
- High (>9) or low (<5) pH[7]
- Infusions containing vesicant drugs (can cause the vessels to become leaky)[5]

Peripheral Parenteral Nutrition

In peripheral access, the catheter tip is located outside of a central vessel[7] Although central access is ideal, peripheral PN may be selected because it is a safer and easier way to access the vasculature, particularly for short-term use.[5] Peripheral PN is typically used for a maximum of 2 to 6 weeks at a time, as the risk of dislocation and complications (e.g., **phlebitis** or inflammation of the vein) is more common than in central PN and the risk increases as dwell time increases.[5,7] An advantage of peripheral PN is that there is evidence that it is associated with a lower risk of catheter-related infections, but this may be due to the shorter dwell time.[5]

Because peripheral PN infuses into the smaller veins of the extremities, the PN formula cannot be as hypertonic as those formulas used in central PN. Formulas should be of low osmolarity, defined as <900 mOsm/L. There is evidence that formulas of higher osmolarity do not increase the risk of phlebitis in the short term, but these formulas may cause a burning sensation.[7,8]

Indications and Contraindications

When evaluating whether a patient is eligible for PN, consider that PN carries a high risk of serious complications. It is also a costly therapy, due to the expense of vascular access devices, monitoring laboratory values, and treating potential complications.[3] While PN has been shown to improve markers of nutritional status, it does not consistently improve clinical outcomes.[3] PN is only clearly indicated for a narrow range of disease states and circumstances and should not be considered a first line of therapy in nutrition support. For these reasons, the expected benefits of PN therapy should outweigh the risks.

The benefits of enteral feeding are significant and every attempt should be made to trial enteral nutrition (EN) therapy before PN is considered.[3] It has been shown that when compared with PN, EN is associated with reduced risk of infection (e.g., pneumonia and central catheter infections) and reduced length of stay in intensive care unit (ICU) patients.[9] EN promotes blood flow to the gut and the maintenance of tight junctions, thereby preventing the gut from becoming leaky and reducing the risk of systemic infection and stress ulcers. EN is also key in maintaining the gut-associated lymphoid tissue, which is important in regulating the systemic immune response.[9] If EN has been attempted but has failed, PN could then be considered.

Despite the preference for EN from a clinical perspective, there are circumstances in which PN would be indicated:

1. EN has been attempted (including trialing different tube placements) but has failed.[3]
2. EN is contraindicated due to a dysfunctional GI tract. Causes of a dysfunctional GI tract include a paralytic ileus, mesenteric ischemia, small-bowel obstruction, a GI fistula distal to the feeding tube tip, and a GI fistula with outputs of greater than 200 mL/day.[3]

The patient's preference should always be considered. Some patients who are prescribed EN may refuse to have a tube placed and prefer to be fed via the parenteral route.[10] A discussion of the risks and benefits of enteral versus parenteral nutrition should occur so that a patient can make an informed decision.

Determining whether a patient is a candidate for PN requires a thorough nutrition assessment, the first step of the nutrition care process (NCP). If a patient cannot meet their nutritional needs through oral intake or EN alone, and is either at risk of malnutrition or is already malnourished, they may be a candidate for PN.[3] The American Society of Parenteral and Enteral Nutrition (A.S.P.E.N.) defines "nutritional risk" as a Nutrition Risk Screening (NRS) 2002 score of ≥5 or a Nutrition Risk in Critically Ill (NUTRIC) score of ≥5.[9] However, the exact length of time that a patient can remain either NPO or without adequate nutrition before negatively impacting clinical outcome is not clearly defined.[3]

Box 1

Guidelines for PN in Critical Illness

While PN is clearly indicated when the gut is nonfunctional, indications for PN in critical illness are less well established. Critically ill patients usually experience a catabolic state and systemic inflammation and may experience increased infectious morbidity, multiple organ dysfunction, prolonged hospitalization, and high risk of mortality.[11] Early nutrition support in the form of EN is recommended to reduce disease severity, reduce the risk of complications, and decrease ICU length of stay.[11] Enteral access should be attempted within 24 to 48 hours of ICU admission if the patient cannot maintain oral intake.[11]

There are, however, cases that necessitate PN as a last resort. PN may be indicated for patients in whom enteral access cannot be obtained or EN is not tolerated, although the timing of PN administration depends on nutrition status.[11]

The 2016 A.S.P.E.N. guidelines on nutrition support of critically ill adults specify that if a patient is at low nutrition risk (e.g., NRS 2002 score of ≤3 or NUTRIC score of ≤5), early PN is associated with minimal benefit or even harm. In these patients, exclusive PN should be withheld for the first 7 days after ICU admission.[11] However, if the patient is at high nutrition risk (e.g., NRS 2002 score of ≥5 or NUTRIC score of ≥5), initiation of PN as soon as possible is associated with improved outcome. Regardless of nutritional risk status, if a patient cannot meet at least 60% of their energy and protein needs through the enteral route, supplemental PN should be considered after 7 to 10 days.[11]

Box 2

Conditions in which PN should be used with caution

- Hemodynamic instability
- Hyperglycemia: Glucose >300 mg/dL
- Azotemia: BUN >100 mg/dL
- Hyperosmolality: Serum osmolality >350 mOsm/kg
- Hypernatremia: Na >150 mEq/L
- Hypokalemia: K <3 mEq/L
- Hyperchloremic metabolic acidosis: Cl >115 mEq/L
- Hypophosphatemia: Phos <2 mg/dL
- Hypochloremic metabolic alkalosis: Cl <85 mEq/L

In addition to assessing tolerance of EN, GI function, and disease state, it is also essential to assess whether the patient could tolerate PN. Patients must meet certain criteria in clinical status, including the ability to tolerate the quantities of fluid, carbohydrate, and protein required. PN should be used with caution in patients with fluid and metabolic imbalances. These conditions are outlined in Box 2.[3]

PRACTICE POINT

Severe hyperglycemia, azotemia, encephalopathy, and hyperosmolality, along with severe fluid and electrolyte imbalances, are associated with poor tolerance of any type of nutrition support, whether it be EN or PN. These abnormalities should be corrected prior to starting nutrition support therapy.[3]

Clinical Controversy

Early versus Late Parenteral Nutrition

A.S.P.E.N. currently recommends delaying administration of PN for 7 to 10 days in critically ill adult patients where enteral nutrition is not feasible, unless they are severely malnourished or at high nutritional risk. Similarly, their recommendations state that in both low- and high-risk patients who are unable to meet greater than 60% of their goal by EN, supplemental PN should be delayed 7 to 10 days. These guidelines are based on evidence that despite an increase in energy and protein intake, there is a lack of clinical benefit associated with early parenteral supplementation. Studies such as that by Heyland confirm the risk of PN use by demonstrating increased infection rates and intensive care unit length of stay as well as cost.

However studies have shown that PN can be used safely. In their study, Doig and colleagues demonstrated that PN use can be safe and also decrease number of days on ventilation, although length of intensive care and hospital stay were not improved. When providing nutrition support therapy, critical review of a patient's nutritional risk and status as well as clinical condition must accompany guidelines for PN use, particularly given that evidence does exist to support a benefit.

Based on the two studies referenced, provide how you might apply evidence-based findings and professional guidelines when providing nutrition support, and when you might determine that early supplemental PN may be indicated. What are the strengths and weaknesses of each study in terms of their design and rigor? How might study population or clinical status impact your conclusion based on these studies?

References

1. Doig GS, Simpson F; Early PN Trial Investigators Group. Early parenteral nutrition in critically ill patients with short term relative contraindications to early enteral nutrition. *JAMA.* 2013;309(20):2130-2138.
2. Heyland DK. Early supplemental parenteral nutrition in critically ill adults increased infections, ICU length of stay and cost. *Evid Based Med.* 2012;17(3):86-87.

If PN is to be used, the next step is determining the venous access site and type of venous access device. Central PN is appropriate when PN is required for longer term use (>2 weeks), peripheral venous access is inadequate, the patient has significant nutrient needs, or the patient is fluid restricted.[3] Peripheral PN may be considered if nutrition support is only needed for a short time frame (up to 2 weeks) if the patient is not a candidate for central PN.[3] Peripheral PN can provide partial or total nutrition, but because the peripheral PN solution is less concentrated, a higher volume must be administered to provide total nutrition. For this reason, a patient who requires fluid restriction (e.g., due to renal disease) would not be a candidate for peripheral PN.[3] In general, patients receiving peripheral PN should be able to tolerate 2 L to 3 L of fluid per day.

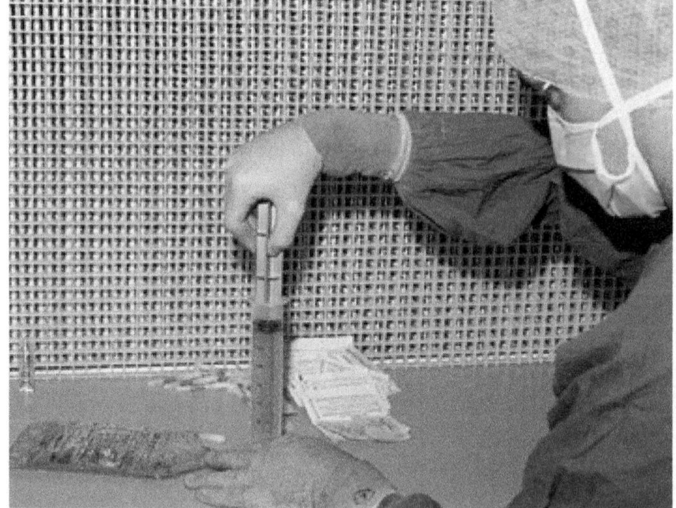

FIGURE 8 **Sterile Preparation of Parenteral Nutrition Formula**

CORE CONCEPT 3

Candidates for parenteral nutrition must be fully evaluated for nutritional risk and nutritional status with adherence to standardized protocols for initiation of parenteral nutrition.

Parenteral Nutrition Formulation

Although there are standard PN formulas, PN solutions in the inpatient setting may be compounded daily and are customizable to the individual needs of the patient (Figure 8).

The components that can be included in the solution are carbohydrate, amino acids, lipids, vitamins, electrolytes, trace minerals, and a number of other specific additives.

Given in the appropriate amounts, the intravenous administration of these components can maintain nutrition status and support life-long term without use of the gastrointestinal tract.

CORE CONCEPT 4

Parenteral nutrition is a hypertonic solution made up of, but not limited to, carbohydrate in the form of dextrose, crystalline amino acids, lipid emulsions, vitamins, minerals, and sterile water.

Carbohydrate

As the primary energy source for the body, the carbohydrate component of PN is critical. It is especially important during times of metabolic stress, when proteins can be catabolized as an energy source at an increased rate, causing negative nitrogen balance.[12] Carbohydrate should always be included in PN because of its protein-sparing effect.[13]

The most commonly used carbohydrate substrate used in PN formulas is dextrose monohydrate, the dextrorotatory form of glucose. In its hydrated form, dextrose provides 3.4 kcal per gram, not 4 kcal per gram like dietary carbohydrates.[1,14]

Commercially, dextrose is available in multiple concentrations ranging from 5% to 70%.[1] Because dextrose is an acidic molecule, the higher concentration solutions are more acidic. According to the United States Pharmacopoeia (USP), dextrose solutions range from pH 3.5 to 6.5. Dextrose solutions greater than 10% concentration are typically reserved for central venous administration because the hypertonicity and acidity of the solution has the potential to cause thrombophlebitis in peripheral veins.[14]

Dextrose infusion can be challenging due to its effect on blood sugar. Infusing dextrose directly into the bloodstream directly raises serum glucose, which commonly leads to hyperglycemia.[1] Appropriate monitoring of serum glucose and intervention of highs and lows beyond acceptable limits must be implemented to avoid more serious complications.

The most common dextrose solution used in parenteral nutrition is 50% dextrose in water (D50W). This concentration supplies 500 grams of dextrose per liter and 1700 kcal per liter. The mathematical process used to equate the grams of dextrose supplied per liter and the calories supplied per liter is shown as follows:

$$\text{50\% dextrose} = \frac{\text{50 grams dextrose}}{\text{100 mL}} \times \frac{\text{1000 mL}}{\text{L}}$$

$$= \frac{\text{500 grams dextrose}}{\text{L}} \times 3.4 \frac{\text{kcal}}{\text{grams dextrose}}$$

$$= \text{1700 kcal}$$

In fluid-restricted patients, more concentrated PN is indicated. A more-concentrated dextrose solution like D60W or D70W is often used in compounding because less volume is required to meet carbohydrate requirements.[14] As an example, if a patient had a daily carbohydrate requirement of 400 grams, the PN formula would require 800 mL of D50W to meet that requirement. In contrast, the PN formula would only require 571 mL of D70W to meet the daily requirement of 400 grams of carbohydrate. This difference of 229 mL could be significant in a fluid-restricted patient.

How many mL of 70% dextrose is needed to provide 400 g dextrose?

$$\text{70\% dextrose} = \frac{\text{70 grams dextrose}}{\text{100 mL}} \times \frac{\text{1000 mL}}{\text{L}}$$

$$\frac{\text{700 grams dextrose}}{\text{1000 mL}} = \frac{\text{400 grams}}{\text{x mL}}$$

$$x = \text{571 mL}$$

Table 2 shows different dextrose solutions available for use in parenteral nutrition, grams of dextrose per liter, kcal per liter, and peripheral versus central access requirement.

Amino Acids

A variety of illnesses and catabolic conditions can disturb the blood amino acid profile, promote a decrease in lean

TABLE 2 DEXTROSE SOLUTIONS

Solution	Grams of Dextrose per Liter (g/L)	Kilocalories per Liter (Kcal/L)	Peripheral versus Central Administration
5% dextrose in water (D5W)	50	170	Peripheral or central
10% dextrose in water (D10W)	100	340	Peripheral or central
20% dextrose in water (D20W)	200	680	Central
30% dextrose in water (D30W)	300	1020	Central
40% dextrose in water (D40W)	400	1360	Central
50% dextrose in water (D50W)	500	1700	Central
60% dextrose in water (D60W)	600	2040	Central
70% dextrose in water (D70W)	700	2380	Central

body mass, and increase body protein requirements. Mixed amino acid formulations that provide both essential and nonessential amino acids are a standard component of complete PN prescriptions to support cell, organ, skeletal, and cardiac, and respiratory muscle functions, as well as wound healing.[15]

Amino acids are supplied through PN in their crystalline form. If oxidized for energy, crystalline amino acids supply 4 kcal per gram. As with other PN components, amino acid solutions are available in different concentrations ranging from 3% to 20%.[14] All commercially available amino acid solutions for PN contain all nine essential amino acids in varying amounts between 38% and 57% of total amino acids. Standard solutions also provide some nonessential amino acids at about 43% to 62% of total amino acids. Nitrogen content varies depending on the concentration of the solution and the amino acid profile.[15]

Specialty amino acid formulations are commercially available for use in certain disease states like renal failure, hepatic encephalopathy, metabolic stress, trauma, thermal injury, and hypercatabolic states. These products are generally more costly than standard formulas and should only be used in patients who meet the intended indications and who are expected to benefit clinically from the specialty amino acid formula.[14] A.S.P.E.N. has published guidelines for the use of these products in clinical practice.[16] **Table 3**

TABLE 3 COMMERCIALLY AVAILABLE CRYSTALLINE AMINO ACID SOLUTIONS

Brand Name, Manufacturer	Type/Indication	Stock Concentrations	Composition
Travasol, Baxter	Standard	3.5%, 4.25%, 5.5%, 8.5%, 10%	Essential amino acids + alanine, glycine, arginine, proline, serine, and tyrosine[15]
Clinisol, Baxter	Standard/fluid restriction	15%	Essential amino acids + alanine, glycine, arginine, proline, glutamic acid, serine, aspartic acid, and tyrosine[17]
ProSol, Baxter	Standard/fluid restriction	20%	Essential amino acids + alanine, glycine, arginine, proline, glutamic acid, serine, aspartic acid, and tyrosine[15]
Aminosyn II, Abbott	Standard	3.5%, 4.25%, 5%, 7%, 8.5%, 10%, 15%	Essential amino acids + alanine, glycine, arginine, proline, glutamic acid, serine, aspartic acid, tyrosine, and histidine[18]
FreAmine III, B.Braun	Standard	8.5%, 10%	Essential amino acids + alanine, glycine, arginine, proline, serine, histidine, and cysteine[19]
HepatAmine, B.Braun	Hepatic failure	8%	Essential amino acids + alanine, glycine, arginine, proline, serine, and histidine[19]
Hepatasol, Baxter	Hepatic failure	8%	Essential amino acids + alanine, glycine, arginine, proline, serine, histidine, and cysteine[17]
FreAmine HBC, B.Braun	Metabolic stress	6.9%	Essential amino acids + alanine, glycine, arginine, proline, serine, and histidine[19]
Aminosyn HBC, Abbott	Metabolic stress	7%	Essential amino acids + alanine, glycine, arginine, proline, serine, tyrosine, and histidine[19]
BranchAmin, Baxter	Metabolic stress	4%	Contains branched chain amino acids only (leucine, isoleucine, and valine)[14]
NephrAmine, B.Braun	Renal failure	5.4%	Contains essential amino acids only[14]
Aminosyn RF, Abbott	Renal failure	5.2%	Contains essential amino acids + arginine[14]
TrophAmine, B.Braun	Infants and young children	6%, 10%	Essential amino acids + alanine, glycine, arginine, proline, glutamic acid, serine, aspartic acid, tyrosine, taurine, and cysteine[15]

provides more information on some of the standard and specialty crystalline amino acid solutions available for use in PN.

Lipids

Energy deficit is a common and serious problem in intensive care unit patients and is associated with increased rates of complications, length of stay, and mortality.[20]

The infusion of lipid injectable emulsions (ILEs) provides a high energy supply, contributes to the prevention of high glucose infusion rates, and is indispensable for supplying the body with essential fatty acids (EFAs).[21]

In the United States, ILE components include an oil source, egg yolk phospholipid as an emulsifier, glycerin to render the formulation isotonic, and sodium hydroxide to adjust the final pH to a range of 6 to 9 (**Table 4**). Historically, the most common oil sources used in ILEs have been soybean oil and safflower oil, which contain long chain triglycerides (LCTs).[14] These oils were used because they are relatively inexpensive, abundant on the market, and effectively deliver nonglucose energy to the body. A disadvantage of soybean and safflower oils is their high levels of omega-6 fatty acid and low levels of omega-3 fatty acid, a ratio that is known to promote systemic inflammation. In an effort to address concerns associated with the soybean oil–based lipid emulsions, alternative sources of fatty acids were and continue to be investigated.[20]

In 2016, the Food and Drug Administration approved SMOFlipid™, which is comprised of four different oils: 30% soybean, 30% medium-chain triglycerides derived from coconut oil, 25% olive oil, and 15% fish oil. SMOFlipid, and others like it, have an improved omega-3:omega-6 ratio that may reduce the risk of harmful changes to the liver, such as **parenteral nutrition associated liver disease (PNALD)** and **hepatic steatosis**, and may preserve antioxidant capacity in critically ill patients. Ideally, this can contribute to better health outcomes such as shorter ICU stays.[22]

ILEs are commercially available in 10% (1.1 kcal per milliliter), 20% (2 kcal per milliliter), and 30% concentrations (2.9 to 3 kcal per milliliter, depending on the manufacturer); however, 30% ILE is not approved for direct intravenous administration. This high concentration is only approved for the compounding of a **total nutrient admixture** (TNA).

A 3 in 1 TNA is a PN formulation that contains 3 macronutrients (dextrose, amino acids, and lipid) in one solution. In addition, PN can be prepared as a 2 in 1 formulation containing 2 macronutrients (dextrose and amino acids) in one solution. When ILEs are infused as separate preparations from dextrose and amino acids as with a 2 in 1 formulation, there is enhanced microbial growth potential because the pH of the lipid emulsion is biologically compatible with bacteria. For this reason, the Centers for Disease Control and Prevention recommends a 12-hour hang time limit for ILE.[23] In contrast, a 3 in 1 TNA containing dextrose, amino acids, and ILE in the same container may be administered over 24 hours because the solution has a pH of 5.6 to 6, which is more likely to inhibit bacterial growth, and the increased total osmolarity with the combination of all three substrates in one container delays/inhibits microbial growth.[14,23]

In practice, lipid is not always given in PN. Although institutions may have their own criteria, it is common to hold lipid when a patient is receiving propofol, which is a short-acting hypnotic sedative provided in a 10% lipid emulsion. Lipids should also be withheld in patients who have an egg or soy allergy, or when they have hypertriglyceridemia prior to the initiation of lipid. According to A.S.P.E.N. guidelines, soybean oil–based ILE should be withheld from or limited in critically ill patients during the first week following initiation of parenteral nutrition to a maximum of 100 grams per week if there is concern for essential fatty acid deficiency. This provision is often divided into two doses of 50 grams or less per week. Alternative ILEs like SMOFlipid may provide outcome benefit over soy-based ILEs.[11]

TABLE 4 COMPOSITION OF PARENTERAL LIPID EMULSIONS

ILE, Manufacturer	Soybean Oil (%)	Safflower Oil (%)	Coconut Oil (%)	Olive Oil (%)	Fish Oil (%)
Intralipid, Fresenius Kabi	100	0	0	0	0
Liposyn II, Hospira	50	50	0	0	0
Lipofundin, B. Braun	50	0	50	0	0
SMOF Lipid™, Fresenius Kabi	30	0	30	25	15
ClinOleic, Baxter	20	0	0	80	0
Omegaven, Fresenius Kabi	0	0	0	0	100

CORE CONCEPT 5

Many lipid emulsions are composed of primarily omega-6 fatty acids and should be provided judiciously given their role in inflammation.

PRACTICE POINT

Most intravenous lipid emulsions contain egg yolk phospholipids as an emulsifying agent and soybean oil as the primary lipid source. For this reason, egg and soy allergies are contraindications of intravenous lipid infusion.

Electrolytes

Parenteral solutions represent a significant portion, if not all, of total daily fluid and electrolyte intake.[1] Maintenance or therapeutic amounts of various electrolytes are added to PN formulations depending on the patient's individual requirements. Acetate and chloride do not have specific ranges for intake; rather, they are adjusted as needed to maintain acid–base balance.[24] Other electrolytes are available in various salt forms as outlined in Table 5. For administration in PN, calcium gluconate and magnesium sulfate are the preferred forms of these electrolytes compared to calcium chloride, calcium gluceptate, and magnesium chloride because they are less likely to produce **physicochemical incompatibilities**, which are physical or chemical changes that can occur in PN leading to precipitation, color changes, or chemical degradation that can compromise the solution.[14]

PRACTICE POINT

Parenteral nutrition formulas that are high in amino acids can contribute to an increase in blood pH. To balance this effect, electrolytes in this situation can be provided as acetate.

Electrolytes are commercially available as individual salts and as combination products for ease in admixing. They are also pre-added to certain stock amino acid solutions or premixed PN formulations.[14]

Multivitamins

In addition to macronutrients and electrolytes, patients receiving PN require vitamins to prevent deficiency and promote optimal health. Clinical practice guidelines include the justification, dosage, and the route of delivery for inclusion of vitamins in patients receiving PN. Guideline adherence ensures optimum nutrition care and improves patient outcomes.

Commercially available vitamin products for parenteral nutrition supplementation include both single and multivitamin infusion products. In 2000, the Food and Drug Administration issued parenteral multivitamin dosing requirements.[14] In accordance with these requirements, parenteral multivitamins include vitamin A, vitamin D, vitamin E, vitamin K, vitamin B1, vitamin B2, vitamin B6, vitamin B12, niacin, folic acid, pantothenic acid, biotin, and vitamin C. One parenteral multivitamin product is available without vitamin K for patients on warfarin anticoagulant therapy.[25] Composition of the standard parenteral multivitamin products available in the United States is included in Table 6.

Single vitamins are used when a patient requires more of a vitamin than a parenteral multivitamin provides. Currently, there are no single vitamin products available for biotin, pantothenic acid, riboflavin, vitamin A, vitamin D, or vitamin E.[14]

Trace Elements

The need for trace elements in long-term parenteral nutrition was realized when patients began to develop deficiency symptoms that were alleviated through trace element supplementation. Some of the deficiencies that developed were copper, zinc, manganese, selenium, chromium, and molybdenum.[27] Of these, copper, zinc, manganese, selenium, and chromium are the most commonly supplemented trace elements in PN formulations. These trace minerals are available in both individual form and various trace element combinations at concentrations safe for use in neonates, pediatrics, and adults.[14] The American Medical Association and A.S.P.E.N. have published recommendations for daily parenteral dose of selenium, zinc, copper, manganese, and chromium, as seen in Table 7.

Other trace elements that are less commonly used in PN but are still available are molybdenum, iodine, and iron. Iron dextran is the only iron product approved for addition to PN. This product should only be added to 2 in 1 dextrose-amino acid formulations as opposed to PN formulas that contain lipid, like a 3 in 1 TNA, because ILEs are disrupted by iron.[14] If iron dextran is administered, strict protocol should be followed and the patient should be closely monitored as anaphylaxis is a potential side effect.[28] Nonetheless, iron is still an essential part of most long-term PN regimens and necessary in order to prevent deficiency.[29]

TABLE 5 COMMERCIALLY AVAILABLE PARENTERAL ELECTROLYTE SALTS

	Chloride	Acetate	Phosphate	Sulfate	Gluconate	Gluceptate
Sodium	X	X	X	–	–	–
Potassium	X	X	X	–	–	–
Calcium	X	–	–	–	X	X
Magnesium	X	–	–	X	–	–

TABLE 6 COMPOSITION OF ADULT PARENTERAL MULTIVITAMIN PRODUCTS AVAILABLE IN THE UNITED STATES[1,26]

Vitamin/Mineral	FDA requirement	MVI-12	MVI-13
Vitamin C (ascorbic acid)	200 mg	200 mg	200 mg
Niacin (niacinamide)	40 mg	40 mg	40 mg
Pantothenic acid (dexpanthenol)	15 mg	15 mg	15 mg
Vitamin E (dl-α-Tocopherol acetate)	10 mg (10 USP units)	10 mg (10 USP units)	10 mg (10 USP units)
Vitamin B6 (pyridoxine)	6 mg	6 mg	6 mg
Vitamin B1 (thiamin)	6 mg	6 mg	6 mg
Vitamin B2 (riboflavin)	3.6 mg	3.6 mg	3.6 mg
Vitamin A (retinol)	1 mg (3300 USP units)	1 mg (3300 USP units)	1 mg (3300 USP units)
Folic acid	600 mcg	600 mcg	600 mcg
Vitamin K (phylloquinone)	150 mcg	0	150 mcg
Biotin	60 mcg	60 mcg	60 mcg
Vitamin D (ergocalciferol)	5 mcg (200 USP units)	5 mcg (200 USP units)	5 mcg (200 USP units)
Vitamin B12 (cyanocobalamin)	5 mcg	5 mcg	5 mcg

TABLE 7 TRACE ELEMENT DEFICIENCIES ASSOCIATED WITH LONG-TERM PARENTERAL NUTRITION[24,27]

Deficiency	Symptoms	A.S.P.E.N. Recommendation
Copper	• Sensory ataxia • Lower extremity spasticity • Paresthesias in extremities • Hypochromic microcytic anemia • Leukopenia • Neutropenia • Hypercholesterolemia • Decreased ceruloplasmin and erythrocyte Cu/Zn • Increased erythrocyte turnover • Abnormal electrocardiographic patterns • Myeloneuropathy	0.3-0.5 mg/day
Zinc	• Inadequate growth • Acrodermatitis • Hypogonadism • Impaired night vision	2.5-5 mg/day

(*continues*)

TABLE 7 TRACE ELEMENT DEFICIENCIES ASSOCIATED WITH LONG-TERM PARENTERAL NUTRITION[24,27] *(Continued)*		
Deficiency	**Symptoms**	**A.S.P.E.N. Recommendation**
Zinc (continued)	• Anorexia • Diarrhea • Alterations in taste and smell • Alopecia • Impaired epithelialization and wound healing • Impaired immune function	
Manganese	• Poor reproductive performance • Congenital abnormalities in offspring • Abnormal bone/cartilage formation • Ataxia • Growth retardation • Defects in lipid/carbohydrate metabolism	60-100 mcg/day
Selenium	• Oxidative injury • Increased susceptibility to mercury poisoning • Altered thyroid hormone metabolism • Increased plasma glutathione levels • Keshan disease	20-60 mcg/day
Chromium	• Weight loss • Hyperglycemia refractory to insulin • Glycosuria • Elevated plasma free fatty acids • Peripheral neuropathy • Hyperlipidemia	10-15 mcg/day
Molybdenum	• Tachycardia • Tachypnea • Visual/mental changes • Elevated methionine • Headache • Lethargy • Nausea • Vomiting	
Iron	• Microcytic hypochromic anemia • Tachycardia • Poor capillary refilling • Fatigue • Sleepiness • Headache • Anorexia • Nausea • Pallor • Impaired ability to maintain body temperature in cold environments • Increased lead absorption • Koilonychia • Glossitis	

Other Additives

Insulin

The development of hyperglycemia during inpatient parenteral nutrition therapy has been independently associated with higher rates of mortality and hospital complications. These observations indicate that prevention and correction of hyperglycemia through modification of nutrient composition or by insulin administration should be strongly considered during PN therapy.[30] Insulin can be administered through sliding scale coverage, subcutaneous injection of long-acting insulin, an intravenous insulin infusion, insulin mixed into the PN formula, or any combination of these. The most common initial regimen for insulin in PN is 1 unit of regular insulin per 10 grams of dextrose. In hyperglycemic patients (glucose >150 mg/dL), the regimen may increase to 1.5 units of regular insulin per 10 grams of dextrose.[31] It is critical to use hospital- or unit-specific protocols for insulin infusions that include careful monitoring blood glucose to allow for proper intervention of both high and low levels.

Medications

Addition of certain medications into PN solutions is generally not advised due to potential for the formation of precipitates, adverse reactions, and disturbances in acid–base balance.[14,31] Medication compatibility with PN often depends on the hydrophilicity or hydrophobicity of the drug/medication and the formulation of the PN solution. Lipid-based (hydrophobic) medications are more likely to be compatible with ILE or TNA, while water-based medications (hydrophilic) are more likely to be compatible with a 2 in 1 dextrose-amino acid solutions.[14] Under current practice standards, pharmacists can admix certain medications into PN solutions; however, medication should never be added after the solution leaves the pharmacy or compounding center (Figure 9).[32]

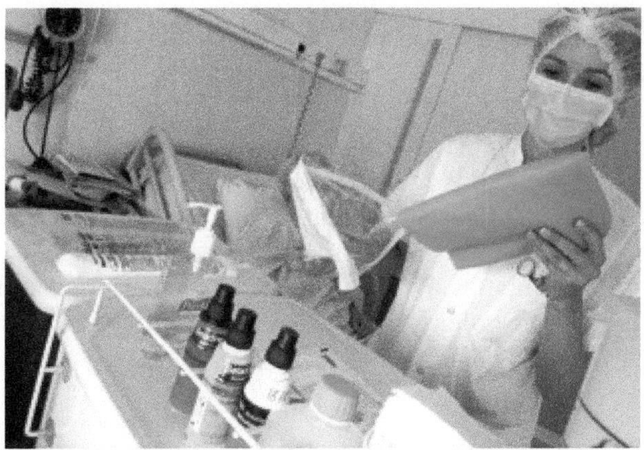

FIGURE 9 **Clinician Preparing to Infuse Patient with Parenteral Nutrition**

PRACTICE POINT

When in doubt about compatibility or safety of a medication or parenteral nutrition additive, seek evidence in existing literature and contact the pharmacist responsible for admixing parenteral solutions at your institution.

Clinical Roundtable

Topic: PN Component Shortages: An Ethical Challenge

Background: PN component shortages have been consistently impacting hospitals and home infusion companies since spring 2010.[33] Since then, every parenteral nutrition component has been in short supply, including ILE, amino acids, vitamins, electrolyte additives, and sterile water.[34] Shortages arise due to issues in the manufacturing process. Because producing PN components and other drugs is a highly controlled process for safety and sterility, there are a limited number of production lines that can meet these requirements. When a problem arises at one of these locations, pharmaceutical companies are responsible for notifying the Food and Drug Administration if a decrease in supply is projected.

Currently, there is no mandatory timeframe to resolve the manufacturing issue. Because the PN drug market is not a particularly profitable one, there is little incentive for pharmaceutical companies to resolve shortages quickly.[35] These shortages pose a significant risk for patients who rely on PN as their sole source of nutrition. If a component is in short supply, clinicians are forced to administer a lower dose, prioritize which patients receive the component, or omit the component entirely. Various deficiencies have been reported as a result of this ongoing issue.[34]

In response to ongoing drug shortages, A.S.P.E.N. created the Parenteral Nutrition Product Shortage Committee as a subcommittee of the Clinical Practice Committee. This group continually disseminates information on current and expected component and drug shortages.[34] They have also developed and published a set of recommendations for managing shortages. The recommendations provide strategies for rationing and conserving products so that drugs and PN components are available for the most critical patients.[33-35]

Roundtable Discussion

Consider a scenario in which there was a PN component shortage at your institution.

1. How would you prioritize which patients would continue to receive PN and which patients would not?
2. What strategies could you use to ensure that as many patients as possible receive adequate nutrition despite the shortage?

Initiation and Progression of Parenteral Nutrition

As stated previously in this chapter, PN is a type of nutrition support that is typically individualized to the needs of the patient. This customization requires knowledge of each of the component parts that compose PN and use of basic mathematics. Calculating the PN prescription and filling out the order form appropriately is often the most intimidating aspect of PN for clinical trainees and novice clinicians. Table 8 provides a commonly used method to calculate a PN prescription. An example of this method is provided in Table 9.

CORE CONCEPT 6

Prescription of parenteral nutrition is based on energy and protein requirements with consideration of fluid specifications and substrate utilization of macronutrients.

TABLE 8 PARENTERAL NUTRITION FORMULA CALCULATION METHOD

For steps where there is more than one way to determine needs, the most commonly used formulas are highlighted in gray.

Determine energy requirements	• Use the standard method utilized by your institution including but not limited to: – Indirect calorimetry – Harris–Benedict equation – Mifflin–St. Jeor predictive equation – Penn State predictive equation – Estimation using kcal/kg
Determine protein requirements and calories from protein	Protein stress factor based on disease state or severity of disease × weight in kg = protein requirement (grams) $\text{protein (gram)} \times 4\ \frac{\text{kcal}}{\text{gram}} = \text{kcal from protein}$
Determine ILE requirements	Does the patient need to receive lipids? No: – If patient is receiving propofol **or** – If patient has hypertriglyceridemia (TG >300 mg/dL) **or** – If patient has egg or soy allergy **or** – If the patient is critically ill and has received PN for fewer than 7 days Yes: If above conditions do not apply and/or if the patient has essential fatty acid deficiency If yes: total energy requirement (kcal) × x% energy from lipid = lipid requirement (kcal) *energy from lipid is typically 30% or less and should not exceed 60% kcal from lipid
Calculate kcal remaining for dextrose	Total energy requirement – [(protein kcal) + (lipid kcal)] = dextrose kcal protein kcal = grams protein × 4 kcals/gram protein
Calculate grams of dextrose	$\text{Dextrose (kcal)} \div 3.4\ \frac{\text{kcal}}{\text{gram}} = \text{dextrose (g)}$
Determine desired total volume	Is the patient fluid restricted? If yes: Aim for 1 L volume of PN or less per day If no: Use predictive equation for fluid, typical PN volumes are 1.2 to 2 per day: $\text{X fluid} \left(\frac{\text{mL}}{\text{kg}}\right) \times \text{weight (kg)} = \text{fluid requirement (mL)}$

TABLE 8 PARENTERAL NUTRITION FORMULA CALCULATION METHOD *(Continued)*

	x is the factor being used to calculate fluid. Typical factors for maintenance fluid needs are listed below: If fluid losses are expected or the nutrition care plan includes home PN, be sure to provide at least maintenance fluid needs. • Young adults: 35 mL/kg body weight • Adults: 30 mL/kg body weight • Older Adults: 25 mL/kg body weight
Calculate component concentration/ volume	Protein (concentration): $\text{protein requirement (g)} \div \text{desired volume of parental nutrition (mL)} \times 1000\ \frac{\text{mL}}{\text{L}}$ $= \text{concentration of amino acid solution } \frac{\text{grams AA}}{\text{L}}$ $\text{grams AA/L} \div 100 \longrightarrow \text{percent AA\%}$ Round to the nearest available amino acid concentration Lipid (volume and gram): $\text{lipid requirement (kcal)} \div \text{ILE concentration } \frac{\text{kcal}}{\text{mL}} = \text{lipid requirement (mL)}$ $\text{lipid volume (mL)} \times \text{ILE concentration } \frac{\text{kcal}}{\text{mL}} \times \frac{\text{1g ILE}}{\text{10 kcal}} = \text{lipid grams (g)}$ ILE volume is considered anhydrous and some may prefer to exclude ILE volume from total fluid volume when providing maintenance fluid requirements. Dextrose (concentration): $\text{dextrose requirement (g)} \div \text{desired volume of parental nutrition (mL)} \times 1000\ \frac{\text{mL}}{\text{L}}$ $= \text{concentration of dextrose solution } \frac{\text{grams}}{\text{L}}$ $\text{grams dextrose/L} \div 100 \longrightarrow \text{percent dextrose\%}$ Round to the nearest available dextrose concentration
Determine goal rate	$\text{Total volume (mL)} \div 24\ \frac{\text{hours}}{\text{day}} = \text{goal rate } \frac{\text{mL}}{\text{hour}}$
Final answer	The PN prescription can be ordered per day or per liter. Per day: Total grams of dextrose per day, total grams of amino acids per day, and total grams of lipid per day = _______ kcal/day, ___________g protein/day Per liter: D(percent concentration of dextrose)AA(percent concentration of amino acid) with (concentration of ILE) ILE at (goal rate) mL/hour = _______ kcal/day, _______ grams protein/day

TABLE 9 PARENTERAL NUTRITION FORMULA CALCULATION METHOD: A SAMPLE CALCULATION

40-year-old male
178 cm, 91 kg
Trauma, hypermetabolic, intubated, sedated, 8 days NPO
All labs within normal limits
Propofol: 20 mL/hour, Maintenance fluid requirement: 114 mL/hour
The hospital utilizes 2 in 1 PN formulations and 20% ILE

Determine energy requirements	Penn State Equation = 2650 kcal per day
Determine protein requirements and calories from protein	Protein stress factor based on disease state or severity of illness $\times$ weight in kg = protein requirement $\frac{g}{kg}$ $\left(1.4\ \frac{g}{kg}\right) \times 91\ \text{kg} = 127$ grams protein/day Protein requirement = 127 grams per day $127\ \text{Protein (gram)} \times 4\ \frac{\text{kcal}}{\text{gram}} = 508$ kcal from Protein
Determine ILE requirements	Does the patient need to receive IV lipids? No: – If patient is receiving propofol **or** – If patient has hypertriglyceridemia (TG >300 mg/dL) **or** – If patient has egg or soy allergy **or** – If the patient is critically ill and has received PN for fewer than 7 days Yes: If above conditions do not apply and/or if the patient has essential fatty acid deficiency No, the patient is receiving propofol at 20 mL/hour. To calculate calories from propofol which is based in 10% ILE: $20\ \frac{\text{mL}}{\text{hr}} \times 24\ \frac{\text{hours}}{\text{day}} = 480\ \frac{\text{mL}}{\text{day}}$ $480\ \text{mL} \times 1.1\ \frac{\text{kcal}}{\text{mL}} = 528\ \text{kcal}$ This is supplying the patient with 528 kcal/day from lipid. If the patient was not receiving propofol, triglycerides were within normal limits, and his goal was set at 20% of total calories, his requirement would be 530 kcal. This is calculated with the following equation: total energy requirement (kcal) $\times$ x% energy from lipid = lipid requirement (kcal) 2650 kcal $\times$ 20% energy from lipid = 530 (kcal) After 14 days of NPO status, if no other lipid source provided, the patient should be given essential fatty acids at a minimum of 2% to 4% of total kcals to prevent essential fatty acid deficiency.
Calculate kcal remaining for dextrose	Total energy requirement (kcal) – (protein (kcal) + lipid (kcal)) = dextrose (kcal) 2650 kcal – (508 kcal + 528 kcal) = 1614 kcal Kcal remaining for dextrose = 1614
Calculate grams of dextrose	$\text{Dextrose (kcal)} \div 3.4\ \frac{\text{kcal}}{\text{gram}} = \text{dextrose (g)}$ $1614\ \text{kcal} \div 3.4\ \frac{\text{kcal}}{\text{gram}} = 475\ \text{grams}$ 475 grams of dextrose/day

TABLE 9 PARENTERAL NUTRITION FORMULA CALCULATION METHOD: A SAMPLE CALCULATION *(Continued)*

Determine desired total volume	$X \text{ fluid} \left(\frac{mL}{kg}\right) \times \text{weight (kg)} = \text{fluid requirement (mL)}$ $30 \left(\frac{mL}{kg}\right) \times 91 \text{ (kg)} = 2730 \text{ mL/day}$ This patient is not on a fluid restriction, so the predictive equation for adults was used. The desired volume of both the patient's maintenance fluid and parenteral nutrition is 2730 mL per day.
Calculate component concentrations/volume	Protein (concentration): $(\text{Protein requirement (g)} \div \text{desired volume of parental nutrition (mL)}) \times 1000 \frac{mL}{L}$ $= \text{concentration of amino acid solution} \frac{grams}{L}$ $(127 \text{ (g)} \div 2730 \text{ (mL)}) \times 1000 = 46.5 \text{ g/L} \rightarrow 4.7\% \text{ amino acid (rounded)}$ Lipid (volume): No ILE required. Sufficient lipid coming from propofol at 20 mL/hour. If the patient was not receiving propofol and required 530 kcal from ILE, the volume of 20% ILE needed to meet his lipid requirement would be calculated as follows: $530 \text{ kcal} \div 2 \frac{kcal}{mL\ ILE} = 265 \text{ mL ILE at 20\% concentration}$ $265 \text{ mL} \times 2 \frac{kcal}{mL} \times \frac{1g\ ILE}{10\ kcal} = 53 \text{ g lipid}$ Dextrose (concentration): $(\text{dextrose requirement (g)} \div \text{desired volume of parental nutrition (mL)}) \times 1000 \frac{mL}{L}$ $= \text{concentration of dextrose solution} \frac{grams}{L}$ $(475 \text{ (g)} \div 2730 \text{ (mL)}) \times 1000 = 174 \frac{g}{L}$ $= 17.4\% \rightarrow 17\% \text{ dextrose (rounded)}$
Determine goal rate	$\text{total volume (mL)} \div 24 \frac{hours}{day} = \text{goal rate} \frac{mL}{hour}$ $2730 \text{ (mL)} \div 24 \frac{hours}{day} = 114 \frac{mL}{hour}$
Final answer	Per day: 475 g dextrose/day, 127 g AA/day with propofol at 20 ml/hr = 2603 kcal/day, 127 grams protein/day Per liter: D17AA4.7 at 114 mL/hour with propofol at 20 mL/hour = 2623 kcal/day, 129 g protein/day Note that when ordering per liter, numbers tend to be rounded leading to slight difference in calculated calories and protein.

Safety Check of Macronutrient Infusion Rates

Due to risk for complications, there are maximum infusion rates set for both lipid and carbohydrate. The maximum lipid infusion rate is 1.7 mg/kg/min, the maximum rate of lipid oxidation.[21]

The maximum glucose infusion rate, also based on glucose oxidation rate in metabolically stressed adult patients, is 5 mg/kg/min.[36]

In order to calculate the glucose infusion rate, convert carbohydrate requirement in grams to milligrams by multiplying by 1000. Then, divide the requirement in milligrams by the weight of the patient in kilograms. Lastly, divide this number by 1440 minutes per day to give the infusion rate of milligrams per kilogram of body weight per minute (Table 10). If the glucose infusion rate is calculated to be greater than the maximum infusion rate, it is highly recommended that the PN formula be adjusted.

CORE CONCEPT 7

Carbohydrate infusion from parenteral nutrition should not exceed 5 mg/kg/min in adults and children over the age of 2 years.

Electrolyte Requirements

It is common that electrolytes are ordered in milliequivalents instead of milliliters in PN solutions. The standard daily electrolyte requirements in milliequivalents are listed in Table 11, although electrolyte levels should be monitored regularly and adjusted as needed. Each component of PN solution contributes to its osmolarity, which ultimately determines into which type of vein (central versus peripheral) the solution can be infused. Refer to Table 12 for the method to calculate osmolarity.

Vitamin and Trace Element Requirements

Typically, the adult dose of multivitamin given per day is 10 mL. If a patient has needs beyond what is provided in MVI-12 or MVI-13, additional may be provided in single-vitamin form. This may add to the total volume of parenteral nutrition provided.[14]

The standard adult dose of the multiple trace elements solution given per day is 5 mL.

When the parenteral nutrition prescription is complete and safety checks have been made in regard to safe infusion rates, an order form must be completed and provided to the pharmacy. Most institutions have their own standard PN order form. It is crucial that the information input into the order form is specific and easily understood so that the formulation is made correctly.

TABLE 10 CALCULATING GLUCOSE INFUSION RATE

$$\text{Carbohydrate requirement (g)} \times 1000\ \frac{\text{mg}}{\text{g}} = \text{requirement (mg)}$$

$$\text{requirement (mg)} \div \text{weight (kg)} = \text{infusion}\ \frac{\text{mg}}{\text{kg body weight}}$$

$$\text{infusion}\ \frac{\text{mg}}{\text{kg body weight}} \div 1440\ \frac{\text{minute}}{\text{day}}$$

$$= \text{infusion rate}\ \frac{\frac{\text{mg}}{\text{kg body weight}}}{\text{minute}}$$

TABLE 11 DAILY ELECTROLYTE REQUIREMENTS[24]

Electrolyte	Daily Parenteral Requirement
Sodium	1-2 mEq/kg
Potassium	1-2 mEq/kg
Chloride	As needed to maintain acid–base balance
Acetate	As needed to maintain acid–base balance
Calcium	10-15 mEq
Magnesium	8-20 mEq
Phosphate	20-40 mmol

TABLE 12 OSMOLARITY CALCULATION

1. Multiply grams of dextrose per liter by 5
2. Multiply grams of amino acids per liter by 8.8
3. Multiply mEq of sodium per liter by 2
4. Multiply mEq of potassium per liter by 2
5. Multiply mEq of calcium per liter by 1.5
6. Multiply mEq of magnesium per liter by 1
7. Add numbers 1 -7 to calculate total osmolarity in mOsm/L

CORE CONCEPT 8

Parenteral nutrition formulations are customizable to the specific needs of each patient or patient population.

CASE STUDY REVISITED

You determine that PN is justified for Alex and are asked to provide Alex's PN prescription.

Questions

1. **Is the provision of lipid as a component of Alex's PN indicated? Justify your answer.**
2. **Calculate a PN prescription for Alex assuming Alex requires 1920 kcal and 85 g protein**
3. **Calculate the glucose infusion rate of your prescription. Does the glucose infusion rate of your prescription follow safe protocol?**

Progression of PN

Before initiating PN, ensure that the patient has stable vital signs and normal fluid and electrolyte balance. Box 2 details clinical scenarios in which PN should be used with caution. Any imbalances should be corrected and addressed either prior to PN initiation or in the PN formula.[3] Shortly after the initiation of PN is a common time for patients to experience fluid and electrolyte disturbances. It is critical for the clinician to monitor the patient closely during this time to reduce the risk of complications and/or slowing the advancement of the PN.

For patients previously on insulin or hypoglycemic agents, or fasting glucose ≥200 mg/dL, dextrose should be limited to approximately 100 g on the first day of PN.[31] However, if a patient's blood glucose exceeds 300 mg/dL, PN should be withheld until glycemic control improves.

Infusion may begin at a low rate (approximately half of energy needs) and gradually advance over 2 to 3 days to minimize the risk of refeeding syndrome, hyperglycemia, and hypervolemia.[3,36,37] Patients at risk of refeeding syndrome should progress at a slower rate over 3 to 4 days.[9] Aim for a glucose infusion rate of no more than 4 to 5 mg/kg/min to minimize the risk of hyperglycemia.[37] In the ICU, glucose infusion rate is typically initially held to 3 to 4 mg/kg/min. Blood glucose should be well controlled before advancing to the goal rate.[3]

Critically ill patients require special considerations for advancement of PN as they are at greater risk for hyperglycemia and insulin resistance. In addition, among some critically ill patients, excessive energy intake is associated with greater risk of infectious morbidity, increased duration of mechanical ventilation, and increased length of stay.[9] Permissive underfeeding (80% of target calorie intake) may be considered. Among obese critically ill patients, permissive underfeeding may be as low as 65% to 70% of target calories.[11] However, as the patient stabilizes, feeding may be advanced to 100% of goal.

Administration of PN may be through **continuous infusion** (over 24 hours) or **cyclical infusion** (10 to 12 hours per day). Hospitalized patients typically receive PN continuously, whereas those on long-term PN usually receive cyclical infusions in order to allow freedom from the pump.

Transitional Feeding

Use of the GI tract is ideal when possible, and so patients may be transitioned from PN to EN or oral intake under careful supervision. Among the critically ill, once a patient is stabilized on PN, EN should be periodically trialed. If transitioning to EN, begin at a slow rate of 30 to 40 mL/hour with a formula appropriate to the patient's needs to assess tolerance. As the volume of EN received increases, the amount of energy provided by PN should decrease accordingly to prevent overfeeding. However, PN should not be terminated until ≥60% of target calories are provided enterally.[9] As with initiating PN, terminating PN should be done gradually to prevent hypoglycemia.

Transitioning from PN to oral intake is a less-predictable process than transitioning from PN to EN due to variations in patients' appetite and motivation to eat. Patients may be introduced first to clear liquids followed by a low-fat, low-fiber, and lactose-free diet. Oral intake should account for approximately 75% of the patient's calorie needs before discontinuing PN. For patients who cannot meet this goal, PN may continue to provide supplementary nutrition.

Parenteral Nutrition Monitoring

Parenteral nutrition is a costly therapy that requires regular clinical monitoring and diligent care of the patient in order to support a good outcome. Nutritional monitoring is needed to determine efficiency of the solution being administered, to discover and prevent complications, and to document changes in the clinical course. Monitoring should preferably be carried out by a nutrition support team, which monitors efficiency and sufficiency of PN with regards to specific endpoints defined by the patient's underlying illness, clinical status, the facilities available in the institution caring for the patient, and patient requests.[11,38]

CORE CONCEPT 9

Parenteral nutrition formulations are customizable to the specific needs of each patient or patient population.

Anthropometrics

Weight monitoring of parenteral nutrition patients is important. Steep, short-term increases and decreases in body weight may indicate changes in fluid status such as dehydration or edema. Intake and output can give further insight to suspected changes in fluid status.

Vital Signs

Vital signs include temperature, blood pressure, pulse, and respiration rate. Temperature is important to monitor in PN patients because fever is an indicator of infection and increases energy requirements. This may change the course of clinical care and PN requirements.

Blood pressure is important to monitor because it reflects hemodynamic stability or instability. If a patient is hemodynamically unstable, he or she may not be able to tolerate PN and require a medical intervention in order to correct the issue.

Heart rate is important to monitor because many electrolyte imbalances, a common occurrence in patients receiving PN, present with changes in pulse and arrhythmias when severe enough.

In PN patients, respiratory quotient is more useful information than respiration rate. The respiratory quotient is the ratio of carbon dioxide eliminated to oxygen consumed. Measurement of respiratory quotient in patients receiving PN is important in the prevention of fat accumulation in the liver and alleviation of potential respiratory distress secondary to excess glucose. Respiratory quotient should ideally be maintained between 0.7 and 1.0 to avoid metabolic disturbances.[39]

Biochemistry

Biochemical monitoring of electrolyte balance, blood glucose, renal function, iron studies, liver function, vitamin and trace element levels is important for both acute and long-term PN. Biochemical markers should be measured and analyzed on a defined, regular basis since attention to and adjustment of biochemical trends can reveal and prevent complications related to parenteral nutrition. Table 13 contains a sample monitoring schedule for anthropometric measurements, vital signs, and biochemical markers.

TABLE 13 SUGGESTED PARENTERAL NUTRITION MONITORING SCHEDULE (*MAY VARY BETWEEN INSTITUTIONS*)

Parameter	Initiation Period	Stable Period	Long-term
Vital signs	3-4x/day	Daily	As needed
Weight	Daily	2x/week	Weekly
Intake and output	Daily	Daily	
Blood glucose	Every 6 hours	Daily	Monthly
Sodium	Daily	Weekly	Monthly
Potassium	Daily	Weekly	Monthly
Chloride	Daily	Weekly	Monthly
Bicarbonate	Daily	Weekly	Monthly
Blood urea nitrogen	Daily	Weekly	Monthly
Creatinine	Daily	Weekly	Monthly
Calcium	Daily	Weekly	Monthly
Magnesium	Daily	Weekly	Monthly
Phosphorus	Daily	Weekly	Monthly
Complete blood count with differential	Weekly	Weekly	Monthly
Liver function tests (ALT and AST)	Weekly	Weekly	Monthly
Triglycerides	Weekly	Weekly	Monthly
Prothrombin time	Weekly	Monthly	4x/year
Prealbumin	Weekly	Monthly	4x/year
Trace element levels	N/A	N/A	4x/year

TABLE 14 NUTRITION-FOCUSED PHYSICAL EXAM IN MONITORING PATIENTS ON PARENTERAL NUTRITION

Physical Sign	Etiology	Parenteral Nutrition Implication
"Tenting" of skin Dry mucosa Poor skin turgor Sunken eyes Decreased urine output	Dehydration	Increase fluid provided through PN if not on restriction
Edema (pitting or abdominal) Dilution per laboratory values Weight gain	Overhydration	Decrease fluid provided through PN by transitioning to more-concentrated solution
Inflammation at the catheter site (swollen, red, or hot to the touch)	Potential infection	Appropriate medical intervention and patient education on proper catheter-site care if applicable
Signs of nutrient deficiency in sites with high cell turnover (hair, skin, mouth, tongue)	Nutrient deficiency	Test to confirm and add to PN prescription to compensate
Changes in clinical status such as intubation/sedation		May require changes to PN prescription

Nutrition-Focused Physical Exam

Nutrition-focused physical exam (NFPE) of patients on PN is a necessary component of monitoring. Physical signs to evaluate in an NFPE, their etiology, and PN implications are further described in Table 14.

Central Venous Access Complications and Their Management

Patients receiving PN are at risk for a wide variety of **catheter-related complications (CRCs)**, beginning at the time of catheter placement. These complications may be mechanical (infectious or noninfectious) or metabolic in nature. Risk of CRCs is impacted by the type of catheter used, the team's procedural experience, the duration of PN therapy, the quality of catheter care, and the patient's underlying disease state.[40] Some complications may be relatively manageable, while others are more serious. For these reasons, careful monitoring by a skilled team is essential. The prevention of many CRCs is possible with strict adherence to evidence-based protocols.[41]

Mechanical Complications

Catheter-related Mechanical Complications

Mechanical complications are related to the insertion of and care for the catheter and can be classified as either infectious or noninfectious. Some complications may develop at the time of catheterization or soon after (e.g., pneumothorax, arterial puncture, air embolism), while others develop over time (e.g., occlusion, infection).[42]

Certain types of venous access devices and their method of securement (e.g., sutures versus suture-less) are associated with more or less frequent occurrence of complications. PICCs and implantable ports are associated with a particularly low rate of mechanical complications, whereas nontunneled catheters are associated with a higher rate of bloodstream infections and symptomatic venous thrombosis.[41] The method of catheter placement also impacts risk of complications. Using ultrasound-guided catheterization can significantly reduce complications such as pneumothorax and catheter-related thrombosis compared to "blind" catheterization that relies on anatomical landmarks.[41,43]

Noninfectious Mechanical Complications

Noninfectious mechanical complications include pneumothorax, arterial puncture, embolism, occlusion, and venous thrombosis. In general, these complications are rare, occurring in 1% to 4% of central catheter placements when access is established by an experienced operator, and potential complications can be identified early on by radiologic and clinical exam.[40]

Pneumothorax Catheterization carries the risk of **pneumothorax**, a puncture in the pleura of the lung leading to air accumulation in the pleural space, resulting in a collapsed lung.[44] Depending on the severity of the pneumothorax, the patient may require a chest tube while the air leak seals. PICCs carry a lower risk of pneumothorax, although they are more likely to be malpositioned.[40]

Arterial puncture In general, the veins used for PN are large and easy for an experienced operator to access. Accidental arterial puncture can occur resulting in complications such as temporary occlusion, pseudoaneurysm, and hematoma. Factors that contribute to the risk of arterial puncture include darkly pigmented skin and anatomical variations such as thoracic outlet syndrome.[45]

Occlusion A **catheter occlusion** is the most common type of noninfectious mechanical complication and is defined as the inability to infuse, flush, and/or aspirate on the venous access device.[5,46] Occlusions can be caused by the precipitation of minerals, medications, and lipids, which then obstruct the catheter. Symptoms include neck vein distension, edema, tingling/pain in the arm and neck, a tight feeling in the throat, and prominent veins of the anterior chest.[5] Occlusions may be cleared via repeated saline flushes.[40] Failing this, flushing with other solutions such as thrombolytics, sodium bicarbonate, hydrochloric acid, and sodium hydroxide can be used. If the catheter cannot be cleared, it may need to be replaced.

Catheter-related venous thrombosis (CRVT) may occur when catheterization damages the vessel wall, activating the coagulation of platelets and fibrin and resulting in a thrombus.[5] This process can begin within minutes of catheter placement. The risk of thrombus development is influenced by the catheter tip location, catheter material, type of PN formula, and length of catheter duration. The major risks of venous thrombosis are the potential for **thrombotic occlusion** (the cannulated vessel is blocked) and **thromboembolism** (the thrombus breaks free and blocks an artery).[5,40] The symptoms of thrombotic occlusion are similar to a catheter occlusion (edema, neck vein distension, tingling of the arm and neck). If the catheter is still functional (i.e., not fully occluded), there is evidence that the catheter should be left in situ rather than removed. Removing the catheter could dislodge any thromboses in contact with the catheter and result in thromboembolism.[46] Thrombolytics injected into the catheter may be used to treat this complication. Currently, there is no universally accepted strategy to prevent CRVT. Commonly used strategies include the use of heparin and heparin-bonded catheters.[40]

Embolism Embolisms are a rare occurrence in which material becomes lodged in an artery, resulting in significant morbidity and mortality.[47] In PN, various types of embolism are possible, including thromboembolism, **catheter embolism**, and **air embolism**.[40] Catheter embolisms can occur if the catheter becomes damaged and a piece of the equipment breaks free. Air embolisms can occur when there is a connection between the air and the cannulated vessel.[47] The pressure gradient drives air into the bloodstream, halting blood flow. Depending on the location of the blockage, embolisms may affect the cardiovascular, pulmonary, and neurological systems.

Phlebitis Phlebitis, or inflammation of the vein, is a relatively common complication in PN and is more common in PICC lines than other forms of access.[40] Inflammation at the exit site often raises suspicion of a bloodstream infection. However, in phlebitis, the inflammation is due to physical or chemical irritation from the catheter as opposed to infection.[40] Unless the exit site is overtly inflamed, and particularly if the patient has a fever, the appearance of the site is not a reliable indicator of catheter-related bloodstream infection.[48]

Infectious Complications

Catheter-related infections may be local or systemic. Local infections include infections of the exit site, tunnel, and port-pocket. They are usually treated by removing the catheter or port and administering a course of systemic antibiotics.[44] An exit-site infection in a tunneled catheter may not necessitate removal of the catheter—rather, frequent dressing changes coupled with a course of antibiotics should be provided.

Conversely, **catheter-related bloodstream infection (CRBSI)**, also called **central line–associated bloodstream infection (CLABSI)**, is a systemic infection and is one of the most serious complications of PN. Not only does it contribute to increased costs per patient, but CRBSI also increases length of stay by approximately 3 weeks and increases mortality by 14% to 40%.[49] CRBSI may lead to **sepsis**, a condition in which the body's normal inflammatory response to infection is amplified.[50] Sepsis can lead to organ dysfunction, hypotension, and death. While it has been understood since the 1970s that PN contributes to the risk of bloodstream infection, PN has recently been identified as an independent risk factor for infection.[51] A proposed mechanism is that the highly concentrated dextrose content of PN increases blood glucose concentrations, which increases the risk of infection, particularly among critically ill patients. The catheter itself also provides a surface on which bacteria can colonize, forming a **biofilm**. Biofilms are particularly resistant to antibiotics, antibodies, and phagocytes because bacteria are protected by a polysaccharide matrix.

CRBSI is characterized by fever, chills, and increased white blood cell count, and the diagnosis is confirmed through positive blood cultures drawn from the catheter lumen(s) and peripherally.[44] Increased bacterial growth in blood drawn from the catheter indicates CRBSI. CRBSI is commonly caused by *Candida* or yeast species, gram-positive bacteria (including *Staphylococcus aureus*, *Staphylococcus epidermis*, and *Enterococcus*), and gram-negative bacteria (including *Pseudomonas*, *Serratia marcescens*, *Klebsiella pneumoniae*, and *Escherichia coli*).[44]

CRBSI is first treated by administering broad-spectrum antibiotics through the catheter in order to avoid catheter removal.[44] However, it is necessary to remove the infected catheter if the patient continues to deteriorate or if blood cultures remain positive.[40,44] Prevention of CRBSI requires following strict guidelines at every point from choosing the appropriate venous access device to caring for the exit site. **Table 15** contains evidence-based strategies for preventing CRBSI.

TABLE 15 POINTS AT WHICH CATHETER-RELATED BLOODSTREAM INFECTION CAN BE PREVENTED[7,5,44]

Time Point	Strategies to Prevent CRBSI
Device selection	• For long-term PN, use tunneled and implanted catheters • Antimicrobial coated catheters are effective for short-term PN • Use single-lumen catheters unless the patient requires multiple ports • If using multiple lumens, one lumen should be reserved exclusively for PN
Catheterization procedure	• Use ultrasound-guided venipuncture • Take maximal barrier precautions during insertion: cap, mask, disposable gown, gloves, and large drape
PN administration and site care	• Enforce a strict hand washing policy • Use 2% chlorhexidine as skin antiseptic • Appropriately dress the exit site • Disinfect hubs, stopcocks, and needle-free connectors • Regularly change administration sets • Use antibiotic-lock or ethanol-lock: catheter lumen is filled with antibiotic solution or ethanol when not in use

CASE STUDY REVISITED

Alex has been on PN for 2 weeks. Below are his weight and his most recent metabolic panel:

Anthropometric Data:

Weight: 68 kg (150 lbs)
Admission weight: 64 kg (141 lbs)

Biochemical Data:

Sodium 133 (135-145 mEq/L)
Potassium 3.7 (3.6-5.0 mEq/L)
Chloride 99 (98-110 mEq/L)
Carbon dioxide 22 (20-30 mEq/L)
Blood urea nitrogen 8 (6-24 mg/dL)
Creatinine 0.4 (0.4-1.3 mg/dL)
Glucose 180 (70-139 mg/dL)
Aspartate transaminase (AST) 110 (10-35 IU/L)
Alanine tranaminase (ALT) 99 (4-36 units/L)
Alkaline phosphatase (ALP) 130 (30-120 units/L)
Direct (conjugated) bilirubin 3.0 (0-0.3 mg/dL)
Total bilirubin 1.9 (0.3-0.9 mg/dL)
Calcium 9 (8.5-10.5 mEq/L)
Phosphorus 3.4 (2.7-4.5 mg/dL)
Magnesium 1.5 (1.3-2.1 mEq/L)
Albumin 3.0 (3.5-5.0 g/dL)

Questions

1. **What is your interpretation of Alex's weight?**
2. **What biochemical labs are concerning?**
3. **How might you alter the PN composition or prescription? Provide specific changes to the initial PN prescription if necessary.**
4. **Are there other options you might consider for feeding Alex?**

Metabolic Complications

Hyper- and Hypoglycemia

It is normal for blood glucose to rise after initiating PN. However, endogenous insulin secretion should bring glucose back to a normal range. Hyperglycemia is the most common metabolic complication of PN. Prolonged, uncontrolled hyperglycemia can lead to nonketotic dehydration, coma, and death.[37] It is usually caused by excessive dextrose infusion, although it can also be a result of the stress response in acutely ill or septic patients. These patients are known to develop insulin resistance, suppressed insulin secretion, and increased gluconeogenesis and glycogenolysis.[37] Patients with diabetes, acute pancreatitis, or on corticosteroid medication are also at risk of hyperglycemia. To prevent hyperglycemia, ensure that dextrose is infused at no higher than 5 mg/kg/min. In addition, identify other potential sources of dextrose or changes in medications (e.g., corticosteroids).[52] Hyperglycemia is treated with insulin, which can be administered subcutaneously, intravenously, or added to the PN formula itself.[37]

Patients receiving PN are typically secreting higher-than-normal levels of insulin due to the high concentration of dextrose in the formula. Abruptly stopping PN infusion can therefore result in reactive hypoglycemia within 15 to 60 minutes.[42] A blood glucose level <70 mg/dL would suggest hypoglycemia.[53] This complication can be prevented by slowly tapering PN over 1 to 2 hours or by infusing 10% dextrose immediately after PN cessation.[42] The safest way to provide and manage insulin therapy is through standardized protocols.

Electrolyte Abnormalities

As discussed in Parenteral Nutrition Formulation, the electrolyte content added to PN is customizable to the patient's needs. Biochemical monitoring should be performed regularly to assess whether a patient requires more or less of particular electrolytes.

When initiating PN, however, severe electrolyte disturbances may be indicative of refeeding syndrome, especially in malnourished patients. Refeeding syndrome is characterized by hypophosphatemia, hypokalemia, and hypomagnesemia in addition to disturbances in glucose metabolism and fluid and sodium balance.[52] Advancing PN gradually over several days and supplementing electrolytes can help to prevent refeeding syndrome.[42]

Electrolyte abnormalities may also result in acid–base disturbances. Arterial blood normally has a pH range of 7.35 to 7.45, and this range should be closely monitored to ensure optimal organ function.[54] Many factors can contribute to disturbances in a patient's acid–base balance, including components of the PN formula. Treatment of acid–base disturbances should address the underlying cause. Acidosis (arterial pH <7.35) may be corrected by decreasing the amount of chloride provided or by providing bicarbonate in the form of acetate (a bicarbonate precursor).[54] Bicarbonate itself should not be added to the PN formula, as it is unstable. Alkalosis (arterial pH >7.45) may be corrected by decreasing the amount of acetate salts provided or replacing any potassium and magnesium deficits.[54]

Hyper- and Hypovolemia

Patients may receive all of their fluid intake from PN alone, but some may also be consuming fluids orally.[55] For these patients, assess whether there have been any changes in oral intake. Hypervolemia, or fluid overload, is likely due to excessive PN or intravenous fluid infusion.[55] Symptoms include weight gain, edema, and shortness of breath. Manage hypervolemia by maintaining or decreasing PN volume, unless fluid overload is severe, in which case PN may need to be discontinued temporarily.[52]

Hypovolemia, or a deficit in the extracellular fluid, can occur in a variety of ways, including ostomy output, diarrhea, fistulae, fever, or diuresis.[55,56] Symptoms include weight loss, decreased urine output, decreased urinary sodium concentration (<15 mEq/L), low blood pressure, muscle cramps, weakness, dizziness, thirst, and dry mouth.[55,56] Hypovolemia may or may not be accompanied by an electrolyte deficit. Repletion with intravenous fluids should take into consideration whether any electrolytes must also be repleted.[56]

Overfeeding

Dr. Jonathan Rhoads, one of the founders of PN, originally described this form of nutrition support as "hyperalimentation" (overfeeding).[57] It was initially believed that malnourished or hypermetabolic patients should be fed much more than their required nutrient needs in order to stimulate an anabolic response. However, it is now recognized that overfeeding increases the risk of complications, particularly bloodstream infections.[58] Overfeeding is more common in the ICU setting because critically ill and septic patients do not metabolize glucose and lipids normally, excess glucose and lipids increase metabolic stress and exacerbate the storage impairments associated with insulin resistance.[59]

Essential Fatty Acid Deficiency

Linoleic acid, an omega-6 fatty acid, and α-linolenic acid, an omega-3 fatty acid, are considered EFAs because they cannot be synthesized by humans.[60] EFA deficiency can develop in infants and children receiving fat-free PN within a few days, and in adults receiving fat-free PN within 2 weeks.[61,62] Clinical signs of essential fatty acid deficiency include hepatomegaly; thrombocytopenia; impaired wound healing; hair loss; and dry, desquamated skin.[60] In order to prevent EFA deficiency in patients receiving fat-free PN, linoleic acid must be administered.[61,62] **Table 16** contains more information on the amount of EFA required to prevent deficiency.

TABLE 16 AMOUNT OF LINOLEIC ACID REQUIRED TO PREVENT ESSENTIAL FATTY ACID DEFICIENCY DURING DIFFERENT STAGES OF THE LIFE CYCLE[61,62]	
Preterm infants	0.25 g/kg/day
Term infants and older children	0.1 g/kg/day
Adults	2%-4% of total calorie intake

Hepatobiliary Complications

There are essentially three types of hepatobiliary disorders associated with PN therapy: **hepatic steatosis**, **cholestasis**, and **cholelithiasis**.[63] These complications can happen without the use of parenteral nutrition; however, when attributable to the usage of PN, these complications are referred to as PN-associated liver disease (PNALD). It is estimated that PNALD develops in 40% to 60% of infants on long-term PN and 15% to 40% of adults on home PN for intestinal failure.[64]

Hepatic steatosis is the accumulation of fat in the liver. Although the development of hepatic steatosis is thought to be multifactorial, the use of soybean lipid emulsions is thought to be one of the largest contributing factors. Although the lipid particles in parenteral soybean oil emulsion mimic the size and structure of chylomicrons, they primarily contain omega-6 fatty acids and triglycerides and are devoid of cholesterol or protein. With reduced cholesterol, lipolysis is limited and the liver is prone to the accumulation of lipid particles. Although steatosis is reversible, it can advance to more serious stages of liver disease, and eventually to cirrhosis, if not appropriately managed.[65]

Cholestasis is a condition of reduced bile flow. This can be caused by any impairment between hepatocytes, which produce bile, and the duodenum, the site where bile is incorporated into the gastrointestinal tract. When bile flow is stopped, the pigment bilirubin escapes into the bloodstream and accumulates. For this reason, the primary indicator of cholestasis is a serum conjugated bilirubin >2 mg/dL. PNALD is initially characterized by cholestasis but can progress to fibrosis and cirrhosis with continued exposure to PN.[66,67]

Cholelithiasis is the presence of gallstones or gallbladder sludge. Gallstones can develop in patients receiving PN due to gallbladder stasis, or inactivity of the gallbladder. When the gallbladder is not stimulated to secrete stored bile, the bile begins to form sludge, which turns into gallstones.[68]

When a patient receiving PN develops hepatobiliary complications, it is necessary to rule out all treatable causes and minimize other risk factors. All potential hepatotoxic medications and herbal supplements should be eliminated. Modifications to the PN regimen that may be helpful include reduction of calories, reduction of ILE dose to <1 g/kg/day, replacement of an omega-6 lipid source with an omega-3 containing lipid source, supplementation of taurine in the infant, and use of cyclic infusion. Initiation of even small amounts of EN and use of ursodiol may be beneficial in stimulating bile flow. In the long-term PN patient with severe and progressive liver disease, intestinal or liver transplantation may be the only remaining treatment option.[63]

CASE STUDY REVISITED

Shortly after surgery, Alex remains on PN, but you believe that he is ready for trial oral feeding. A liquid diet is ordered, which he appears to tolerate well, and his PN is tapered. Two days later, Alex develops a fever, abdominal distention, and diarrhea. A CT scan reveals an enterocolonic fistula between the distal ileum and ascending colon. The surgeon determines that Alex will require further surgery to repair the fistula but advises waiting 3 to 6 months to allow the densest peritoneal adhesions to resolve. Until then, Alex will need to remain NPO and continue receiving PN. After another week in the hospital, Alex's fever, distention, and diarrhea have resolved and he is ready to be discharged on home PN.

Questions

1. **What questions would you ask to determine whether Alex would be able to independently manage home PN?**
2. **Describe three common complications associated with long-term PN. What symptoms and lab values would you monitor?**

Home Parenteral Nutrition

Indications and Access

Home parenteral nutrition (HPN) is becoming an increasingly common therapy. It is estimated that approximately 300 patients are placed on HPN in the United States each year.[69] The indications for HPN are similar to those for hospitalized patients. These patients have long-term (≥2 weeks) intestinal failure, cannot meet their nutritional needs through the enteral route alone, and can be treated outside of the acute care setting.[3,70] However, HPN is not recommended for terminally ill patients with a short life expectancy.[71] A.S.P.E.N. provides guidelines related to the ethical issues of nutrition support in end of life.[72]

Because hospitalization is no longer necessary, indications for HPN involve further considerations. Is the patient, family, or caregiver capable of administering PN? Is the home environment safe for PN? Will the patient's insurance cover HPN-related costs?

PRACTICE POINT

In the United States, the federal-level health insurance program Medicare will only cover HPN-related costs if it is documented that the patient's GI tract is nonfunctional, the condition is "permanent" (i.e., at least 90 days of therapy are needed), and the patient cannot tolerate EN.

In terms of type of venous access indicated for HPN, current guidelines recommend tunneled catheters or implanted ports.[69,70] As discussed earlier in this chapter, CRBSIs are one of the most common complications associated with catheters. PICCs have been shown to carry a lower risk of CRBSI in the hospital setting, but this has not yet been shown definitively in the home setting.[69] In addition, placement of PICCs do not have the potential for some of the serious mechanical complications associated with tunneled catheters, including pneumothorax and accidental arterial puncture.[73] Recent studies have assessed the feasibility of PICCs for HPN and have found that, overall, PICCs are associated with the same incidence of complications as traditional forms of access.

HPN is usually administered on a cyclic schedule. The infusion rate is controlled by an automatic pump that gradually increases the rate over the first 30 minutes, administers the total volume over 12 to 15 hours, then gradually tapers over the last 30 minutes.[70] Many patients choose to infuse overnight in order to allow freedom from the pump for daytime activities. The downside of nighttime infusion is frequent urination, so some patients may choose daytime infusion to ensure a better night's sleep.[74]

Once it has been established that a patient will return home on PN, it is essential to involve a interprofessional team to assist in the transition. This team may include a doctor, specialized nurse, dietitian, and pharmacist.[70] In reality, however, few HPN patients in the United States receive care from interprofessional nutrition support teams due to healthcare-cost restraints.[71] A psychologist and/or social worker may also be needed, depending on how HPN affects the patient's personal and social life. The primary goals of patient/caregiver education are to promote the patient's independence, improve their quality of life, and make living with HPN as normal as possible.[75]

HPN is a complex therapy that requires intensive education and training. Patients/caregivers must learn how to administer the PN formula, care for the IV site, and identify and address complications. Several factors can affect a patient's level of success in managing HPN. These include health literacy (performing basic reading and math skills in a healthcare environment), socioeconomic status, knowledge of the English language (or dominant language), and age (older than 65 years is associated with poorer health literacy).[75]

It can be difficult to assess HPN a patient's quality of life as it is affected both by HPN itself and the underlying disease state. Quality of life (QOL) is defined as "enjoying life" and "being able to do what you want to do when you want to do it."[76] Assessments of HPN patients' QOL have found that the poorest QOL is experienced during the first year, particularly if the patient was previously well.[55] QOL tends to improve with time. Strong self-esteem, spousal and family support, and financial security are associated with improved quality of life.[55,76]

Factors that negatively contribute to quality of life include frequent catheter-related infections; the inability to work and loss of income (although some patients can continue to work); decreased social interactions; lack of energy and stamina; the inconvenience of the catheter, tubing, and pump; and the rigidity of the infusion schedule.[55,76]

Transitioning to HPN can be an intense, stressful experience. Patients will have different attitudes in how they approach this new phase of their life. The infusion schedule can be particularly challenging. Some patients may be able to maintain a relatively spontaneous lifestyle and learn to adjust their infusion schedule accordingly, while others may feel burdened by a strict infusion schedule. Successful patients will acknowledge that their lives have changed, but will learn to redefine their "new normal." It can be helpful for patients to focus on what they can still do while on HPN, rather than what they cannot do.[76]

Prognosis of HPN

Retrospective cohort studies have found that the 5-year survival rate for patients on HPN range from 58% to 83%.[77] Because there are a wide variety of conditions that may necessitate HPN, the most influential and variable effect on survival rate is the underlying disease state.[55] For example, patients with cancer may have an expected survival of several months, whereas patients with Crohn's disease can expect to measure survival in decades. In the overwhelming majority of cases, death of a patient on HPN is due to the underlying disease and not a complication of HPN, particularly for patients on HPN for <1 year. As the length of HPN use increases, so does the risk of serious complications such as sepsis, liver failure, and thrombosis. Among long-term HPN patients, complications account for 15% to 20% of deaths.[55,77] Additional factors that influence prognosis of patients on HPN include the following:[55]

- Age (better prognosis amongst younger patients)
- Experience of supervising clinician
- Use of narcotics (associated with increased incidence of sepsis)
- Peer-support and education programs (associated with decreased incidence of sepsis)

While some patients will remain on life-long HPN, others may be able to transition off of HPN to an oral diet. Depending on the length and type of bowel that remains intact, patients with short-bowel syndrome may undergo a process known as adaptation. If the colon remains intact, absorption improves over 1 to 3 years, and with dietary counseling, patients may be able to reduce PN or transition off of PN entirely.[78] Recent studies have found that adaptation may even occur up to 5 years after onset of intestinal failure[77]

CORE CONCEPT 10

Parenteral nutrition may be a long-term or even life-long therapy for some patients.

Chapter Summary

Parenteral nutrition is a life-sustaining therapy for individuals with a nonfunctional GI tract who cannot consume nutrition through oral intake or enteral nutrition. It may be used to sustain patients before they are able to resume oral or enteral intake, whereas for those who have permanent GI dysfunction, it may be used for decades. PN is a highly complex therapy that requires careful calculation of nutrient needs, strict hygienic practices when administering PN and caring for the catheter site, and constant monitoring for complications. An experienced, interprofessional team is ideal for managing PN.

Key Terms

parenteral nutrition (PN), hypertonic, asepsis, central parenteral nutrition, peripheral parenteral nutrition, venipuncture, exit site, thrombophlebitis, extravasation, central venous catheter (CVC), peripherally inserted central catheter (PICC), phlebitis, parenteral nutrition associated liver disease (PNALD), hepatic steatosis, total nutrient admixture (TNA), physicochemical incompatibility, continuous infusion, cyclical infusion, catheter-related complication (CRC), pneumothorax, catheter occlusion, catheter-related venous thrombosis (CRVT), thrombotic occlusion, thromboembolism, catheter embolism, air embolism, catheter-related bloodstream infection (CRBSI), central line associated bloodstream infection (CLABSI), sepsis, biofilm, cholestasis, cholelithiasis.

References

1. Mahan KL E-SS, Raymond JL, Krause MV. *Krause's Food & the Nutrition Care Process.* 13th ed. St. Louis, MO.: Elsevier/Saunders; 2012.
2. Dudrick SJ. History of parenteral nutrition. *J Am Coll Nutr.* 2009;28(3):243-251.
3. Mirtallo JM, Patel M. Overview of parenteral nutrition. In: Mueller CM, ed. *The A.S.P.E.N. Adult Nutrition Support Core Curriculum.* 2nd ed. Silver Spring, MD: American Society for Parenteral and Enteral Nutrition; 2012:232-244.
4. Dudrick SJ, Wilmore DW, Vars HM, Rhoads JE. Long-term total parenteral nutrition with growth, development, and positive nitrogen balance. *Surgery.* 1968;64(1):134-142.
5. Krzywda EA, Andris DA, Edmiston CE. Parenteral access devices. In: Mueller CM, ed. *The A.S.P.E.N. Adult Nutrition Support Core Curriculum.* 2nd ed. Silver Spring, MD: American Society for Parenteral and Enteral Nutrition; 2012:265-283.
6. Derenski K, Catlin J, Allen L. Parenteral nutrition basics for the clinician caring for the adult patient. *Nutr Clin Pract.* 2016;31(5):578-595.
7. Pittiruti M, Hamilton H, Biffi R, MacFie J, Pertkiewicz M, ESPEN. ESPEN Guidelines on Parenteral Nutrition: Central venous catheters (access, care, diagnosis and therapy of complications). *Clin Nutr.* 2009;28(4):365-377.
8. Boullata JI, Gilbert K, Sacks G, et al. A.S.P.E.N. clinical guidelines: parenteral nutrition ordering, order review, compounding, labeling, and dispensing. *JPEN J Parenter Enteral Nutr.* 2014;38(3):334-377.
9. McClave SA, Martindale R, Taylor B, Gramlich L. Appropriate use of parenteral nutrition through the perioperative period. *J Parenter Enteral Nutr.* 2013;37(5 Suppl):73S-82S.
10. Muscaritoli M, Molfino A, Laviano A, Rasio D, Rossi Fanelli F. Parenteral nutrition in advanced cancer patients. *Crit Rev Oncol Hematol.* 2012;84(1):26-36.
11. McClave SA, Taylor BE, Martindale RG, et al. Guidelines for the provision and assessment of nutrition support therapy in the adult critically ill patient: Society of Critical Care Medicine (SCCM) and American Society for Parenteral and Enteral Nutrition (A.S.P.E.N.). *JPEN J Parenter Enteral Nutr.* 2016;40(2):159-211.
12. Şimşek T, Şimşek HU, Cantürk NZ. Response to trauma and metabolic changes: posttraumatic metabolism. *Turk J Surg.* 2014;30(3): 153-159.
13. Bolder U, Ebener C, Hauner H, et al. Carbohydrates – Guidelines on Parenteral Nutrition, Chapter 5. *Ger Med Sci.* Vol 72009.
14. Barber JR, Sacks GS. Parenteral nutrition formulations. In: Mueller CM, ed. *The A.S.P.E.N. Adult Nutrition Support Core Curriculum.* 2nd ed. Silver Spring, MD: The American Society for Parenteral and Enteral Nutrition; 2012:245-264.
15. Yarandi SS, Zhao VM, Hebbar G, Ziegler TR. Amino acid composition in parenteral nutrition: what is the evidence? *Curr Opin Clin Nutr Metab Care.* 2011;14(1):75-82.
16. A.S.P.E.N. Board of Directors and the Clinical Guidelines Task Force. Guidelines for the use of parenteral and enteral nutrition in adult and pediatric patients. *JPEN J Parenter Enteral Nutr.* 2002;26(1 Suppl):1sa-138sa.
17. 15% Clinisol [package insert]. Deerfield, IL: Baxter Healthcare Corporation; 2006. https://dailymed.nlm.nih.gov/dailymed/archives/fdaDrugInfo.cfm?archiveid=2629.

18. Aminosyn II with Electrolytes [package insert]. Lake Forest, IL: Hospira, Inc.; 2004. https://www.accessdata.fda.gov/drugsatfda_docs/label/2005/019683s027lbl.pdf.
19. Friedman M. *Absorption and utilization of amino acids*. Vol 2. Boca Raton, FL: CRC Press; 1989.
20. Calder PC, Jensen GL, Koletzko BV, Singer P, Wanten GJ. Lipid emulsions in parenteral nutrition of intensive care patients: current thinking and future directions. *Intensive Care Med*. 2010;36(5):735-749.
21. Adolph M, Heller AR, Koch T, et al. Lipid emulsions – Guidelines on Parenteral Nutrition, Chapter 6. *Ger Med Sci*. 2009;7.
22. Antebi H, Mansoor O, Ferrier C, et al. Liver function and plasma antioxidant status in intensive care unit patients requiring total parenteral nutrition: comparison of 2 fat emulsions. *JPEN J Parenter Enteral Nutr*. 2004;28(3):142-148.
23. O'Grady NP, Alexander M, Burns LA, et al. Guidelines for the Prevention of Intravascular Catheter-related Infections. Clinical Infectious Diseases: An Official Publication of the Infectious Diseases Society of America. 2011;52(9):e162-e193.
24. Mirtallo J, Canada T, Johnson D, et al. Safe practices for parenteral nutrition. *JPEN J Parenter Enteral Nutr*. 2004;28(6):S39-70.
25. Clark SF. Vitamins and trace elements. In: Mueller CM, ed. *The A.S.P.E.N. Adult Nutrition Support Core Curriculum*. 2nd ed. Silver Spring, MD: The American Society for Parenteral and Enteral Nutrition; 2012:121-151.
26. M.V.I.-12 [package insert]. Westborough, MA: AstraZeneca; 2004.
27. Itokawa Y. Trace elements in long-term total parenteral nutrition. *Nihon Rinsho Jpn J Clin Med*. 1996;54(1): 172-178.
28. Rampton D, Folkersen J, Fishbane S, et al. Hypersensitivity reactions to intravenous iron: guidance for risk minimization and management. *Haematologica*. 2014;99(11):1671-1676.
29. Forbes A. Iron and parenteral nutrition. *Gastroenterology*. 2009;137 (5 Suppl):S47-54.
30. Gosmanov AR, Umpierrez GE. Management of hyperglycemia during enteral and parenteral nutrition therapy. *Curr Diab Rep*. 2013;13(1): 155-162.
31. Mirtallo J, Canada T, Johnson D, et al. Safe practices for parenteral nutrition. *JPEN J Parenter Enteral Nutr*. 2004;28(6): S39-70.
32. Hadaway LC. Administering parenteral nutrition with other I.V. drugs. *Nursing*. 2005;35(2):26.
33. Drug Shortages Update. A.S.P.E.N. website. https://www.nutritioncare.org/News/Product_Shortages/Drug_Shortages_Update/. Accessed January 31, 2017.
34. Mirtallo JM. The drug shortage crisis. *JPEN J Parenter Enteral Nutr*. 2011;35(4):433.
35. Product Shortages. A.S.P.E.N.website. http://www.nutritioncare.org/public-policy/product-shortages/. Accessed January 31, 2017.
36. Burke JF, Wolfe RR, Mullany CJ, Mathews DE, Bier DM. Glucose requirements following burn injury. parameters of optimal glucose infusion and possible hepatic and respiratory abnormalities following excessive glucose intake. *Ann Surg*. 1979;190(3):274-285
37. Kumpf VJ, Gervasio J. Complications of parenteral nutrition. In: Mueller CM, ed. *The A.S.P.E.N. Adult Nutrition Support Core Curriculum*. 2nd ed. Silver Spring, MD: The American Society for Parenteral and Enteral Nutrition; 2012; 284-297.
38. Hartl WH, Jauch KW, Parhofer K, Rittler P. Complications and Monitoring – Guidelines on Parenteral Nutrition, Chapter 11. *Ger Med Sci*. Vol 72009.
39. Hematology ASo. Sickle Cell Anemia. http://www.hematology.org/Patients/Anemia/Sickle-Cell.aspx. Accessed May 4, 2017.
40. Ghabril MS, Aranda-Michel J, Scolapio JS. Metabolic and Catheter Complications of Parenteral Nutrition. *Curr Gastroenteroly Rep*. 2004;6:327-334.
41. Cotogni P, Barbero C, Garrino C, et al. Peripherally inserted central catheters in non-hospitalized cancer patients: 5-year results of a prospective study. *Support Care Cancer*. 2015;23(2):403-409.
42. Ukleja A, Romano MM. Complications of parenteral nutrition. *Gastroenterol Clin N A*. 2007;36:23-46.
43. Cavanna, L, Civardi, G, Vallisa D, et al. Ultrasound-guided central venous catheterization in cancer patients improves the success rate of cannulation and reduces mechanical complications: A prospective observational study of 1,978 consecutive catheterizations. *World J Surg Oncol*. 2010;8(91).
44. Hamilton C. Vascular access. In: Charney P, Malone AM, eds. *ADA Pocket Guide to Parenteral Nutrition*: Chicago, IL: Academy of Nutrition and Dietetics; 2007:33-51.
45. Lirk P, Keller C, Colvin J, et al. Unintentional arterial puncture during cephalic vein cannulation: case report and anatomical study. *Br J Anaesth*. 2004;92(5):740-742.
46. Brandt CF, Tribler S, Hvistendahl M, et al. Home parenteral nutrition in adult patients with chronic intestinal failure: catheter-related complications over 4 decades at the main Danish Tertiary Referral Center. *JPEN J Parenter Enteral Nutr*. 2017;41(7):1178-1187
47. McCarthy CJ, Behravesh S, Naidu SG, Oklu R. Air embolism: Practical tips for prevention and treatment. *J Clin Med*. 2016;5(11).
48. Safdar N, Maki DG. Inflammation at the insertion site is not predictive of catheter-related bloodstream infection with short-term, noncuffed central venous catheters. *Crit Care Med*. 2002;30(12):2632-2635.
49. Fonseca G, Burgermaster M, Larson E, Seres DS. The relationship between parenteral nutrition and central line–associated bloodstream infections: 2009–2014. *JPEN J Parenter Enteral Nutr*. 2017:1-5.
50. Prasad, P, ed. Sepsis in adults. Dynamed website. http://www.dynamed.com/topics/dmp~AN~T115805/Sepsis-in-adults. Updated July 28, 2017. Accessed October 2, 2017.
51. Beghetto MG, Victorino J, Teixeira L, de Azevedo MJ. Parenteral nutrition as a risk factor for central venous catheter–related infection. *JPEN J Parenter Enteral Nutr*. 2005;29(5):367-373.
52. Roberts S. Initiation, advancement, and acute complications. In: Charney P, Malone AM, eds. *ADA Pocket Guide to Parenteral Nutrition*: Chicago, IL: Academy of Nutrition and Dietetics; 2007:76-102.
53. Olveira G, Tapia MJ, Ocon J, et al. Hypoglycemia in noncritically ill patients receiving total parenteral nutrition: a multicenter study. (Study group on the problem of hyperglycemia in parenteral nutrition; Nutrition area of the Spanish Society of Endocrinology and Nutrition). *Nutrition*. 2015;31(1):58-63.
54. Ayers P, Warrington L. Diagnosis and treatment of simple acid-base disorders. *Nutr Clin Prac*. 2008;23(2):122-127.
55. Howard L. Home Parenteral nutrition: Survival, cost, and quality of life. *Gastroenterology*. 2006;130(2):S52-S59.
56. Rhoda KM, Porter MJ, Quintini C. Fluid and electrolyte management. *JPEN J Parenter Enteral Nutr*. 2011;35(6):675-685.
57. Vinnars E WD. History of parenteral nutrition. *JPEN J Parenter Enteral Nutr*. 2003;27(3):225-231.
58. Jeejeebhoy KN. Total parenteral nutrition: potion or poison? *Am J Clin Nutr*. 2001;74:160-163.
59. Griffiths RD. Too much of a good thing: the curse of overfeeding. *Crit Care*. 2007;11(6):176.
60. Jeppesen PB, Hoy CE, Mortensen PB. Essential fatty acid deficiency in patients receiving home parenteral nutrition. *Am J Clin Nutr*. 1998;68(1):126-133.

61. ESPEN. Guidelines of Pediatric Parenteral Nutrition 4. Lipids. *J Ped Gastroenterol Nutr.* 2005;41(2):S19-S27.

62. Morlion B. Update on Parenteral Lipids: Therapeutic Goals. www.espen.org/presfile/Morlion-2-010902-web.doc. Updated September 14, 2017. Accessed October 2, 2017.

63. Kumpf VJ. Parenteral nutrition-associated liver disease in adult and pediatric patients. *Nutr Clin Pract.* 2006;21(3):279-290.

64. Xu ZW, Li YS. Pathogenesis and treatment of parenteral nutrition-associated liver disease. *Hepatobiliary Pancreat Dis Int.* 2012;11(6):586-593.

65. Nandivada P, Carlson SJ, Chang MI, Cowan E, Gura KM, Puder M. Treatment of parenteral nutrition-associated liver disease: the role of lipid emulsions. *Adv Nutr.* 2013;4:711-717.

66. Cholestasis. Merckmanuals.com. http://www.merckmanuals.com/home/liver-and-gallbladder-disorders/manifestations-of-liver-disease/cholestasis. Accessed September 30, 2017.

67. Guglielmi FW, Regano N, Mazzuoli S, et al. Cholestasis induced by total parenteral nutrition. *Clin Liver Dis.* 2008;12(1):97-110, viii.

68. Cholelithiasis. Merckmanuals.com. http://www.merckmanuals.com/professional/hepatic-and-biliary-disorders/gallbladder-and-bile-duct-disorders/cholelithiasis. Published August 2016. Accessed September 30, 2017.

69. Botella-Carretero JI, Carrero C, Guerra E, et al. Role of peripherally inserted central catheters in home parenteral nutrition: a 5-year prospective study. *JPEN J Parenter Enteral Nutr.* 2013;37(4):544-549.

70. Wanten G, Calder PC, Forbes A. Managing adult patients who need home parenteral nutrition. *BMJ.* 2011;342:d1447.

71. Kumpf VJ, Tillman EM. Home parenteral nutrition: Safe transition from hospital to home. *Nutr Clin Prac.* 2012;27(6):749-757.

72. Barrocas A, Geppert C, Durfee SM, et al. A.S.P.E.N. Ethics Position Paper. *Nutr Clin Prac.* 2010;25(6):672-679.

73. Christensen LD, Rasmussen HH, Vinter-Jensen L. Peripherally inserted central catheter for use in home parenteral nutrition: a 4-year follow-up study. *JPEN J Parenter Enteral Nutr.* 2014;38(8):1003-1006.

74. Hamilton C, Austin T. Home parenteral nutrition. In: Charney P, Malone AM, eds. *ADA Pocket Guide to Parenteral Nutrition.* Chicago, IL: Academy of Nutrition and Dietetics; 2007:118-146.

75. Gifford H, DeLegge M, Epperson LA. Education methods and techniques for training home parenteral nutrition patients. *Nutr Clin Prac.* 2010;25(5):443-450.

76. Winkler MF, Hagan E, Wetle T, Smith C, O'Sullivan Maillet J, Touger-Decker R. An exploration of quality of life and the experience of living with home parenteral nutrition. *JPEN J Parenter Enteral Nutr.* 2010;34(4):395-407.

77. Dibb M, Soop M, Teubner A, et al. Survival and nutritional dependence on home parenteral nutrition: Three decades of experience from a single referral centre. *Clin Nutr.* 2017;36(2):570-576.

78. Van Gossum A, Cabre E, Hebuterne X, et al. ESPEN Guidelines on Parenteral Nutrition: gastroenterology. In: Mueller CM, ed. *The A.S.P.E.N. Adult Nutrition Support Core Curriculum.* 2nd ed. Silver Spring, MD: American Society for Parenteral and Enteral Nutrition; 2012:415-437.

ndex

I

J

K

L

M